DERMATOPATHOLOGY

A Practical Guide to Common Disorders

DERMATOPATHOLOGY

A Practical Guide to Common Disorders

GEORGE F. MURPHY, M.D.
Herman Beerman Professor of Dermatology
Professor of Pathology
University of Pennsylvania
Philadelphia, Pennsylvania

With special assistance in photomicrography by Arlene Herzberg, M.D.

W.B. SAUNDERS COMPANY
A Division of Harcourt Brace & Company
Philadelphia   London   Toronto   Montreal   Sydney   Tokyo

W.B. SAUNDERS COMPANY
A Division of
Harcourt Brace & Company

The Curtis Center
Independence Square West
Philadelphia, Pennsylvania 19106

Library of Congress Cataloging-in-Publication Data

Murphy, George F. (George Francis)

Dermatopathology / George F. Murphy.—1st ed.

p. cm.

ISBN 0–7216–2418–9

1. Skin—Diseases.   2. Skin—Pathophysiology.   I. Title.
[DNLM: 1. Skin Diseases—pathology.   2. Skin—pathology.
WR 140 M978d 1995]

RL96.M87   1995

616.5—dc20

DNLM/DLC   94–6843

DERMATOPATHOLOGY   ISBN 0–7216–2418–9

Last digit is the print number: 9   8   7   6   5   4   3   2   1

At the outset of a project such as this,
there are many cheerleaders and supporters.
At the end, there are few.
My wife, Sharon, and my daughters, Erin and Emily,
provided love and encouragement to the very end,
and thus are responsible for the accomplishment
of what would otherwise have been an impossible task.
To them, I am profoundly indebted.

This book is also dedicated to the extended family of patients
suffering from as yet undiagnosed skin diseases
in the hope that they will benefit from this effort.

Contributors

Rosalie Elenitsas, M.D.
Pigmented Lesion Specialty Group, Department of Dermatology, University of Pennsylvania, Philadelphia, Pennsylvania
Diagnostic Methodology: Immunofluorescence

Michael H. Goldschmidt, M.Sc., B.V.M.S., M.R.C.V.S.
Professor, Veterinary Pathology, and Head, Surgical Pathology, University of Pennsylvania School of Veterinary Medicine, Philadelphia, Pennsylvania
Comparative Dermatopathology

Suzanne M. Jacques, M.D.
Assistant Professor, Department of Pathology, Wayne State University School of Medicine, Detroit, Michigan; Associate Pathologist, Hutzel Hospital and Institute for Women's Medicine, Detroit, Michigan
Dermatopathology of Anogenital Skin

Christine Jaworsky, M.D.
Assistant Professor, University of Pennsylvania Medical School, Philadelphia, Pennsylvania; Staff Physician, Hospital of the University of Pennsylvania, Philadelphia, Pennsylvania
Diagnostic Methodology: Immunofluorescence; Dermatopathology of Hair; Dermatopathology of Nails

W. Dwayne Lawrence, M.D.
Associate Professor, Department of Pathology, Wayne State University School of Medicine, Detroit, Michigan; Chief of Pathology, Hutzel Hospital and Institute for Women's Medicine, Detroit, Michigan
Dermatopathology of Anogenital Skin

William C. Lloyd, III, M.D.
Clinical Assistant Professor, Department of Ophthalmology, University of Texas Health Science Center, San Antonio, Texas
Dermatopathology of the Ocular Adnexa

Kenneth L. Piest, M.D.
Assistant Professor and Director, Oculoplastic, Orbit, and Oncology Service, Department of Ophthalmology, University of Texas Health Science Center, San Antonio, Texas
Dermatopathology of the Ocular Adnexa

Neil W. Savage, M.D.Sc., Ph.D.
Senior Lecturer in Oral Pathology and Oral Pathologist, Department of Dentistry, University of Queensland Dental School, Brisbane, Queensland, Australia; Consultant Oral Pathologist, Royal Brisbane Hospital, Brisbane, Queensland, Australia
Dermatopathology of Oral Mucosa

Laurence J. Walsh, B.D.Sc., D.D.Sc., Ph.D.
Senior Lecturer in Preventive Dentistry and Periodontology, University of Queensland Dental School, Brisbane, Queensland, Australia; Dental Officer, Bone Marrow Transplant Unit, Royal Brisbane Hospital, Brisbane, Queensland, Australia
Dermatopathology of Oral Mucosa

Allan E. Wulc, M.D.
Assistant Professor and Chief of Oculoplastic and Orbital Surgery, Scheie Eye Institute/University of Pennsylvania, Philadelphia, Pennsylvania
Dermatopathology of the Ocular Adnexa

Preface

Why another text in dermatopathology? Perhaps the best answer is found in repeated complaints of the *residents* and *fellows* we have trained over the past years. They aver the following: (1) many existing texts in dermatopathology are not ''user-friendly''; they require considerable previous knowledge of the field in order to be utilized effectively; (2) too much attention is devoted to disorders seldom or never encountered in daily practice; and (3) the formats of some present resources are not logical, and do not follow the manner and methods inherent in visual diagnosis through the microscope. Over the past several years, we have attempted to analyze these criticisms with the goal of identifying potential means of partially rectifying these limitations. Thoughts, conclusions, and the resultant approaches presented in this text are summarized below.

Existing texts in dermatopathology are not user-friendly; they require considerable previous knowledge of the field in order to be utilized effectively. Today, when an experienced dermatopathologist encounters a lichenoid infiltrate with a vaguely granulomatous appearance, prominence of endothelium lining associated vessels, and occasional plasma cells, a silver stain is ordered and additional clinical history with regard to serologic evaluation for secondary syphilis is obtained. In a similar way, when the same seasoned diagnostician encounters a frankly granulomatous infiltrate with associated panniculitis, neutrophilic abscess formation with zonal necrosis, and vascular and epithelial injury or necrosis, it is realized that these findings do not fit well into conventional patterns of noninfectious granuloma formation or panniculitis. Accordingly, further clinical history is taken and stains are ordered to exclude deep mycotic infection. Prior knowledge that the histologic features of both cases are likely to portend infection would also prompt reference to chapters that deal with infectious diseases of skin in many standard texts of dermatopathology. However, when first undertaking the study of dermatopathology, which section in a text should be consulted? In the first instance, not suspecting syphilis, one might have turned to descriptions of lichen planus, erythema multiforme, or lupus erythematosus. In the second case, chapters dealing with sarcoidosis, primary panniculitis, or granulomatous vasculitis might have been consulted. Although such exercises have didactic merit, they emphasize a limitation of many existing texts in facilitating efficient identification of pertinent diagnostic information based solely on initial evaluation of the slide, not extensive previous knowledge of the subject.

Although several recent texts have attempted to ameliorate this problem by presenting approaches based on pattern analysis for inflammatory dermatoses, no single volume has dealt with this issue in a comprehensive manner. Perhaps this is not possible, in view of the complexity of dermatopathology. Yet, just as computers have become accessible to the general public, so, too, should textbooks of pathology of specialized areas be friendly to their users. Accordingly, this text has attempted to group disorders according to the most common classes and patterns of their morphologic expression. For example, there is, in fact, no single chapter that focuses exclusively on the multitude of cellular and architectural patterns of expression that constitute cutaneous infection. Rather, the pathologist who encounters a benign verrucous epithelial neoplasm will read about human papillomavirus as a cause in the chapter dealing with benign epidermal tumors, whereas infectious granulomas will be discussed under the chapter concerned with granulomatous dermatitis, and infections in which neutrophils predominate will be grouped in the chapter on granulocytic dermatitis. Such a system, however imperfect, has the advantage of directing the diagnostician who is not armed with substantial prior knowledge to the section likely to contain relevant information.

Too much attention is devoted to disorders seldom or never encountered in daily practice. In an effort to be comprehensive, many medical texts devote considerable time and space to rare disorders that are infrequently or never encountered by the dermatopathologist. Although this approach has its place in reference-style compendia, it detracts from the practical utility of books intended to guide the diagnostician through the complex nuances and variations inherent in the differential recognition of common diseases of the skin. Moreover, many texts provide such detail about rare and exotic disorders that significant prose and visual information are devoted to these entities. Books so cluttered may be difficult to use and inherently inefficient for the daily practice of dermatopathology. In the present text, each chapter focuses on a limited number of common disorders for each diagnostic category. Collectively, the text thus embraces the majority of the diagnoses made annually in a large dermatopathology practice, such as the one at the University of Pennsylvania. A subsidiary section entitled ''rare disorders'' is included in each chapter to make note of those conditions that may mimic their more common counterparts and to provide references for further reading. In this way, variant forms of the common inflammatory pattern of spongiotic dermatitis or acquired nevocellular nevi are provided with appropriately extensive coverage, whereas relatively rare conditions such as the dermatitis of Wiskott-Aldrich syndrome or so-called ''minimal deviation melanoma'' are dealt with in an abbreviated fashion.

On the other hand, some existing dermatopathology texts often fail to include or de-emphasize diagnostic information concerning commonly encountered diagnostic challenges in the areas of pathology of hair, nails, oral mucosa, ocular adnexa, the genital region, and even comparable diseases affecting animal skin (not uncommonly, practicing pathologists are consulted by veterinarians regarding interpretation of animal skin biopsies). This effort, therefore, attempts to include these categories in the hope that this text may also be useful to those concerned with cutaneous pathology in dentistry and oral medicine, obstetrics and gynecology, ophthalmology, and veterinary medicine.

The formats of many available resources are not logical and do not follow the manner and methods inherent in visual diagnosis through the microscope. When a dermatopathologist approaches an unknown slide, a defined yet often unconscious series of analytic steps occur. First, the slide is observed at scanning, mid-range, and high objective lens magnifications. During this process, different areas of the slide are viewed as it is moved on the stage, a process permitting constant comparison and contrast with what has already been seen as well as with stored, more remote mental images of similar visual information from other cases. At this juncture, an algorithmic approach has already been enacted based upon quantity or quality of histologic features (e.g., type and degree of scale abnormality, pattern and composition of an infiltrate, and presence, extent, and degree of dysplasia), which allows greater and greater restriction of diagnostic possibilities. Finally, these possibilities are limited to several categories or diagnostic entities that may be further refined based on clinical parameters (clinical-pathologic correlation) or other available data. During this analytic process, guidance may be sought from a text in dermatopathology. Ideally, such a text should ''see and think'' the way the dermatopathologist does—at varying magnifications; by comparisons and contrasts; at times, in color; and by use of an algorithm. But how many really do?

This present effort was inspired by the chapter on ''The Skin'' in the last three editions of *Robbins Pathologic Basis of Disease*. Because this book was written with medical students in mind, its clear and focused style has become applicable to and useful for all students of medicine worldwide, regardless of level of training. In this text, we have furthered this task in the hope that this first and admittedly imperfect attempt will test the waters for what seems to be a logical and self-evident approach to the teaching of dermatopathology. Accordingly, we provide comparative photographic panels and simple tables to illustrate temporal evolutionary characteristics, differential diagnostic points, and architectural and cytologic features of lesions. A color atlas and teaching slide set will be produced for those who find these added dimensions useful. Algorithms are used where appropriate to assist in honing down differential diagnostic features and providing a practical approach that imitates the way we think when confronted with a diagnostic problem. Finally, an effort has been made to incorporate helpful clues that are passed down as a verbal tradition but that may not have been promulgated widely. Such ''pearls,'' as they are called, have grown by accretion over time and are of considerable value; yet they remain partially encased as a result of their tendency to be transmitted by tongue rather than by script.

The result of the approach outlined above is the book that immediately follows. Accordingly, it is entitled *Dermatopathology. A Practical Guide to Common Disorders*. If it proves to be a practical, user-friendly approach to most of the skin diseases encountered by dermatologists and pathologists in daily practice, this first attempt will have begun to succeed. But this is only a beginning, for texts are not static entities that grow only by the number of disorders they list. They must evolve and change like the lesions they describe. Thus, if this first edition survives to the point whereby we vigorously modify its contents in accord with the rapidly evolving needs of the specialty of dermatopathology, it will have been a success.

GEORGE F. MURPHY, M.D.

Acknowledgments

Preparation of this text was made possible by the photomicrographic assistance of Dr. Arlene Herzberg, who during her fellowship at the University of Pennsylvania, selected and recorded the images of thousands of examples of common cutaneous lesions for portrayal in these pages. Ms. Diana Whitaker-Menezes and Mr. Brett Telegan prepared the photographic plates with care and precision. The photographic archives of the Department of Dermatology of the University of Pennsylvania, assembled and maintained by Mr. William Witmer, yielded extraordinary clinical examples that permitted a degree of gross-microscopic correlation unprecedented in existing texts of dermatopathology. This text owes a significant debt to the chapter that spawned its creation, ''The Skin,'' in Cotran, K, and Robbins, *Robbins Pathologic Basis of Disease.* I joined this effort, now in its fifth edition, more than a decade ago at the invitation of my respected mentor and friend, Martin C. Mihm. With his guidance and encouragement, the chapter grew into a nidus for the crystallization of this present work and indeed has directly inspired the philosophy and many of the thoughts expressed in this book. Cooperation of the Armed Forces Institute of Pathology in making available illustrative and written material from the first two volumes of the third series of ''Fascicles'' also contributed to the genesis and quality of this undertaking. In particular, some of the descriptive text from Fascicle 1, *Non-Melanocytic Tumors of the Skin,* has been reorganized and adapted to the present text so that this material could be shared with a larger audience. The support and guidance of my friend and colleague, David E. Elder, is acknowledged in this and many other didactic ventures in which I have been involved. Finally, the input of Drs. Rosalie Elenitsas, Michael Goldschmidt, Suzanne M. Jacques, Christine Jaworsky, Dwayne Lawrence, William C. Lloyd, III, Kenneth L. Piest, Neil W. Savage, Laurie Walsh, and Allan E. Wulc in formulating chapters not usually found in dermatopathology texts has added significantly to the novel and we hope useful nature of this work.

Contents

I

Basic Nomenclature, Structure, and Methods

1

Structure, Function, and Reaction Patterns

DEFINITIONS AND GENERAL CONSIDERATIONS

The skin is composed of three layers: the epidermis, the dermis (Fig. 1–1), and the subcutaneous fat. The epidermis is composed of keratinocytes, Langerhans cells, melanocytes, and Merkel cells. The dermis, which is separated from the epidermis by a basement membrane, contains fibroblasts and highly dendritic cells, which express coagulation Factor XIIIa, mast cells, phagocytic and antigen-presenting macrophages, nerve fibers, and endothelial cells. Adipocytes predominate in subcutaneous fat. A summary of salient structural and functional considerations for these various cell types is provided in Table 1–1.

An equally important component of skin is adnexal epithelium, which consists of pilar and related sebaceous structures as well as apocrine and eccrine glands. Sebaceous glands lubricate the skin surface; apocrine glands are a source of protective and attractive scents, particularly in lower vertebrates; and eccrine glands are critical for temperature regulation. In Chapters 12, 21, and 22, anatomic issues pertaining to these structures are discussed.

Diagnostic Terms

Hyperkeratosis: Increased thickness of the stratum corneum, as in a clavus.

Parakeratosis: Retention of keratinocyte nuclei in the stratum corneum, as in psoriasis.

Hypergranulosis: Thickening of the stratum granulosum, as in lichen simplex chronicus.

Hypogranulosis: Thinning or absence of the stratum granulosum, as in psoriasis.

Acanthosis: Thickening of the viable epidermal layer, predominantly involving the stratum spinosum, as in a verruca.

Atrophy: Thinning of the epidermal layer with loss of rete ridges, as in lupus erythematosus.

Dyskeratosis: Abnormal or premature keratinization, as in squamous cell carcinoma.

Apoptosis: Programmed or pathologically accelerated cell degeneration and death due to endonuclease-mediated nuclear degeneration, as in involuting hair follicles.

Spongiosis: Epidermal intercellular edema, resulting in widened intercellular spaces, as in acute eczematous dermatitis.

Acantholysis: Dissolution of intercellular junctions resulting in rounded, detached keratinocytes, as in pemphigus.

Vacuolar degeneration: Lucent cytoplasmic vacuoles, often within basal cells, as in erythema multiforme.

Squamatization: Transformation of normally rounded basal cells to polyhedral cells resembling those of stratum spinosum, as in lichen planus.

Munro microabscess: Focal collection of neutrophils within parakeratotic stratum corneum, as in psoriasis.

Impetiginization: Diffuse infiltration of stratum corneum by neutrophils, serum, and bacteria, as in impetigo.

Pautrier microabscess: Discrete collection of atypical lymphocytes within a relatively nonspongiotic epidermal layer.

Spongiform pustule: Focal collection of neutrophils in the upper stratum spinosum, as in psoriasis.

Epidermotropism: The process whereby cells, usually T lymphocytes, migrate into the epidermal layer; such cells are referred to as being epidermotropic.

Mucinosis: Infiltration of epithelial intercellular spaces, as in follicular mucinosis, or dermal collagen, as in lupus erythematosus, by stringy, particulate, blue-grey mucopolysaccharides.

Colloid body: An anucleate residua of a keratinocyte that has been incorporated into the papillary dermis, as in lichen planus.

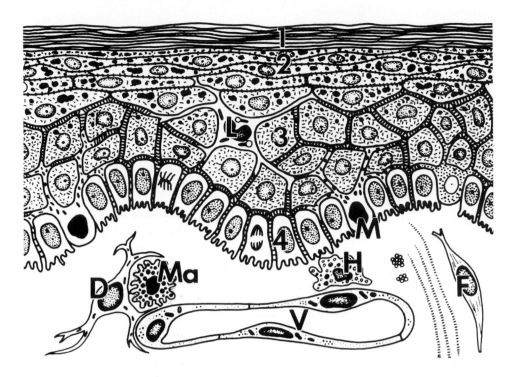

Figure 1–1. Normal human skin. The epidermis is composed of four layers of keratinocytes: the stratum corneum (1), the stratum granulosum (2), the stratum spinosum (3), and the stratum basalis (4). Within the midepidermis are dendritic Langerhans cells (L), and admixed within the stratum basalis are pigment-producing melanocytes (M). The underlying collagenous dermis contains microvessels (V), fusiform fibroblasts (F), histiocytes (H), dendrocytes (D), and granule-containing mast cells (Ma).

Pigment incontinence: Loss of epidermal melanin pigment into superficial dermal macrophages, as in postinflammatory hyperpigmentation.

Sclerosis: Abnormal collagen deposition, as in keloids.

Elastosis: Abnormal superficial dermal deposition of grey, homogeneous elastin, as in actinic change.

Desmoplasia: Proliferation of fibroblasts, often associated with invasive tumors, as in sclerosing basal cell carcinoma.

Fibrinoid necrosis: Deposition of pink-purple, granular, refractile fibrin in vessel walls, as in leukocytoclastic vasculitis.

Necrobiosis: Mucinous, fibrinoid, or sclerotic alteration of connective tissue, as in forms of palisaded granulomatous dermatitis.

Dysplasia: Nuclear and cytoplasmic alterations intermediate between benign-reactive and anaplastic, as in dysplastic nevi.

Anaplasia: Variation in nuclear size, dense and clumped heterochromatin, and nuclear contour angulation typical of malignant cells, as in metastatic melanoma.

GROSS PATHOLOGY

The gross or clinical pathology of skin disease is the basis for the discipline of diagnostic dermatology. Clinical terms to describe gross pathology should accompany specimens and are often useful adjuncts in diagnosis using clinicopathologic correlation.

Table 1–1. STRUCTURE AND FUNCTION OF CELLS IN THE EPIDERMIS, DERMIS, AND SUBCUTIS

CELL TYPE	LOCATION	FEATURES	FUNCTION
Keratinocyte	Entire epidermis	Tonofilaments	Keratin production
		Desmosomes	Cytokine production
Melanocyte	Basal cell layer	Melanosomes	Melanin production and transfer
Langerhans cell	Midepidermis	Birbeck granule	Antigen presentation
Merkel cell	Basal cell layer	Neurosecretory granules	? Mechanoreceptor
Fibroblast	Throughout dermis	Spindle cell	Collagen and elastin production
		Procollagen	
Dermal dendrocyte	Superficial dermis	Factor XIIIa	? Wound healing
			? Antigen presentation
Endothelial cell	Superficial and deep vascular plexuses	Weibel-Palade bodies	Leukocyte adhesion
		Factor VIII	Microcoagulation
Mast cell	Perivascular space	Scroll-containing secretory granules	Modulation of vessel permeability and leukocyte-endothelial binding
Macrophage	Perivascular space and throughout dermis	Lysosomes	Phagocytosis and antigen presentation
Nerve fiber	About vessels and adnexae	Neurosecretory granules and neurofilaments	Afferent and efferent impulses and sensory perception; ? Immunomodulation
Adipocyte	Subcutis	Cytoplasmic lipid	Mechanical cushion and energy storage

Clinical Terms

Papule: An elevated, often dome-shaped solid lesion less than 1 cm in diameter, as in acne.

Nodule: An elevated, deep, often dome-shaped solid lesion with a palpable inferior contour, as in an epidermal inclusion cyst.

Vesicle: An elevated, fluid-filled lesion less than 0.5 cm in diameter, as in herpes simplex.

Bulla: An elevated, fluid-filled lesion more than 0.5 cm in diameter, as in bullous pemphigoid.

Macule: A relatively flat zone of hyperpigmentation or erythema, as in lentigo maligna.

Patch: A relatively flat zone of erythema, often with abnormal scale, as in pityriasis rosea.

Plaque: A raised, circumscribed lesion occupying a relatively large area of skin, often associated with erythema and scaling, as in psoriasis.

Poikiloderma: Relatively flat zones of epidermal thinning imparting a finely wrinkled texture; hyperpigmentation; hypopigmentation; and prominent, dilated vessels visible beneath the epidermal surface, as in some early forms of cutaneous T-cell lymphoma.

Erythroderma: Cutaneous erythema covering most or all of the body surface, as in generalized seborrheic dermatitis.

Wheal: A rounded or flat-topped, pale pink elevation which usually disappears within 24 hours, as in hives.

Pustule: A circumscribed elevation of the skin formed by aggregated inflammatory cells, as in folliculitis.

Crust: Admixture of serum, blood, and inflammatory exudate on the cutaneous surface, producing granular, yellow-brown, dried material, as in impetigo.

Gyrate and circinate: Lesions that form rounded, polycyclic, arcuate borders, as in erythema annulare centrifugum.

Collarette: A fine line of scale that closely follows an advancing erythematous border, as in dermatophytosis.

Telangiectasia: Prominent, dilated, tortuous blood vessels visible through the superficial dermis and epidermis, as in discoid lupus erythematosus.

Umbilication: A central crater or indentation, usually within a papule or nodule.

Follicular plugging: Dilated follicular ostia containing keratotic debris and sometimes melanin, as in a comedone or discoid lupus.

Hide-bound: Inability to freely move the dermis over underlying fascial planes, as in progressive systemic sclerosis.

Dermal atrophy: Diffuse or discrete regions of dermal thinning, as in aging or atrophoderma.

REGIONAL ANATOMY

It is critical to recognize regional anatomic characteristics in skin biopsy specimens to prevent potential misinterpretation of normal variations as pathology. Table 1–2 summarizes some of the more common pitfalls.

STRUCTURE, FUNCTION, AND REACTION PATTERNS

A comprehensive understanding of the structure and function of normal skin and recognition of its extensive yet finite repertoire of responses to exogenous and endogenous injury and mutagenic stimuli are fundamental to the practice of dermatopathology. For example, most inflammatory dermatoses are typified by a constellation of reaction patterns, which collectively permit diagnostic recognition and sometimes even prediction of etiology. Similarly, neoplasms involve architectural and cytologic perturbations grounded in normal cutaneous anatomy.

In this section, normal anatomic and functional relationships are briefly reviewed, with specific reference to their diagnostic utility in evaluating commonly encountered pathologic conditions affecting the skin. The goals of this chapter are to (1) define structural and functional relations that assist in the biopsy diagnosis of certain skin diseases; (2) introduce characteristic patterns whereby skin normally reacts to various pathologic stimuli; and (3) introduce and use nomenclature that facilitates practical application of concepts advanced in the subsequent chapters. In this section, discussion is limited to keratinizing skin of normal, nonparamucosal or mucosal surfaces. Anatomic considerations for regionally characteristic conditions affecting epithelium of the nail bed, oral mucosa, ocular conjunctiva and adnexae, and anogenital skin are considered in chapters specifically addressing these issues.

Epidermal Keratinocytes

Keratinocytes are cells that form the most superficial layers of the skin (i.e., surface epidermis). These cells are responsible for synthesis of the tough structural protein keratin. Keratinocytes now are recognized as synthesizing sources of immunologically active cytokines. Indeed, if these cells had been named after this discovery, they might have been termed cutaneous "cytokinocytes"! Keratinocytes serve as primary intermediates between the internal fibrovas-

Table 1–2. REGIONAL DIFFERENCES IN HUMAN SKIN AND RELATED DIAGNOSTIC PITFALLS

SITE OR TYPE OF SKIN	EPIDERMAL AND ADNEXAL PATTERN	POTENTIAL ERROR
Acral skin	Thick, compacted stratum corneum; thick stratum granulosum; elongated rete	Lichen simplex chronicus
Paramucosa and mucosa	Diminished, compacted, or absent stratum corneum; diminished or absent stratum granulosum; pale, glycogenated cytoplasm	Ichthyosis, psoriasis, pale cell acanthoma
Eyelid	Thin epidermis; basaloid buds and small, rudimentary hairs	Atrophy, basal cell carcinoma
Nose	Numerous, well-developed sebaceous glands	Sebaceous hyperplasia
Axilla	Admixed pilosebaceous units and apocrine glands	Nevus sebaceus

cular milieu of the underlying dermis and the external environment. Keratin is a resilient, protective protein that forms the outermost scaly layer that shields the body from harmful environmental stimuli. Keratinocytes are also recipients of brown melanin pigment produced by nearby melanocytes, which allows uniform distribution of this endogenous sunscreen throughout the epidermal layer. Cytokines produced by epidermal keratinocytes are fundamental to the regulation of cutaneous inflammatory responses, protecting the body from harmful exogenous antigens and potentially assisting in recognizing endogenous neoantigens on mutated cells.

At scanning magnification, the epidermis appears as a well-demarcated layer of eosinophilic cells on the surface of the superficial dermis (Fig. 1–2). On closer inspection, it is apparent that the cells that form the uppermost layers of the epidermis are radically different from those that form the lower layers. This distinction is the result of epidermal maturation, a phenomenon that results in the genesis of terminally differentiated keratinizing cells that form the most superficial anucleate layer, the stratum corneum. The normal stratum corneum from truncal skin shows a characteristic basket-weave architecture, a pattern that changes dramatically according to normal regional anatomic variation and in response to injury (Fig. 1–3). Cells that form the stratum corneum are flattened, anucleate, keratin-filled plates that are fused together to form protective surface scale.

Directly beneath the stratum corneum is a layer that is normally several cells thick and is composed of nucleated, flattened keratinocytes that are slightly smaller in radial diameter than the cells of the overlying stratum corneum.

These small flattened keratinocytes contain small, variably shaped, dark blue keratohyalin granules; accordingly, this layer is named the stratum granulosum. These cytoplasmic granules appear to contribute to assembly of the cell envelope, composed of the protein involucrin, that typifies terminal epidermal differentiation. The thickest epidermal layer lies immediately below the stratum granulosum and is termed the stratum spinosum because of its spiny appearance. This is a result of the prominence of intercellular attachment plaques (i.e., desmosomes) that are present throughout all of the epidermal layers (Fig. 1–4). Cells composing the stratum spinosum are smaller than those that lie above and have a polyhedral contour in situ.

The lowermost epidermal layer is the stratum basalis, a single layer of round to vertically ovoid cells. These cells rest upon a subjacent basement membrane, which joins the epidermis to the dermis below. Unlike the cells of other layers, the cells of the stratum basalis are capable of continuous replication, resulting in self-renewal of the entire epidermis on a monthly basis (i.e., generally between 26 and 42 days). The undersurface of the epidermis forms a honeycomb of rete ridges, which interdigitate with dermal papillae of the adjacent papillary dermis.

The thickness and architecture of the epidermis varies considerably according to body site (see Fig. 1–3). The density, morphology, and composition of adnexal downgrowths of the epidermal layer also change according to anatomic location. Diagnostic recognition of these differences is fundamental to determining whether tissue is expressing normal regional variation or true pathologic alteration. It therefore is

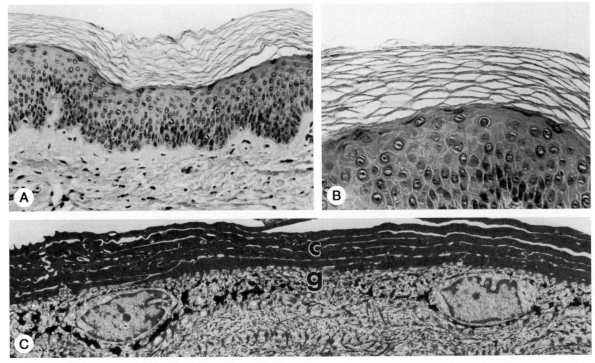

Figure 1–2. Normal human epidermis, truncal skin. **(A)** The epidermal layer is composed of discrete cell populations that undergo orderly, gradual upward maturation from the stratum basalis to form the overlying stratum spinosum, stratum granulosum, and stratum corneum. Rete ridges undulate with underlying dermal papillae along the base of the epidermal layer. **(B)** The normally anucleate stratum corneum shows a characteristic basket-weave appearance, and subtle perturbations in underlying nucleated keratinocytes are translated into diagnostically informative abnormalities of this horny layer. **(C)** Ultrastructurally, the transition from the stratum granulosum (g) to the stratum corneum (c) is quite dramatic and correlates with terminal differentiation and the formation of involucrin-rich cell envelopes.

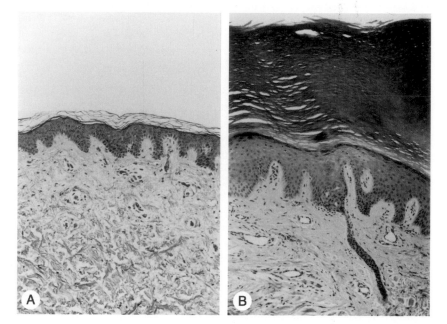

Figure 1–3. Comparison of normal cutaneous architecture in **(A)** back and **(B)** palm. There are marked differences in epidermal and stratum corneum thickness, in degree of compaction of stratum corneum, and even in texture and vascularity of the underlying dermal connective tissue. A longitudinally sectioned eccrine duct is observed in **B;** eccrine glands occur in much higher density on the palm than on truncal skin.

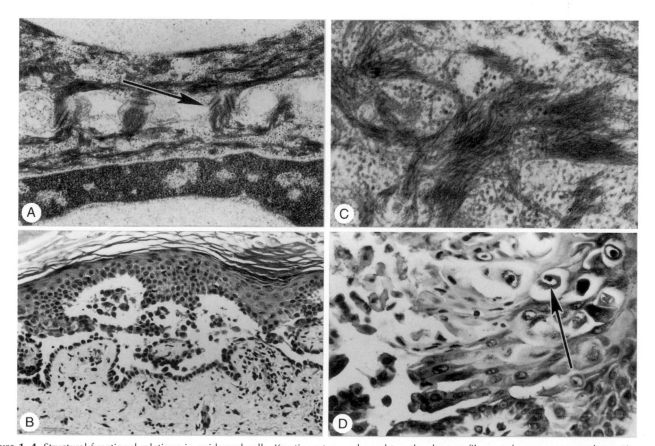

Figure 1–4. Structural-functional relations in epidermal cells. Keratinocytes are bound together by tonofilament-desmosome complexes **(A;** *arrow*) that span the peripheral cytoplasm and plasma membranes of adjacent cells. Compromise of these adhesion sites results in cleft or blister formation due to dyshesion **(B),** a process termed acantholysis. Keratinocyte cytoplasm is progressively filled with keratin intermediate filaments (i.e., tonofilaments; **C**) as these cells mature. Aberrant or premature expression of these structural proteins produces dense, hypereosinophilic cells **(D;** *arrow*), a process termed dyskeratosis.

imperative to evaluate all skin specimens within the context of the known anatomy of normal skin at the site of the biopsy. Moreover, normal physiologic alterations may also account for confusion. Common examples of this include the universal thinning of the epidermal layer associated with advanced age, a finding that could be interpreted as pathologically relevant atrophy when associated with underlying inflammation, and racially determined darkly pigmented skin, which may superficially mimic a freckle or lentigo as a result of prominent melanization of the stratum basalis.

The ultrastructural features of the epidermis that are relevant to diagnostic dermatopathology include detection of desmosomes, intermediate filaments, and phagocytized melanosomes. Desmosomes are specialized laminated attachment plaques that bind together the plasma membranes of adjacent keratinocytes (see Fig. 1–4). Desmosomes consist of two outer, electron-dense, thick bands, and three inner thin bands arranged in a parallel array. Between the inner bands is the glycocalyx, or intercellular cement substance, which is the presumed site of injury in pemphigus. Smaller, structurally less complex hemidesmosomes assist in anchoring the inferior surface of the basal cell plasma membrane to the adjacent basement membrane. Detection of desmosomes is particularly important in the ultrastructural confirmation of poorly differentiated or spindle cell squamous cell carcinomas, which may mimic amelanotic melanoma and lymphoma or mesenchymal neoplasia, respectively. Although desmosomes cannot be detected at routine light microscopy, their presence may often be inferred by detection of spiny intercellular junctions.

Intermediate filaments, which are also called tonofilaments when found in keratinocytes, are clustered aggregates of cytoplasmic fibrils 7 to 8 nm in diameter (see Fig. 1–4). While many of these filaments are continuous with the attachment plaques of desmosomes, others appear to lie free within the cytoplasm. Most of these filaments represent intracytoplasmic keratin protein, and their distribution throughout the cell results in a cytoskeleton integral to formation and preservation of cell shape and structural stability. Keratin-type intermediate filaments are characteristic of keratinocytes, although they are not entirely specific, and cells such as Merkel cells may display prominent perinuclear clusters of keratin-type intermediate filaments within their cytoplasm.

Epidermal intermediate filaments correlate with expression of cytoplasmic keratin, and commercially available antibodies to keratin are routinely employed to establish epidermal origin of certain poorly differentiated cutaneous neoplasms. Involucrin, a marker of terminal squamous differentiation, has shown promise in the differentiation of certain squamous cell carcinomas from keratoacanthomas (see Chap. 11), but routine use awaits further testing.

Melanosome complexes are membrane-bound aggregates of melanized, electron-dense melanosomes within the cytoplasm of keratinocytes, macrophages, or phagocytic tumor cells. In normal epidermis, these complexes result from physiologic pigment donation from nearby melanocytes, and they tend to be diffusely distributed within the epidermal layer. The tendency for keratinocytes to package melanosomes in small aggregates, as opposed to solitary organelles, is characteristic of the skin of Caucasians and those of Asian descent, whereas transmitted melanosomes remain solitary within keratinocytes of those of African descent and in Australian aborigines. Diagnostically, it is important to recognize that cells other than melanocytes may contain melanin pigment, thereby minimizing the possibility for misdiagnosis of melanoma based on ultrastructure of a poorly differentiated malignancy that has nonspecifically phagocytized this pigment. Solitary melanosomes in early stages of melanization, on the other hand, are typical of cells of melanocytic derivation (see following discussion of melanocyte structure).

Epidermal hyperplasia (Fig. 1–5) may be diffuse or preferentially favor the stratum granulosum (hypergranulosis), stratum spinosum (acanthosis), or stratum basalis (basaloid hyperplasia). It is manifested by increased epidermal thickness for body site, by abnormal keratinization, and often but not invariably, by increased numbers of mitotic figures within and above the stratum basalis. Epidermal hyperplasia involving the stratum spinosum may take the form of endophytic expansion of rete ridges to similar (regular acanthosis) or differing (irregular acanthosis) horizontal levels within the superficial dermis. Accurate characterization of acanthosis is imperative, because it greatly facilitates diagnostic recogni-

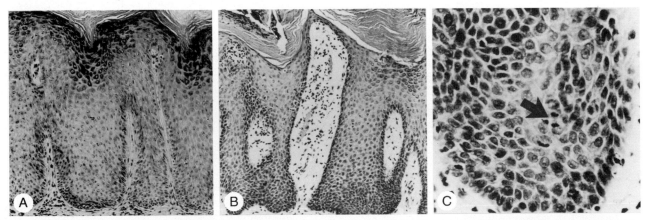

Figure 1–5. Epidermal hyperplasia, or acanthosis. **(A)** As a result of chronic exogenous trauma (e.g., rubbing, irritation), the stratum spinosum, stratum granulosum, and stratum corneum may become markedly thickened. Note the associated prominence of enlarged rete ridges. **(B)** In response to poorly defined endogenous stimuli, acanthosis is also characteristic of established psoriasis, although in this case there is thinning and loss of the stratum granulosum and retention of pyknotic nuclei into the scale (i.e., parakeratosis). There also is associated upward enlargement of dermal papillae. **(C)** Hyperplasia is often but not invariably associated with increased mitotic activity, particularly above the stratum basalis *(arrow).*

tion of a number of commonly encountered dermatoses. For example, regular acanthosis with hypogranulosis of psoriasis is distinct from irregular acanthosis with hypergranulosis of lichen simplex chronicus. The features of the latter are separable from chronic active eczematous dermatitis, which also displays spongiosis. Wedge-shaped hypergranulosis with acanthosis is more commonly seen in lichen planus than in lupus erythematosus, which rarely may exhibit hypertrophic epidermal changes. Acanthosis may be accompanied by *reactive atypia* (i.e., variability in nuclear size and nucleolar prominence in the presence of uniformly finely dispersed chromatin and a delicate nuclear membrane), particularly in the setting of repeated attempts at re-epithelialization (e.g., at the edge of an ulcer). Reactive atypia must be differentiated from keratinocyte proliferation accompanied by *dysplasia* (i.e., variability in nuclear size and nucleolar prominence in the presence of irregularly coarsely dispersed chromatin and a thickened nuclear membrane as a result of chromatin condensation), as is commonly encountered in actinic keratoses and squamous cell carcinomas.

Abnormalities in keratinization (Fig. 1–6) may represent one of the most subtle diagnostic abnormalities detectable at the light microscopic level (e.g., in the setting of ichthyosis), or may be so gross as to produce the spouting of a clinically apparent, ram-like cutaneous horn. Normal basket-weave stratum corneum is referred to as *orthokeratotic* scale. When the stratum corneum is increased in thickness, the term hyperorthokeratotic is used, and when the cells that form the layer come to lie closer together, the modifier *compact* is used. Thus, whereas ichthyosis may show only compact orthokeratotic scale, lichen simplex chronicus is characterized by a compact hyperorthokeratotic stratum corneum. Retention of nuclei into the scale is termed *parakeratosis,* a process that may be exquisitely focal and mound-like, as in pityriasis rosea, or diffuse and confluent, as in untreated, active psoriasis and advanced actinic keratoses. In general, hyperorthokeratosis is associated with underlying hypergranulosis, and parakeratosis is associated with underlying diminution in thickness of the stratum granulosum, although exceptions exist. Abnormalities in the stratum corneum do not always correlate with an underlying proliferative defect, because impaired desquamation may also result in retention of altered scale. Recognition of normal stratum corneum overlying an inflammatory infiltrate associated with epidermal injury usually signifies that the lesion is days or hours old (e.g., erythema multiforme) and testifies to the sensitivity of scale as an eventual indicator of even subtle chronic perturbations of underlying epidermal cells (e.g., guttate parapsoriasis). It is important to remember that the normal stratum corneum of palm and sole skin would represent strikingly compacted

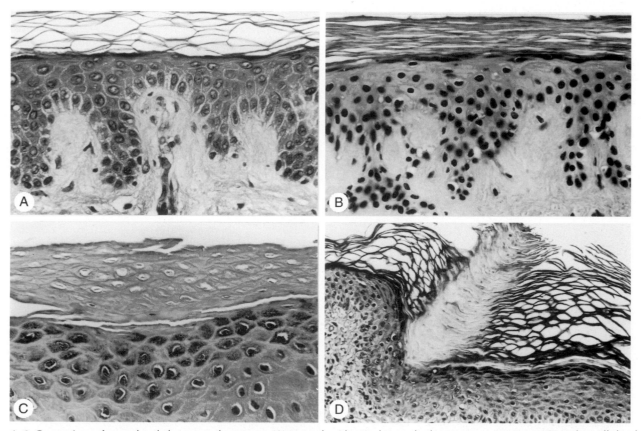

Figure 1–6. Comparison of normal and aberrant scale patterns. **(A)** Normal epidermis shows a basket-weave stratum corneum and a well-developed pattern of interdigitating rete ridges and dermal papillae. **(B)** Poorly fixed skin may result in artifactual distortion of the normal scale pattern, producing compacted orthokeratosis similar to that seen in certain forms of ichthyosis. **(C)** Early hyperkeratosis is characterized by compaction of scale and residua of degenerated nuclei. **(D)** Parakeratosis is characterized by retention of pyknotic nuclei into the stratum corneum. It is discretely localized to a small zone of underlying hypogranulosis, permitting side-by-side comparison with normal scale. This extremely focal, column-like zone of parakeratosis is referred to as a cornoid lamella.

hyperorthokeratosis if it occurred on the trunk, and any form of stratum corneum or stratum granulosum formation is abnormal for true mucosal epithelium.

Although epidermal keratinization normally occurs on the skin surface, keratin may be produced prematurely by underlying cells in certain pathologic circumstances. In invasive squamous cell carcinoma, small concentric lamellae of keratin aberrantly produced within the tumor are referred to as *keratin pearls.* Individual keratinocytes prematurely undergoing keratinization acquire cytoplasmic eosinophilia inappropriate for their level within the epidermis. This phenomenon, termed *dyskeratosis,* is different from the cellular degeneration and necrosis that result in cytoplasmic hypereosinophilia due to pH and water shifts or that are usually accompanied by an inflammatory insult and evidence of nuclear degeneration.

Epidermal atrophy (Fig. 1–7) connotes thinning of the epidermis. As noted previously, some degree of atrophy accompanies normal senescence, although physiologic thinning may be accelerated by substances such as prolonged application of potent topical steroids. Chronic destruction of the stratum basalis commonly eventuates in epidermal atrophy (e.g., discoid lupus erythematosus). Early atrophy is first evidenced by gradual loss of the normal epidermal rete ridge pattern. Advanced atrophy may result in a clinically semi-

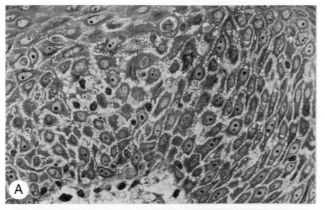

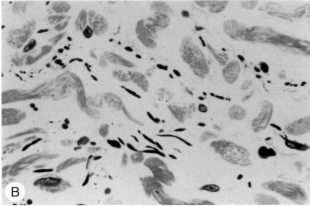

Figure 1–8. Spongiosis and dermal edema. **(A)** The widened intercellular spaces and prominence of spiny intercellular attachment sites result in a spongy appearance. **(B)** Similar widening of intercollagenous spaces occurs in the underlying dermis. Epidermal spongiosis and dermal edema are characteristic of acute contact hypersensitivity reactions, whereas pure dermal edema is more typical of urticaria.

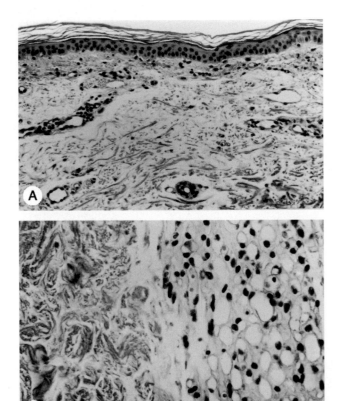

Figure 1–7. (A) Epidermal, dermal, and **(B)** subcutaneous atrophy. The epidermal layer is only three cells thick, and rete ridges are entirely absent. Dermal collagen fibers are abnormally thin and pale, and even subcutaneous fat is atrophic. These atrophic changes were elicited by chronic topical application of a potent fluorinated steroid; similar alterations are associated with senescence. Epidermal atrophy occurs independent of mesenchymal atrophy in certain cytotoxic dermatoses (e.g., discoid lupus erythematosus).

transparent, easily wrinkled epidermal layer reduced to only several cell layers thick.

The accumulation of plasma fluid in the intercellular spaces of the epidermis results in widened intercellular spaces and a prominent display of stretched intercellular junctions (Fig. 1–8). This spongy appearance is the basis for the term *spongiosis* and permits broad classification of a diverse array of inflammatory dermatoses that share this feature (see Chap. 3). The prototype of spongiotic dermatitis is allergic contact dermatitis. Pathophysiologically, spongiosis usually occurs in disorders characterized by increased permeability of superficial dermal venules and migration of lymphocytes into the epidermis. Epidermal hyperplasia or acanthosis is often seen in combination with spongiosis of subacute to chronic duration (weeks to months). Progression of spongiosis results in traumatic disruption of desmosomes and the formation of fluid-filled intraepidermal or subepidermal vesicles. The absence of spongiosis may be as diagnostically critical as its detection, as is the case in psoriasis and in the early phases of cutaneous T-cell lymphoma.

Acantholysis is the process whereby desmosomal attachments are lost or compromised, resulting in defective intercellular adhesion within the epidermis (see Fig. 1–4). The result generally is blister formation that occurs spontaneously or in association with minor trauma. Acantholytic cells within the stratum spinosum lose their angulated, polyhedral contour and characteristically become rounded up. Unlike spongiosis, which mechanically disrupts membrane attachment sites potentially killing cells that constitute the perimeter of the forming blister, precisely localized lysis of desmosomal plaques produces an acantholytic cell which may persist for some time as a rounded epithelial cell floating in nutrient-rich plasma filtrate. Pemphigus vulgaris is an example of immunologically mediated acantholysis. Keratinocytes genetically or neoplastically altered to produce faulty intercellular attachments also may exhibit acantholysis (e.g., as in Darier disease and in certain invasive squamous cell carcinomas). These acantholytic cells also frequently show associated dyskeratosis (so-called *acantholytic dyskeratosis*). Acantholytic and dyskeratotic cells may appear as small, seed-like ovoid cells with densely eosinophilic cytoplasm and pyknotic nuclei (''corps grains'') when they occur in the uppermost epidermal layers, or as larger, rounded acantholytic cells with characteristic perinuclear halos (''corps ronds'') when they occur in the midepidermis. Extensive acantholysis in squamous cell carcinoma may produce gland-like spaces resulting in confusion with adenocarcinoma, unless the acantholytic process is accurately recognized.

Although cell replication is balanced in part by surface desquamation, keratinocytes are also individually eliminated by the process of *apoptosis*. Apoptosis refers to necrosis of individual cells within the epidermis, often within the stratum spinosum. Affected cells show cytoplasmic eosinophilia and nuclear pyknosis. The earliest degenerative alterations involve the nucleus, however, and consist of programmed cell death mediated by endonucleases. Frequently, these cells are in apposition to or are partially engulfed by adjacent mononuclear cells. Ultrastructurally, these phagocytic cells are macrophages capable of digestion of necrotic keratinocytes. Rare apoptotic cells are physiologically normal, although their presence is increased after certain forms of radiation and chemotherapy, and in the setting of cytotoxic or cytokine-mediated epidermal injury. Apoptotic cells may also be incorporated into the superficial dermis, where they appear as anucleate, rounded eosinophilic bodies (i.e., colloid bodies) that stain for epidermal amyloid and contain immuno-globulin on immunofluorescence examination. Colloid body formation is typical of lichen planus, and may assist in the diagnosis of this condition.

Cytotoxic alteration refers to degeneration and necrosis of keratinocytes in association with inflammatory infiltrates composed of lymphocytes with cytotoxic capabilities (Fig. 1–9). Some forms of cytotoxic injury may involve apoptosis, whereas others (e.g., those due to cell membrane lysis) involve primary extranuclear insult. Acute cytotoxic injury frequently results in vacuolar degeneration of germinative cells that form the stratum basalis. This finding is of diagnostic significance in disorders such as lupus erythematosus, erythema multiforme, and fixed drug eruptions. Other manifestations of cytotoxic injury include increased numbers of apoptotic cells, which may be present singly or in small clusters. When mononuclear cells are radially arranged about apoptotic cells, this phenomenon is referred to as satellitosis, a finding of diagnostic significance in acute graft-versus-host disease and certain other forms of cytotoxic dermatitis. Chronic manifestations of cytotoxic injury include epidermal atrophy, abnormalities in stratum corneum formation, and reorganization of the stratum basalis into more angulated, keratinized, polyhedral cells, which is often referred to as squamatization. The latter feature is a characteristic finding in lichen planus.

Subtle *ischemic injury* may produce mild basal cell layer vacuolization or an increase in the number of apoptotic cells within the midepidermis. Marked ischemia, on the other hand, may result in full-thickness necrosis of the epidermis as well as blister formation as a result of dermal-epidermal separation. Ischemia must be differentiated from other forms of epidermal injury that result in similar zones of full-thickness epidermal necrosis (e.g., second- and third-degree burns). Electrical injury may produce extensive necrosis, although the tendency for keratinocyte nuclei to become elongated and arranged in parallel is a characteristic feature that usually permits diagnostic recognition of this type of insult.

Swelling of keratinocytes (Fig. 1–10) (hydropic degeneration) may result from fluid shifts, cytopathic effects of viral infection, or nutritional and metabolic imbalance. The net result is cellular enlargement and cytoplasmic pallor. In

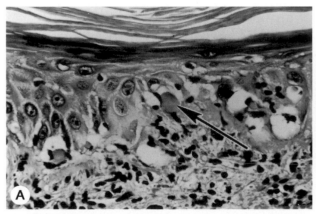 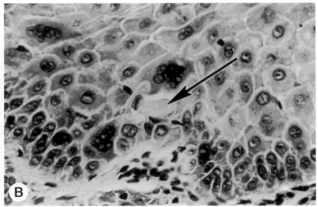

Figure 1–9. Cytotoxic alteration. **(A)** Numerous degenerating and necrotic keratinocytes appear as hypereosinophilic bodies *(arrow)* in the lower epidermal layers of the skin of this patient, who has dermatitis associated with an influx of lymphocytes with cytotoxic capabilities. Keratinocytes undergoing vacuolar degeneration are also prominent. Incorporation of apoptotic bodies into the superficial dermis (i.e., colloid body formation) may occur in some dermatoses. **(B)** Occasional apoptotic cells are observed within normal epidermis *(arrow)*. Note the adjacent multinucleated keratinocyte, a phenomenon of no pathologic significance when not associated with evidence of causation (e.g., herpes virus).

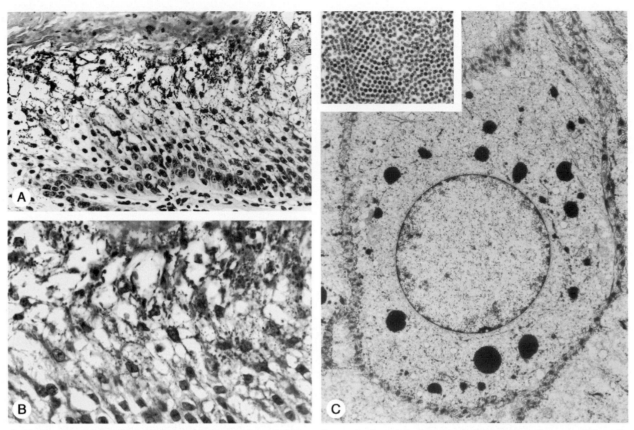

Figure 1–10. Keratinocyte lysis and swelling. **(A, B)** In epidermolytic hyperkeratosis, there is ballooning and dissolution of upper epidermal cells as a result of faulty maturation. **(C)** In patients who have human papillomavirus infection, cells of the upper epidermal layers show electron-lucent cytoplasm and diminished tonofilament expression for this level by electron microscopy and are recognized as koilocytes by light microscopy. There are intranuclear viral inclusions *(inset)* and characteristically rounded contours of enlarged keratohyaline granules within the cytoplasm.

human papillomavirus infection of epidermal keratinocytes, cell swelling and associated nuclear changes produce diagnostically important *koilocytes* within the superficial epidermal layers. Maturational disturbances may result in frank lysis of keratinocytes, resulting in cellular clearing and dyshesion. An example of this phenomenon is epidermolytic hyperkeratosis, in which lytic defects involving superficial keratinocytes are associated with excessive scale formation and expression of enlarged keratohyaline and trichohyaline granules by affected cells.

Melanocytes

In tissue sections stained with hematoxylin and eosin (H&E), melanocytes are relatively imperceptible. At high magnification, melanocytes may be detected along the stratum basalis by virtue of the clear pericellular spaces that result as an artifact of tissue fixation. The structural basis for this is the shrinkage of their cell bodies, which contract freely since they are not anchored to adjacent basal keratinocytes by desmosomal attachments. Compared to the larger and more open nuclei of keratinocytes, melanocytes have small, dense, ovoid nuclei—another distinguishing feature at the light microscopic level. The cytoplasm of melanocytes is pale, pink, and difficult to visualize in routine preparations.

Melanin pigment is infrequently detected in melanocytes by light microscopy. When melanin is observed, particularly in heavily pigmented individuals, it tends to be distributed diffusely throughout the basal keratinocytes of the epidermis.

There is a normal tendency for melanocytes to grow exclusively within the basal cell layer, and suprabasal melanocytes are seldom encountered. There are approximately 5 to 10 melanocyte cell bodies per linear millimeter of epidermis, although regional variation is common. Hyperplastic melanocytes may initially appear to represent vacuolated basal keratinocytes on cursory inspection (Fig. 1–11).

By electron microscopy, melanocytes show a relatively electron-lucent cytoplasm that is free of tonofilaments (Fig. 1–11*C*). Numerous thin dendrites extend from the cell bodies, insinuating themselves upward between keratinocytes of the stratum spinosum and stratum granulosum. The characteristic feature of melanocytes is a cytoplasmic organelle termed the *melanosome*. This is a 0.3- to 0.8-μm-wide, membrane-bound, ellipsoid structure with a characteristic internal periodicity formed by membranes upon which tyrosinase-dependent melanization occurs. As this enzymatic process takes place, melanosomes become progressively electron-dense. Eventually, melanosomes are transported to melanocytic dendrites and expelled into the cytoplasm of adjacent keratinocytes, a process known as pigment donation. This mechanism results in diffuse dispersion of pigment within keratinocytes, which results in an endogenous sunscreen that partially protects against deleterious effects of ultraviolet radiation. Within keratinocytes, melanosomes of Caucasians and those of Asian descent become packaged, with several melanosomes enclosed within a limiting membrane. Melanosomes within keratinocytes of those of African descent tend to reside as solitary organelles (unpackaged) within the keratinocyte cytoplasm.

Ultrastructural detection of melanosomes is an accepted method of establishing the diagnosis of amelanotic malignant melanoma. Because a variety of cell types may phagocytize melanin pigment, detection of immature melanosomes in formative stages of melanization is required to infer melanocytic lineage at an ultrastructural level. Early melanosomes tend to be relatively electron-lucent but exhibit characteristic internal periodicity. Mature melanosomes tend to be electron-dense, and periodicity may be partially or completely obscured.

There are a number of special diagnostic techniques that facilitate the study of melanocytes. For example, the Fontana-Masson stain renders melanosomes intensely dark gray to black, facilitating their detection by light microscopy in situations in which defective synthesis or pigment donation is suspected. The dopa enzyme histochemical stain requires frozen tissue, and is capable of detecting cells and organelles that contain tyrosinase. This approach may be helpful in the evaluation of certain forms of albinism. Although not entirely specific for melanocytes, antibodies to S100 protein (Fig. 1–

11B) are routinely used for melanocyte enumeration (e.g., in the evaluation of vitiligo) and in conjunction with panels of antisera to epithelial and lymphoreticular antigens in the evaluation of poorly differentiated tumors. A melanoma-associated antibody termed HMB-45 has become available. This antibody does not react with normal melanocytes or most melanocytic nevi, but with melanoma cells principally of the non–spindle cell type. It is not entirely specific for melanoma, however. Both S100 protein and HMB-45 are applicable to formalin-fixed, paraffin-embedded tissue sections.

Melanocytic hyperplasia connotes an increase in melanocyte number and represents a very common event. Whereas simple lentigos show melanocytic hyperplasia, freckles do not. Hyperplastic melanocytes generally proliferate within the stratum basalis. Advanced lentigos may show striking increases in the number of basal cell layer melanocytes with otherwise normal cytologic features. This mode of hyperplasia is frequently referred to as *lentiginous* (Fig. 1–11A), and may occur de novo, in response to chronic actinic exposure, or in association with evolving melanocytic nevi.

Melanocytic dysplasia is a cytologic term that, for cells of the melanocytic series, refers to varying degrees of nuclear contour irregularity, variation in nuclear size and shape, and coarse aggregation of chromatin within nuclei and in apposition to the nuclear membrane. Melanocytic dysplasia must

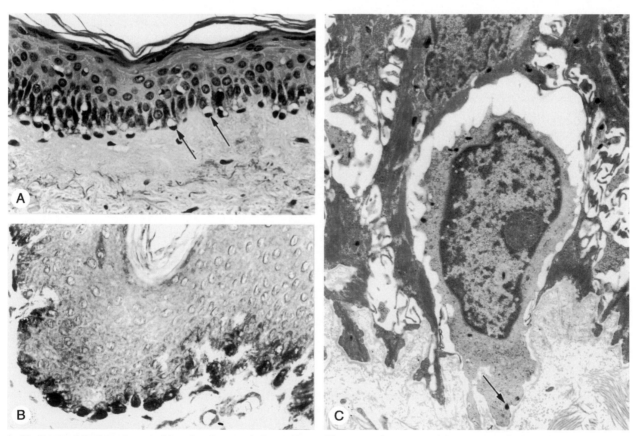

Figure 1–11. Routine histology, immunohistochemistry, and ultrastructure of human melanocytes. **(A)** In patients who have lentiginous melanocytic hyperplasia, melanocytes are prominently displayed along the stratum basalis as cells with ovoid, dense nuclei; unapparent cytoplasm; and pericellular clear spaces due to cytoplasmic contraction *(arrows)*. **(B)** Immunohistochemistry for S100 protein further defines the normal basal distribution of these cells. **(C)** Ultrastructural examination shows melanocytes have relatively electron-lucent cytoplasm devoid of tonofilaments; note solitary melanosomes *(arrow)*.

be differentiated from reactive melanocytic atypia, a phenomenon which may be seen at sites of inflammation, fibrosis, or in actively growing or hormonally stimulated lesions. As is the case for keratinocytes, reactive melanocytic atypia is characterized by nuclear enlargement without significant angulation or irregularity of nuclear contour, prominent nucleoli, and a finely distributed, uniform chromatin pattern bordered by a delicate, thin, uniform nuclear membrane. Dysplasia may occur de novo, particularly in sites of chronic sun exposure, or it may be seen in association with melanocytic nevi. Many dermatologists believe that the dysplastic lentiginous component of nevi represents a precursor cellular pool for the genesis of malignant melanoma.

The concept of *nevic cell transformation of melanocytes* is important, because these commonly encountered lesions are composed of melanocytic cells that differ significantly from normal melanocytes with respect to both cytology and architecture. Nevic cells are round, display variable quantities of pale pink cytoplasm, and may be heavily pigmented. These cells do not possess dendrites, and their nuclei are larger and less uniformly dense than those of melanocytes. Unlike melanocytes, which grow and persist normally within the stratum basalis of the epidermis, nevic cells proliferate in small clusters or nests both within the epidermis and, over time, within the dermis.

Malignant transformation of cells of the melanocytic series is generally heralded by progressive dysplasia, which may be detected at a morphologic level. Although exceptions exist (see Chap. 12), malignant melanocytes generally contain large, highly pleomorphic nuclei with one or more eosinophilic nucleoli, and coarsely clumped heterochromatin. Melanin production, when present, is aberrant, producing a coarsely granulated cytoplasm. Unlike normal melanocytes, which grow radially within the lower epidermis, and nevus cells, which grow in uniform small nests within the lower epidermis and dermis, melanoma cells proliferate within all

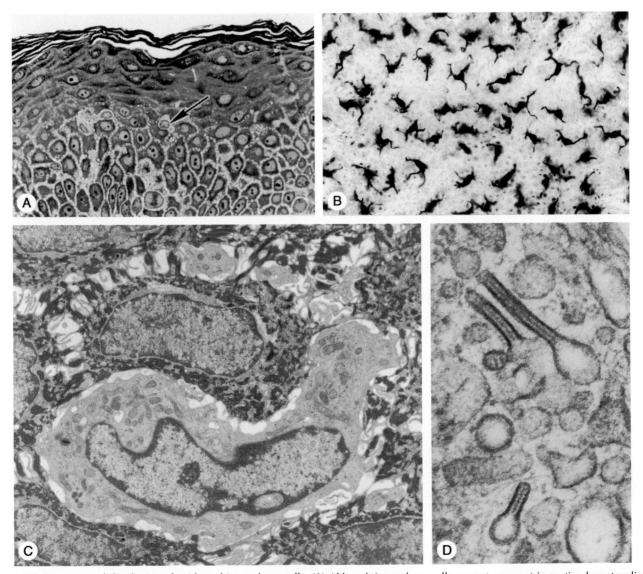

Figure 1–12. Structure and distribution of epidermal Langerhans cells. **(A)** Although Langerhans cells are not apparent in routine hematoxylin and eosin–stained sections, in 1-μm-thick, plastic-embedded sections, they appear as midlevel epidermal clear cells *(arrow).* **(B)** Like melanocytes, Langerhans cells and associated dendrites are uniformly distributed throughout the epidermal layer for efficient coverage of the epidermal surface (ATPase enzyme histochemistry of epidermal sheet viewed en face). **(C)** Ultrastructurally, Langerhans cells have relatively electron-lucent cytoplasm and vaguely infolded nuclear contours and contain tennis racket–shaped Birbeck granules **(D).**

levels of the epidermis. Upon reticular dermal invasion, melanoma cells show inexorable downgrowth, which over time eventuates in metastases.

Langerhans Cells

Langerhans cells are predominantly located in the midportion of the stratum spinosum and, like underlying melanocytes, extend elaborate dendritic processes toward the epidermal surface (Fig. 1–12). These cells are remarkably uniformly distributed in a highly efficient manner that leaves no region of the epidermal surface free of the presence of a nearby dendrite. Routine H&E-stained sections do not permit detection of Langerhans cells; ultrastructural and immunohistochemical methods are required for their definitive identification. One-micron-thick, plastic-embedded sections (Fig. 1–12A) render Langerhans cells apparent as midepidermal clear cells, although migrant histiocytes may mimic this picture.

On ultrastructural examination (Fig. 1–12C, D), Langerhans cells are characterized by eccentric, frequently infolded nuclei; relatively clear cytoplasm; absence of cell junctions; and specific cytoplasmic granules termed Birbeck granules. These organelles are plate-like disks with variably sized, round vacuoles at one end. In cross section, Birbeck granules frequently appear as tennis racquet–like structures with an internal zipper-like periodic striation within the handle. Although Birbeck granules have proven useful in the ultrastructural detection of Langerhans cells and their proliferative counterparts (i.e., histiocytosis X cells), their function remains an enigma. They appear to form in association with endocytotic, clathrin-coated pits at the plasma membrane surface. Cells with all ultrastructural features of Langerhans cells, but without Birbeck granules upon serial sectioning, have been referred to as indeterminate cells.

Like melanocytes, Langerhans cells show cytoplasmic reactivity for S100 protein. They are also characterized by ATPase reactivity (Fig. 1–12B), as well as by the display of the CD1a cell surface epitope in fresh frozen tissue preparations. This latter antigen may be defined by antibodies such as OKT6 or Leu 6 and represents a highly specific marker for the detection of Langerhans cells and histiocytosis X cells. Although fresh frozen tissue is required for this purpose, tissue transported in immunofluorescence transport medium (i.e., Michel medium) has proved adequate for immunohistochemical detection of the CD1a epitope.

Functionally, Langerhans cells are important primarily as antigen presenters to T cells during the evolution of cell-mediated immune responses in skin. Focal occurrences of Langerhans-cell hyperplasia, referred to as Langerhans-cell microgranulomas, may produce small clusters of mononuclear cells in the epidermis in the setting of florid immune responses. Such clusters must not be confused with Pautrier microabscesses of cutaneous T-cell lymphoma. Tumoral proliferations of Langerhans cells occur in histiocytosis X (see Chap. 14).

Merkel Cells

Merkel cells are poorly understood cells that, in lower vertebrates, probably subserve neurosensory function in as-

sociation with the pilar apparatus. In humans, these neuroendocrine cells are located individually along the basal cell layer, where they are detected by light microscopy only with the use of immunohistochemical techniques (Fig. 1–13A). The significance of Merkel cells lies in the rare occurrence of primary neuroendocrine carcinoma (see Chap. 11).

Merkel cells ultrastructurally contain small, dense core–type neurosecretory granules (Fig. 1–13B). These granules are uniform in size, membrane-bound, and considerably smaller than melanosomes and lysosomes. Merkel cells also contain characteristic perinuclear aggregates of keratin-type intermediate filaments, and their plasma membranes display desmosomes akin to keratinocytes. Unlike epithelial cells, however, Merkel cells contain neuron-specific enolase and occasionally are documented ultrastructurally in apposition to unmyelinated nerve fibers (Fig. 1–13B).

Cutaneous Adnexae

Hair Follicles

Hair follicles are specialized downgrowths of the epidermis (Fig. 1–14). Their importance in diagnostic dermatopathology lies in (1) their involvement in inflammatory and neoplastic diseases (e.g., lupus erythematosus, cutaneous T-cell lymphoma); (2) the tendency of certain adnexal neoplasms to recapitulate follicular ontogeny and differentiation; and (3) their participation in certain inflammatory and non-

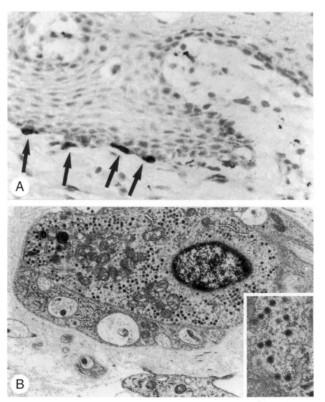

Figure 1–13. Epidermal neuroendocrine or Merkel cells. **(A)** Neuroendocrine cells are present in small numbers in normal epidermis and require immunohistochemical probes for their detection within the stratum basalis *(arrows).* **(B)** These cells characteristically contain small, membrane-bound, dense core–type granules *(inset).*

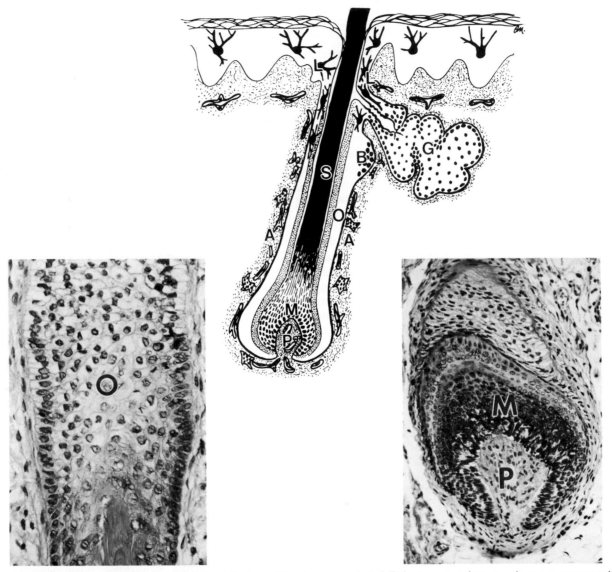

Figure 1–16. Schematic representation and correlative histology of human anagen hair follicle. Important features relevant to common follicular tumors and inflammatory diseases include hair papillae (P), hair matrix cells (M) surrounding follicular papillae (see lower right for correlative histology), glycogenated outer root sheath (O, see lower left for correlative histology), hair shafts (S), follicular stem cell bulge (B), sebaceous gland (G), perifollicular connective adventitia (A) rich in blood vessels and mast cells and contiguous with papillary dermal collagen, and Langerhans cells (L) that are concentrated within the infundibular epithelium, as well as evenly distributed in the interfollicular epidermis.

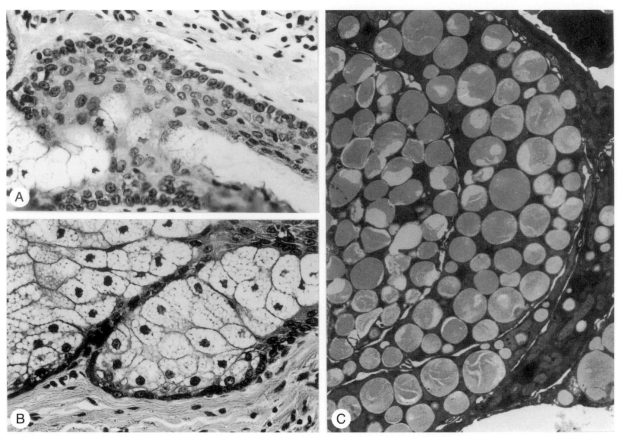

Figure 1–17. Sebaceous duct and lobule. **(A)** The sebaceous duct has a corrugated, eosinophilic lining that is recapitulated in the walls of steatocystomas. **(B)** The lobule is composed of large polyhedral epithelial cells containing clear lipid vacuoles bordered by a single layer of nonlipidized basaloid cells. Scalloped nuclear borders result from compression by vacuoles. **(C)** These vacuoles contain homogeneous grey material on ultrastructural examination, a technique that may be helpful in evaluation of sebaceous carcinoma, even after retrieval from paraffin blocks.

Eccrine Glands

Eccrine glands originate as pores on the epidermal surface which, for unknown reasons, form corkscrew-like spiraling ducts that course through the epidermal layer (i.e., the acrosyringium). These ducts are lined by a thin mantle of hyalinized eosinophilic material (i.e., cuticle) which stains positively with periodic acid–Schiff (PAS) stain. This is a helpful feature in determining eccrine ductular differentiation in certain neoplasms. The eccrine duct becomes straight as it courses downward into the dermis. The terminal eccrine gland (Fig. 1–18) is coiled and consists of a single layer of cuboidal epithelial cells that exhibit lighter-staining cytoplasm than the more darkly staining cytoplasm of the cells that compose the eccrine duct. The outer mantle of the secretory coil is rimmed by myoepithelial cells embedded in a vascular adventitia replete with unmyelinated nerves and mast cells.

Apocrine Glands

Apocrine ducts generally originate in the upper portion of the hair follicle, although direct origination of ducts on the epidermal surface has been documented. The apocrine duct, similar to the eccrine duct, communicates with the apocrine gland and secretory coil, which is composed of cuboidal epithelium showing characteristic ''decapitation''

secretion (Fig. 1–19A, B). Apocrine glands are concentrated at specific body sites, such as axillae, the anogenital region, and the periumbilical area. The occurrence of apocrine glands at anomalous loci (e.g., scalp) generally signifies specific pathology (e.g., nevus sebaceus). The architectural and tinctorial differences in cytoplasmic staining between eccrine, apocrine, and sebaceous glands permit differentiation among cutaneous secretory glands with respect to subtle histologic characteristics (Fig. 1–20). For example, eccrine glands have pale eosinophilic cytoplasm, whereas apocrine glands have finely granular, intensely eosinophilic cytoplasm. Sebaceous glands, on the other hand, have finely vacuolated cytoplasm in which individual vacuoles often indent the nuclear contour. These features may be of assistance in identifying differentiation pathways in neoplasms of adnexal derivation.

Basement Membrane Zone

The epidermal-dermal basement membrane zone (BMZ) represents the structural cement that anchors the epidermal layer to the leathery underlying dermis. The normal BMZ is composed of a thin layer of compacted protein that defines the lower limits of the basal cell layer (Fig. 1–21A); this zone can be identified by PAS stain. Immunocytochemical data has revealed that this region is enriched for specialized struc-

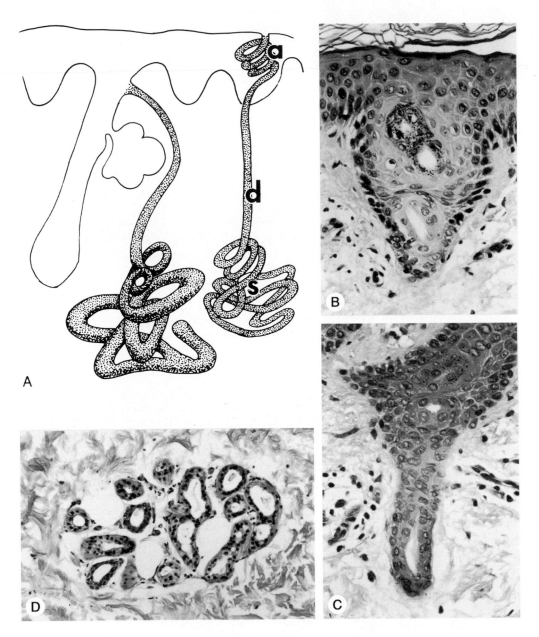

Figure 1–18. Schematic representation and correlative histology of the human eccrine apparatus. **(A)** The eccrine gland consists of a coiled secretory segment (s), a straight intradermal duct (d) that ascends toward the epidermal layer, and a coiled terminal duct or acrosyringium (a) which traverses the epidermal layer and terminates on the skin surface. The acrosyringium is lined by a thin mantle of eosinophilic material (i.e., cuticle). **(B)** Acrosyringium. **(C)** Superficial portion of dermal eccrine duct. **(D)** Secretory coil.

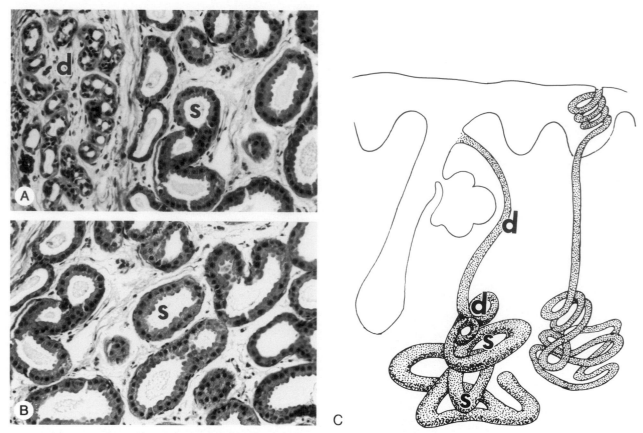

Figure 1–19. Schematic and correlative histology of the human apocrine apparatus. **(A–C)** The apocrine secretory coil (s) is larger and composed of more dilated glands than its eccrine counterpart. The apocrine duct (d) courses upward from the coil toward the superficial dermis, where it most often empties into a follicular orifice. In cross section, the apocrine duct resembles the eccrine duct.

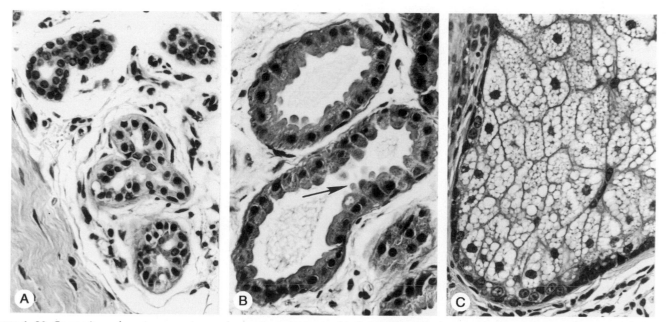

Figure 1–20. Comparison of eccrine, apocrine, and sebaceous secretory epithelium. **(A)** Unlike the eccrine duct, the eccrine secretory coil is lined by cuboidal epithelium with a pale, often vacuolated cytoplasm and surrounded by a thin mantle of myoepithelial cells. The vessels surrounding the duct and coil are contiguous with the superficial vascular plexus, which separates papillary from reticular dermis. **(B)** The epithelium lining the apocrine coil has granular, eosinophilic cytoplasm and protuberant lumenal membranes that appear to bud into the lumen (decapitation- or apocrine-type secretion; *arrow*). **(C)** The sebaceous gland is composed of vacuolated, lipidized epithelial cells bordered by a single layer of nonlipidized basaloid cells at the perimeter. Lipid vacuoles characteristically indent the nuclear membrane, producing a scalloped nuclear contour.

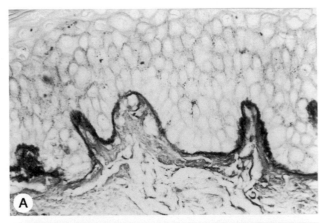

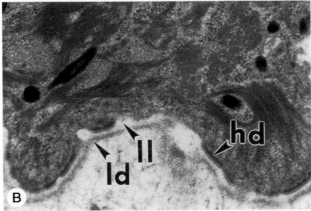

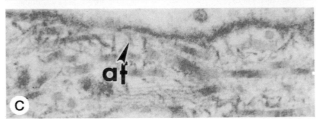

Figure 1–21. Normal epidermal basement membrane zone. **(A)** This PAS stain demonstrates the thin, uniform basement membrane that normally separates the epidermal and dermal layers. **(B and C)** Ultrastructurally, this membrane is composed of a lamina lucida (ll), lamina densa (ld), and anchoring fibrils (af). Hemidesmosomes (hd) bind basal keratinocytes to the basement membrane.

tural proteins such as bullous pemphigoid antigen and laminin. These proteins appear to facilitate normal epidermal-dermal attachment. Ultrastructurally, the BMZ is comprised of a dense lamina (i.e., lamina densa), which is separated from the inferior border of the basal cell plasma membrane by a uniform, thin, clear zone (i.e., lamina lucida). The lamina lucida is deceptively vacuous; it contains bullous pemphigoid antigen and probably other visually elusive proteins critical to epidermal-dermal bonding. The basement membrane (i.e., lamina densa and lamina lucida) is linked to the overlying epidermis by hemidesmosomes (Fig. 1–21B) and to the underlying dermis by anchoring fibrils. Defects in integral components of basement membrane structures may result in specific pathology, as is the case in bullous pemphigoid (bullous pemphigoid antigen) and epidermolysis bullosa dystrophica (anchoring fibrils).

Microvessels and Related Cells

The *superficial microvascular plexus* divides the papillary dermis from the reticular dermis (Fig. 1–22); therefore, it is an important landmark in distinguishing level II from level III melanoma (see Chap. 12). This plexus also contains postcapillary venules, which are critical targets of inflammatory cells that become adherent to endothelial cells in the cutaneous immune response (see Chap. 7). From this plexus emanate capillary loops that extend upward into each dermal papilla, supplying nutrients to the nearby avascular epidermal layer (Fig. 1–23A, B). These vascular loops may undergo hyperplasia in the setting of chronic stasis dermatitis, and the delicate, felt-like papillary dermal matrix in which they are embedded may transform to vertically oriented strands of collagen as a result of chronic excoriation (Fig. 1–23C, D). The reticular dermis and subcutis are separated by a horizontal plexus of venules and arterioles termed the deep vascular plexus. This plexus is linked to its superficial counterpart by vertically oriented vessels that course, often at angles, through the reticular dermis at irregular intervals. Vessels that supply septa that separate lobules of underlying subcutaneous fat communicate with those of the deep vascular plexus.

The dermal microvasculature is surrounded by a sparse complement of immunologically important cells, including Factor XIIIa–containing dermal dendrocytes, phagocytic and antigen-presenting macrophages, and mast cells. These cells probably collaborate to coordinate antigen presentation, induction of cellular inflammation, wound healing, and hemostasis in the immediate perivascular microenvironment. In this regard, it has been determined that mast cells may trigger adhesive events between circulating leukocytes and endothelial cells that result in certain forms of angiocentric cutaneous inflammation. One of the triggers for mast cell activation and degranulation, resulting in the local release of granule mediators such as histamine, heparin, serine proteinases, and cytokines, are neuropeptide molecules within unmyelinated axons that surround perivascular mast cells (Fig. 1–24). These axons contain neuropeptides such as substance P, which is capable of rapidly liberating the contents of nearby mast cells, setting into motion a cascade of molecular events that eventuate in leukocyte-endothelial adhesion. In addition, small fibers from these neural plexuses innervate sensory receptors responsible for the critically important sensations of cutaneous pain, pressure, and temperature perception (Fig. 1–24).

Extracellular Dermal Matrix

The dermis is predominantly composed of the tough structural protein collagen, the primary component in animal hide or leather. Fibroblasts, the source of collagen production, are present in relatively low numbers throughout the dermal matrix. Collagen within the dermis is quite heterogeneous and specialized with regard to its molecular structure. The papillary dermis is composed primarily of type III collagen, whereas the reticular dermis is composed of type I collagen. Basement membranes about dermal vessels and

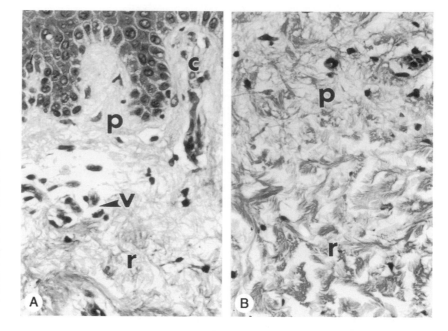

Figure 1–22. Superficial microvascular plexus and comparison of papillary and reticular dermal structure. **(A)** The superficial microvascular plexus (v) represents an anatomic boundary between papillary dermis (p) and reticular dermis (r). Cells that surround this plexus include mast cells (1 to 3 per vessel profile), macrophages, and dermal dendrocytes. Capillary loops (c) emanating from this plexus extend vertically into dermal papillae and are conduits for nutrients that supply the avascular epidermal layer. **(B)** The papillary dermis (p) is composed of type III collagen and is formed by thin, interwoven strands. The reticular dermis (r) is composed of type I collagen and is formed by relatively thick collagen bundles.

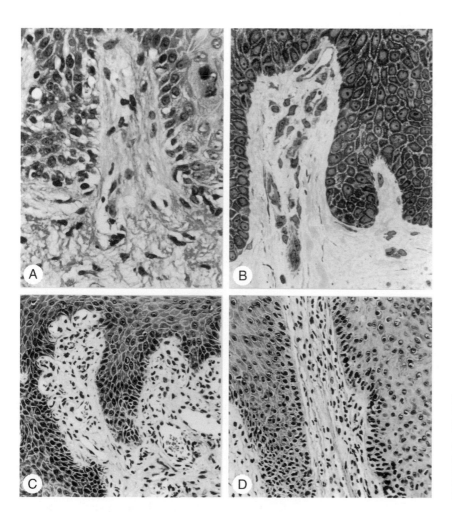

Figure 1–23. Dermal papillae and associated microvessels. The delicate capillary loops and surrounding papillary dermal collagen seen in **(A)** routine and **(B)** 1-μm sections of normal skin undergo dramatic alterations in patients with conditions such as **(C)** stasis dermatitis and **(D)** lichen simplex chronicus. In stasis dermatitis, superficial vessels become ectatic and tortuous, and in lichen simplex chronicus, collagen thickens and aligns in a vertical array.

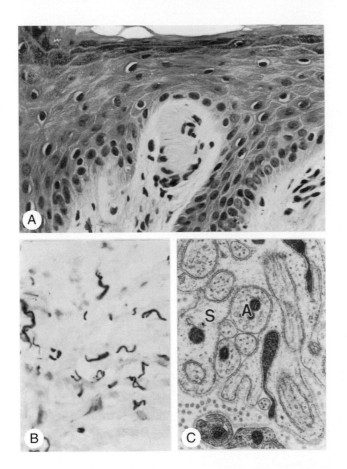

Figure 1–24. Dermal nerve fibers and associated sensory receptors. **(A)** Meissner corpuscles within the superficial dermis represent touch receptors. **(B)** Unmyelinated nerve fibers, stained immunocytochemically for the neural cell adhesion molecule, are closely associated with vascular plexuses and adnexal structures. **(C)** Ultrastructure of unmyelinated dermal nerve fibers. Axons (A) are enveloped by Schwann cell cytoplasm (S).

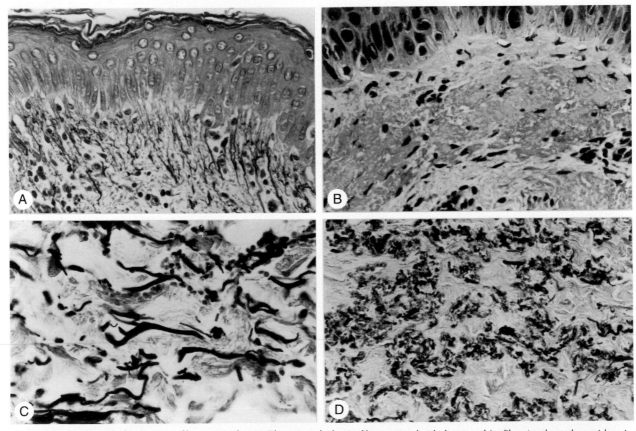

Figure 1–25. Human dermal elastic tissue fiber network. **(A)** The normal elastic fiber network *(dark grey, thin fibers)* tethers the epidermis to the reticular dermis. **(B)** Solar elastosis *(clumped, pale grey material in central portion of panel)* replaces the normal elastic fiber network. **(C)** Reticular dermal elastic fibers are normally present amid collagen bundles. **(D)** Pathologically altered reticular dermal elastic fibers are seen in a patient who has pseudoxanthoma elasticum. (**C** and **D,** Verhoeff-van Gieson elastic fiber stains.)

forming the dermal-epidermal interface contain type IV collagen, whereas anchoring fibrils that tether the epidermal basal lamina to the papillary dermis are composed of type VII collagen.

The papillary dermis also contains thin elastic fibers that traverse this layer in vertical array and appear to anchor the epidermis with respect to the underlying superficial reticular dermis (Fig. 1–25A). It is not surprising, therefore, that when these exquisitely delicate and intricate fibers are replaced by coarse, amorphous deposits of abnormal elastin due to chronic solar exposure (Fig. 1–25B), diminished recoil and actinic ageing (i.e., surface wrinkles) ensue. The elastic fibers that normally course through the reticular dermis are thick, branching strands that tend to be horizontally oriented (Fig. 1–25C). Pathologic conditions such as pseudoxanthoma elasticum may provoke profound alterations even in these most resilient components of the dermal extracellular matrix, resulting in marked fraying and fragmentation (Fig. 1–25D).

An often overlooked but major component of the dermal extracellular matrix is the mucopolysaccharide ground substance present between collagen and elastin fibers. Ground substance is apparent only as minute, particulate, grey-blue particles and strands on routine light microscopy (see Fig. 1–27B). Ground substance often is appreciated only after it has become markedly increased, as in lupus erythematosus, granuloma annulare, and pretibial myxedema. Special stains help-

ful for detection of mucopolysaccharides include alcian blue (pH 2.5), colloidal iron, and mucicarmine.

Pathologic alterations in the extracellular matrix occur frequently, and recognition of related alterations is critical to formulation of an accurate diagnosis. Collagen fibers undergo hyperplasia in the setting of hypertrophic scars (Fig. 1–26A), and individual bundles become hypertrophied and hyalinized in the poorly understood yet common condition of keloid formation (Fig. 1–26B). Diffuse hyalinization and hypertrophy of collagen with encroachment on adnexae and subcutaneous fat is characteristic of scleroderma (Fig. 1–26C). Sclerosis and edema of collagen in association with tumoral proliferation of hyperplastic vessels is the pattern seen in pyogenic granulomas (Fig. 1–26D). In all of these hyperplasias and hypertrophies of extracellular matrix and related cells, characteristic clinical lesions evolve, and their histologic identification depends on recognition of these basic reaction patterns of extracellular matrix proliferation and deposition.

Degeneration of extracellular matrix elements also occurs commonly, and there are several basic reaction patterns. Mucinous degeneration with necrobiosis is a poor term, because extracellular matrix is not living (bio), and therefore it cannot die (necro). A typical disorder in which this pattern is observed is granuloma annulare (Fig. 1–27A, B). In mucinous degeneration of the extracellular matrix, there is pallor

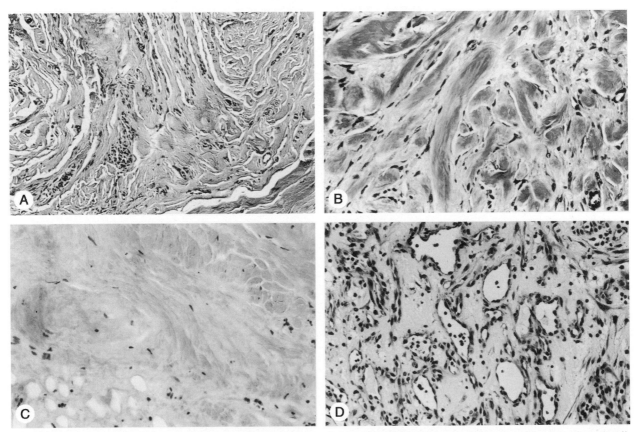

Figure 1–26. Common reaction patterns of dermal collagenous matrix: Sclerosis and proliferation. **(A)** In hypertrophic scars, dermal collagen is replaced by whirling parallel arrays of collagen fibers and proliferating vessels. **(B)** Keloids are characterized by glassy, intensely eosinophilic bands of collagen interspersed with pale, thin fibers. **(C)** Scleroderma typically shows pale pink, homogenized collagen containing few nucleated cells. **(D)** Pyogenic granulomas are typified by congeries of dilated, proliferating vessels within a pale, edematous, often inflamed collagenous stroma.

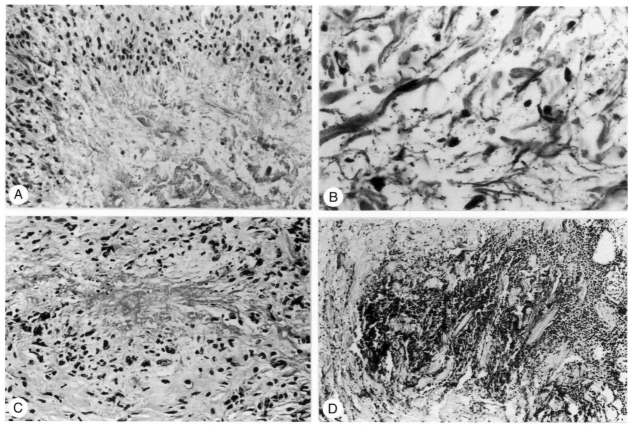

Figure 1–27. Common reaction patterns of dermal collagenous matrix: Degeneration. **(A)** Particulate, mucinous necrobiosis of collagen takes place in patients who have granuloma annulare. **(B)** Higher magnification of **A** shows stringy, particulate mucin strands admixed with thin collagen fibers. **(C)** Granular (i.e., fibrinoid) collagen degeneration of the rheumatoid nodule is present in the central portion of the panel. **(D)** Glassy collagen bundles entrapped in darkly stained aggregates of inflammatory cells (eosinophils) are known as flame figures.

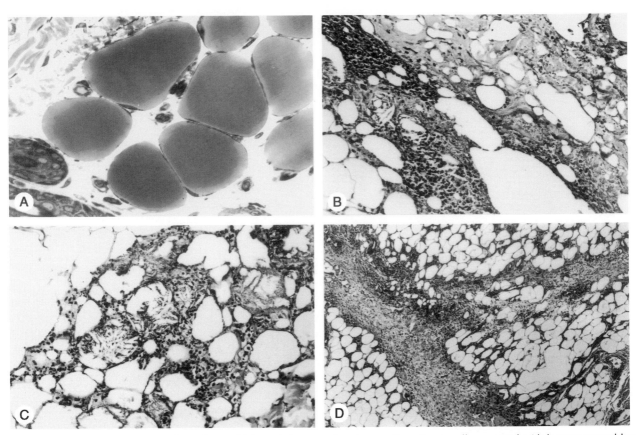

Figure 1–28. Subcutaneous fat: Patterns of reaction and injury. A 1-μm section shows adipocytes as cells engorged with homogeneous blue lipid with compressed nuclei at the cell perimeter. **(B)** Atrophy and liquefactive necrosis of adipocytes within a lobule in lupus panniculitis. **(C)** Aggregates of basophilic inflammatory cells are associated with crystallization of lipid within adipocytes in subcutaneous fat necrosis of the newborn. **(D)** Septa that separate fat lobules are prominently infiltrated by basophilic aggregates of inflammatory cells in patients who have septal panniculitis (i.e., erythema nodosum); the less cellular zone in the involved septum represents early fibrosis.

of collagen fibers associated with mucin deposits manifested as particulated, string-like, pale blue-grey fibers between collagen bundles. Fibrinoid degeneration of collagen is characteristically seen in rheumatoid nodules. In these nodules, zones of collagen acquire a deep red, refractile quality typical of extravasated fibrin (Fig. 1–27C). Collagen bundles may also become eosinophilic as a result of exposure to potent proteolytic enzymes, such as those produced by eosinophils. Degeneration of collagen bundles associated with degranulating eosinophils is observed in eosinophilic cellulitis (i.e., Well syndrome) (see Chap. 8). In this disorder, irregular arrays of deeply eosinophilic collagen bundles resemble flames, and thus have been termed "flame figures" (Fig. 1–27D). This is a diagnostic feature of assistance in the recognition of eosinophilic cellulitis, although similar findings may be seen in insect bites containing numerous eosinophils.

Subcutaneous Fat

The subcutaneous fat is both a cushion to prevent mechanical injury as well as a storage depot for high-potency energy sources. Fat is stored in adipocytes, which are enormously distended cells that comprise the majority of cells in mature (i.e., adult) adipose tissue (Fig. 1–28A). Adipocytes are best observed with glutaraldehyde fixation and plastic embedding. With this technique, the intracytoplasmic stores

of fat do not dissolve, but appear as homogeneous, dense, storage globules (Fig. 1–28A). Adipocytes are arranged in sheet-like lobules separated by thin, fibrous septa in which course nutrient vessels. These septa anchor the deepest limits of the reticular dermis to underlying fascia, with an intervening cushion of subcutaneous lobules formed by masses of adipocytes. Degeneration of adipocytes is observed as a consequence of inflammation, as in lupus panniculitis, in which these cells undergo coagulative and liquefactive necrosis (Fig. 1–28B). Lipids may also crystallize into needle-like arrays in certain disorders, such as subcutaneous fat necrosis of the newborn (Fig. 1–28C). Inflammation of the subcutaneous fat may result in either a septal or lobular panniculitis, and preferential involvement of either of these architectural domains is of profound diagnostic significance (Fig. 1–28D).

SELECTED REFERENCES

Lever WF, Schaumburg-Lever G. Histopathology of the Skin, 7th ed. Philadelphia: JB Lippincott, 1990:9.

Murphy GF, Elder DE. Atlas of Tumor Pathology. Non-Melanocytic Tumors of the Skin. Washington, DC: AFIP Press, 1991:2.

Murphy GF, Mihm MC Jr. The skin. *In* Cotran RS, Kumar V, Robbins SL, eds. Robbins Pathologic Basis of Disease, 4th ed. Philadelphia: WB Saunders, 1989:1277.

Stenn KS, Bhawan J. The normal histology of the skin. *In* Farmer ER, Hood AF, eds. Pathology of the Skin. Norwalk, CT: Appleton & Lange, 1990:3.

2

Diagnostic Methodology: Immunofluorescence

Rosalie Elenitsas, Christine Jaworsky, and George F. Murphy

DEFINITIONS AND GENERAL CONSIDERATIONS

This chapter briefly discusses the available special diagnostic techniques and provides a practical guide for commonly encountered immunofluorescence patterns in skin. Techniques other than direct immunofluorescence required for diagnosis of specific disorders will be discussed in detail in those chapters. With the historic development of diagnostic immunofluorescence techniques for evaluation of lupus erythematosus and certain vesiculobullous disorders, dermatopathology has paved the way for the growing use of special diagnostic techniques in pathology as a whole. Although virtually all laboratories employ histochemistry as an adjunct to routine hematoxylin-and-eosin (H&E) sections, many are not capable of providing immunostaining or ultrastructural studies. However, growing numbers of referral laboratories provide these services on receipt of appropriately fixed or preserved tissue samples, making these specialized approaches readily available when diagnostic problems arise.

Of critical importance in the use of special diagnostic techniques is an educated approach to the strengths and limitations as well as to the relative specificity and sensitivity of the tests in question. Overinterpretation or underinterpretation of information derived from special diagnostic techniques is potentially more limiting than the failure to employ these approaches. The remainder of this chapter provides a summary of those techniques that are of greatest assistance in diagnostic dermatopathology and contains practical advice regarding the selection, interpretation, and overall clinical utility of those techniques.

Routine Histochemistry

Routine histochemistry stains are generally used for chemical detection of inorganic substances such as iron, calcium, and silver; polysaccharides (periodic acid–Schiff [PAS] stain, with and without diastase digestion); mucopolysaccharides (alcian blue stain); mast cell metachromasia (Giemsa reagent); lipids (oil-red-O stain); extracellular matrix elements (Weigert elastic stain); organisms (Ziehl-Neelsen stain for acid-fast bacilli); and certain enzymes (dopa reagent). Figure 1–25A, C depicts histochemical stains for elastic fibers, and Figure 1–12B demonstrates enzyme histochemistry. Although these stains provide important information in the evaluation of many skin disorders, they should be used with discretion and not be overused. For example, superficial fungi within the stratum corneum may often be detected without the aid of PAS stain, and when required for detection of viable fungi, either a PAS or silver stain, but not both, is usually sufficient. Nonviable fungi in deep mycotic infections may be silver-positive and PAS-negative. Alternatively, the epidermal basement membrane thickening that

Table 2–1. COMMON HISTOCHEMICAL STAINS

HISTOCHEMICAL STAIN	STRUCTURE OR SUBSTANCE IDENTIFIED	REPRESENTATIVE DISORDERS
Periodic acid–Schiff	Glycogen (diastase sensitive)	Clear cell neoplasms
	Mucopolysaccharides	Granuloma annulare
	Fungi	Dermatophytosis
	Basement membranes	Lupus erythematosus
Alcian blue (pH 2.5)	Acid mucopolysaccharides	Dermal mucinosis
Giemsa and toluidine blue	Metachromatic cytoplasmic granules (mast cells)	Urticaria pigmentosa
Oil-red–O	Lipid (frozen tissue)	Sebaceous carcinoma
Masson trichrome	Collagen	Connective tissue nevus
Verhoff-van Gieson	Elastin	Pseudoxanthoma elasticum
Fontana-Masson	Melanin	Macular hypopigmentation and hyperpigmentation
Methenamine silver	Fungi	Deep mycoses
	Donovan bodies	Granuloma inguinale
Brown-Brenn	Bacteria	Gonococcemia
Fite	Acid-fast bacilli	Lupus vulgaris
		Leprosy
Congo red	Amyloid	Macular amyloid
		Systemic amyloidosis

accompanies established lesions of lupus erythematosus often requires the PAS stain for visualization. A partial listing of histochemical stains frequently used in routine dermatopathology practice is provided in Table 2–1.

The majority of histochemical stains may be performed on formalin-fixed, paraffin-embedded tissue sections. Enzyme histochemistry, however, usually requires cryostat sections of fresh frozen tissue. The 3,4-dihydroxyphenylalanine (dopa) stain permits detection of cells with tyrosinase activity and has proven to be useful in identification and quantification of epidermal melanocytes. Methods to detect enzymes such as succinic dehydrogenase and amylophosphorylase, which are normally present in embryonic and adult cutaneous appendages, have been used to classify various appendage tumors and as an adjunct to the diagnosis of their malignant counterparts (see Chap. 12).

Paraffin Immunohistochemistry[1, 2]

Paraffin immunohistochemistry is used for detection by immunoperoxidase methods of tissue antigens preserved after formalin fixation and paraffin embedding. Immunoperoxidase detection involves incubation of tissue sections with the relevant antibody (usually polyclonal for paraffin immunohistochemistry) to the target antigen (generally cytoplasmic proteins), followed by application of a biotinylated or peroxidase-linked secondary antibody directed against the target-specific antibody probe. The antigen-bound antibody-antibody complex is identified and localized by using either avidin-biotin or peroxidase-antiperoxidase enzyme detection systems, whereby horseradish peroxidase is linked to the growing ''sandwich'' of layered antibodies. The complex is then incubated with an enzyme substrate (aminoethyl carbazole or an insoluble chromagen such as diaminobenzidine), which on reaction with the peroxidase becomes red or brown at sites of antibody-antigen reactivity. This approach, unlike fluorescence-based methods of antibody localization, produces a permanent record in which the signal does not fade or dissipate over time. Examples of paraffin immunohistochemistry include antibody stains for S100 protein (melanocytes and Langerhans cells), keratin proteins (epithelial

cells), carcinoembryonic antigen (some gland-forming epithelial tumors); chromogranin (neuroendocrine tumors); desmin (smooth muscle); Factor VIII–associated antigen (endothelium); α_1-antichymotrypsin (histiocytic tumors); and vimentin (mesenchymal and fibroblastic proliferations). None of these antibodies is entirely specific, and results must be interpreted within the context of a comprehensive panel of reagents. These reagents are especially informative when evaluating poorly differentiated neoplasms. For example, a panel that combines screening for cytokeratins, S100 protein, melanocyte-associated HMB-45, and leukocyte common antigen is helpful in the differential diagnosis of amelanotic melanoma, lymphoma, and carcinoma. Figure 1–11B depicts an example of paraffin immunohistochemistry.

Cell Marker Analysis[1, 3]

Cell marker analysis is used primarily for T- and B-lymphocyte typing and for detection of antigenic abnormalities in early evolutionary stages of cutaneous T-cell lymphoma. Because monoclonal antibodies are used and cell surface antigens are fragile, unlike cytoplasmic antigens detected by polyclonal antibodies in paraffin immunohistochemistry, frozen sections of nonfixed tissue are most often employed. Specifically, exposure to formaldehyde solution may alter cell surface markers; therefore, fresh tissue in cold physiologic saline or routine immunofluorescence transport medium (e.g., Michel medium) is necessary for cell-typing studies. The immunophenotype of T-cell lymphoma often involves loss of one or more pan–T-cell maturation markers defined by Leu 1, 4, and 5 antibodies, and a CD4 : CD8 (Leu 3 : Leu 2) ratio of more than 6 to 1 (Fig. 2–1). The immunophenotype of B-cell lymphoma often involves preferential or exclusive expression of either kappa or lambda immunoglobulin light chains.

One-Micron Section Analysis and Diagnostic Electron Microscopy[3–5]

One-micron sections are generated from glutaraldehyde-fixed tissue embedded in plastic resin and sectioned at one

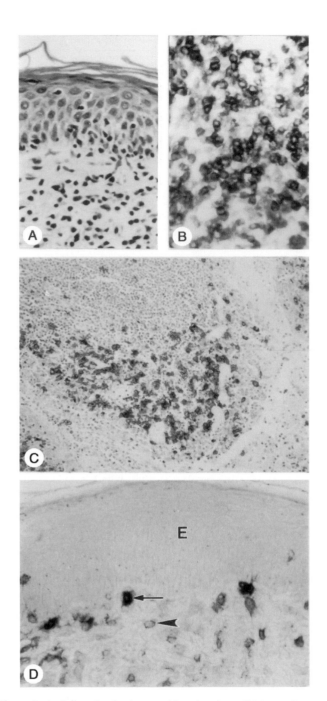

Figure 2–1. Cell typing by immunohistochemistry. **(A)** In routine sections, these relatively small lymphocytes appear bland, although they are diffusely infiltrating the papillary dermis and have begun to migrate into a relatively nonspongiotic epidermal layer. **(B)** T-cell typing reveals more than 90% of these cells to be of the CD4 helper-inducer T-cell subset, consistent with a clonal proliferation of this functional class of T cells. **(C)** Aggregates of Ki-1-positive cells in the dermal component of lymphomatoid papulosis. **(D)** Double immunohistochemical labeling using two chromagens; dark cells *(arrow)* are natural killer cells, light cells *(arrowhead)* are cytotoxic-suppressor cells. (E, epidermis.)

sixth the thickness of conventional paraffin sections. The result is a high-resolution image under higher power lenses that makes possible the detection of subtle nuclear membrane characteristics (e.g., Sézary cells), microvascular injury (e.g., urticarial vasculitis), and anomalies in organelles (e.g., macromelanosomes) not possible in routine sections (Fig. 2–2).

Diagnostic electron microscopy is well suited to confirmation of histogenesis in poorly differentiated tumors (e.g., detection of premelanosomes or epithelial junctional complexes) or as an adjunct to the diagnosis of different forms of epidermolysis bullosa. Figure 2–2A, B depicts the 1-μm-section technique and diagnostic electron microscopy, and Table 2–2 provides examples of the use of diagnostic electron microscopy in dermatopathology practice.

In Situ Hybridization[1, 6]

In situ hybridization involves detection of mRNA or DNA when detectable quantities of protein antigen are not present for conventional immunohistochemical evaluation. Typing of oncogenic forms of papillomavirus is possible using in situ hybridization. Detection of other infectious agents (e.g., human immunodeficiency virus, cytomegalovirus) is also possible, and oncogene expression may also be defined by this technology. Figure 2–3 shows in situ hybridization for human papillomavirus (HPV).

Tools used in localization of genes responsible for certain diseases include DNA hybridization and restriction enzyme analysis in combination with karyotypic analysis. In viral diseases such as genitoanal warts, a strong association has been established between infection by HPV types 16 and 18 and the subsequent development of neoplasia of affected skin as well as the uterine cervix. The gross appearance of these lesions is of limited predictive value for estimation of viral type. Although the degree of dysplasia associated with unequivocal HPV cytopathic change can be indicative of infection with HPV type 16 or 18, lack of dysplasia does not exclude this possibility. Immunohistochemistry has not been helpful in this setting, because antibodies against type-specific capsid proteins are not normally produced. Molecular viral probes fill a significant void as diagnostic tools. Hybridization reactions permit evaluation of viral DNA replication, degree of viral integration, and specific transforming regions of viruses. With such techniques, it has been shown that genitoanal verrucae are primarily induced by HPV types 6, 11, 16, and 18, of which the latter two have prognostic significance in the future development of carcinoma.

Standardized kits are available that enable laboratories to perform in situ hybridization as if it were a routine stain. Such approaches rely upon admixtures of molecular probes (e.g., probes for HPV types 6 and 11; 16 and 18; and 31, 33, and 35) as well as the appropriate secondary reagents for chromogenic detection of the hybridization reaction. However, caution must be exercised so that overprotection resulting from less stringent conditions does not result in designation of ordinary condylomas as having oncogenic potential.

An innovative approach to the detection of HPV is the polymerase chain reaction (PCR). This technique permits detection of as few as 20 viral copies of DNA in sections of paraffin-embedded tissue, and analysis can be performed within 24 hours, in contrast to the more time-consuming technique of in situ DNA hybridization. In PCR, target DNA sequences are selectively amplified through repeated cycles of denaturation, annealing with oligomer primers complementary to flanking regions of the target sequence, and primer extension with DNA polymerase 1. Detectable quantities of target DNA increase exponentially as a function of

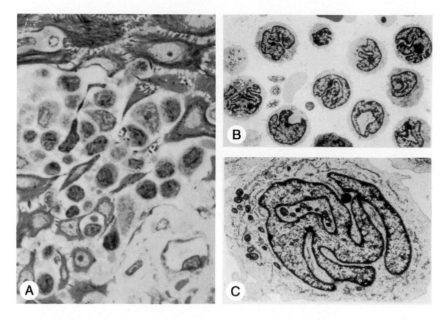

Figure 2–2. One-micron sections and transmission electron microscopy. **(A)** In early cutaneous T-cell lymphoma, lymphocytes infiltrating the epidermis display markedly infolded nuclear membranes when viewed in 1-μm sections. **(B, C)** These cells in skin or in buffy coat preparations from peripheral blood have characteristic cerebriform contours of Sézary-Lutzner cells. Computer-assisted image analysis of such ultrastructural images has been used to quantify the degree of nuclear complexity and to show that such cells are different from activated T cells, which also may exhibit some degree of nuclear irregularity.

the number of cycles, thus enabling detection with labeled complementary oligomers. This rapid and sensitive technique has already been applied to the detection of HPV types 16 and 18 in cervical biopsy specimens, and these viral subtypes have correlated with dysplasia.

Direct Immunofluorescence[7–9]

Direct immunofluorescence is a method of visualizing tissue deposits of immune reactants that have become bound to target cells and matrix molecules in vivo. This approach involves detection of antigen in a frozen section of a skin biopsy specimen by the application of fluorescein isothiocyanate (FITC)-labeled antibody of desired specificity. Fresh tissue is generally provided immediately after biopsy on saline-soaked gauze on an ice slurry delivered within 2 hours of biopsy, or alternatively, after placement into Michel transport medium, which preserves immunoreactants for at least

several weeks, in our experience. Tissue is gently washed prior to embedding and freezing in a viscous, soluble, embedding medium (e.g., Tissue-Tek O.C.T. Compound, Miles Inc., Elkhart, IN) and cryostat sections are then reacted for 30 minutes in a moist chamber with various antisera such as antibodies to IgG, IgA, IgM, complement, and fibrinogen linked to FITC. After incubation, sections are rinsed in buffer and examined by epifluorescence microscopy. This technique is widely used as an adjunct in the diagnosis of connective tissue diseases and vesiculobullous disorders. With minor modification, the same basic technique has been applied effectively in the detection of various infectious agents.

Indirect Immunofluorescence[7–9]

Indirect immunofluorescence is used to determine titers of circulating immunoglobulins in the serum of a patient with

Table 2–2. EXAMPLES OF THE USE OF DIAGNOSTIC ELECTRON MICROSCOPY IN DERMATOPATHOLOGY

DISORDER	ULTRASTRUCTURAL FINDING(S)	DIAGNOSTIC PROBLEM
Epidermolysis bullosa	Basal layer cytolysis (simplex) Lamina lucida split (junctional) Split beneath lamina densa (dystrophic)	Differential diagnosis and classification of congenital blistering disease
Histiocytosis X	Langerhans cell granules	Histiocytic or xanthomatous infiltrate
Spindle cell melanoma	Premelanosomes	Spindle cell carcinoma Primary sarcoma Atypical fibroxanthoma
Neuroendocrine carcinoma	Dense core–type granules; perinuclear intermediate filaments	Lymphoma Metastatic small cell carcinoma
Eccrine or apocrine carcinoma	Embryonic duct formation; characteristic secretory granules	Metastatic adenocarcinoma
Fabry disease	Laminated cytoplasmic endothelial inclusions	Ordinary angiokeratoma Other storage diseases
Soft tissue sarcoma	Actin-type filaments (leiomyosarcoma) Dilated, rough endoplasmic reticulum (fibrosarcoma) Axon-like dendrites and pericellular basement membrane (malignant neural tumor) Weibel Palade bodies (angiosarcoma) Lysosomes, fibroblasts (malignant fibrous histiocytoma)	Differential diagnosis and classification according to histogenesis

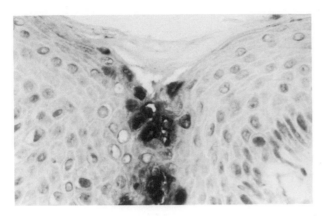

Figure 2–3. In situ hybridization for human papillomavirus. The labeled genomic probe is seen as zones of deep purple staining over virally infected nuclei. This probe was specific for human papillomavirus types 6 and 11, which are the common cause of condylomata.

bullous disorders such as pemphigus vulgaris and bullous pemphigoid. For this analysis, serum is separated from a sample of venous blood, serially diluted with buffered saline admixed with bovine serum albumen, and incubated with cryostat sections of a target tissue containing the relevant target molecules (e.g., monkey esophagus, normal human skin). Sections are gently rinsed, and FITC-linked antiserum to human immunoglobulin is applied to define sites of in vitro serum antibody binding. By fluorescence microscopy, zones of reactivity are designated as present or absent, and the endpoint is represented by the dilution at which reactivity ceases. A typical report would read ''epidermal intercellular immunoglobulin deposition detected to and including a dilution of 1 : 160.'' Such a report could be helpful as an adjunct to diagnosis or in the assessment of disease activity or response to treatment. The linkage between disease activity is generally tighter in pemphigus than in pemphigoid, and occasionally, circulating autoantibodies may be detected in individuals without evidence of primary vesiculobullous disease.

An important application of indirect immunofluorescence is in the evaluation of epidermolysis bullosa acquisita (EBA) (see Chap. 5). This nonheritable disorder differs clinically from classical forms of epidermolysis bullosa (EB) and resembles an autoimmune disorder more than a primary mechanobullous disorder. Direct immunofluorescence shows deposits of IgG and other immunoreactants in linear array along the epidermal basal lamina in 25 to 50% of patients, a pattern that is indistinguishable from bullous pemphigoid. Differentiation of the two disorders relies on a strategy whereby the substrate for indirect immunofluorescence is normal human skin split along the dermal-epidermal junction via preincubation in 1 mol/L sodium chloride. This results in segregation of lamina lucida and associate bullous pemphigoid antigen on the epidermal roof and type IV collagen and lamina densa along the dermal base. When this split substrate is reacted with the patient's serum, bullous pemphigoid antibodies will decorate the epidermal side, whereas autoantibodies in EBA will localize to the dermal side. Split skin preparations, as well as immunologic mapping of native antigens at sites of blister formation to define the molecular site of the lesion, continue to provide important diagnostic insights into classification and pathogenesis of commonly encountered vesiculobullous disorders involving the skin.

BIOPSY TECHNIQUE

For direct immunofluorescence, precision and site selection are of critical importance. The following guidelines should be applied:

1. Early lesions should be sampled.
2. The edges of lesions, particularly when blistering is present, are most useful.
3. At least one third of the biopsy specimen should include perilesional skin.
4. Never biopsy the base of an ulcer or the center of a blister.
5. If the epidermis separates from the dermis, submit both in separate, labeled containers.
6. Place specimens immediately into Michel transport medium, never in fixative.
7. If transport medium is not available, cover specimen with gauze soaked in physiologic saline, place in ice slurry, and transport immediately to immunofluorescence laboratory for processing.

SPECIMEN HANDLING

Specimens placed in Michel transport medium are suitable for immunofluorescence testing for days after biopsy, permitting triage by mail. On receipt, specimens are washed in buffer, rapidly frozen in O.C.T. Compound, and sectioned at 4- to 6-μm intervals in a cryostat. At least two specimens are mounted per slide, along with known positive controls for the antibodies being used. A representative panel of standard antibodies would include antibodies to IgG, IgM, IgA, C3, and fibrin. Once staining is complete, slides are kept refrigerated in the dark to prevent dissipation of the fluorescein label, which may occur within several days of staining. Timely review of freshly stained slides is mandatory, because fluorescence intensity is, by convention, semiquantified according to a 1+ to 4+ grading system. Typical patterns of immunofluorescence for commonly encountered disorders are summarized in Table 2–3.

DIRECT AND INDIRECT IMMUNOFLUORESCENCE

Autofluorescence

Before specific patterns of immune reactant deposition can effectively be interpreted, autofluorescence intrinsic to skin sections must be fully appreciated. Within the dermis, the most common pattern of autofluorescence is produced by elastic fibers within the reticular dermis (Fig. 2–4). In normal skin, these form bright green, glassy fibers of uniform caliber evenly dispersed among reticular dermal collagen bundles. In chronically sun-damaged skin, elastic fibers become clumped and coalescent, particularly within the uppermost regions of the dermis. In the deep dermis and subcutis, inter-

Table 2–3. USEFUL DIRECT IMMUNOFLUORESCENCE PATTERNS IN SKIN

SITE OF DEPOSIT	CHARACTER	DISORDER	SIGNIFICANCE
Stratum corneum	Loculated, homogeneous	Acute to subacute spongiotic dermatitis	Loculated serum, scale-crust
Stratum corneum	Focal, granular, with parakeratosis	Psoriasis	At Munro microabscesses, ? primary or secondary
Intercellular	Fine, uniform, fish-net	Pemphigus family	Anti-intercellular cement autoantibodies
Intercellular	Coarse, irregular	Spongiotic dermatitis	Nonspecific serum leakage
Nuclear	Homogeneous, granular, nucleolar	Connective tissue disorders	Autoimmunity; may not have clinical relevance
Basement membrane	Linear, C3 predominates	Pemphigoid family	Autoantibody to bullous pemphigoid antigen
Basement membrane	Linear, IgG predominates	Epidermolysis bullosa acquisita	Autoantibody to basement membrane component
Basement membrane	Linear, IgA predominates	Linear IgA disease	Autoantibody to basement membrane component
Basement membrane	Granular IgG	Lupus erythematosus	Membrane attack complex
Papillary dermis	Granular IgA	Dermatitis herpetiformis	Gluten-immune complexes
Microvessels (venules)	Granular C3, IgG	Hypersensitivity, vasculitis	Immune complexes
Microvessels (venules)	Granular IgA	Henoch-Schönlein purpura	Immune complexes
Microvessels (venules)	Homogeneous IgG, albumen	Porphyria cutanea tarda	Vascular injury
Vessels (arteries)	Granular, segmental	Polyarteritis nodosa	Immune complexes

nal elastic lamina of small- to medium-sized arteries show similar fluorescence, a finding that must not be confused with granular deposition of FITC-labeled antibody in the setting of vasculitis, such as in cutaneous polyarteritis nodosa. Basement membranes may also emit autofluorescence in some specimens, producing the false impression of linear antibody deposition along the dermal-epidermal interface or within superficial vessel walls (Fig. 2–5). Nuclear autofluorescence may be prominent in certain biopsy specimens, and must be differentiated from true antinuclear antibody deposits (Fig. 2–5). In general, autofluorescence produces a glassy, homogeneous pattern of fluorescence that will be variably present in all sections, irrespective of the specific antibody or complement component being evaluated. Moreover, negative controls in which the antibody-FITC conjugate has been entirely omitted will also maintain the native autofluorescence pattern.

Nonspecific Staining

Nonspecific staining refers to either nonimmunologic binding of FITC-antibody complexes to tissue components, or to specific binding that does not correlate with a defined immune-mediated disorder. Examples of the latter include the aggregation of immune reactants within the stratum corneum in disorders characterized by scale-crust and the localization of immune reactants into the intercellular spaces of the epidermal layer in conditions characterized by spongiosis (Fig. 2–6A, B). The clue to these nonspecific patterns is the presence of all or most immunoglobulin classes being evaluated in these foci (e.g., IgG, IgM, IgA, C3, and fibrin). The ability to recognize these nonspecific patterns and to confirm their identity by correlation with routine histology is important because some may mimic primary immune-mediated dermatoses (e.g., the spongiotic pattern of intercellular immune reactant accumulation may resemble cell membrane deposition in pemphigus). In the dermis, immune reactants may be detected as geographic zones of fluorescence about blood vessels (Fig. 2–6C). This nonspecific pattern indicates

increased vascular permeability and may be seen in a broad range of dermatitides. In early evolutionary stages, in which most of the fluorescence is clustered in the perivascular space, care must be taken to distinguish this pattern from granular deposits confined exclusively to the vessel wall, which correlate with necrotizing vasculitis. In the setting of a specific immune-mediated disorder, all immunoglobulin subclasses should not be indiscriminately deposited, as is generally the case for nonspecific immunoreactivity patterns. A common pattern of nonspecific binding observed in the dermis is the reactivity of FITC-antibody conjugate to the plasma membranes of inflammatory cells within the superficial dermis (Fig. 2–6D). This phenomenon is mediated in part by antibody binding to Fc membrane receptors, and may preferentially involve only one of the FITC-antibody components of the panel. Although the cells so outlined tend to be round and of uniform size and the fluorescence restricted to a thin, homogeneous rim about the cell perimeter, at times this pattern may mimic vasculitis in transverse sections through small, superficial dermal vessels.

Linear Basement Membrane Staining[10–24]

Pemphigoid

Bullous pemphigoid (Fig. 2–7) is a nonscarring, blistering disorder seen predominantly in the elderly population. It presents as tense bullae frequently on an erythematous or urticarial base with a predilection for the flexural regions of the body. Approximately one third of patients also have oral involvement. The bullous pemphigoid antigen is a group of glycoproteins produced by keratinocytes; it is a constituent of normal squamous epithelium. The antigen is composed of a major 230-kD antigen and a minor 180-kD protein. Serum from patients with both localized and generalized bullous pemphigoid have antibodies that immunoprecipitate the 230-kD antigen.

Routine histopathology characteristically reveals a subepidermal blister with eosinophils that are associated with the dermal-epidermal junction in nearly 100% of patients (Fig. 2–7). It is of critical importance to recognize and differentiate the linear pattern from the granular staining seen in lupus erythematosus. Linear staining often has an undulant, glassy quality that has been likened to ribbon candy. IgG is the most common immunoglobulin seen, occurring in 45 to 90% of patients. IgM and IgA also may be present in 25 to 30% of patients and are usually of lesser intensity. IgD and IgE have also been detected rarely. In general, the intensity of C3 staining is far greater than that of IgG or other immunoglobulins, a feature that may be helpful in excluding EBA from the differential diagnosis. Indirect immunofluorescence using the patient's serum will produce a linear basement membrane pattern of reactivity in appropriate substrates, such as monkey esophagus (Fig. 2–8A), and will decorate substrates that have been split via salt solutions at the dermal-epidermal junction along the epidermal portion, which contains the lamina lucida–associated bullous pemphigoid antigen.

False-negative immunofluorescence in patients with bullous pemphigoid has been reported in biopsy specimens from

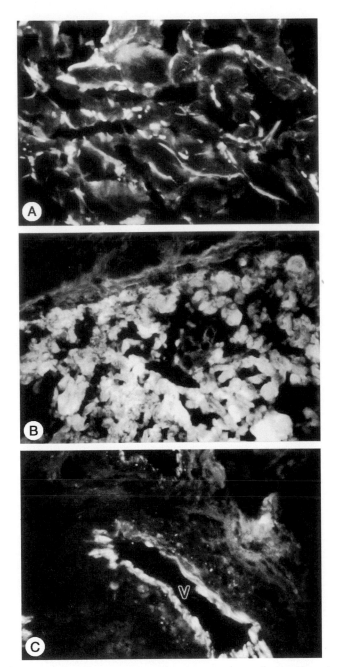

Figure 2–4. Autofluorescence patterns commonly confused with positive staining. Autofluorescence for **(A)** reticular dermal elastic fibers, **(B)** elastotic material in the papillary dermis of sun-damaged skin, and **(C)** elastic lamina of a muscular dermal artery. The glassy quality of the vessel wall staining in **C** differentiates this pattern from true immune complex deposition, which tends to be granular. The patchy autofluorescence of elastotic material is characteristic, and should not be mistaken for colloid bodies or true antibody deposits. (V, vessel.)

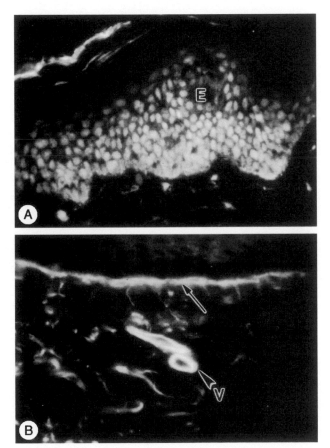

Figure 2–5. Nuclear and basement membrane zone autofluorescence. **(A)** This pattern of nuclear fluorescence within the epidermal layer (E) may be the result of intrinsic nuclear autofluorescence or specific or nonspecific binding of antibodies to nuclear proteins. **(B)** Basement membrane zone autofluorescence affecting the dermal-epidermal junction *(arrow)* and an underlying vessel wall (V). Weak linear basement membrane staining could be erroneously interpreted, although the universal expression of this pattern on all basement membranes, including those of dermal vessels, is an important clue indicating that this pattern represents autofluorescence.

basal cell vacuolization (see Chap. 5). The histology may be confused with a number of other disorders, including EBA, old lesions of dermatitis herpetiformis, herpes gestationis, vesicular insect-bite reactions, and vesicular drug eruptions. Moreover, pruritic clinical variants may be nonvesicular and mimic any cause of urticaria. Direct immunofluorescence in skin biopsy specimens of bullous pemphigoid patients reveals strong, continuous, linear deposition of complement at

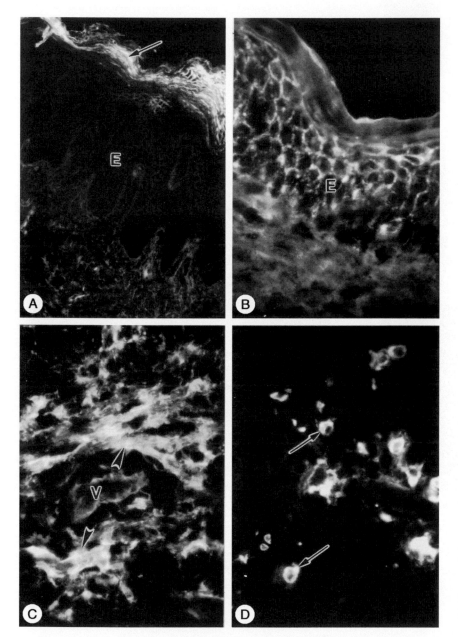

Figure 2–6. Nonspecific patterns of immune reactant deposition within the epidermis. **(A)** Although immunoglobulins and complement within the stratum corneum of the epidermis (E) may be associated with psoriasis, impetigo, scale or crust formation, and loculated serum transmitted into the scale in patients who have resolving spongiotic dermatitis, all may produce a similar picture. **(B)** Active spongiotic dermatitis may result in leakage of immune reactants into the intercellular spaces of the surface epidermis (E) or adnexal epithelium, resulting in a pattern that mimics cell membrane staining in patients who have pemphigus. In such instances, all antibody classes (i.e., IgG, IgA, IgM) are generally detected, in contrast to preferential expression of one antibody class (IgG), which suggests a specific reaction. **(C)** Immune reactants and fibrin commonly are deposited in the perivascular space *(arrowheads)* (V, vessel). This is indicative of increased vascular permeability but is not representative of a diagnostically specific pattern. **(D)** Nonspecific binding of immunoglobulins via Fc-receptor interactions with plasma membranes of inflammatory cells *(arrows)* must be distinguished from specific staining of immune complexes in the walls of small venules.

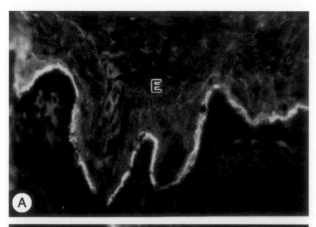

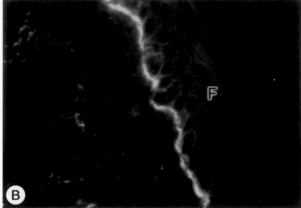

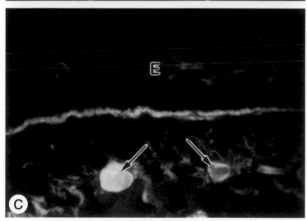

Figure 2–7. Linear basement membrane staining: pemphigoid. **(A)** The linear staining seen in the subepidermal basal lamina of perilesional skin is usually most intense for C3 and has a glassy, ribbon-like quality. An identical pattern is present in herpes gestationis. **(B)** Similar staining may also be present about the adnexal epithelium (F, follicular infundibulum). **(C)** Recurrent involvement of a lesional site with repeated basal cell–layer injury followed by re-epithelialization may result in colloid body formation *(arrows)* in addition to typical linear basement membrane zone reactivity. Colloid bodies characteristically stain diffusely for immunoglobulin (particularly IgM) and complement. In new lesions, the presence of colloid bodies in the setting of linear basement membrane zone staining for C3 also raises the possibility of herpes gestationis. (E, epidermis.)

the lower extremities, and it has been suggested that biopsy specimens from flexural sites may produce the most accurate results. Biopsy specimens of blistered skin or old lesions that have begun to re-epithelialize may yield discontinuous staining or negative results because the basement membrane has been destroyed. A biopsy adjacent to a new blister is optimal. Specimens from patients in remission or on corticosteroid or other immunosuppressive therapy also may fail to show deposition of immunoreactants.

Electron microscopy has shown disintegration of basement membrane and fragmentation of anchoring fibrils, anchoring filaments, and hemidesmosomes. Immune reactants have been localized to the upper lamina lucida by immunoelectron microscopy.

Herpes gestationis (HG), a relatively rare vesiculobullous disorder that occurs in pregnant women and during the puerperium, may produce a histologic and direct immunofluorescence picture that is indistinguishable from pemphigoid. Therefore, this diagnosis is made largely on clinical parameters. Perilesional skin most commonly reveals C3 and other complement components in linear array along the dermal-epidermal junction. Immune deposits also may be present in the walls of cutaneous vessels. Linear C3 is a consistent finding; linear IgG, usually of lesser intensity, is also seen in 30 to 50% of cases. Similar direct immunofluorescence findings are also seen in the neonates of affected mothers, regardless of whether or not the infant has clinical lesions. Immunoelectron microscopy reveals C3 deposition within the lamina lucida, as observed in patients with pemphigoid. IgG is also located in the lamina lucida, but it tends to concentrate near the dermal side of the basal cell plasma membrane and hemidesmosomes. In most cases, indirect immunofluorescence fails to identify anti–basement membrane zone antibodies in the serum of herpes gestationis patients, probably because the concentration of circulating autoantibody is below the level of sensitivity of the technique. Sera from affected individuals contains a substance that is capable of fixing C3 to the basement membrane zone of normal human skin. This antibody identifies the HG factor, which is a complement-fixing factor also present in cord serum from infants of affected patients.

In cicatricial pemphigoid, also known as benign mucosal pemphigoid, patients develop subepidermal blisters on mucosal surfaces, predominantly the oral and conjunctival skin. Skin lesions are present in 10 to 30% of patients. The Brunsting-Perry type of cicatricial pemphigoid is characterized by localized, scarring lesions, frequently on the scalp, without mucosal involvement. On direct immunofluorescence, these changes are similar to those seen in bullous pemphigoid, revealing linear, ribbon-like deposition of C3 at the dermal-epidermal junction. IgG is the most common of the immunoglobulins that may be detected in addition to C3. Immunoelectron microscopy has localized the immune reactants to the lower portion of the lamina lucida.

Epidermolysis Bullosa Acquisita

Epidermolysis bullosa acquisita (EBA) is an acquired, adult-onset, bullous disease characterized by skin fragility, trauma-induced blisters, healing with scars and milia, and possible scarring alopecia and oral dystrophy. Typical blisters are noninflammatory clinically and show an acral distribution. A subgroup of EBA patients present with widespread inflammatory disease resembling bullous pemphigoid. Oral involvement may be seen in 30 to 50% of these patients.

Routine histology reveals subepidermal blister formation with minimal inflammation. The inflammatory variant

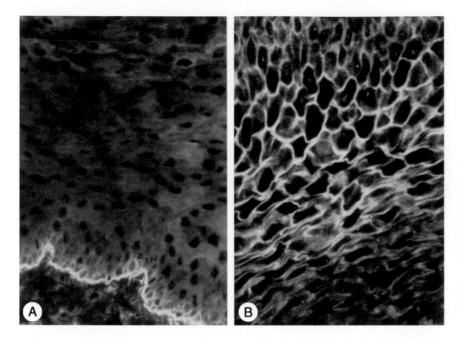

Figure 2–8. Indirect immunofluorescence in **(A)** pemphigoid and **(B)** pemphigus. **(A)** Serum from patients with active pemphigoid may contain antibodies to the bullous pemphigoid antigen also expressed within the lamina lucida of monkey esophagus. Serum incubated with sections of esophagus and then stained with fluorescein isothiocyanate (FITC)-labeled antibodies to human immunoglobulin produce a linear staining pattern identical to that observed by direct immunofluorescence of lesional or perilesional skin. **(B)** In pemphigus, circulating antibodies bind to intercellular spaces within the esophageal epithelium, resulting in a characteristic fishnet pattern.

generally shows a superficial dermal infiltrate with a predominance of neutrophils. Direct immunofluorescence of perilesional skin reveals a broad, homogeneous, linear band of IgG and C3 at the basement membrane zone in nearly all cases. IgA, IgM, C1q, C4, factor B, and properidin have also been described with a much lower frequency. IgG is the most intense immunoreactant, and generally, all four subclasses of IgG are found in patients with EBA. IgG deposits have also been detected in oral and esophageal mucosa of patients who do not have mucosal disease clinically. Immunopathologically, EBA may be difficult to differentiate from bullous pemphigoid, cicatricial pemphigoid, and herpes gestationis. The presence of linear IgG deposition that is stronger in intensity compared to the deposition of C3 favors a diagnosis of EBA. Definitive diagnosis, however, frequently requires immunoelectron microscopy or indirect immunofluorescence using sodium split skin specimens, in which the serum autoantibody localizes to the dermal portion of the split skin. Ultrastructural analysis reveals a band of amorphous material beneath the lamina densa, corresponding to the accumulation of immunoglobulins and complement. Direct immunoelectron microscopy also reveals immune complexes below the lamina densa.

The EBA antigen has been identified as a large glycoprotein in the lamina densa that develops at 8–10 weeks of human gestation. Two bands are identified by gel electrophoresis (PAGE) in sera of patients with EBA; the major band represents a 290-kD protein of type VII collagen, and the 145-kD band is the noncollagenous C-terminal glycoprotein domain of the type VII collagen.

Linear IgA Dermatosis

Linear IgA bullous dermatosis is a pruritic skin disease that frequently presents with vesicles and bullae in clusters. Because of histologic similarities, the differential diagnosis usually includes dermatitis herpetiformis. Clinically, linear IgA bullous dermatosis differs from dermatitis herpetiformis by the lack of gluten-sensitive enteropathy, less mucosal involvement, no association with HLA B8 and HLA DR3 antigens, and less clinical response to dapsone therapy. Drug-induced linear IgA disease has been reported in association with captopril, vancomycin, diclophenac, and cefamandole. Chronic bullous dermatosis of childhood is thought to be the same disease as linear IgA disease, both clinically and immunopathologically.

Histology shows a subepidermal blister in association with neutrophils aligning the dermal-epidermal junction. By definition, direct immunofluorescence reveals linear deposition of IgA in the basement membrane zone. C3 and IgG may also be present, but generally stain with less intensity. If the staining intensity of C3 is stronger than IgA, a diagnosis of bullous pemphigoid should be considered. Immunoelectron microscopy has localized these deposits to the lamina lucida, sub–lamina densa, or both. PAGE of the serum of patients with linear IgA disease identifies a 97-kD band in both dermal and epidermal skin extracts; it is suggested that this antigen is produced and secreted by fibroblasts and subsequently binds to the lamina lucida. The serum of these patients may contain circulating IgA anti–basement membrane zone antibodies. IgA antiendomysial antibodies, which may be seen in dermatitis herpetiformis, are absent.

Granular Basement Membrane and Papillary Dermal Staining[25–33]

Lupus Erythematosus

Cutaneous lesions of lupus erythematosus (LE; Fig. 2–9) include a spectrum of disease including discoid (chronic cutaneous) LE, subacute cutaneous LE, and acute LE (usually systemic). The majority of patients have photodistribution of skin lesions and frequently have circulating antinuclear antibodies. Lesional skin biopsy specimens reveal granular deposition of immunoreactants at the basement

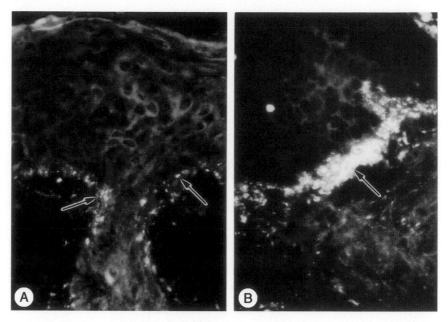

Figure 2–9. Lupus erythematosus. **(A)** Although the epidermal layer shows homogeneous autofluorescence, the bright, shiny quality of the granular deposits *(arrows)* of IgG at the dermal-epidermal junction in this biopsy specimen of nonlesional skin is easily discerned. **(B)** Lesional skin shows even more pronounced granular deposits *(arrow)*. Other antibody classes and complement also may be present. Positive lupus band tests must show continuous, strong staining along the dermal-epidermal junction. The occurrence of a positive band in nonlesional skin is an indicator of systemic disease.

membrane zone; demonstration of these immunoglobulins by immunofluorescence constitutes a positive lupus band test (Fig. 2–9).

Immunofluorescence findings in biopsy specimens of lesions of LE may be completely negative or may show the presence of multiple immunoglobulins and complement. The finding of granular IgG, IgA, and IgM in a single biopsy specimen is highly suggestive of LE. Although frequently only one immunoglobulin is seen in an early, evolving lupus band test, the presence of only one immunoglobulin may be a nonspecific finding. Both IgG and IgM have been reported as the most significant and frequent immunoglobulin. There are a number of reasons for false-positive LE band tests; the more common reasons relate to frequently encountered forms of dermatitis, such as rosacea, or simply are the result of chronic sun exposure of facial skin. The requirement of a strong, continuous band of immune reactant deposition as a pattern in which fine granularity, coarse granularity, or thready or stippled fluorescence predominates, will assist in discriminating true-positive band tests from apparent bands resulting from accretion of immune reactants along the basement membrane zone.

The presence or absence of immunoglobulins in LE depends on several factors: (1) the type of skin lesion (acute, subacute, chronic); (2) duration of the lesion; (3) the site of biopsy; and (4) the previous or concurrent administration of topical and/or systemic therapy. The overall prevalence of a positive lupus band test is approximately 50 to 90%. New lesions are frequently negative, whereas lesions present for more than 3 months are likely to be positive. The presence of a positive lupus band test in clinically normal, non–sun-exposed skin is suggestive of systemic disease. The incidence of such a positive lupus band test has been reported to be as high as 91% in patients with active LE and 33% in those with inactive disease. It has also been suggested that this finding may be indicative of renal involvement, although this has not been well substantiated.

Granular deposits along the dermal-epidermal junction have been localized by electron microscopy in the dermal aspect of the basal lamina with extension into the papillary dermis in patients with LE. Similar deposits may involve the basement membrane zone of follicular infundibula and are occasionally seen in the walls of small dermal venules.

A unique immunofluorescence staining pattern may be seen in patients with subacute cutaneous LE. This pattern consists of a particulate deposition within the lower epidermis and upper papillary dermis. This pattern may be seen in both lesional and nonlesional skin. A similar pattern has been seen in human skin grafted onto immunosuppressed mice that have been infused with anti-Ro/SSA autoantibodies.

Lupus profundus, also known as lupus panniculitis, is a subset of LE with lesions preferentially located on the face, buttocks, upper arms, and thighs. Routine histology reveals a lobular panniculitis that may have dermal and epidermal changes of discoid LE. Approximately 70% of these patients have a positive direct immunofluorescence with immunoglobulin and/or C3 deposition at the basement membrane. IgM has been reported to be the most common immunoglobulin in patients with this subgroup of LE. These patients may also show granular deposition of IgM or complement in dermal blood vessels.

Dermatitis Herpetiformis

Dermatitis herpetiformis (DH; Fig. 2–10) is an autoimmune blistering disease that produces intensely pruritic, grouped, erythematous papulovesicles on skin, particularly overlying extensor surfaces. Accordingly, the clinical differential diagnosis may range from contact allergy and drug eruptions to the urticarial and pruritic forms of pemphigoid. Routine histology reveals aggregates of neutrophils and fibrin within dermal papillae, associated with subepidermal vesicles that form by the confluence of microvesicles that evolve over adjacent dermal papillae. The histology may sometimes be ambiguous, leading to confusion with pemphigoid, linear IgA disease, and even neutrophilic dermatitis.

Direct immunofluorescence is generally confirmatory in cases of DH, revealing granular deposits of IgA with or

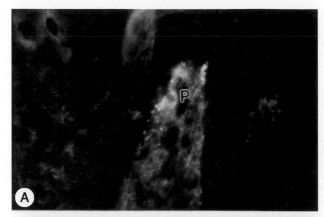

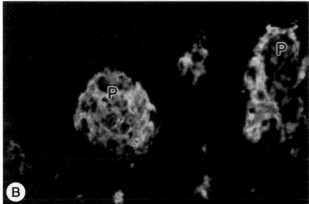

Figure 2–10. Dermatitis herpetiformis. **(A)** Granular staining for IgA within the dermal papilla (P) is readily observed in a developing lesion. At times, anchoring fibrils are outlined by the antibody deposits. In older lesions, granular staining may diffuse along the dermal-epidermal interface, mimicking a positive lupus band test. Unlike the pattern in lupus erythematosus, however, the granular pattern in dermatitis herpetiformis remains accentuated in the papillae and is predominated by antibody deposits of the IgA subclass. **(B)** In a late lesion, aggregated fibrin demarcates each dermal papilla (P).

without fibrin within dermal papillae (Fig. 2–10). Very early lesions reveal fine, barely perceptible strands of fluorescence for IgA at the very tips of dermal papillae. Late lesions may disclose granular reactivity relatively evenly distributed along the dermal-epidermal junction in a pattern that mimics a positive lupus band test. However, in such instances, the predominant immunoglobulin subclass in DH is consistently IgA. Positive direct immunofluorescence results are observed in 85 to 90% of patients affected with DH, although step sections through biopsy specimens in certain cases may be required to increase yield due to focality of the deposits. False-negative results may also occur when a biopsy specimen includes predominantly lesional tissue and insufficient quantities of perilesional skin. In fact, perilesional skin or even normal buttock skin may disclose IgA deposits even in patients undergoing clinical remission.

The immunopathogenesis of DH involves production of IgA-class antibodies to connective tissue components of the gastrointestinal tract (i.e., antiendomysial antibodies). These antibodies occur in 70 to 80% of patients with DH and in a somewhat lower percentage of patients with celiac disease. They have also been detected in cases of other enteropathies. Patients with DH or celiac disease also have antigliadin and

antigluten antibodies of the IgA subclass, which have been shown to cross-react with reticulin fibers. This latter phenomenon may be responsible for the deposition of IgA in the tips of dermal papillae, where reticulin fibers are concentrated.

Cell Membrane Staining[34–38]

Pemphigus

Pemphigus (Fig. 2–11) refers to a group of autoimmune blistering diseases involving skin and mucous membranes. There are several different clinical variants, all of which have circulating antibodies against epithelial intercellular substance. All of these variants have in common the histologic findings of intraepithelial acantholysis and deposition of immunoglobulins in the intercellular spaces.

Pemphigus vulgaris, the most common of the subgroups, shows intercellular deposition of IgG in nearly 100% of patients with active disease. The immunoreactant deposition is in a fine, uniform, fish-net or honeycomb pattern (Fig. 2–11). A similar pattern is reproduced in monkey esophagus when patient serum is evaluated by indirect immunofluorescence (see Fig. 2–8B). C3 may be detected alone or in addi-

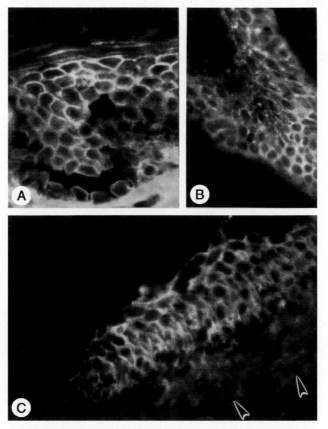

Figure 2–11. Pemphigus. **(A)** A fish-net pattern of cell membrane IgG deposition preferentially stains the lower one half of the epidermal layer in this characteristic biopsy specimen of experimentally induced pemphigus vulgaris. Note the early suprabasal acantholysis. **(B)** Follicular epithelium may show a similar staining pattern. **(C)** In superficial forms of pemphigus, staining is accentuated along the membranes of keratinocytes within the uppermost epidermal layers, where acantholysis and incipient sloughing of rounded individual cells may also be observed. (*Arrowheads*, dermal-epidermal junction.)

tion to IgG in up to 50% of cases. However, intercellular complement binding without IgG has been reported in normal skin of patients without pemphigus. IgA and IgM are seen in addition to IgG less frequently, in approximately 30 to 50% of cases.

Immunoelectron microscopy reveals immunoglobulin deposition on the cell surface of keratinocytes without extension into the cytoplasm of cells. The antigenic binding site of pemphigus vulgaris antibodies is a 130-kD glycoprotein (i.e., the pemphigus vulgaris complex), which is linked to plakoglobin, an 85-kD protein found in both adherens junctions and desmosomes.

In pemphigus foliaceus, or superficial pemphigus, the antigen complex is desmoglein 1, a 160-kD desmosomal core glycoprotein that is linked to plakoglobin. Direct immunofluorescence shows intercellular deposition of IgG and C3 indistinguishable from that of pemphigus vulgaris. Frequently, however, the staining is predominantly in the superficial epidermal layers. Brazilian pemphigus foliaceus, or fogo selvagum, which is endemic in rural South America, is clinically and pathologically indistinguishable from other cases of pemphigus foliaceus. These patients also have autoantibodies that bind to the same desmoglein 1 protein.

In Senear-Usher syndrome, or pemphigus erythematosus, patients develop scaly, erythematous lesions in a photodistribution. Direct immunofluorescence is similar to that of pemphigus vulgaris and pemphigus foliaceus, but additionally, there is granular deposition of IgG and C3 at the dermal-epidermal junction, such as that seen in a positive lupus band test. These immunoreactants have been demonstrated on facial lesions and sun-exposed skin. Although coexistent systemic LE and pemphigus have been reported, patients with Senear-Usher syndrome generally do not develop systemic LE with visceral organ involvement. Positive antinuclear antibodies (ANA) are present in approximately 30% of these patients. These ANA may produce a false-negative indirect immunofluorescence for circulating pemphigus antibodies due to an interference phenomenon termed the prozone effect.

Pemphigus vegetans occurs in two clinical subtypes: the Neumann type, which has a more aggressive course, and the Hallopeau type, which tends to be less severe. Histopathology shows pseudoepitheliomatous hyperplasia, intraepidermal abscesses of eosinophils, and suprabasal acantholysis. Immunofluorescence, however, is indistinguishable from that of pemphigus vulgaris. Pemphigus herpetiformis shows intercellular deposition of IgG and C3 similar to pemphigus vegetans on direct immunofluorescence.

A recently described entity characterized by circulating and/or in vivo bound IgA antibodies to intercellular substance has been termed IgA pemphigus, intraepidermal neutrophilic IgA dermatosis, or intercellular IgA vesiculopustular dermatosis (IAVPD). Immunopathology reveals deposition of IgA in pattern similar to that of pemphigus. Recent immunoblot analysis suggests that IAVPD is a different entity than pemphigus.

With regard to differential diagnosis, Hailey-Hailey disease and Grover disease (i.e., transient acantholytic dermatosis) consistently have negative direct immunofluorescence results. However, nonspecific fluorescence of acantholytic cells may be seen and should not be confused with true staining of the intercellular spaces. Drug-induced pemphigus may be indistinguishable on routine histology from pemphigus vulgaris or, more commonly, pemphigus foliaceus. Direct immunofluorescence is usually negative, but may show staining of the intercellular substance, frequently of the basal cell layer. True intercellular staining must be distinguished from the nonspecific leakage of immunoreactants in spongiotic dermatitis (see Fig. 2–6B). In eczematous processes, many or all of the immunoreactants producing this pattern are seen, in addition to nonspecific fluorescence of loculated serum of a scale-crust.

Colloid Body Reactivity[39, 40]

Acute Cytotoxicity

In acute forms of cytotoxic dermatitis, such as erythema multiforme, the basement membrane zone is often disrupted and irregular due to basal cell layer cytolysis (Fig. 2–12A). Generally, this disruption is associated with formation of intraepidermal necrotic cells that nonspecifically take up immunoglobulin, predominantly of the IgM subclass. Foci of granular immune reactant deposition may also be observed along the dermal-epidermal interface and within the walls of

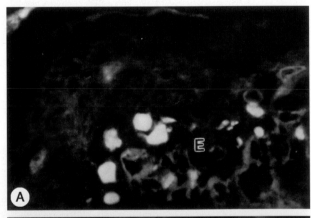

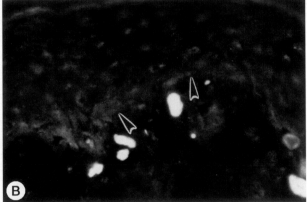

Figure 2–12. Colloid body formation: erythema multiforme and lichen planus. **(A)** In acute cytotoxic dermatitis (i.e., erythema multiforme), apoptotic cells within the epidermis (E) take up immunoglobulin, particularly IgM, and are detected as intensely stained homogeneous round zones above a vacuolated basal cell layer. **(B)** In chronic cytotoxic dermatitis (i.e., lichen planus), such cells often are incorporated into the superficial dermis (*arrowheads,* basement membrane region); colloid bodies are signified by globular zones of predominantly IgM deposition directly beneath the dermal-epidermal junction.

small, superficial vessels. Although foci involving the epidermal basement membrane zone may resemble the findings in LE, those of acute cytotoxicity tend to be discontinuous and of erratic intensity. In addition to erythema multiforme, the previously mentioned alterations have been described in pityriasis lichenoides et varioliformis acuta and in acute graft-versus-host disease.

Chronic Cytotoxicity

Lichen planus, the prototypical disorder for chronic, non–antibody-mediated cytotoxic attack along the dermal-epidermal junction, is characterized by the presence of numerous colloid bodies (i.e., globular degenerating and necrotic keratinocytes) containing immunoglobulin and complement within the papillary dermis (Fig. 2–12B). Although these bodies are not pathognomonic for lichen planus, they are highly suggestive if found in large quantities. Their identification is particularly helpful when evaluating erosive lichen planus of the oral cavity, in which routine histology is a less sensitive indicator of this disorder than of keratinizing epidermis.

Colloid bodies may be found in small numbers in clinically normal skin, as may other inflammatory dermatoses, which may or may not be lichenoid. This is especially true when there is chronic degeneration of the basal layer, such as in LE. Colloid bodies are also commonly seen in lesions of bullous pemphigoid. As is the case in acute forms of cytotoxic dermatitis, focal granular deposits of immunoglobulin (predominantly IgM) may be detected along the dermal-epidermal junction in lichen planus. Discontinuous linear deposits of IgG and C3 have also been noted rarely.

Vascular Reactivity[41–50]

Vasculitis

Necrotizing vasculitis (i.e., leukocytoclastic vasculitis) is characterized histologically by destruction of small dermal venules associated with leukocytoclasia, fibrinoid degeneration of the endothelial wall, and extravasation of erythrocytes. Deposition of immunoglobulins and complement in vessel walls can be detected by direct immunofluorescence and may aid in diagnosis if routine histology is equivocal. This deposition is felt to be a result of increased vascular permeability associated with circulating immune complexes in antigen excess.

Characteristically, granular deposition of complement and/or one or more immunoglobulins is seen within the walls of small, superficial vessels (i.e., postcapillary venules; Fig. 2–13). It is important to ascertain that the immunoglobulin deposition is within vessel walls and not in vascular lumina or in the perivascular space. However, fibrin frequently is detected in the perivascular region. Although this finding is not diagnostic for vasculitis, it suggests increased vascular permeability and possible vascular damage (see Fig. 2–6C). Leukocytoclastic vasculitis secondary to various causes (e.g., systemic lupus erythematosus, rheumatoid arthritis, drug-induced, cryoglobulinemia, livedo vasculitis, hepatitis-associated vasculitis) may also show similar results on direct immunofluorescence.

Timing of skin biopsy to detect vasculitis is critical, because the immune deposits are transitory. The highest yield of detected deposits is in skin lesions that have been present for 18 to 24 hours. Lesions that have been present for more than 48 hours will likely produce negative results. Vascular

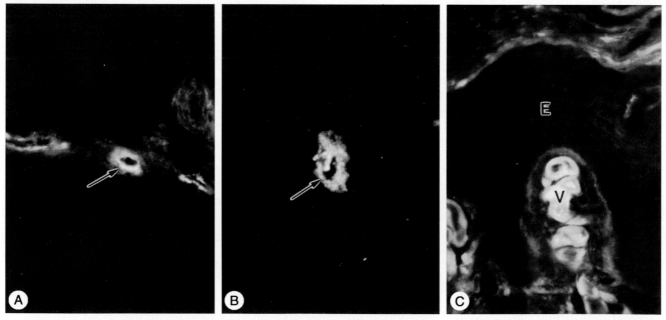

Figure 2–13. Vascular staining. **(A)** Small vessels within dermal papillae show granular deposits of IgG exclusively localized to their walls *(arrow).* **(B)** A similar pattern of deposition is seen for C_3 in an underlying superficial dermal venule. **(C)** In porphyria, there is characteristic widening of small vessel walls (V) by homogeneous, glassy deposits of immunoglobulins (IgG) and albumen. Like vasculitis, the staining is localized precisely to vessel walls, as opposed to the vessel wall staining that accompanies increased permeability (e.g., in urticaria or spongiotic dermatitis). The character of staining, however, is very different: granular in vasculitis and homogeneous in porphyria. (E, epidermis.)

deposition of immunoreactants is not always diagnostic of leukocytoclastic vasculitis; it has been noted in other inflammatory dermatoses such as erythema multiforme. Immunofluorescence findings should always be correlated with clinical history and/or changes on routine histology.

Henoch-Schönlein purpura (HSP) is a specific subset of leukocytoclastic vasculitis in which IgA is the most prominent of the immunoglobulins. Although IgM, IgG, and complement may also be present, IgA usually has the strongest staining intensity. A diagnosis of HSP should be suspected if granular vascular staining with IgA is detected in the absence of all other immunoreactants. Patients with HSP have increased levels of circulating IgA immune complexes and may also have deposition of IgA in renal glomeruli as well as in blood vessels of the gastrointestinal mucosa. These changes correlate with the clinical manifestations of hematuria and abdominal pain frequently seen in this patient population.

Patients with urticarial vasculitis have persistent urticarial skin lesions that last for longer than 24 hours and resolve with purpura or hyperpigmentation. These patients may have associated connective tissue diseases and/or hypocomplementemia. Direct immunofluorescence of these skin lesions is indistinguishable from that of biopsy specimens of leukocytoclastic vasculitis from other causes. Roughly two thirds of patients with urticarial vasculitis will have vascular staining with either immunoglobulins or complement.

Polyarteritis nodosa is a form of vasculitis involving medium-sized arteries of the skin associated with palpable purpura as well as punched-out cutaneous ulcers. These patients may or may not have associated systemic involvement including the kidneys, liver, heart, and gastrointestinal tract. Histology reveals panarteritis in the deep dermis and subcutaneous tissue. Immunopathologic studies have shown IgM, C3, and fibrin deposition within vessel walls. Deposition of immunoreactants in small superficial vessels has also been noted, as has the complete absence of immune deposits.

Porphyria

The cutaneous hallmarks of patients with porphyria cutanea tarda are skin fragility and subepidermal blisters with minimal inflammation on sun-exposed surfaces. Direct immunofluorescence characteristically shows homogeneous deposition of immunoreactants in papillary dermal blood vessels (Fig. 2–13C). These vessels appear doughnut-shaped with thickened walls, probably secondary to reduplicated basement membrane material. IgG is found most commonly; however, IgM, IgA, complement, and fibrinogen have been detected less frequently. Approximately 50% of patients with porphyria cutanea tarda may show similar vascular staining in clinically normal skin. Cytoid bodies, although a nonspecific finding, are also frequently noted in biopsy specimens

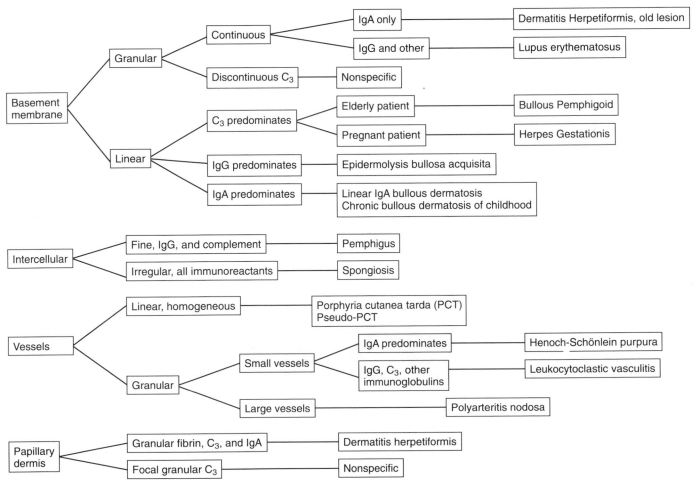

Figure 2–14. A practical algorithm for using direct immunofluorescence to diagnose skin conditions.

from these patients. Similar immunofluorescence findings may be seen in other types of porphyria (e.g., erythropoietic protoporphyria, variegate porphyria, coproporphyria) as well as in drug-induced pseudoporphyria.

CONCLUSION

This chapter is a review of special diagnostic techniques available as diagnostic adjuncts in dermatopathology and provides a practical overview of diagnostic immunofluorescence evaluation of the skin. Although this approach is not comprehensive, and exceptions exist to every rule, based upon analysis of basic immunofluorescence patterns, it is possible to create an algorithm for conceptual understanding of the diagnosis of dermatologic disorders and to facilitate analysis of many immune-mediated skin disorders. Figure 2–14 provides a basis for the more salient branch points in determining the diagnostically significant differences in commonly encountered patterns of direct cutaneous immunofluorescence.

SELECTED REFERENCES

1. Jaworsky C, Murphy GF. Special techniques in dermatology. Arch Dermatol 1989;125:963.
2. Taylor CR. Immunomicroscopy: A Diagnostic Tool for the Surgical Pathologist. Philadelphia: WB Saunders, 1986.
3. Murphy GF, Mihm MC, eds. Lymphoproliferative Disorders of the Skin. Boston: Butterworths, 1986.
4. Murphy GF, Harrist TJ, Mihm MC. Reaction patterns in the skin and special dermatopathologic techniques. In: Moschella SL, Hurley HJ, eds. Dermatology. Philadelphia: WB Saunders, 1985:104.
5. Murphy GF, Dickerson GR, Harrist TJ, Mihm MC. The role of diagnostic electron microscopy in dermatology. In: Moschella SL, ed. Dermatology Update. New York: Elsevier, 1982:355.
6. Duvic M. In situ hybridization. Clin Dermatol 1991;9:129.
7. Beutner EH, Chorzelski TP, Kumar VJ. Immunopathology of the Skin, 3rd ed. New York: John Wiley & Sons, 1987.
8. Black MM, Thomas RH, Bhogal B. The value of immunofluorescence techniques in the diagnosis of bullous disorders: A review. Clin Exp Dermatol 1983;8:337.
9. Harrist TJ, Mihm MC. Cutaneous immunopathology. Hum Pathol 1979;10:625.
10. Lever WF. Pemphigus and Pemphigoid. Springfield, IL, Charles C Thomas, 1965.
11. Woodley DT, Briggaman RA, O'Keefe EJ, et al. Identification of the skin basement membrane autoantigen in epidermolysis bullosa acquisita. N Engl J Med 1984;310:1007.
12. Logan RA, Bhogal BS, Das A, et al. Localization of bullous pemphigoid antibody: An indirect immunofluorescence study of 288 cases using a split skin technique. Br J Dermatol 1987;117:471.
13. Briggaman RA, Gammon WR, Woodley DT. Epidermolysis bullosa acquisita of the immunopathological type (dermolytic pemphigoid). J Invest Dermatol 1985;85:795.
14. Kelly S, Cerio R, Bhogal BS, et al. The distribution of IgG subclasses in pemphigoid gestationis: HG factor is an IgG1 autoantibody. J Invest Dermatol 1989;92:695.
15. Provost TT, Yaoita H, Katz SI. Herpes gestationis. In: Beutner EH, Chorzelski TP, Bean SF, eds. Immunopathology of the Skin, 2nd ed. New York: John Wiley & Sons, 1979:273.
16. Jablonska S, Chorzelski TP, Maciejowska E, et al. Immunologic phenomena in herpes gestationis: Their pathologic and diagnostic significance. J Dermatol 1975;2:149.
17. Harrington CI, Bleehen SS: Herpes gestationis: Immunopathological and ultrastructural studies. Br J Dermatol 1979;100:389.
18. Jordon RE, Heine KG, Tappeiner G, et al: The immunopathology of herpes gestationis. Immunofluorescence studies and characterization of the ''HG factor.'' J Clin Invest 1976;57:1426.
19. Gammon WR, Kowalewski C, Chorzelski TP, et al. Direct immunofluorescence studies of sodium chloride–separated skin in the differential diagnosis of bullous pemphigoid and epidermolysis bullosa acquisita. J Am Acad Dermatol 1990;22(4):664.
20. Woodley DT, Burgeson RE, Lunstrum G, et al. Epidermolysis bullosa acquisita antigen is the globular carboxyl terminus of type VII procollagen. J Clin Invest 1988;81:683.
21. Chorzelski TP, Jablonska S. Evolving concept of IgA linear dermatosis. Semin Dermatol 1988;7:225.
22. Pothupitiya GM, Wojnarowska F, Bhogal BS, Black MM. Distribution of the antigen in adult linear IgA disease and chronic bullous disease of childhood suggests that it is a single and unique antigen. Br J Dermatol 1988;118:175.
23. Wojnarowska F, Marsden RA, Bhogal BS, Black MM. Chronic bullous disease of childhood, cicatricial pemphigoid and linear IgA disease of adults. J Am Acad Dermatol 1988;19:792.
24. Willsteed E, Bhogal BS, Black MM, McKee P, Wojnarowska F. Use of 1M NaCl split skin in the indirect immunofluorescence of the linear IgA bullous dermatoses. J Cutan Pathol 1990;17(3):144.
25. Hood AF. Pathology of cutaneous lupus erythematosus. Adv Dermatol 1988;3:153.
26. Burnham TK, Fine G. The immunofluorescent band for lupus erythematosus. I. Morphologic variations of the band of localized immunoglobulins at the dermal-epidermal junction in lupus erythematosus. Arch Dermatol 1969;99:413.
27. Kobayasi T, Asboe-Hansen G. Ultrastructure of systemic lupus erythematosus skin. Acta Derm Venereol (Stockh) 1973;57:417.
28. Igarashi R, Morohashi M, Koizumi F, et al. Immunofluorescence study of cutaneous blood vessels of 16 patients with systemic lupus erythematosus. Acta Derm Venereol (Stockh) 1981;61:219.
29. Natali PG, Tan EM. Experimental skin lesions in mice resembling systemic lupus erythematosus. Arthr Rheum 1973;16:579.
30. Halberg P, Ullman S, Jorgensen F. The lupus band test as a measure of disease activity in systemic lupus erythematosus. Arch Dermatol 1982;118:572.
31. Sanchez NP, Peters MS, Winkelmann RK. The histopathology of lupus erythematosus panniculitis. J Am Acad Dermatol 1981;5:673.
32. Van der Meer JB. Granular deposits of immunoglobulins in the skin of patients with dermatitis herpetiformis: An immunofluorescent study. Br J Dermatol 1969;81:493.
33. Chorzelski TP, Beutner EH, Sulej J, et al. IgA-endomysium antibody: A new immunological marker of dermatitis herpetiformis and coeliac disease. Br J Dermatol 1984;111:395.
34. Ioannides D, Hytiroglou R, Phelps RG, Bystryn JC. Regional variation in the expression of pemphigus foliaceus, pemphigus erythematosus, and pemphigus vulgaris antigens in human skin. J Invest Dermatol 1991;96(2):159.
35. Hodak E, David M, Ingber A, et al. The clinical and histopathological spectrum of IgA-pemphigus—report of two cases. Exp Dermatol 1990;15(6):433.
36. Beutner EH, Lever WF, Witebsky E, et al. Autoantibodies in pemphigus vulgaris: Response to an intercellular substance of epidermis. J Am Med Assoc 1965;192:682.
37. Beutner EH, Jordan RE. Demonstration of skin antibodies in sera of pemphigus vulgaris patients by indirect immunofluorescent staining. Proc Soc Exp Biol Med 1964;117:505.
38. Cowin P, Kapprell H-P, Franke WW, et al. Plakoglobin: A protein common to different kinds of intercellular adhering junctions. Cell 1986;46:1063.
39. Sobel S, Miller R, Shatin H. Lichen planus pemphigoides: Immunofluorescence findings. Arch Dermatol 1976;112:1280.
40. Lang PG, Maize JC. Coexisting lichen planus and bullous pemphigoid or lichen planus pemphigoides. J Am Acad Dermatol 1983;9:133.
41. Tappeiner G, Jordon RE, Wolff K. Circulating immune complexes in necrotizing vasculitis. In: Wolff K, Winkelmann RK, eds. Vasculitis. Philadelphia: WB Saunders, 1980:68.
42. Mackel SE, Jordon R. Leukocytoclastic vasculitis. Arch Dermatol 1982;118:296.
43. Kauffmann RH, Herrmann WA, Meyer CJ, et al. Circulating IgA-immune complexes in Henoch-Schönlein purpura. Am J Med 1980;69:859.
44. Baart de la Faille-Kuyper EH, Kater L, Kooiker CJ, Dorhout Mees EJ. IgA deposits in cutaneous blood-vessel walls and mesangium in Henoch-Schönlein syndrome. Lancet 1973;1:892.

45. Levinsky RJ, Barratt TM. IgA immune complexes in Henoch-Schönlein purpura. Lancet 1979;2:1100.
46. Zone JJ, LaSalle BA, Provost TT. Induction of IgA circulating immune complexes after wheat feeding in dermatitis herpetiformis patients. J Invest Dermatol 1982;78:375.
47. Mehregan DR, Hall MJ, Gibson LE. Urticarial vasculitis: A histopathologic and clinical review of 72 cases. J Am Acad Dermatol 1992;26:44.
48. Goslen JB, Graham W, Lazarus GS. Cutaneous polyarteritis nodosa: Report of a case associated with Crohn's disease. Arch Dermatol 1983;119:326.
49. Diaz-Perez JL, Schroeter AL, Winkelmann RK. Cutaneous periarteritis nodosa: Immunofluorescence studies. Arch Dermatol 1980;116:56.
50. Chen KR. Cutaneous polyarteritis nodosa: A clinical and histopathological study of 20 cases. J Dermatol 1989;16:429.

II

Inflammatory Dermatoses

3

Spongiotic Dermatitis

DEFINITIONS AND GENERAL CONSIDERATIONS[1]

Spongiotic dermatitis is a category representing a diverse group of cutaneous disorders sharing the common finding of spongiosis within the epidermal layer. The term spongiosis derives from the absorbent sponge, which originates as the porous connective tissue skeleton of marine animals of the phylum Porifera. In spongiotic dermatitis, the dermal-epidermal junction is abnormally permeable to plasma and proteins liberated from superficial venules, and in a sponge-like manner, fluid accumulates predominantly within intercellular spaces separating keratinocytes. In early or mild spongiotic dermatitis, widened intercellular spaces within the epidermal layer impart a spongy appearance to the stratum spinosum, often accompanied by intraepidermal accumulation of benign lymphocytes as they migrate from their initial perivenular location (Fig. 3–1). This reaction pattern is in contrast to urticaria, in which the dermal-epidermal junction is not permissive to upward dissipation of occasionally pronounced dermal edema and inflammatory cell infiltration, and to epidermotropic cutaneous T-cell lymphoma, in which intraepithelial lymphocytic migration and proliferation occurs in the relative absence of spongiosis.

The vague term *eczematous dermatitis* is frequently used to refer to spongiotic processes. Generally, this term refers to a clinical condition characterized by a pruritic, erythematous, oozing, papulovesicular dermatitis which, with chronicity, may evolve to scaling, lichenified plaques. However, numerous disorders may show these features in the absence of the histologic finding of spongiosis. Eczematous dermatitis therefore fails to describe adequately the temporal or clinicopathologic parameters required for its qualification as a meaningful descriptive term, and will not be used in this chapter.

GROSS PATHOLOGY[2-4]

The clinical appearance of spongiotic dermatitis depends both on its evolutionary stage and its cause. Early phases of lesion evolution (i.e., <24 hours) may resemble urticarial plaques, with only faint associated erythema and without epidermal changes. After several days, *acute lesions* show increasing erythema, often accompanied by small, solitary to confluent vesicles filled with clear, yellow fluid (Fig. 3–2). At this juncture, patients usually complain of marked pruritus. *Subacute lesions* (i.e., days to several weeks) demonstrate persistent erythema, little or no vesiculation, and increased scale formation. Excoriation undoubtedly plays a role in inducing superimposed primary irritant reactive epidermal alterations. Bacterial superinfection may result in the honey-colored crust typical of impetigo. *Chronic lesions* (i.e., months to years) are predominated by induration and scale, and marked erythema and vesiculation are not observed. The lichenified plaques of lichen simplex chronicus represent an example of this final common pathway for spongiotic dermatitides. Because spongiosis is not prominent in chronic lesions, they will be considered separately in the chapter concerned with psoriasiform dermatitis (see Chap. 4).

Allergic contact dermatitis occurs at sites of hapten entry into the epidermal layer (see Pathogenesis), and therefore is often precisely localized to sites of environmental contacts (e.g., jewelry, leather, clothing). On the other hand, *seborrheic dermatitis*, a poorly understood form of low-grade spongiotic dermatitis presumably caused in part by endogenous factors, characteristically occurs in seborrheic areas (e.g., scalp, eyebrows, nasolabial creases, midline chest, intertriginous areas). A comprehensive review of the clinical features of the various forms of spongiotic dermatitis is beyond the scope of this chapter; other sources contain this information. However, appreciation of certain clinical fea-

49

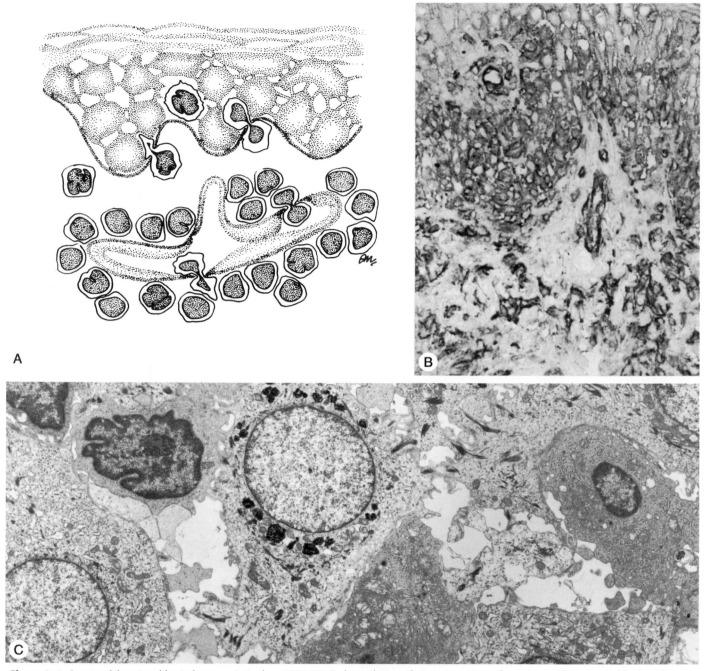

Figure 3–1. Structural-functional basis for spongiotic dermatitis. **(A)** Early evolution of acute spongiotic dermatitis is characterized by lymphocyte epidermotropism. The intercellular spaces of the epidermis are widened by edema fluid derived from hyperpermeable venules within the underlying superficial vascular plexus. This vascular event is accompanied by initial accumulation of lymphocytes and other inflammatory cells within the perivascular space of superficial and sometimes deep dermal venules. Lymphocytes also characteristically migrate into the overlying spongiotic epidermal layer. **(B)** Patterns of lymphocytic trafficking in spongiotic dermatitis are partially determined by the expression of adhesion molecules by skin cells. An immunohistochemical preparation of a specimen from a patient who has early acute spongiotic dermatitis shows reactivity for intercellular adhesion molecule-1 (ICAM-1) by keratinocytes, endothelial cells, and dermal dendritic immune cells and fibroblasts. ICAM-1 binds lymphocytes, and its expression correlated precisely with sites of lymphocyte migration in this biopsy specimen. **(C)** Ultrastructural studies confirm widened intercellular spaces within the epidermis in a patient who has spongiotic dermatitis. Several lymphocytes may also be seen within the prominent, expanded gaps separating adjacent keratinocytes. Disruption of intercellular junctions (i.e., desmosomes) may eventuate in microvesicles and clinical blisters.

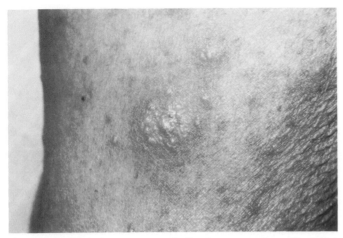

Figure 3–2. Clinical appearance of allergic contact dermatitis. Initial erythema and induration have evolved to form vesicles filled with clear yellow fluid. These vesicles resulted from intercellular edema within the epidermal layer (i.e., spongiosis) that traumatically destroyed intercellular attachments. In time, the vesicles will rupture and dry, and if the inflammatory stimulus remains, persistent erythema and abnormal scale formation will supervene (subacute to chronic spongiotic dermatitis).

tures in spongiotic dermatitis is fundamental to formulation of an accurate clinicopathologic diagnosis, because clinical signs may be more specific or suggestive than histologic findings. Thus, the diagnosis of spongiotic dermatitis consistent with allergic contact dermatitis generally relies on confirmatory histology of spongiosis in the setting of an appropriate set of clinical parameters. Table 3–1 summarizes salient gross pathologic and histologic features that are commonly of assistance in clinicopathologic diagnosis and classification of spongiotic disorders.

GENERAL HISTOLOGY AND TEMPORAL EVOLUTION

Common to all forms of acute spongiotic dermatitis are intercellular edema within the epidermis or follicular epithelium and some degree of associated inflammatory infiltrate. Intercellular edema may be first detected as slight pallor of the epidermal layer at scanning magnification as a result of incorporation of clear edema fluid (Fig. 3–3). As fluid accumulates, intercellular bridges are stretched, and as a consequence, appear abnormally prominent. Ultimately, cell-cell junctions are broken, producing small microvesicles that enlarge and merge to become the fluid-filled vesicles appreciated clinically. Interepithelial cell edema is invariably accompanied by leukocytic infiltration that originates about postcapillary venules lined by prominent (i.e., activated) endothelial cells. This *vasocentric* phase progresses rapidly to an *epidermotropic* response, whereby lymphocytes and occasionally eosinophils migrate across the dermal-epidermal junction into the fluid-filled intercellular spaces separating epidermal or follicular keratinocytes. The immune and cellular mechanisms responsible for these structural alterations are outlined in Pathogenesis. In time, epidermal hyperplasia ensues (Fig. 3–4), resulting in acanthosis and abnormal scale formation (i.e., hyperorthokeratosis and parakeratosis). As lesions enter into subacute and chronic stages with the advent of hyperplasia, spongiotic changes often become progressively less apparent (Table 3–2). Persistence of lymphocytes in the papillary dermis and superimposed excoriation frequently result in papillary dermal fibrosis, an additional marker of chronicity. The temporal evolution of spongiotic dermatitis is summarized schematically in Figure 3–5.

Table 3–1. CLINICAL VARIANTS OF SPONGIOTIC DERMATITIS

| | DISTINGUISHING FEATURES | |
VARIANT	Clinical	Histologic
Allergic contact dermatitis	Sites of antigen contact	Langerhans cell microgranulomas; eosinophils may be numerous
Atopic dermatitis	Flexural involvement in childhood	Epidermal hyperplasia; eosinophils may be sparse
Nummular dermatitis	Coin-like patches and plaques on arms and legs	Pin-point microvesicles with mild spongiosis
Seborrheic dermatitis	Oily, scaling dermatitis of scalp, facial folds, midback, and chest	Subacute spongiotic dermatitis with scale and rare neutrophils in dermis or in scale
Dyshidrotic eczema	Vesicles on palms and/or soles	Prominent intraepidermal microvesicles in acral skin
Id reaction	Association with primary dermatitis, often with fungal or bacterial component; stasis	Numerous eosinophils in dermal infiltrate
Pityriasis rosea	Ovoid patches and plaques following skin lines	Mound-like parakeratosis; papillary dermal hemorrhage
Guttate parapsoriasis	Ovoid patches and plaques, resistant to therapy	Mound-like parakeratosis; no hemorrhage
Photoallergic dermatitis	Photo distribution	Fading of lymphoid infiltrate from superficial to mid-dermal vessels; endothelial vacuolization
Spongiotic drug eruption	Often diffuse involvement	Superficial and deep infiltrate; perivascular eosinophils
Spongiotic insect-bite reaction	Grouped papulonodules	Wedge-shaped infiltrate; eosinophilic spongiosis; interstitial eosinophils

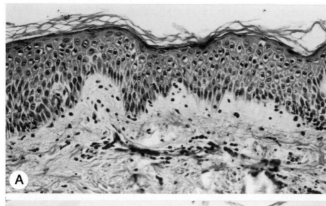

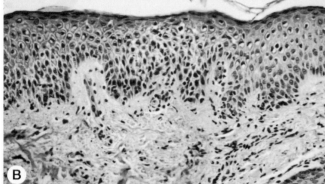

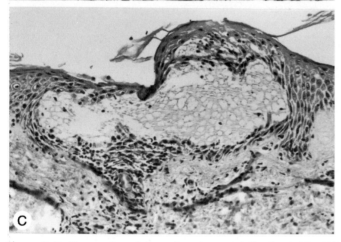

Figure 3–3. Temporal evolution of acute spongiotic dermatitis. **(A)** Edema fluid initially accumulates within the papillary dermis, similar to urticaria. Edema within the dermis is subtle, but it may be appreciated as a band of pallor beneath the basement membrane zone of the epidermis. **(B)** As lymphocytes begin to accumulate about superficial venules and migrate into the epidermal layer, associated spongiosis is observed as focal regions of epidermal pallor resulting from the increased area occupied by widened intercellular spaces. **(C)** Traumatic lysis of intercellular junctions as spongiosis becomes more pronounced results in intraepidermal microvesicles filled with pink, proteinaceous, serum transudate.

HISTOLOGY OF SPECIFIC DISORDERS

Allergic Contact Dermatitis[5, 6]

- SUPERFICIAL PERIVASCULAR LYMPHOCYTIC INFILTRATE
- PAPILLARY DERMAL EDEMA
- VARIABLE SPONGIOSIS AND MICROVESICULATION
- EPIDERMOTROPIC LYMPHOCYTES
- LANGERHANS CELL MICROGRANULOMAS
- VASOCENTRIC AND EPIDERMOTROPIC EOSINOPHILS
- EPIDERMAL HYPERPLASIA, HYPERKERATOSIS AND PARAKERATOSIS WITH CHRONICITY
- SUPPORTIVE CLINICAL HISTORY AND GROSS PATHOLOGY

Allergic contact dermatitis (ACD) invariably occurs at sites where hapten or antigen has challenged an already primed T-cell response (see Pathogenesis). Accordingly, the clinical features of ACD are often sufficient for diagnosis without need for confirmatory biopsy. In certain instances, however, ACD may clinically mimic conditions such as herpetic or superficial fungal infection, drug eruption, bullous impetigo, or causes of erythroderma, and biopsy of an active,

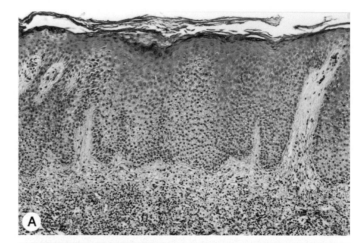

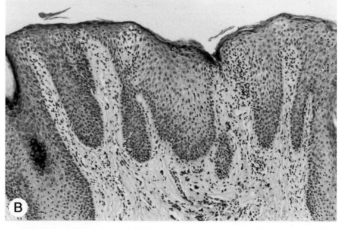

Figure 3–4. Subacute to chronic evolutionary stages of spongiotic dermatitis. **(A)** Persistent perivenular dermal mononuclear cell infiltrate is associated with striking overlying epidermal hyperplasia and mild hyperkeratosis in the subacute to chronic lesions of spongiotic dermatitis. The central portion of the epidermis shows slight pallor, which correlates with residual spongiosis. The dermal papilla to the right contains delicate, vertically oriented, parallel strands of collagen, which is evidence of early lichen simplex chronicus, undoubtedly resulting from repeated excoriation. **(B)** Chronic spongiotic dermatitis has little evidence of antecedent spongiosis and is dominated by changes of lichen simplex chronicus, including irregular acanthosis, hyperkeratosis and parakeratosis, and vertically oriented fibrosis within dermal papillae.

Table 3–2. NATURAL EVOLUTION OF SPONGIOTIC DERMATITIS

HISTOLOGIC ALTERATION	TEMPORAL PHASE		
	Acute	Subacute	Chronic
Spongiosis	+ + +	+ +	+
Vesiculation	+ to + + +	−	−
Epidermal hyperplasia	+	+ +	+ + +
Papillary dermal fibrosis	−	−	+ to + + +
Epidermotropism	+ to + + +	+	−
Endothelial activation*	+ + +	+ to + +	−
Hyperkeratosis and parakeratosis	−	− to +	+ + to + + +

*Defined as bulging of endothelial cells into venular lumina.
+ + +, marked; + +, moderate; +, slight; − absent.

early lesion should be performed and submitted for histologic analysis. Sampling of subacute-to-chronic plaques of ACD may produce confusing patterns as the result of superimposed bacterial superinfection, hyperplasia, and primary irritant effects.

At scanning magnification, acute lesions of ACD are characterized by a superficial perivascular lymphocytic infiltrate with variable associated edema of the papillary dermis discerned as pallor of subepidermal collagen bundles (Fig. 3–6). The epidermis may be of normal thickness for the anatomic site or may show mild irregular acanthosis. Compared to adjacent, uninvolved epidermis, the epithelial layer also may demonstrate pallor due to intercellular edema or frank intraepidermal microvesiculation. Although these changes establish the diagnosis of spongiotic dermatitis, closer inspection at higher magnification is required to determine whether features compatible with ACD are present (see Fig. 3–6). These include: (1) the finding of eosinophils about superficial venules and occasionally within the spongiotic epidermal layer (i.e., eosinophilic spongiosis) in association with epidermotropic lymphocytes; and (2) intraepidermal microgranulomas consisting exclusively of Langerhans cells or an admixture of Langerhans cells and lymphocytes. Hyperplastic Langerhans cells are larger than lymphocytes, exhibit pale but visible cytoplasms, and have a characteristic infolded nucleus containing relatively scant quantities of heterochromatin. Stains for S100 protein occasionally are of assistance in confirming the presence of Langerhans cell microgranulomas. Their prominence in certain biopsy specimens relates to immune mechanisms involved in antigen presentation and cytokine regulation of the superficial delayed hypersensitivity response that underlies the histologic reaction pattern of ACD.

Spongiosis may also involve follicular infundibula in ACD, and in the clinical variant termed follicular eczema, intercellular edema may exclusively affect the pilar apparatus. Certain antigens and haptens, such as nickel, appear to

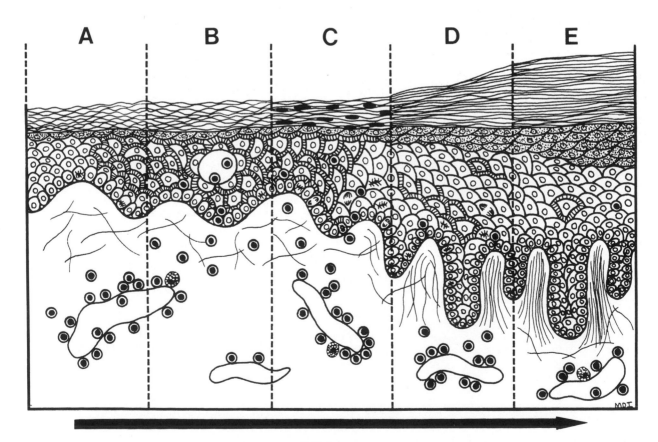

Time

Figure 3–5. Evolutionary stages of spongiotic dermatitis. **(A)** Initial perivascular infiltration is followed within 24 to 48 hours by **(B)** papillary dermal edema and spongiosis with microvesicle formation. **(C)** Abnormal scale, including parakeratosis, follows, along with progressive epidermal **(D)** hyperplasia and **(E)** hyperkeratosis. Chronic excoriation results in vertically oriented fibrosis of dermal papillae (i.e., lichen simplex chronicus). See Chapter 4 for further discussion of psoriasiform evolutionary phases of spongiotic dermatitis.

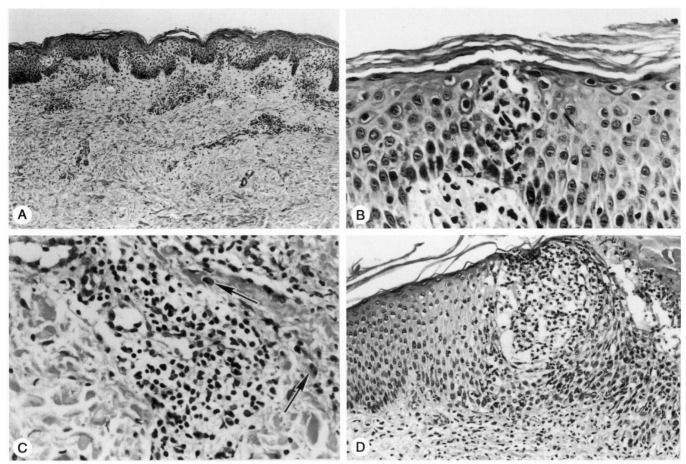

Figure 3–6. Allergic contact dermatitis (ACD). **(A)** At scanning magnification, a superficial perivascular inflammatory infiltrate is associated with a focally spongiotic epidermal layer evidenced by numerous regions of tinctorial pallor. **(B)** Epidermotropism of lymphocytes into spongiotic foci of the epidermal layer is observed at higher magnification. Several cells in this aggregate display infolded nuclear contours and abundant quantities of pale pink cytoplasm. These foci represent aggregates of hyperplastic Langerhans cells (i.e., Langerhans cell microgranuloma), a frequent finding in ACD. **(C)** The perivascular inflammatory infiltrate in ACD consists of lymphocytes, monocytes, and often eosinophils *(arrows)* located about postcapillary venules. Spaces between perivenular collagen bundles are abnormally accentuated as a result of superficial dermal edema. **(D)** In some cases of ACD, eosinophils may be so numerous as to form intraepidermal micropustules (i.e., eosinophilic spongiosis). The finding of eosinophilic spongiosis itself, however, is not specific and has a broad differential diagnosis that includes certain insect-bite reactions, pemphigoid, and, rarely, pemphigus and the vesicular stage of incontinentia pigmenti.

have a peculiar proclivity to stimulate follicular immune responses. The gross pathology of this variant, however, may be confused with other follicular diseases (e.g., inflammatory keratosis pilaris). Accordingly, clinical history is critical to a diagnostic approach, which may include multiple serial sections, for documentation of follicular spongiosis.

Although the histologic findings alone in ACD are not entirely specific beyond categorization as spongiotic dermatitis, with chronicity, they become even less diagnostic. This is because epidermal hyperplasia and secondary alterations resulting from excoriation supervene. Careful scrutiny for residual eosinophils and foci of epidermal or follicular spongiosis, in concert with the appropriate clinical parameters, may be of assistance in suggesting a diagnosis of subacute-to-chronic ACD in such situations. In general, clinicians should be encouraged to biopsy lesions that are early in their clinical evolution, and to avoid sites of refractory dermatitis that have within 3 to 4 weeks been partially treated with topical corticosteroids, which serve to confound further the histology of ACD.

Atopic Dermatitis[7, 8]

- SUPERFICIAL PERIVASCULAR LYMPHOCYTIC INFILTRATE
- EPIDERMAL HYPERPLASIA, HYPERKERATOSIS, AND PARAKERATOSIS COMMON
- MILD PAPILLARY DERMAL EDEMA AND FIBROSIS
- VARIABLE SPONGIOSIS
- EPIDERMOTROPIC LYMPHOCYTES
- EOSINOPHILS VARIABLY OBSERVED
- SUPPORTIVE CLINICAL HISTORY AND GROSS PATHOLOGY

Atopic dermatitis is a genetically inherited form of spongiotic dermatitis in which skin appears to be hypersensitive to many immunologic (i.e., antigen- and hapten-dependent) and nonimmunologic stimuli. The disease generally begins in infancy and childhood, and may persist throughout adult life. Flexural creases are typically preferentially affected, and this chronic disease is known for the production of extraordinary pruritus. It is therefore not surprising that biopsy specimens almost invariably reflect the consequences of lesion persistence over time (i.e., epidermal hyperplasia, abnormal scale formation, and the sequelae of repeated excoriation).

For the previously stated reasons, the histopathology of atopic dermatitis is nonspecific and reflects only a subacute-to-chronic spongiotic reaction pattern. Diagnosis is best rendered after careful consideration of both clinical and histologic data. At scanning magnification, the majority of biopsy specimens of atopic dermatitis will display variable degrees of irregular epidermal hyperplasia (Fig. 3–7), with only slight pallor of the epidermal or papillary dermal regions, the result of mild intercellular and interstitial edema, respectively. On closer inspection, the inflammatory infiltrate, like that of ACD, is superficial, perivascular, and exhibits occasional foci of single-cell epidermotropism into mildly spongiotic epidermal foci. Eosinophils, however, may be difficult to detect or entirely absent (Fig. 3–7). With chronicity, the papillary dermis displays fibrosis, which initially is manifested as coarsely textured collagen and eventually assumes the stromal features of lichen simplex chronicus (see Chap. 4). Accumulation of fibrin and inflammatory cell debris within a thickened stratum corneum is frequently encountered and is likely to represent the sequela of repeated excoriation and bacterial superinfection.

Primary Irritant Dermatitis[9, 10]

- SPARSE SUPERFICIAL PERIVASCULAR LYMPHOCYTIC INFILTRATE
- PAPILLARY DERMAL EDEMA IN ACUTE STAGES
- PAPILLARY DERMAL FIBROSIS IN CHRONIC STAGES
- EPIDERMAL HYPERPLASIA AND HYPERKERATOSIS PREDOMINATE OVER SPONGIOSIS
- NO CLINICAL EVIDENCE OF CONTACT ALLERGY OR ATOPIC DIATHESIS

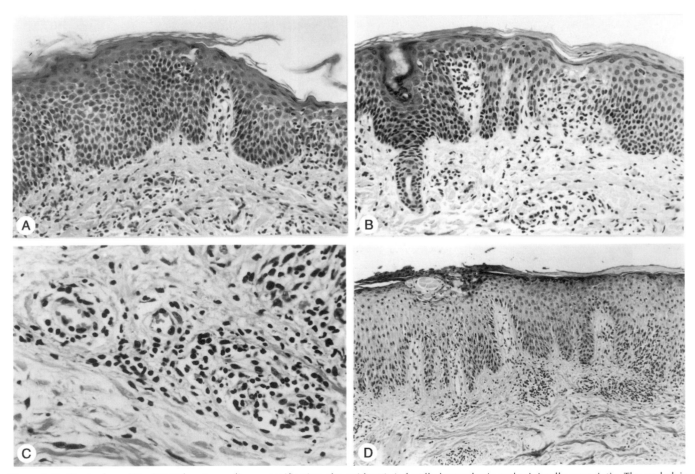

Figure 3–7. Atopic dermatitis. **(A)** At low-to-medium magnification, the epidermis is focally hyperplastic and minimally spongiotic. The underlying papillary dermis contains a sparse, perivascular, lymphocytic infiltrate. **(B)** Single-cell epidermotropism by lymphocytes into a mildly and focally acanthotic and spongiotic epidermal layer is observed in this biopsy specimen from a patient who has atopic dermatitis. In both **A** and **B,** the stratum corneum is diffusely abnormal, exhibiting compacted hyperorthokeratosis or parakeratosis. These features, within the context of a low-grade spongiotic process, indicate the chronicity that typifies the histology of atopic dermatitis. **(C)** The inflammatory infiltrate about superficial venules is composed predominantly of lymphocytes and occasional monocytes; eosinophils are rarely encountered. As in allergic contact dermatitis, spaces separating perivenular collagen bundles are enlarged due to interstitial edema. **(D)** Atopic dermatitis with associated lichen simplex chronicus resulting from excoriation. Features of active atopic dermatitis include a superficial, perivascular, lymphocytic infiltrate; superficial dermal edema with dilated lymphatic lumens; and mild focal spongiosis. Pronounced epidermal hyperplasia, vertically oriented fibrosis within dermal papillae, and early scale-crust formation (i.e., loculated serum and inflammatory cells within abnormal stratum corneum) represent evidence of superimposed chronic recurrent trauma.

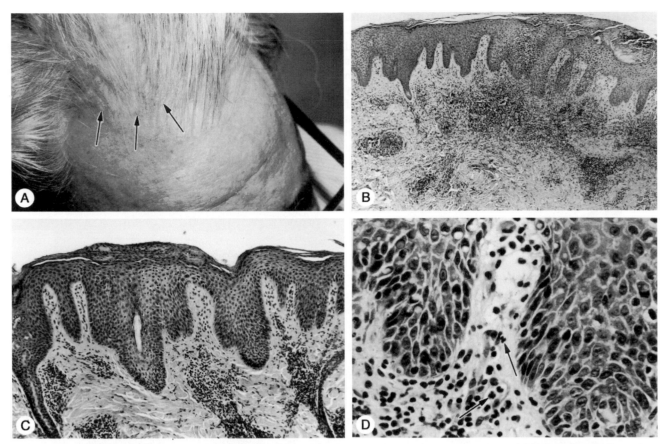

Figure 3–10. Seborrheic dermatitis. **(A)** The gross pathology of this common condition typically is observed as subtle zones of erythema and scaling involving hair-bearing skin (edges of this subtle plaque defined by *arrows*). The scale has an oily consistency and tan-yellow color, a helpful feature in differentiating this condition from psoriasis. **(B, C)** An active lesion of seborrheic dermatitis demonstrates an admixture of mild spongiosis and irregular psoriasiform hyperplasia, broad zones of parakeratotic scale containing occasional neutrophils, and a superficial perivascular inflammatory infiltrate within an edematous papillary dermis. **(D)** On closer inspection, scattered neutrophils *(arrows)* may be identified within pale dermal papillae expanded by interstitial edema.

it is important that the pathologist is assured of a biopsy specimen of active seborrheic dermatitis in a pristine state, without modification by recent application of topical steroids, which can render a difficult diagnosis impossible.

Dyshidrotic Eczema[15]

- SUPERFICIAL PERIVASCULAR LYMPHOCYTIC INFILTRATE
- WELL-FORMED INTRAEPIDERMAL VESICLES IN ACRAL SKIN

One of many examples of misnomers in dermatologic disease, dyshidrotic eczema is not a disturbance of eccrine sweat production, nor is it a specific eczematous disorder. Rather, it represents a form of pruritic, vesicular hand and foot dermatitis without apparent external cause, or occasionally it is associated with atopic disease, dermatophyte infection, or contact allergy. Superinfected vesicles may form pustules that may mimic pustular psoriasis and pustulosis palmaris et plantaris.

At scanning magnification, diagnosis of dyshidrotic dermatitis (i.e., hand or foot eczema) is facilitated by recognition of well-formed, intraepidermal, spongiotic vesicles beneath the normally thickened stratum corneum of acral skin (Fig.

3–11). It is conjectured that microvesicles are well-developed as a result of prolonged retention within the relatively thick epidermal and horny layers that typify palm and sole skin. The inflammatory infiltrate is typically superficial and composed of mononuclear cells, although neutrophils and eosinophils may occasionally be found. Lymphoid exocytosis is generally restricted to spongiotic areas. Even with chronicity, evidence of intraepidermal serum extravasation may be detected in the stratum corneum overlying a nonspongiotic, hyperplastic epidermis.

After a diagnosis of dyshidrotic dermatitis is established, easily identified causes should be excluded. A detailed clinical history should assist in excluding atopic dermatitis. History and patch testing are appropriate screening maneuvers for contact hand and foot allergy. Periodic acid–Schiff (PAS) stain will aid in excluding dermatophytes.

Id Reaction[16]

- MILD, NONSPECIFIC, SPONGIOTIC DERMATITIS
- COEXISTENCE OF FOOT OR LEG DERMATITIS, DERMATOPHYTOSIS, OR STASIS

The id reaction, perhaps better termed *autosensitization spongiotic dermatitis* (ASD), is a peculiar disorder that prin-

Table 3–3. DIFFERENTIAL DIAGNOSIS OF SEBORRHEIC DERMATITIS, ALLERGIC CONTACT DERMATITIS (ACD), AND EARLY PSORIASIS

	SEBORRHEIC DERMATITIS	ACD	PSORIASIS
Spongiosis	Mild	Mild to marked	Absent
Hypogranulosis	Absent	Absent	Present
Eosinophils	Absent	Present	Absent
Lymphoid epidermotropism	Minimal	Mild to marked	Minimal
Capillary alterations*	Absent	Absent	Present

*Defined as dilated and tortuous capillary loops within edematous dermal papillae.

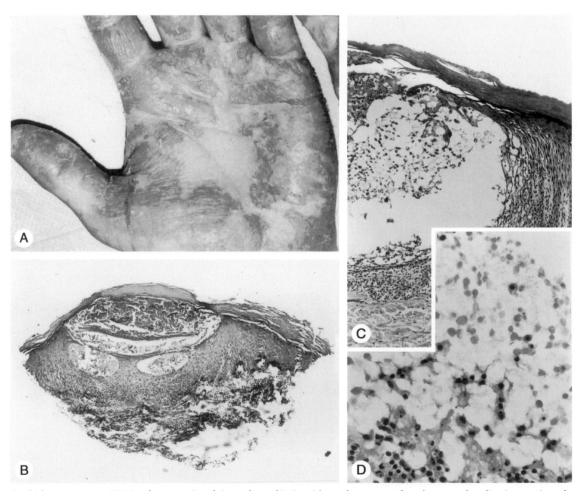

Figure 3–11. Dyshidrotic eczema. **(A)** Hand eczema involving palmar skin is evidenced as zones of erythema and scaling in a setting of superimposed atrophy resulting from chronic steroid use. Small vesicles are present in the erythematous regions. **(B)** A typical biopsy specimen of dyshidrotic eczema demonstrates a well-formed intraepidermal fluid-filled vesicle that is readily appreciated at scanning magnification. The acral origin of the skin sample is indicated by the uniformly thick, compacted stratum corneum that extends to cover adjacent, relatively uninvolved skin. **(C)** The blister roof may be thin or necrotic, and overlying or adjacent scale should be examined to exclude fungi as a cause. The inflammatory infiltrate is predominantly lymphocytes, although occasional neutrophils and eosinophils are detected in some lesions. **(D)** The blister cavity contains proteinaceous fluid that may condense in fixed tissue to form drop-like aggregates. Over time, secondary impetiginization may result in inflammatory cell influx into the cavity, producing confusion with other forms of dermatitis exhibiting primary subcorneal pustules.

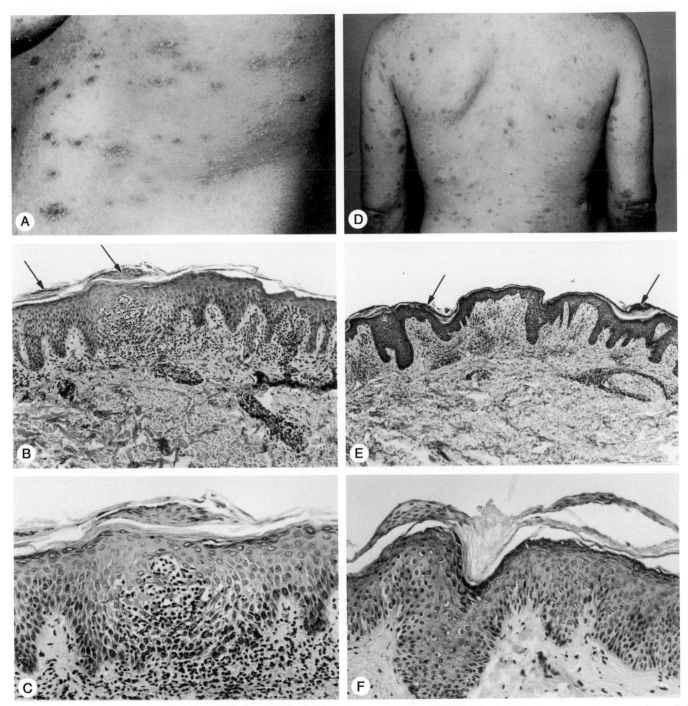

Figure 3–12. Comparison of **(A–C)** pityriasis rosea and **(D–F)** guttate parapsoriasis. **(A)** Oval plaques of pityriasis rosea are in a typical parallel arrangement along long axes of skin folds, as if along the branches of a fir tree when viewed sagitally from the back. Each plaque is pale pink to orange and has delicate, adherent scale, which is often most pronounced at the periphery. **(B)** Scanning magnification of pityriasis rosea demonstrates the characteristic superficial perivascular lymphocytic infiltrate underlying a mildly hyperplastic and spongiotic epidermal layer. Discrete pulses of parakeratotic scale *(arrows)* are evident at this level of magnification. **(C)** Higher magnification of pityriasis rosea. Note the zone of lymphoid epidermotropism associated with overlying, tightly compacted parakeratotic scale. Free erythrocytes within the papillary dermis are frequently associated with such zones of epidermotropism and assist in differentiating pityriasis rosea from its close mimic, guttate parapsoriasis. **(D)** The gross pathology of guttate parapsoriasis closely resembles that of pityriasis rosea, although a tree-like distribution pattern is not characteristic of guttate parapsoriasis. Individual plaques are small and digitate in appearance, and should not be confused with the ambiguously named, yet unrelated large-plaque parapsoriasis, which is a dysplasia of T-cell lineage. **(E)** At low power, guttate parapsoriasis has an appearance that is difficult to distinguish from pityriasis rosea. There is a superficial perivascular lymphocytic infiltrate, irregular epidermal hyperplasia with mild spongiosis, and mounds of parakeratotic scale *(arrows)*. **(F)** Changes within the epidermis and stratum corneum in guttate parapsoriasis are nearly identical to those in pityriasis rosea. Epidermotropism is minimal, however, and primary papillary dermal hemorrhage is not observed. Nonetheless, the two disorders often require persistent clinical observation for differentiation; guttate parapsoriasis is a chronic disorder, whereas pityriasis rosea usually resolves within months after onset.

cipally affects the hands and forearms of patients with a pre-existing primary focus of dermatitis elsewhere on the body surface. This primary focus often takes the form of leg or foot dermatitis complicated by dermatophytosis or stasis. Although the histology of ASD is described only as a nonspecific mild spongiotic dermatitis, the immunopathology of this fascinating phenomenon is bound to yield provocative findings. The practical diagnosis of ASD relies on recognition of mild spongiotic dermatitis in the appropriate clinical setting. Such disorders underscore the importance of the clinicopathologic approach in establishing accurate diagnoses of certain inflammatory skin disorders.

Pityriasis Rosea[17–19]

- SPARSE, SUPERFICIAL, PERIVASCULAR LYMPHOCYTIC INFILTRATE
- MILD, SUBACUTE SPONGIOTIC DERMATITIS
- DISCRETE, MOUND-LIKE FOCI OF PARAKERATOSIS
- FOCAL PAPILLARY DERMAL HEMORRHAGE

Pityriasis rosea (PR) is a relatively common dermatitis of unknown etiology. Lesions may be mimicked clinically by secondary syphilis, guttate parapsoriasis, and nummular eczema, and consequently, biopsies are frequently performed. Multiple lesions may be preceded by a larger, solitary herald patch (see Chap. 4). Individual plaques that ensue are salmon-colored, slightly elevated, and display a fine, adherent, peripheral scale. Typically, patches and plaques are arranged in a fir tree–like pattern on trunk skin (Fig. 3–12A–C), although some individuals present with a more acral distribution (i.e., inverted PR). Whereas PR is self-limiting within months, guttate parapsoriasis is refractory to treatment and may persist for years.

The pattern of PR is that of a mild, subacute, spongiotic dermatitis (Fig. 3–12B, C). In contrast to secondary syphilis, plasma cells are not observed, and endothelial cells, although activated, seldom demonstrate luminal obliteration. A characteristic finding in PR is the presence of small foci of tightly compacted parakeratotic scale forming mound-like configurations (Fig. 3–12C). Frequently, the affected scale will appear to be desquamating from the underlying epidermis. This scale pattern is unusual in nummular dermatitis and seborrheic dermatitis, although it may occur; it is characteristically seen, however, in guttate parapsoriasis. A potentially differential feature is the occasional presence of small foci of papillary dermal hemorrhage in PR. An algorithm for the diagnosis of subacute spongiotic dermatitis, including PR and its mimics, is offered in Figure 3–13.

Guttate Parapsoriasis[20]

- SPARSE, SUPERFICIAL, PERIVASCULAR LYMPHOCYTIC INFILTRATE
- MILD, SUBACUTE SPONGIOTIC DERMATITIS
- DISCRETE, MOUND-LIKE FOCI OF PARAKERATOSIS

Guttate parapsoriasis and PR are differentiated primarily by their clinical features; both are low-grade subacute spongiotic dermatitides that may look virtually identical under the microscope. Guttate parapsoriasis refers to a persistent, nonpruritic, recalcitrant dermatitis that is generally distributed over the trunk and proximal extremities as small, drop-like pink-tan plaques covered by scant adherent scale (Fig. 3–12D). Alternative names include small plaque parapsoriasis and superficial digitate dermatosis. Like psoriasis, guttate parapsoriasis may occur as small plaques, demonstrates a chronic course, and may be recalcitrant to treatment. However, here the similarity ends; guttate parapsoriasis is not a variant of psoriasis, but rather a low-grade spongiotic dermatitis of unknown cause. Moreover, guttate parapsoriasis is entirely distinct from patch- and early plaque-stage cutaneous T-cell lymphoma, which regrettably has been referred to as parapsoriasis of the large plaque type (i.e., parapsoriasis en plaques) (see Chap. 14).

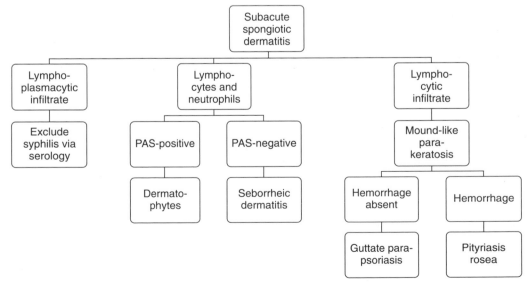

Figure 3–13. Algorithmic approach to subacute spongiotic dermatitis, particularly those cases that may mimic pityriasis rosea and guttate parapsoriasis.

At scanning magnification, guttate parapsoriasis is identical to PR, demonstrating mild epidermal hyperplasia and spongiosis accompanied by a superficial perivascular lymphocytic infiltrate (Fig. 3–12E). Upon closer inspection, foci of mound-like parakeratotic scale, again similar to that of PR and occasionally also encountered in other forms of spongiotic dermatitis, is observed (Fig. 3–12F). In contrast to PR, guttate parapsoriasis seldom demonstrates superficial dermal hemorrhage. However, in examples of PR in which hemorrhage cannot be detected, biopsy specimens may be indistinguishable from those of guttate parapsoriasis, and occurrence or absence of clinical resolution may be the determining factor in designation of lesions as PR or guttate parapsoriasis.

It is important to emphasize that the characteristic scale pattern of guttate parapsoriasis and PR is frequently only focally present, and multiple levels may be required in order to segregate low-grade, spongiotic dermatitis into these categories. Guttate parapsoriasis and PR virtually never demonstrate plasma cells in their infiltrates, and affected vessels show only moderate endothelial prominence. Examples of secondary syphilis without plasma cells that closely mimic guttate parapsoriasis and PR both clinically and histologically have been observed, although such lesions generally demonstrated some degree of basal cell layer vacuolization. Accordingly, serologic exclusion of secondary syphilis should be recommended when this entity is a clinical diagnostic possibility, even when the corresponding histopathology suggests guttate parapsoriasis or PR.

Photoallergic Dermatitis, Spongiotic Type[21, 22]

- SUPERFICIAL AND MID-DERMAL PERIVASCULAR LYMPHOCYTIC INFILTRATE WITH OCCASIONAL EOSINOPHILS
- INFILTRATE DIMINISHES GRADUALLY IN INTENSITY WITH DEPTH
- ENDOTHELIAL PROMINENCE AND VACUOLIZATION
- VARIABLE SPONGIOSIS AND LYMPHOID EPIDERMOTROPISM

Photoallergic dermatitis occurs in a number of clinically distinctive types, including polymorphous light eruption and solar urticaria, phototoxic dermatitis, and photoallergic spongiotic dermatitis. Whereas polymorphous light eruption and solar urticaria result primarily from angiocentric infiltration with variable papillary dermal edema, and phototoxic dermatitis is a form of exaggerated sunburn, photoallergic spon-

giotic dermatitis is akin to a delayed hypersensitivity response with epidermal involvement similar to that seen in ACD (Table 3–4). Photoallergic spongiotic dermatitis may result when topically applied substances (e.g., perfumes) or ingested agents (e.g., certain drugs) are rendered antigenic in exposed skin by ultraviolet light, evoking an initially vesicular and eventually scaling dermatitis. Deposition of plant material (e.g., pollen) carried by wind may also elicit this condition upon exposure to sunlight (i.e., phytophotodermatitis).

Clinically, photoallergic dermatitis is confined to sites of solar irradiation, and the gross pathology is frequently of considerable assistance in making the correct diagnosis (Fig. 3–14A). Biopsy of involved skin (Fig. 3–14B) will demonstrate at scanning magnification a superficial and at least mid-dermal perivascular inflammatory infiltrate composed predominantly of lymphocytes with occasional eosinophils (Fig. 3–14C, D). A helpful diagnostic feature is the finding that the infiltrate gradually diminishes in intensity with depth (i.e., grades off). Another clue to the diagnosis is the presence of prominent endothelial cells with vacuolated cytoplasm lining involved dermal venules (Fig. 3–14E). The overlying epidermal layer shows spongiosis and lymphoid epidermotropism to variable degree. The histologic findings in photoallergic spongiotic dermatitis are not entirely specific, and validation by appropriate clinical history is required in the majority of cases to establish accurate diagnosis. Photo patch testing may be of further diagnostic assistance when gross and microscopic pathology together fail to reveal definitive alterations.

Spongiotic Drug Eruption[23]

- SUPERFICIAL AND DEEP PERIVASCULAR LYMPHOCYTIC INFILTRATE WITH PERIVASCULAR EOSINOPHILS
- PAPILLARY DERMAL AND PERIVASCULAR EDEMA
- VARIABLE, OFTEN MILD SPONGIOSIS AND LYMPHOID EPIDERMOTROPISM
- SCALE ABNORMALITIES WITH CHRONICITY

Literally any ingested agent capable of being perceived as a foreign antigen in the form of a hapten-protein complex may elicit a spongiotic drug eruption. This form of dermatitis often presents as a diffusely erythematous or morbilliform rash several days after administration of the offending agent. In some cases, photoactivation is required to elicit clinical lesions, and this variant could also be appropriately considered under the category of photoallergic dermatitis. Although

Table 3–4. DIFFERENTIAL DIAGNOSTIC FEATURES OF FORMS OF PHOTOALLERGIC DERMATITIS

	CLINICAL	EPIDERMIS	INFILTRATE
Photoallergic, spongiotic type	Vesicular, scaling	Spongiosis	Superficial and mid-dermal; grades off
Phototoxic	Erythema	Dyskeratosis	Minimal
Polymorphous light eruption	Papules, plaques	Minimal change	Superficial and deep; papillary dermal edema
Urticarial	Plaques	Minimal change	Minimal; edema predominates

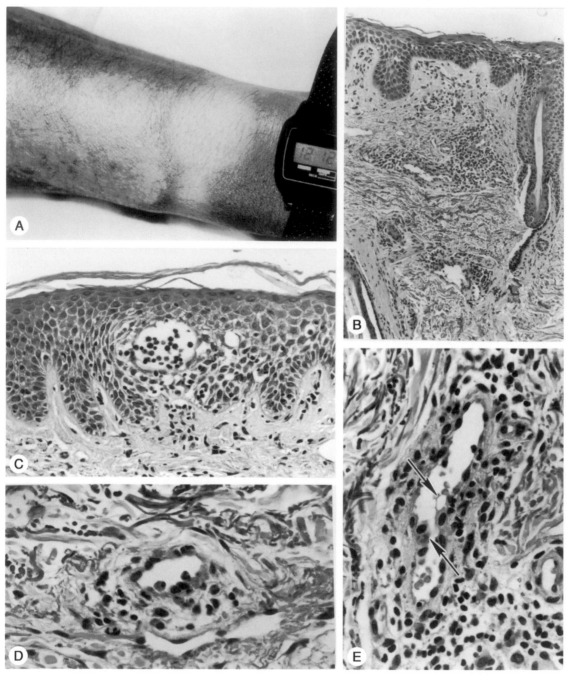

Figure 3–14. Photoallergic dermatitis. **(A)** In this clinical example of photoallergic dermatitis, induration, erythema, pruritus, and early vesiculation occurred 24 hours after modest exposure to sunlight. Skin remains normal only in protected regions such as the zone shielded by the wristwatch. **(B)** The inflammatory infiltrate in photoallergic dermatitis often involves both superficial and mid-dermal vessels, and gradually diminishes (i.e., grades off) with increasing depth. **(C)** Spongiosis and lymphoid epidermotropism are similar to that encountered in allergic contact dermatitis; the former is an important discriminating feature in excluding polymorphous light eruption and photoexacerbated lupus erythematosus, which generally are devoid of spongiosis. **(D)** The early inflammatory infiltrate of photoallergic dermatitis involves postcapillary venules and often consists of an admixture of lymphocytes and eosinophils. Note the eosinophil margination to enlarged endothelial cells and the perivascular elastosis typical of chronically sun-exposed skin. **(E)** A helpful feature in the diagnosis of photoallergic dermatitis is prominent endothelial cells with apparently vacuolated cytoplasm *(arrows)*.

spongiotic dermatitis is caused by certain drugs, it is important to remember that the gross pathology may be highly variable, ranging from predominantly urticarial to frankly vesicular manifestations. It should also be emphasized that drug ingestion is associated with a wide range of dermatitides with highly variable histologic patterns, including cytotoxic dermatitis and panniculitis (see Chaps. 6 and 10).

At scanning magnification, spongiotic drug eruptions appear as superficial and deep perivascular infiltrates associated with variable superficial dermal edema (Fig. 3–15A). Spongiosis may be minimal. In contrast to photoallergic dermatitis, the inflammatory components of drug eruptions that develop independent of irradiation generally do not diminish in intensity with extension into the deep dermis. In fact, vessels of the subcutaneous fat are frequently involved. At higher magnification, eosinophils, in addition to lymphocytes and monocyte-macrophages, are present within the perivascular space (Fig. 3–15B). Unlike insect-bite reactions, however, eosinophils within intervascular collagen are not conspicuous. The epidermis may show only minimal areas of spongiosis and lymphoid epidermotropism (Fig. 3–15C).

The possibility of spongiotic drug eruption should be considered whenever a biopsy specimen shows a superficial and deep angiocentric inflammatory infiltrate with eosinophils, particularly when spongiosis is minimal. Careful history is required to elicit evidence of a potentially offending agent, particularly because routine and over-the-counter preparations may not be considered and reported by affected individuals (e.g., aspirin, oral contraceptives). The timing of clinical rash to drug administration is usually within several days, about the same time as is required for the development of delayed-type hypersensitivity after challenge. Although sensitization is required, reactions may develop in some individuals months or even years after repeated use.

Spongiotic Insect-Bite Reaction[24, 25]

- WEDGE-SHAPED ARCHITECTURE
- ANGIOCENTRIC INFILTRATE AT PERIPHERY, CONFLUENT INFILTRATE AT CENTER
- LYMPHOHISTIOCYTIC INFILTRATE WITH EOSINOPHILS
- EOSINOPHILS WITHIN INTERVENULAR INTERSTITIUM
- PUNCTUM WITH FOCAL EPIDERMAL NECROSIS AND PERIPHERAL SPONGIOSIS
- OCCASIONAL EOSINOPHILIC SPONGIOSIS
- BENIGN LYMPHOID HYPERPLASIA AND FIBROSIS WITH CHRONICITY

Spongiotic insect-bite reactions are common causes of spongiotic dermatitis in routine dermatopathology practice. Often referred to as arthropod-bite reactions, the term insect bite is preferred for spongiotic reactions because bites and stings of many members of the phylum Arthropoda do not produce the histology described (e.g., many spiders and crustaceans). The reaction is the result of the direct injection of foreign protein producing a predominantly dermal delayed hypersensitivity reaction. The spongiotic component of the reaction is often appreciated only histologically, and accordingly, the initial gross impression may range from urticaria

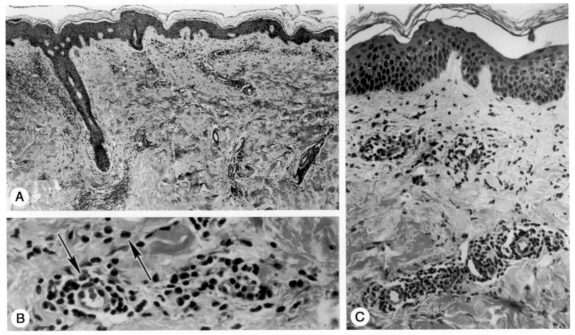

Figure 3–15. Spongiotic drug eruption. **(A)** At scanning magnification, the inflammatory infiltrate in many spongiotic drug eruptions involves both superficial and deep dermal vessels. As opposed to photoallergic dermatitis, the degree of angiocentric infiltration does not diminish with increasing depth. **(B)** Eosinophils *(arrows)* are often numerous within the mononuclear cell infiltrates of spongiotic drug eruptions. **(C)** The epidermis is minimally spongiotic in this early lesion; in time, focal microvesiculation indistinguishable from that seen in allergic contact dermatitis may develop in some lesions, although many lesions show only slight spongiotic change during the entirety of their evolution. Note that the cuff of inflammatory cells about the lowermost vessel in the reticular dermis is actually more pronounced than that surrounding the more superficial vessel within the pale, edematous papillary dermis.

to pityriasis lichenoides to erythema nodosum and nodose forms of vasculitis.

A characteristic feature of spongiotic insect-bite reactions at low-power magnification is the tendency to form a wedge-shaped infiltrate within the superficial and deep dermis (Fig. 3–16A). This infiltrate is angiocentric at the periphery and tends toward coalescence at the center. The overlying epidermis may demonstrate a small, centrally located, indented zone lined by necrotic cells and inflammatory debris (Fig. 3–16B). This represents the punctum through which the proboscis or stinger injected the offending protein. The adjacent epidermis may show variable hyperplasia and spongiosis, with occasional frank microvesiculation and eosinophilic spongiosis (such as that seen in allergic contact dermatitis) (see Fig. 3–3).

At medium-to-high magnification, the inflammatory infiltrate is noted to be composed of activated lymphocytes, histiocytes, and frequently, large numbers of eosinophils

(Fig. 3–16C, D). A helpful diagnostic feature is the tendency for these inflammatory cells to diffusely infiltrate collagen bundles of the intervenular interstitium, often in a fashion similar to the early histiocytic response in granuloma annulare. When degranulating eosinophils are numerous at these sites, they may surround zones of hypereosinophilic, degenerating collagen (i.e., flame figures), similar to that seen in eosinophilic cellulitis (i.e., Well syndrome). In occasional cases of exuberant inflammatory responses to insect bites, focal vasculitis with fibrin thrombus formation, or striking dermal mucinosis may be detected. Rarely, small granulomatous foci responding to birefringent particles of chitinous insect mouth parts may be observed. With chronic immunologic stimulation by foreign proteins refractory to proteolytic degradation (i.e., persistent insect-bite reaction), benign lymphoid hyperplasia and fibrosis supervene. Such lesions may clinically and histologically mimic lymphoma (see Chap. 14).

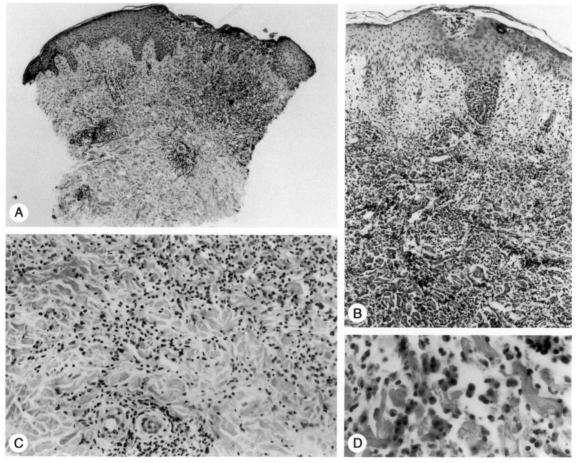

Figure 3–16. Spongiotic insect-bite reaction. **(A)** The architecture of this spongiotic insect-bite reaction is angiocentric at the edge *(left)* and confluent in the center *(right)*. This, combined with the depth of infiltration (frequently into the subcutis), imparts a wedge-like shape that is helpful in making this diagnosis at scanning magnification. **(B)** The central portion of an insect bite may contain a dell lined by necrotic and inflammatory cells and representing a residual punctum through which foreign protein was injected. Note the spongiosis, papillary dermal edema, and almost tumoral (i.e., lymphocytoma-like) confluent inflammatory infiltrate composed of activated mononuclear cells, eosinophils, and occasionally granulomas reacting to retained birefringent chitinous fragments. **(C)** At the edge of the infiltrate depicted in **B,** inflammatory cells infiltrate the dermal matrix as streams of cells, a pattern reminiscent of granuloma annulare and focally observed in many insect-bite reactions. **(D)** Numerous eosinophils are present among the inflammatory cells that infiltrate the intervenular connective tissue. This loss of angiocentric distribution by eosinophils is a helpful feature in the diagnosis of insect-bite responses.

Dermatophytosis[26]

- MILD, NONSPECIFIC, SUPERFICIAL PERIVASCULAR LYMPHOID INFILTRATE WITH OCCASIONAL EOSINOPHILS
- MILD SPONGIOSIS
- "SANDWICHED" PARAKERATOSIS AND HYPERKERATOSIS
- PAS-POSITIVE HYPHAE IN STRATUM CORNEUM

Dermatophytosis may mimic both the gross and histologic pathology of noninfectious spongiotic dermatitis. It should be suspected whenever a biopsy specimen of a low-grade, subacute dermatitis shows mild, nonspecific spongiotic changes in the absence of obvious clinical cause. Tinea probably elicits a mild, indolent contact hypersensitivity response as a result of incorporation of protein excretory and possibly secretory products into the stratum corneum. Hydration of scale may facilitate detection of these potential antigens by immune skin cells that incite delayed hypersensitivity. Hence, frequently hydrated intertriginous regions may be particularly prone to the inflammatory sequelae of dermatophytosis. Lesions typically present as pink erythematous plaques with central clearing and peripheral scale (Fig. 3–17A).

Aside from the findings of mild contact dermatitis with minimal spongiosis, histologic changes in dermatophytosis may be extremely protean. An important clue is the finding of focal parakeratotic scale alternating with compacted hyperkeratotic scale (Fig. 3–17B). This abnormality may produce a sandwich-like effect within the scale and be associated with the accumulation of occasional neutrophils. Although fungi may be visible in routine preparations, variability in staining among laboratories frequently necessitates the use of the PAS stain for confirmation. In such preparations, hyphal forms are present within the affected scale (Fig. 3–17C). Proteinaceous material and inflammatory debris may also stain positively with PAS; therefore, definitive criteria for hyphal morphology must be met, including branching and septation. Lesions partially treated prior to biopsy may harbor ballooned and distorted hyphal forms or too few organisms to permit diagnosis. Therapy should be discontinued, and lesions resampled at least 2 to 3 weeks after cessation in such instances. Biopsies should only be encouraged and performed if simpler and more economical approaches (e.g., KOH preparations) fail to yield definitive diagnostic information.

Rare Disorders

- INCONTINENTIA PIGMENTI, VESICULAR STAGE[27]
- FAMILIAL LEINER DISEASE[28]
- HYPERIMMUNOGLOBULIN E SYNDROME[29]
- WISKOTT-ALDRICH SYNDROME[30]
- PAPULAR ACRODERMATITIS OF CHILDHOOD[31]
- TOXIC SHOCK SYNDROME[32]

The literature is replete with less common conditions associated with or characterized by spongiotic dermatitis in varying stages of lesional evolution, and the list provided previously is undoubtedly incomplete. This section in this chapter and in subsequent chapters is provided to re-emphasize that the stated approach and objectives of this text are not comprehensive. References for further reading regarding these specific rare disorders are provided.

Incontinentia pigmenti is an X-linked, dominantly inherited condition to which homozygous male patients tend to succumb in utero. Lesser-affected female patients show clinical evolution through three stages: a vesicular stage occurring shortly after birth; a period when lesions exhibit verrucous epidermal hyperplasia; and a time when hyperpigmentation predominates. Biopsy during the vesicular stage discloses spongiotic dermatitis characterized by a superficial perivascular lymphocytic infiltrate, with eosinophils that often infiltrate the overlying epidermal layer. Overt intraepidermal microvesicles may contain eosinophils and are often associated with small zones of dyskeratosis, an important clue to this diagnosis (Fig. 3–18).

Spongiotic dermatitis associated with immunodeficiency may be encountered in the settings of familial Leiner disease, hyperimmunoglobulin E syndrome, Wiscott-Aldrich syndrome, and the seborrheic dermatitis of AIDS discussed previously. *Familial Leiner disease* is characterized by usually fatal immunodeficiency in infants with spongiotic dermatitis and features of seborrheic dermatitis, diarrhea, wasting, and infections. In *hyperimmunoglobulin E syndrome*, defective neutrophil chemotaxis and high serum elevations of IgE are associated with an atopic dermatitis–like skin rash. *Wiskott-Aldrich syndrome* is an X-linked, recessive disorder affecting male children, with deficits in cellular and humoral immunity and spongiotic lesions with atopic features.

Papular acrodermatitis of childhood (i.e., Gianotti-Crosti syndrome) is a viral exanthem usually resulting from transcutaneous or transmucosal passage of hepatitis B virus. In addition to hepatitis and lymphadenopathy, affected individuals have an acute-to-subacute spongiotic dermatitis that is histologically similar to mild allergic contact or atopic dermatitis.

Toxic shock syndrome is produced by *Staphylococcus aureus* toxins often elaborated after prolonged use of superabsorbent vaginal tampons by menstruating women. The disorder is initially identified by fever, hypotension, and diffuse, sunburn-like erythema characterized by a superficial mixed inflammatory infiltrate containing both neutrophils and eosinophils in addition to mononuclear cells. Spongiosis with associated neutrophil infiltration and necrotic keratinocytes and occasional subepidermal blisters may be observed.

PATHOGENESIS[33–35]

The prototype of spongiotic dermatitis is ACD in its various stages of clinical evolution. ACD may be experimentally reproduced and studied as the sequential evolution of delayed hypersensitivity reactions induced by topical application of potent sensitizers like dinitrochlorobenzene. It is known that initial application of intact antigen or hapten that combines with endogenous protein to form antigen is mediated by epidermal Langerhans cells. These cells take up antigen by endocytosis and migrate through lymphatics from skin to draining lymph nodes. There, they present processed antigenic signals to helper T cells, which then become sensitized to proliferate and become immunologically activated

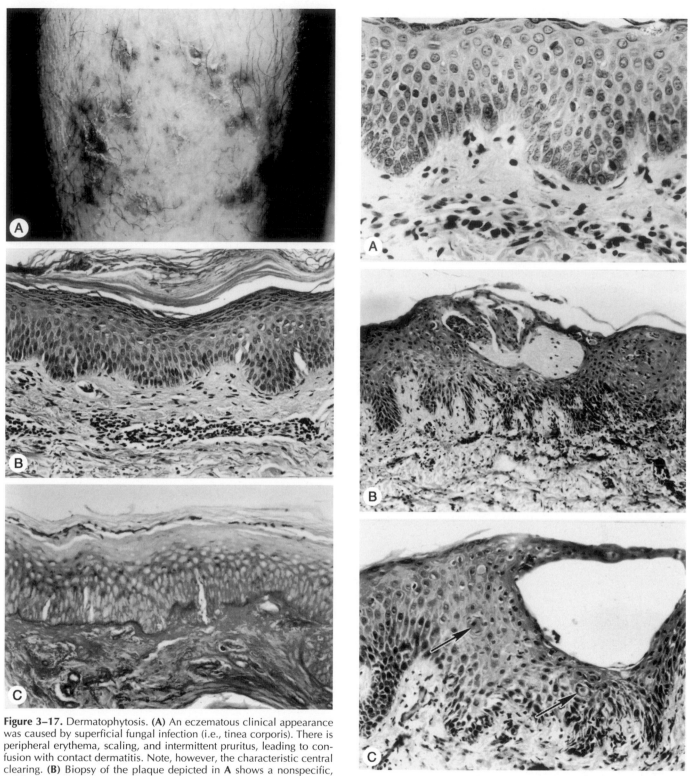

Figure 3–17. Dermatophytosis. **(A)** An eczematous clinical appearance was caused by superficial fungal infection (i.e., tinea corporis). There is peripheral erythema, scaling, and intermittent pruritus, leading to confusion with contact dermatitis. Note, however, the characteristic central clearing. **(B)** Biopsy of the plaque depicted in **A** shows a nonspecific, mild spongiotic dermatitis. The zones of vertically alternating parakeratosis and compacted orthokeratosis, giving a laminated "sandwich-like" appearance to the stratum corneum, provide a clue regarding the underlying cause of these apparently nondiagnostic changes. **(C)** Periodic acid–Schiff stain reveals numerous hyphal forms within the stratum corneum, confirming the diagnosis of a low-grade spongiotic response evoked by dermatophytosis.

Figure 3–18. Incontinentia pigmenti, spongiotic-vesicular stage. **(A)** An early lesion shows only mild spongiosis and a nonspecific superficial lymphocytic infiltrate. **(B)** An advanced lesion has a typical, well-formed intraepidermal vesicle overlying a superficial infiltrate composed of mononuclear cells, eosinophils, and rare basophils. **(C)** A clue to the diagnosis is the finding of early zones of dyskeratosis *(arrows)* within the vesiculated epidermal layer.

(e.g., capable of lymphokine production) on re-exposure to the specific antigen. It may take many repeated exposures to some antigens before sensitization occurs. About 2 weeks after successful sensitization, the primed T cells are ready to respond when challenged.

Topical challenge by antigen in a previously sensitized individual may initiate a complex cascade of events. Within several hours and possibly within minutes after challenge, dermal mast cells about superficial blood vessels are induced to degranulate, resulting in discharge of their preformed mediators in the vicinity of postcapillary venules. Endothelial cells contract as a result of mast cell histamine release, and mast cell cytokines aid in the induction of endothelial glycoproteins that promote adhesive interactions between circulating sensitized T cells and the vessel surface. Mast cell proteases potentially play a role in facilitating subsequent T-cell diapedesis across the vessel wall, and it is even possible that heparin impedes formation of microthrombi during this process. Once liberated into the skin, the primed antigen-specific T cells may respond to the antigen by release of cytokines, which amplify the inflammatory infiltrate by recruiting even more mononuclear cells.

By 24 hours after challenge, significant numbers of T cells may be observed about superficial dermal venules. Until this point, the ongoing tissue changes may be relatively unapparent clinically. During the subsequent 2 to 3 days, progressive movement of T cells into the epidermis, facilitated by lymphokine-mediated induction of adhesive glycoproteins such as intercellular adhesion molecule-1 on keratinocytes, is associated with progressive erythema, spongiosis, and vesiculation clinically. The association of T-cell epidermotropism with spongiosis raises the possibility that factors associated with the induction phases of inflammation (e.g., protease release) and passage of inflammatory cells across the normally intact dermal-epidermal junction may, in concert, be responsible for the accumulation of intercellular edema within the epidermal layer. The epidermotropism of early cutaneous T-cell lymphoma may actually represent intraepidermal T-cell proliferation rather than dermal-epidermal trafficking, hence the relative absence of spongiosis (see Chap. 14).

Responses to injected antigens are probably similar to those of topical antigens, but it is likely that most of the antigenic signals are communicated to T cells by native populations of dermal dendritic immune cells rather than epidermal Langerhans cells. This may be why contact allergy evokes prominent epidermal changes as opposed to the preponderantly dermal alterations that typify delayed hypersensitivity to circulating or injected proteins (e.g., drug eruptions, insect-bite reactions). For most disorders of the spongiotic dermatitis group, the exogenous or endogenous antigens that stimulate their respective immune reaction patterns are yet to be discovered. It is also important to remember that this discussion has centered on *normal* immune responses to proteins perceived as antigenic. In immunocompromised patients, provocative stimuli may differ from those

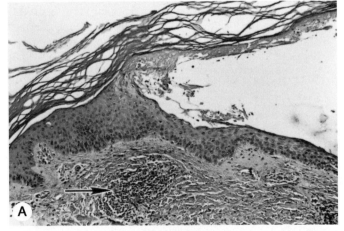

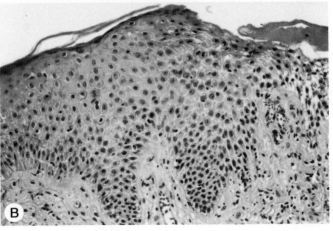

Figure 3–19. Resolving spongiotic dermatitis. **(A)** Although acute spongiotic dermatitis may progress to subacute and chronic stages, an alternative pathway is spontaneous or iatrogenic resolution. Lesions biopsied during resolution stages may not be recognized as representing a spongiotic process. This large intraepidermal vesicle has a necrotic roof; the base is formed by a regenerating epidermal layer devoid of spongiosis. The only clue to the inciting cause is the persistent angiocentric infiltrate of lymphocytes and eosinophils *(arrow)* within the superficial dermis. **(B)** A lesion similar to that in **A** in which the necrotic roof has been sloughed. At the edge of the previous blister *(right side of field)*, a small area of residual spongiosis is retained.

that are antigenic to normal skin. Moreover, the patterns, cytologic composition, and time course of hypersensitivity reactions may vary from the aforementioned responses.

DIFFERENTIAL DIAGNOSIS

Recognition of spongiotic dermatitis depends on documentation of inflammation associated with spongiosis. False-negative diagnoses for this entity arise when either or both are not fully appreciated. A common cause of this is the lesion that has been treated with topical corticosteroids, partially abrogating the inflammatory response and rendering spongiotic change subtle. Such lesions should be left untreated for several weeks before biopsy, and a full history of how lesions have been therapeutically manipulated should always be obtained. Occasionally, acute spongiotic dermatitis will spontaneously involute without progression to subacute and chronic stages. When such inactive lesions are sampled, the only evidence of vesicular dermatitis may be the necrotic residua of a blister roof above a fully re-epithelialized, relatively nonspongiotic base (Fig. 3–19). Close inspection at high magnification of regions of the base still associated with inflammation generally will reveal foci of spongiosis, confirming the nature of the antecedent inflammatory insult. Another common cause of false-negative diagnoses is the biopsy of lesions that have evolved into chronic phases predominated by hyperplasia. Evidence of preceding spongiosis may be detected in many such cases by documentation of pulses of loculated serum within the stratum corneum (Fig. 3–20A). This finding indicates the former presence of intercellular fluid that has been transmitted into the superficial epidermal layers as the spongiotic component subsided.

False-positive diagnoses must be differentiated from *epithelial mucinosis, reticular degeneration,* and *acantholysis* (Fig. 3–20B). Epithelial mucinosis is a phenomenon that may primarily affect hair follicles in the relative absence of inflammation (i.e., alopecia mucinosa) or that may be secondary to intraepidermal or intrafollicular accumulation of malignant cells in T-cell lymphoma. Epithelial mucinosis results from enhanced synthesis of hyaluronic acid which is deposited between keratinocytes, imparting widened intercellular spaces similar to that seen in spongiosis. Whereas the fluid of spongiosis appears as empty or clear spaces in routine tissue preparations, mucin is detectable as pale blue-grey particles that stain more prominently with alcian blue.

Reticular degeneration is caused by collapse of keratinocyte membranes in the absence of intercellular fluid. Although this may produce widened intercellular spaces and prominent intercellular bridges, the size of individual keratinocytes is reduced. This is in contrast to spongiosis, in which keratinocytes are either normal in diameter or even expanded as a result of concomitant intracellular fluid. Reticular degeneration is most commonly the result of the cytopathic effect of certain viruses, such as those of the herpesvirus group.

Acantholysis is characterized by primary instability or lysis of intercellular cement at the level of desmosomal attachment sites. Acantholytic cells become rounded, and intercellular bridges become *less* conspicuous than normal. Acantholytic cells also tend to exhibit hypereosinophilic cytoplasms, the result of faulty or premature keratinization or premature cell death. Acantholysis is most commonly seen as nonspecific, as a genetically inherited tendency for aberrant epidermal maturation, or as the result of immunologically mediated lysis of intercellular attachment sites.

After a diagnosis of spongiotic dermatitis has been established, it may be difficult to classify lesions further based on histology alone. Correlative clinical information and gross pathology are therefore of paramount importance in the accurate diagnosis of spongiotic dermatitis. Often, subtle histologic alterations provide important clues that assist in cor-

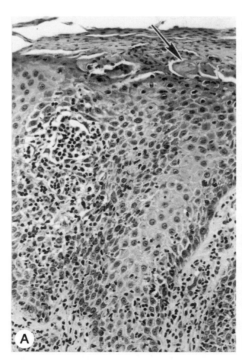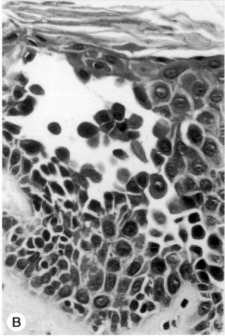

Figure 3–20. False-negative and false-positive diagnosis of spongiotic dermatitis. **(A)** False-negative. In this chronic dermatitis, only acanthosis and inflammation persists. An important clue that this lesion had been preceded by a spongiotic process is the presence of loculated serum *(arrow)* that has not yet been shed within the stratum corneum. **(B)** False-positive. Acantholysis must be differentiated from spongiosis and microvesicle formation. The former is characterized by rounded cells with hypereosinophilic (i.e., dyskeratotic) cytoplasm. Prominent (i.e., stretched) intercellular bridges, the hallmark of spongiosis, are not observed in acantholysis, even in the earliest stages, which here are appreciated as widened intercellular spaces.

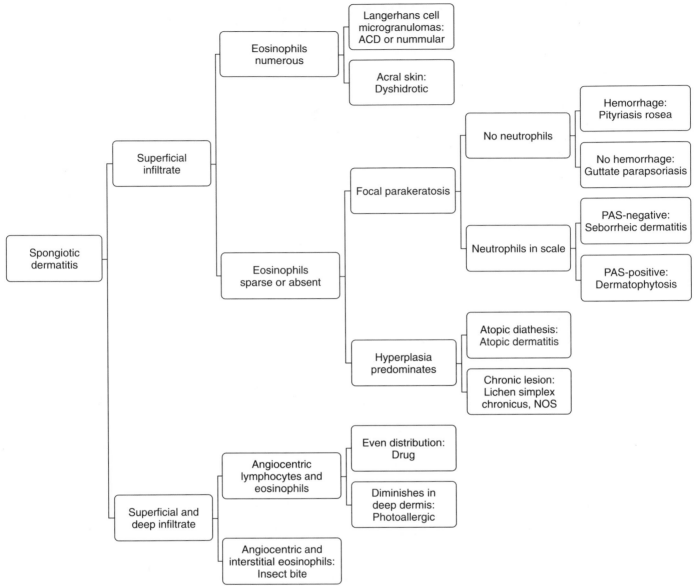

Figure 3–21. An algorithmic approach to the differential diagnosis of spongiotic dermatitis. (ACD, allergic contact dermatitis; NOS, not otherwise specified; PAS, periodic acid–Schiff stain).

roborating clinical and gross impressions. Figure 3–21 provides one of many possible approaches to assessing the histopathology of the more commonly encountered members of the spongiotic dermatitides. This simplified approach has obvious limitations, but it presents a point of departure on which diagnostic refinements may be superimposed, and lesions may be initially screened and subsequently correlated with critically important clinical information.

SELECTED REFERENCES

1. Leider M, Rosenblum M. A Dictionary of Dermatologic Words, Terms, and Phrases. West Haven, CT: Dome Laboratories/Miles Laboratories, 1976:140.
2. Cronin E. Contact Dermatitis. Edinburgh, Scotland: Churchill Livingstone, 1980.
3. Fisher AA. Contact Dermatitis, 3rd ed. Philadelphia: Lea & Febiger, 1986.
4. Fitzpatrick TB, Eisen AZ, Wolff K, et al. Dermatology in General Medicine. New York: McGraw-Hill, 1987.
5. Dvorak HF, Mihm MC, Dvorak AM. Morphology of delayed type hypersensitivity in man. J Invest Dermatol 1976;67:391.
6. Ackerman AB, Breza TS, Capland L. Spongiotic simulants of mycosis fungoides. Arch Dermatol 1974;109:218.
7. Mihm MC, Soter NA, Dvorak HF, et al. The structure of normal skin and the morphology of atopic eczema. J Invest Dermatol 1976;67:305.
8. Lever WF, Schaumburg-Lever G. Histopathology of the Skin. Philadelphia: JB Lippincott, 1990:105.
9. Ackerman AB. Histologic Diagnosis of Inflammatory Skin Disease. Philadelphia: Lea & Febiger, 1978.
10. Kouskoukis CE, Scher RK, Ackerman AB. The problem of features of lichen simplex chronicus complicating the histology of diseases of the nail. Am J Dermatopathol 1984;6:45.
11. Braun-Falco O, Petry G. Feinstruktur der Epidermis bei chronischem nummularem Ekzem. Arch Klin Exp Dermatol 1966;222:219.
12. Pinkus H, Mehregan AH. The primary histologic lesion of seborrheic dermatitis and psoriasis. J Invest Dermatol 1966;46:109.
13. Metz J, Metz G. Zur Ultrastruktur der Spongiose beim allergischen Kontaktekzem. Dermatologica 1970;141:315.

14. Mathes BM, Douglas MC. Seborrheic dermatitis in patients with acquired immunodeficiency syndrome. J Am Acad Dermatol 1985;13:947.

15. Kutzner H, Wurzel RM, Wolff HH. Are acrosyringia involved in the pathogenesis of "dyshidrosis"? Am J Dermatopathol 1986;8:109.

16. Abell E. Spongiotic dermatitis. In: Farmer ER, Hood AF, eds. Pathology of the Skin. Norwalk, CT: Appleton & Lange, 1990:74.

17. Panizzon R, Bloch PH. Histopathology of pityriasis rosea Gilbert: Qualitative and quantitative light-microscopic study of 62 biopsies of 40 patients. Dermatologica 1985;165:551.

18. Bunch LW, Tilley JC. Pityriasis rosea: A histologic and serologic study. Arch Dermatol 1961;84:79.

19. Verbov J. Purpuric pityriasis rosea. Dermatologica 1980;160:141.

20. Hu CH, Winkelmann RK. Digitate dermatosis: A new look at symmetrical small plaque parapsoriasis. Arch Dermatol 1973;107:65.

21. Willis I, Kligman AM. The mechanism of photoallergic contact dermatitis. J Invest Dermatol 1968;51:378.

22. Harber LC, Baer RL. Pathogenic mechanisms of drug-induced photosensitivity. J Invest Dermatol 1972;58:327.

23. Fellner MJ, Prutkin L. Morbilliform eruptions caused by penicillin: A study of electron microscopy and immunologic tests. J Invest Dermatol 1970;55:390.

24. Shaffer B, Jacobson C, Beerman H. Histopathologic correlation of lesions of papular urticaria and positive skin test reactions to insect antigens. Arch Dermatol 1954;70:437.

25. McNutt NS. Cutaneous lymphohistiocytic infiltrates simulating malignant lymphoma. In: Murphy GF, Mihm MC Jr, eds. Lymphoproliferative Disorders of the Skin. Boston: Butterworths, 1986:257.

26. Gottlieb GJ, Ackerman AB. The "sandwich sign" of dermatophytosis. Am J Dermatopathol 1986;8:347.

27. Epstein S, Vedder JS, Pinkus H. Bullous variety of incontinentia pigmenti (Bloch-Sulzberger). Arch Dermatol Syph 1951;65:557.

28. Jacobs JC, Miller ME. Fatal familial Leiner's disease. Pediatrics 1975;49:225.

29. Stanley J, Perez D, Gigli I, et al. Hyperimmunoglobulin E syndrome. Arch Dermatol 1973;108:806.

30. Rosen FS. The primary immunodeficiencies: Dermatologic manifestations. J Invest Dermatol 1976;67:402.

31. Gianotti F. Papular acrodermatitis of childhood and other papulovesicular syndromes (review). Br J Dermatol 1979;100:49.

32. Hurwitz RM, Ackerman AB. Cutaneous pathology of the toxic shock syndrome. Am J Dermatopathol 1987;7:563.

33. Streilein JW, Bergstresser PR. Two antigen presentation pathways, only one of which requires Langerhans cells, lead to the induction of contact hypersensitivity. J Invest Dermatol 1983;80:302.

34. Lewis RE, Buchsbaum M, Whitaker D, Murphy GF. Intercellular adhesion molecule expression in the evolving human cutaneous delayed hypersensitivity response. J Invest Dermatol 1989;93:672.

35. Klein LM, Lavker RM, Matis WL, Murphy GF. Degranulation of human mast cells induces an endothelial antigen central to leukocyte adhesion. Proc Natl Acad Sci USA 1989;86:8972.

4
Psoriasiform Dermatitis

DEFINITIONS AND GENERAL CONSIDERATIONS

Psoriasiform dermatitis is adapted from the word psoriasis which derives from the Greek words for a condition (-iasis) of itching (psor-). Although the pathogenesis of pruritus is not as yet understood, the term is an appropriate one. This is because disorders that eventuate in psoriasiform dermatitis may itch at some stages of their clinical evolution, and because chronic scratching of pruritic skin invariably results in psoriasiform changes. True psoriasis is a disorder that may be clinically and histologically confused with other forms of psoriasiform dermatitis. Although psoriasis is the prototype for this family of epidermal reaction patterns, significant differences in gross appearance, clinical behavior, and histologic evolution exist among members of the entire family of psoriasiform dermatitides.

As discussed in Chapter 1, epidermal thickening generally correlates with an increased number of keratinocytes as a result of heightened proliferative rate, alterations in cell cycle, or decreased surface shedding. Preferential, although generally not exclusive, involvement of various epidermal layers has given rise to the terms basaloid hyperplasia, acanthosis (hyperplasia of the stratum spinosum), hypergranulosis (hyperplasia of the stratum granulosum), hyperkeratosis, and parakeratosis. In psoriasiform disorders, one or more epidermal layers may become diminished in prominence or entirely absent whereas adjacent layers become markedly thickened. The prototype for disorders characterized by epidermal hyperplasia is psoriasis, and considerable attention is devoted in daily practice to differentiation of true psoriasis from other disorders that may recapitulate some, but not all, of its clinical and histologic features.

Accurate diagnostic recognition of psoriasiform dermatitis is important, because differentiation among psoriasis, chronic irritant dermatitis, and psoriasiform changes associated with underlying tumors or infection depends on histologic recognition of salient and reproducible features. The treatments for disorders that produce psoriasiform changes clinically and histologically may be quite different, and when specifically and appropriately targeted at accurately diagnosed diseases, such therapies are often quite effective.

Although the cellular and molecular biology of psoriasiform dermatitis is beyond the scope of this chapter, it deserves brief mention. The inciting events that precipitate psoriasiform changes frequently involve inflammation and dysregulation of cytokines and growth factors instrumental to the maintenance of normal epidermal proliferation. Aberrant molecular signals may be influenced by genetic factors, particularly in situations such as true psoriasis and its variants, and in the setting of chronic lesions of atopic dermatitis. Growing appreciation of the proinflammatory pathways and associated epidermal cytokine dysregulation that accompany various forms of psoriasiform dermatitis should foster more complete understanding of the endogenous and environmental factors that govern keratinocyte proliferation.

GROSS PATHOLOGY

Psoriasiform dermatitis is predominated clinically by excessive scale. As such, it often appears as a plaque with a rough, irregular, scaling, tan- to skin-colored surface. Hyperkeratotic scale (i.e., thickened scale without retained nuclei) often is tan-yellow to light brown, as seen in a callus. Parakeratotic scale (i.e., scale with retained nuclei) is frequently silver-white, as in psoriasis. Because inflammation is frequently the underlying cause of psoriasiform dermatitis, erythema and induration often precede and accompany the zone of excessive scale formation. In acute lesions of psoriasis, pustules may be present within these erythematous plaques. Early lesions of psoriasiform dermatitis may be predominated by inflammatory changes of erythema and edema, and scale abnormalities may be inconspicuous.

Table 4–1. COMMON CLINICAL DISORDERS WITH PSORIASIFORM GROSS PATHOLOGY

Chronic seborrheic dermatitis	Superficial fungal infection
Chronic eczema	Patch or plaque cutaneous T-cell
Psoriasis	lymphoma
Confluent lichen planus	Localized stasis dermatitis
Squamous cell carcinoma in situ	Certain epidermal nevi

Because a number of common cutaneous diseases may mimic the gross features of psoriasiform dermatitis, the history provided with a biopsy specimen may contain a number of seemingly misleading suggestions based on clinical differential diagnosis alone. Table 4–1 summarizes some of the more frequently encountered disorders that appear in such clinical differentials.

GENERAL HISTOLOGY AND TEMPORAL EVOLUTION

A histologic feature common to all forms of psoriasiform dermatitis is epidermal hyperplasia, with or without a characteristic inflammatory component. This hyperplasia is so characteristic that many diagnoses may be made based on the nature of the proliferative response within the four epidermal strata (i.e., basalis, spinosum, granulosum, and corneum). Table 4–2 emphasizes some of these simple differential features.

There are many diagnostic nuances that confound differentiation of the diseases that produce psoriasiform dermatitis; these will be addressed in detail in the sections dealing with specific disorders. Some complicating factors are the temporal evolution of lesions and the corresponding stages at which tissue sampling is performed. As was demonstrated in Chapter 3, the evolutionary stage of spongiotic dermatitis greatly influences its generic histologic appearance. This is also the case with psoriasiform dermatitis. Figure 4–1 demonstrates the evolutionary phases of a psoriatic plaque. Sampling at any of these stages would greatly influence diagnostic interpretation. Superimposed treatment at any juncture can produce a confusing mix of normal and abnormal findings that may prevent definitive diagnosis unless precise information concerning the gross pathology, clinical behavior, and details of treatment regimen accompanies the biopsy specimen.

HISTOLOGY OF SPECIFIC DISORDERS

Psoriasis[1-7]

- FOCAL TO DIFFUSE PARAKERATOTIC SCALE
- FOCAL TO DIFFUSE HYPOGRANULOSIS
- ACANTHOSIS WITHOUT SPONGIOSIS
- REGULAR (EVEN) DOWNWARD ELONGATION OF RETE RIDGES
- SUPRABASAL MITOSES
- THINNING OF SUPRAPAPILLARY EPIDERMAL PLATE

- EDEMA AND UPWARD ENLARGEMENT OF DERMAL PAPILLAE
- DILATATION AND TORTUOSITY OF DERMAL CAPILLARIES
- NEUTROPHILS IN UPPER EPIDERMAL LAYERS

As mentioned previously, the term psoriasis derives from Latin and Greek word elements meaning a condition of itching. Although some psoriatic lesions are indeed pruritic, many are not. The derivation of the term psoriasis perhaps underscores the confusion that sometimes exists between this disorder and chronic eczematous processes in which repeated excoriation aids in the induction of epidermal hyperplasia.

Most commonly, psoriasis manifests as solitary or multiple erythematous plaques with characteristic adherent, silvery white scale. Lesions preferentially occur on distal extremities and sites of trauma. Traumatic removal of scale may result in minute bleeding points (i.e., Auspitz sign), which are a result of the pathologic proximity of capillary loops in dermal papillae to overlying stratum corneum. The predilection for occurrence of psoriatic plaques on the extensor surfaces, particularly the elbows, knees, and knuckles, and other sites of frequent trauma has been attributed to the Koebner phenomenon, in which new lesions may be mechanically induced. Mucosal involvement is rare, although paramucosal lesions (e.g., preputial, perianal) are occasionally encountered. Nail involvement characterized by thickening, separation, and discoloration and pitting of the plate is noted in certain patients (see Chap. 21). Nail changes may occur with or without the associated deformity of underlying bones that may mimic rheumatoid joint disease. Extensive psoriasis may involve the entire body surface and represents one of many causes of erythroderma. Acute, eruptive lesions may have a pustular component (i.e., pustular psoriasis), which frequently predominates over scale formation and produces somewhat arcuate configurations (Fig. 4–2A). Oral mucosal involvement (see Chap. 23) has been rarely reported. Geographic tongue is thought to be a localized manifestation of psoriasis. Because of the plethora of gross pathologic manifestations of psoriasis, clinical differentials accompanying submitted biopsy specimens may be diverse. Some of the

Table 4–2. PATTERNS OF EPIDERMAL HYPERPLASIA IN COMMON FORMS OF PSORIASIFORM DERMATITIS

STRATUM	ABNORMALITY	EXAMPLE
Corneum	Parakeratosis	Psoriasis
	Hyperkeratosis	Lichen simplex chronicus
Granulosum	Decreased	Psoriasis
	Increased	Lichen simplex chronicus
Spinosum	Increased; many mitoses	Psoriasis
	Increased; few mitoses	Lichen simplex chronicus
Basalis	Rete regular	Psoriasis
	Rete irregular	Lichen simplex chronicus
	Basaloid or squamoid hyperplasia	Inductive (DF)*
	Squamoid hyperplasia	Inductive (GCT)†

*DF, dermatofibroma with overlying psoriasiform changes.
†GCT, granular cell tumor with overlying psoriasiform changes.

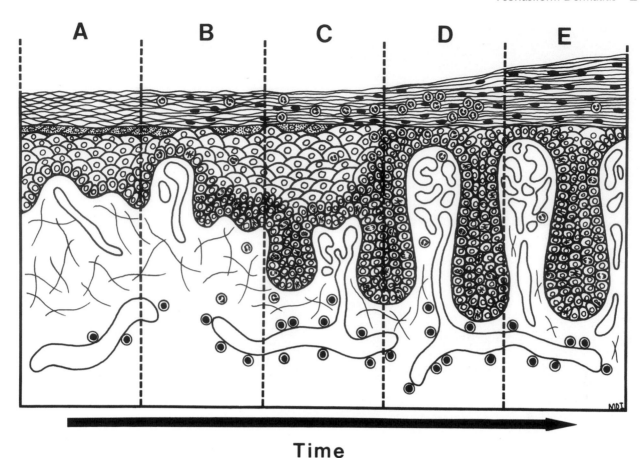

Time

Figure 4–1. Temporal evolution of psoriasiform dermatitis: Psoriasis. **(A, B)** The earliest manifestations of psoriasis involve subtle basal cell hyperplasia and focal parakeratosis, which evolve into **(C)** an initially irregular epidermal hyperplasia (i.e., rete ridges extending unevenly into the underlying dermis) with parakeratosis containing occasional neutrophils and associated hypogranulosis. **(B)** Even in early stages, capillary loops within dermal papillae may be ectatic and slightly tortuous, and there is a sparse-to-moderate mononuclear cell infiltrate about superficial venules. **(D, E)** In established lesions, basaloid hyperplasia becomes regular (i.e., even, downward extension of hyperplastic rete), and dermal papillae are edematous and extend upward to lie in close proximity to diffusely parakeratotic scale, often containing clustered neutrophils. Capillary loops within these hyperplastic papillae are markedly tortuous and ectatic at this juncture, and the stratum granulosum is generally absent.

more commonly encountered differential diagnostic considerations to rule out include the following:

- Chronic eczematous dermatitis and lichen simplex chronicus
- Pityriasis rubra pilaris
- Confluent lichen planus
- Seborrheic dermatitis
- Patch-stage cutaneous T-cell lymphoma
- Squamous cell carcinoma in situ
- Pustular dermatoses and infections

Early or Eruptive Psoriasis

The histopathology of early or partially treated psoriasis may be extraordinarily subtle. Only slight epidermal hyperplasia is observed, and the even and regular downward elongation of rete ridges typical of advanced lesions is not present (Fig. 4–2C, D). Slight spongiosis may be observed and cause confusion with eczematous processes. Small foci of hypogranulosis may occur with associated bursts of parakeratosis, although multiple cuts through the tissue block at different levels may be required to detect these regions. In eruptive or guttate lesions, small collections of neutrophils may be ob-

served beneath (spongiform pustules) or within (Munro microabscesses) the parakeratotic stratum corneum. However, because the typical hyperplasia of psoriasis has not yet developed, such findings may prompt special stains to exclude superficial fungi or bacteria. The underlying superficial dermis is relatively noninflamed, and dermal papillae contain slightly ectatic capillary loops. Acute lesions of pustular psoriasis will have arcuate arrays of pustules at the periphery of erythematous plaques (Fig. 4–2A). Subcorneal pustule formation generally predominates over the degree of established epidermal hyperplasia (Fig. 4–2B, C).

Established Active Psoriasis

Established plaques of active psoriasis demonstrate focal-to-diffuse parakeratosis, often containing clusters of neutrophils. This parakeratosis corresponds to the characteristic silvery white scale that covers established plaques (Fig. 4–3A). Unlike the superficially similar scale of impetiginized actinic keratoses, the scale of psoriasis contains thin, pale, delicate nuclei, as opposed to plump, "dysplastic" nuclei containing dark, clumped chromatin (Fig. 4–3B, C). The granular cell layer in established psoriasis is absent beneath

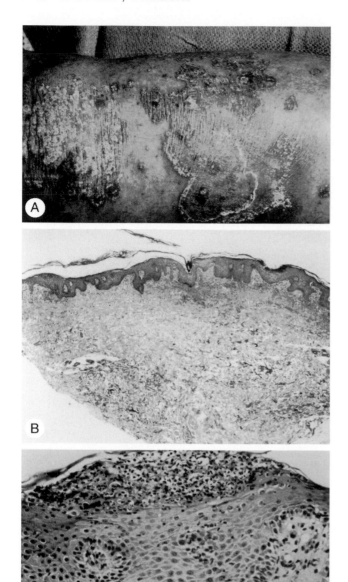

Figure 4–2. Psoriasis, eruptive and pustular lesions. **(A)** The clinical picture is predominated by arcuate and grouped pustules superimposed upon boggy, erythematous plaques. Scale is not a predominant feature. **(B)** At scanning magnification, there is irregular acanthosis, the impression of a basophilic superficial perivascular infiltrate, and clear evidence of early scale abnormality characterized by compaction and exfoliation. **(C)** At higher magnification, subcorneal and intracorneal pustules formed by aggregated neutrophils are observed. The stratum granulosum is diminished, and the dermal papilla *(right)* contains a prominent, ectatic capillary loop.

loops are dilated and considerably more tortuous than normal. A similar vascular reaction pattern is also seen in stasis dermatitis and in association with clear cell acanthoma.

The dermal inflammatory infiltrate is usually superficial, perivascular, and composed of lymphocytes with or without small numbers of admixed neutrophils; it is of secondary diagnostic importance. Although it is generally true that spongiosis is not present in psoriasis, excoriated lesions and early, eruptive plaques may demonstrate foci of mild intercellular epidermal edema. Recalcitrant lesions may be biop-

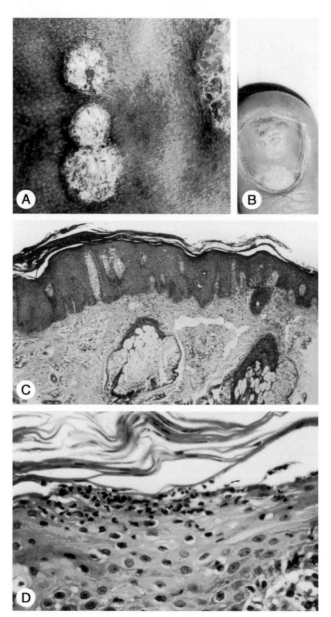

Figure 4–3. Psoriasis, established lesions. **(A)** Well-demarcated plaques are typically covered by adherent, silvery scale. **(B)** Nail involvement often includes surface pitting and thickening and discoloration of the nail plate. **(C)** The biopsy specimen is predominated by regular epidermal hyperplasia and compacted scale which focally appears to lift off of the epidermal surface. The normal coalescence (i.e., fusion) of rete ridges is accentuated in this biopsy showing established basaloid hyperplasia. **(D)** At higher magnification, the absence of stratum granulosum, the compacted parakeratotic scale, and the infiltration of the upper stratum spinosum by neutrophils (i.e., spongiform pustule formation) are all apparent.

parakeratotic foci, and the epidermis displays acanthosis without spongiosis; suprabasal mitoses; and even, regular downward extension of rete ridges as the result of basaloid hyperplasia at rete tips (Fig. 4–3B). Aggregation of neutrophils within the uppermost layers of the hyperplastic stratum corneum is a helpful diagnostic sign and is indicative of active disease (Fig. 4–3C). Dermal papillae are edematous and may even appear to be swollen. The included capillary sied after partial treatment with potent topical steroids, obscuring some of the diagnostic features listed previously. Early or incompletely evolved lesions may also show only partial histologic evolution. The focal presence of parakeratosis, intraepithelial neutrophils, and typical vascular alterations are required to make a positive diagnosis in such instances. In equivocal situations, lesions are described in a note with the recommendation that resampling be performed after cessation of therapy for 3 to 4 weeks or that a more fully evolved, untreated plaque be biopsied. Established lesions of pustular psoriasis are characterized by well-formed subcorneal pustules, as is the case in more acute, eruptive counterparts, discussed previously. Although fully evolved psoriasiform hyperplasia may not be apparent, vascular alterations are typically present.

The most commonly encountered problem is distinguishing true psoriasis from psoriasiform dermatitis (e.g., chronic eczematous processes). Classic teaching emphasizes the regularity or evenness of rete hyperplasia in psoriasis versus the irregularity of this process in chronic dermatosis. The presence or absence of capillary alterations within dermal papillae may be more consistently useful, however, provided that associated stasis, which may produce similar vascular changes, is excluded.

Unfortunately, there are no reliable diagnostic adjuncts to routine histology in the diagnosis of psoriasis. Attempts have been made to use immunophenotyping of dermal lymphoid infiltrates, electrophoretic analysis of psoriatic scale, and immunofluorescence for this purpose. With direct immunofluorescence there is localization of immune reactants to the stratum corneum of psoriatic skin. However, this pattern may also be seen in certain examples of spongiotic dermatitis and in the setting of bacterial impetiginization.

Numerous studies have attempted to discern the pathophysiology of this common disorder with little success. Debate persists regarding whether the initial lesion is within the dermis or epidermis, with proponents of the latter speculating that unregulated epidermal proliferation akin to alterations seen in epithelial neoplasia is fundamentally involved. The occurrence of lesions on cutaneous sites prone to trauma and the accepted clinical observation that disease in some patients worsens with neuropsychiatric stress raises the possibility that cutaneous nerves and the cells that they may influence directly (e.g., mast cells) could in some way participate in lesion initiation. A growing body of data indicate that the neuropeptide, substance P, which may degranulate mast cells, is involved in the early formation of psoriatic plaques. Aside from releasing vasoactive peptides that augment microvascular permeability, substance P–stimulated mast cells have also been shown to induce the expression of adhesion molecules for circulating leukocytes on microvascular endothelial cells. Neutrophils so liberated might then traffic toward chemotactic molecules within the psoriatic epidermis, such as the leukotriene LTB$_4$, which is increased in psoriatic stratum corneum.

Subsequent stimulation of keratinocyte proliferation is somewhat conjectural, although several studies suggest that pathologic induction of quiescent, noncycling basal cells, which normally reside in G1 and G2 phases of the cell cycle, may be responsible for the development of an enlarged, mitotically active pool. Other factors that have been suggested as possible causes of deranged cell kinetics include loss of contact inhibition for replication by virtue of a pathologically diminished keratinocyte surface coat and dysregulation of cyclic nucleotide ratios within the epidermal layer. Figure 4–4 summarizes some of the relevant interactions with regard to the possible pathogenesis of psoriasis.

Reiter Syndrome[8]

- EPIDERMAL AND DERMAL ALTERATIONS OF ACTIVE PSORIASIS
- OFTEN LARGE SUBCORNEAL PUSTULES
- ASSOCIATED ARTHRITIS, URETHRITIS, AND CONJUNCTIVITIS

One reason to include a brief discussion of Reiter syndrome in this section is to emphasize the critical role of the dermatopathologist in clinicopathologic patient care and diagnosis. Recognition of the potential for associated extracutaneous pathology based on a skin biopsy may save patients and clinicians unnecessary evaluation, treatment, and anxiety over what may appear to be unrelated and enigmatic signs and symptoms. Reiter syndrome usually affects men (>90%) in the third to fourth decades of life. Genetic and infectious factors have been implicated in the possible pathogenesis of this condition, which may also affect internal organs such as those of the gastrointestinal, cardiovascular, and musculoskeletal systems. The triad of urethritis, arthritis (Fig. 4–5B), and conjunctivitis is typical. Clinically, cutaneous lesions vary among erythematous papules and plaques covered by scale and pustules on acral skin (i.e., keratoderma blennorrhagicum; Fig. 4–5A); classic psoriasiform lesions elsewhere on the body surface; erythematous penile papules and plaques with central clearing (i.e., balanitis circinata); and transient oral mucosal erosions or hyperkeratotic glossitis resembling geographic tongue.

Histologically, the typical epidermal and dermal changes of psoriasis are observed, although dermal edema and the neutrophilic inflammatory component may be more marked in Reiter syndrome (Fig. 4–5C, D). The observation of large intracorneal pustules in the absence of a typical clinical history of eruptive or pustular psoriasis should raise the possibility of Reiter syndrome, particularly in young to middle-aged men.

Lichen Simplex Chronicus[9]

- HYPERORTHOKERATOSIS PREDOMINATES
- HYPERGRANULOSIS
- IRREGULAR EPIDERMAL HYPERPLASIA WITH MINIMAL SPONGIOSIS
- SUPRAPAPILLARY PLATE NORMAL OR THICKENED
- VERTICAL STREAKING OF PAPILLARY DERMAL COLLAGEN
- DERMAL CAPILLARIES PROMINENT, NOT TORTUOUS

Lichen simplex chronicus is perhaps one of the most common disorders represented in biopsy specimens. In early evolutionary phases, it takes the form of spongiotic dermatitis of the primary irritant type (see Chap. 3). With chronicity,

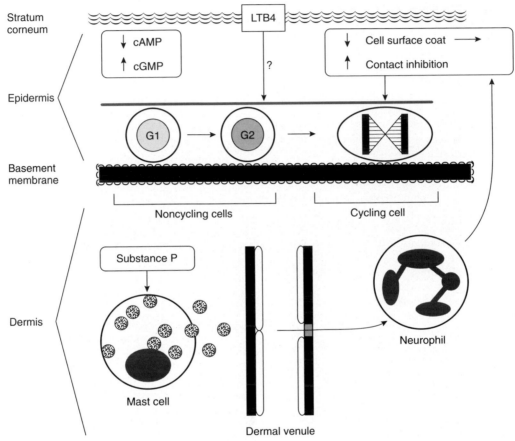

Figure 4–4. Possible pathogenetic mechanisms in psoriasis. Proposed mechanisms that may contribute to the evolution of psoriasis are potentially active at the level of epidermal proliferation as well as dermal inflammation. Alterations in normal levels of cyclic nucleotides, such as cyclic AMP and GMP, as well as the potential contribution of the leukotriene LTB_4, may produce shifts in cell cycling in favor of basal cell division. Within the dermis, it has been hypothesized that proinflammatory neuropeptides, such as substance P, may play a contributory role by provoking mast cell degranulation, thus releasing activators of endothelium and promoting recruitment of leukocytes to endothelial-lined vessels and ultimately into the epidermis. Inflammatory cells may then contribute to alterations in the keratinocyte surface that impair contact inhibition of cell replication, further propagating the proliferative process.

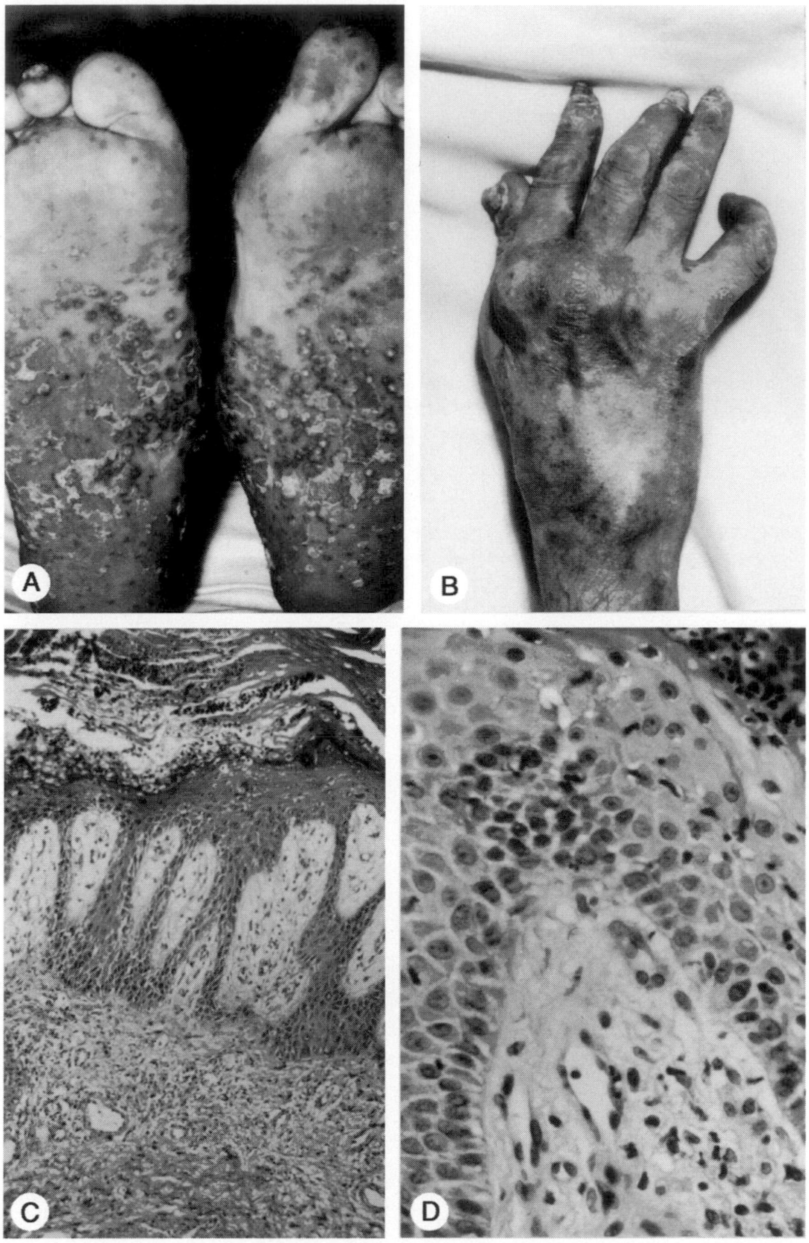

Figure 4–5. Reiter syndrome. **(A)** Clinically, lesions include erythematous papules and plaques covered by scale and pustules on acral skin (i.e., keratoderma blennorrhagica); classic psoriasiform lesions elsewhere on the body surface; erythematous penile papules and plaques with central clearing (i.e., balanitis circinata); and transient oral mucosal erosions or hyperkeratotic glossitis resembling geographic tongue. **(B)** Associated arthritis is similar to psoriatic arthritis occurring in the absence of Reiter syndrome. **(C, D)** Histologically, the typical epidermal and dermal changes of psoriasis are observed, although dermal edema and the neutrophilic inflammatory component may be more marked. Note the prominent intracorneal accumulations of neutrophils **(C)** and the dilated, tortuous vessels within edematous dermal papillae **(D)**. The observation of large intracorneal pustules in the absence of a typical clinical history of eruptive or pustular psoriasis should raise the possibility of Reiter syndrome, particularly in young boys to middle-aged men.

it is represented by irregular psoriasiform hyperplasia, which results in hyperkeratotic and verrucous plaques (Fig. 4–6A) that may mimic true psoriasis, lichen planus, or even cutaneous T-cell lymphoma. Localized regions of lichen simplex chronicus may produce nodular, hyperkeratotic foci known as prurigo nodularis (i.e., ''picker's nodule''). Any site of chronic pruritus and excoriation is subject to the development of lichen simplex chronicus. A classic location for typical lesions is the posterior neck, and lichen simplex chronicus superimposed upon primary dermatitis is a frequently encountered challenge to diagnostic interpretation. The term neurodermatitis to describe chronic irritant dermatitis and lichen simplex chronicus is a clinical designation that may imply imagined rather than real pruritus. Therefore, the use of this term in dermatology is discouraged.

Histologically, the characteristic features of lichen simplex chronicus include acanthosis with irregular, uneven, downward elongation of rete ridges; hypergranulosis; and compacted hyperorthokeratosis (Fig. 4–6B). The underlying dermal papillae are also abnormally prominent and elongated and contain coarse streaks of collagen fibers which are in perpendicular alignment to the epidermal surface. There is often a variable mononuclear cell infiltrate about vessels within the superficial dermis. Some lesions will demonstrate a verrucous epidermal architecture, producing confusion with old verrucae and keratoses. Lichen simplex chronicus, however, invariably fades gradually into the adjacent normal epidermal layer, a feature helpful in distinguishing verrucous variants from true epidermal neoplasms. Such verrucous lesions of lichen simplex chronicus may be best designated simply as verrucous epidermal hyperplasia.

Pseudoepitheliomatous Hyperplasia[10]

- EPIDERMAL CHANGES OF LICHEN SIMPLEX CHRONICUS

- DERMAL-EPIDERMAL JUNCTION JAGGED
- DERMAL-EPIDERMAL JUNCTION MAY BE DEEPLY ENDOPHYTIC
- REACTIVE ATYPIA
- ASSOCIATED INFLAMMATION, FIBROSIS, NEARBY ULCERATION

Unlike lichen simplex chronicus, the related process of pseudoepitheliomatous or pseudocarcinomatous hyperplasia generally occurs spontaneously in the absence of repeated mechanical trauma. A characteristic site for the development of pseudoepitheliomatous hyperplasia is at the edge of a chronic ulcer (Fig. 4–7A), where the epidermal layer is presumably under the constant stimulation of inflammatory cytokines and growth factors. Because epithelial carcinomas may be the cause of ulceration, it is critical to differentiate secondary pseudoepitheliomatous hyperplasia at an ulcer edge from primary epidermal malignancy.

At scanning magnification (Fig. 4–7A), pseudoepitheliomatous hyperplasia has many of the characteristics of lichen simplex chronicus, namely acanthosis with pronounced epidermal thickening, hypergranulosis, and compact hyperkeratosis (Fig. 4–7B). The inferior margin, however, is characterized not by an undulant, smooth, irregular dermal-epidermal interface, but by a jagged, angulated, complex interface separating the reactive epidermis from the inflamed and fibrotic underlying dermis. Although the basal cell layer exhibits reactive atypia, true dysplasia is not observed (Fig. 4–7C). The distinction between reactive atypia of keratinocytes and dysplasia is of critical diagnostic importance, and salient comparative features are therefore summarized in Table 4–3. Pseudoepitheliomatous hyperplasia, as would be expected, also fails to show other markers of true invasion and malignancy, such as intralymphatic and perineural spread and single-cell infiltration between collagen bundles.

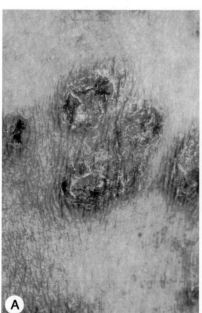
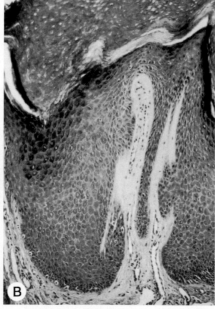

Figure 4–6. Lichen simplex chronicus and prurigo nodularis. **(A)** Multiple nodules and plaques covered by scale also show evidence of hyperpigmentation and recent excoriation. **(B)** Histologically, in addition to irregular psoriasiform acanthosis and hyperkeratosis, there is a markedly *increased* stratum granulosum and typical, vertically oriented fibrosis (i.e., streaking) within dermal papillae.

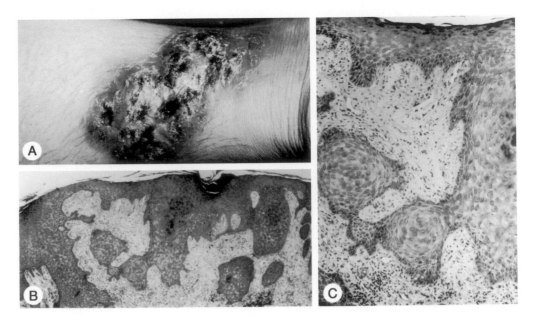

Figure 4–7. Pseudoepitheliomatous hyperplasia adjacent to chronic ulcer. **(A)** A multifocal ulcer with zones of fibrosis and hyperkeratosis producing a tumor-like plaque. This lesion was self-induced. **(B)** Reactive epidermal hyperplasia adjacent to one of the ulcerated foci. Note the jagged inferior border, which raises the possibility of superficially invasive squamous cell carcinoma. **(C)** At higher magnification, the associated dermis is markedly fibrotic and inflamed. Significant dysplasia or single-cell invasion is not present in the epithelial elements.

Pityriasis Rubra Pilaris[11, 12]

- FOLLICULAR PLUGGING AND ERYTHEMA
- ERYTHRODERMIC PLAQUES
- SHARP DEMARCATION WITH ISLANDS OF UNINVOLVED SKIN
- PSORIASIFORM EPIDERMAL HYPERPLASIA
- ALTERNATING PARAKERATOSIS AND ORTHOKERATOSIS
- FOLLICULAR PLUGGING AND SHOULDER PARAKERATOSIS

Pityriasis rubra pilaris is a disorder characterized by follicular and interfollicular erythema and abnormal scale formation. A number of clinical variants exist, and children as well as adults may be affected. Interfollicular involvement is characterized by erythematous coalescent plaques with sharply demarcated zones of sparing (Fig. 4–8A). Follicular lesions show punctate erythema and infundibular keratotic plugs (Fig. 4–8B). Hyperkeratosis of the palms and soles, as well as scaling of scalp skin, may also be observed. Certain patients may develop near-total body involvement. Therefore pityriasis rubra pilaris is one of several disorders that may cause a clinical erythroderma, including generalized psoriasis, atopic and allergic spongiotic dermatitis, seborrheic dermatitis, and cutaneous T-cell lymphoma.

Histologically, there is irregular psoriasiform hyperplasia with minimal spongiosis (Fig. 4–8C). The scale overlying interfollicular and within follicular infundibular epithelium is variably thickened and lacks the normal basket-weave configuration. Interfollicular scale characteristically demonstrates focal parakeratosis, which alternates as discrete pulses in both horizontal and vertical planes within the thickened and compacted orthokeratin. Plugged follicles also may show parakeratosis, which often is localized precisely at the interfaces between the surface epidermis and the follicular orifice (i.e., "shoulder parakeratosis"). The associated inflammatory infiltrate is composed predominantly of mononuclear cells about superficial dermal vessels. Occasional neutrophils may percolate into the superficial epidermal layers, although the degree of neutrophilic participation is not constant and is not of the degree encountered in active psoriasis.

Pityriasis Rosea, Herald Patch[13, 14]

- PSORIASIFORM PLAQUE LARGER THAN SUCCEEDING LESIONS
- PSORIASIS-LIKE EPIDERMAL HYPERPLASIA
- FOCAL PARAKERATOSIS AND PAPILLARY DERMAL HEMORRHAGE
- SUPERFICIAL AND MID-DERMAL LYMPHOCYTIC INFILTRATE

A peculiar characteristic of pityriasis rosea (see Chap. 3) is the development of a relatively large, salmon-colored, scaling plaque prior to the development of the characteristic, smaller, ovoid lesions (Fig. 4–9A). Because this initial lesion is a harbinger of what is to come, it has been referred to as the herald patch of pityriasis rosea. The lesion may produce considerable confusion, however, both clinically and histologically, because it exhibits considerably more psoriasiform epidermal hyperplasia than its successors, leading to confusion with other forms of psoriasiform and chronic spongiotic dermatitis.

At scanning magnification, the herald patch of pityriasis rosea is characterized by slightly irregular psoriasiform hyperplasia accompanied by a superficial and sometimes deep

Table 4–3. CYTOLOGIC DIFFERENCES BETWEEN REACTIVE KERATINOCYTIC ATYPIA AND DYSPLASIA

	REACTIVE ATYPIA	DYSPLASIA
Nuclear size	Relatively uniform	Variable
Nuclear shape	Round to ovoid	Angulated contour
Nuclear membrane	Thin, uniform	Thick, irregular
Heterochromatin	Delicate, evenly dispersed	Clumped, uneven
Nucleolus	Prominent	Prominent
Mitotic rate	Often high	Often high
Atypical mitosis	Infrequent	Frequent

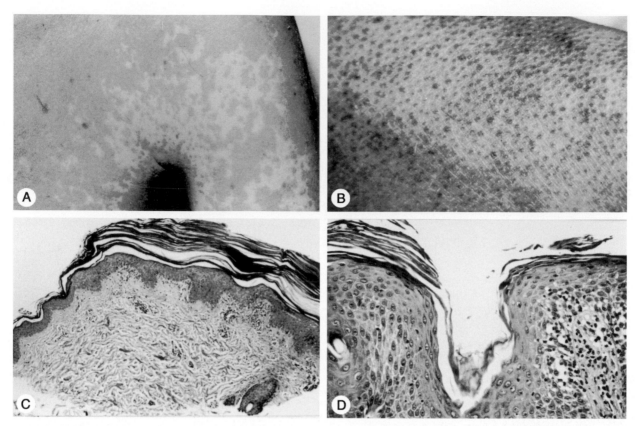

Figure 4–8. Pityriasis rubra pilaris. **(A)** Interfollicular involvement, showing erythrodermic plaques with sharply defined islands of sparing. **(B)** Follicular involvement, with erythematous follicular papules with small central keratotic plugs. **(C)** Biopsy of edge of interfollicular erythema demonstrates normal skin *(left one third)* juxtaposed with lesional skin *(right two-thirds)*. The lesion is characterized by slightly irregular psoriasiform epidermal hyperplasia and compact hyperkeratosis. **(D)** Scale devoid of neutrophilic infiltration (an important sign of psoriasis) and showing subtle zones of nuclear retention (parakeratosis) which alternate with orthokeratotic scale in both vertical and horizontal planes. The accentuation of parakeratosis at the orifice of a follicular infundibulum (i.e., shoulder parakeratosis) is a typical feature of pityriasis rubra pilaris.

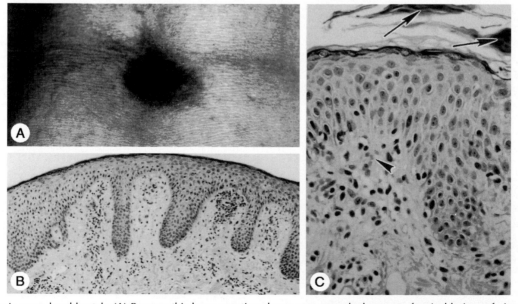

Figure 4–9. Pityriasis rosea, herald patch. **(A)** Because this large, eruptive plaque may precede the onset of typical lesions of pityriasis rosea, it may be biopsied to rule out psoriasis. In lightly pigmented individuals, the plaque is often salmon-colored; in darkly pigmented patients, it may be hyperpigmented, as depicted in **A. (B)** Biopsy specimen of the herald patch, which is really a plaque, shows psoriasiform epidermal hyperplasia without neutrophils in the stratum corneum, as would be typical of true psoriasis. **(C)** There is focal parakeratosis *(arrows)*, and focal papillary dermal hemorrhage *(arrowhead)*, as may also be seen in ordinary pityriasis rosea (see Fig. 3–12 *B,C*). The inflammatory infiltrate is brisk and is composed of lymphocytes about superficial and mid-dermal vessels. The presence of epidermal hyperplasia and the depth of the inflammatory infiltrate are the primary histologic features that distinguish herald patch from subsequent lesions of pityriasis rosea.

perivascular lymphocytic infiltrate (Fig. 4–9B). At higher magnification, there is focal, tightly compacted parakeratosis, similar to that which may be seen in regular pityriasis rosea (Fig. 4–9C). Moreover, there may also be superficial dermal hemorrhage and slight epidermal spongiosis. Unlike the condition in psoriasis, the vessels within dermal papillae are neither tortuous nor ectatic. Moreover, dermal papillae, although potentially edematous and thus widened, do not extend upward, producing marked thinning of the suprapapillary plate, as is characteristically seen in established psoriasis.

Psoriasiform Stasis Dermatitis[15]

- VARIABLE EPIDERMAL HYPERPLASIA
- DERMAL FIBROSIS
- SUPERFICIAL DERMAL VESSEL PROLIFERATION

Stasis dermatitis may produce a plethora of clinical alterations; therefore, it is frequently biopsied to exclude other conditions. This is particularly true because stasis dermatitis may at times result in localized changes that resemble an individual nodule or inflammatory plaque. Although some lesions of stasis dermatitis are associated with epidermal atrophy, resulting in a delicate, cigarette-paper–like surface,

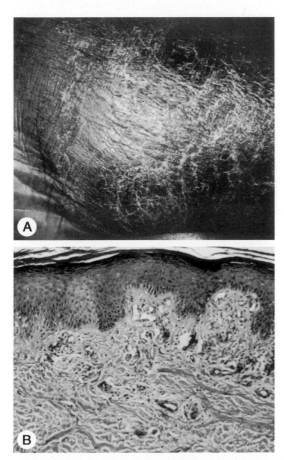

Figure 4–10. Stasis dermatitis with psoriasiform features. **(A)** Clinical presentation of stasis dermatitis as scaling, hyperpigmented plaques on the lower extremity. **(B)** Irregular epidermal hyperplasia predominates at scanning magnification. Dermal papillae are fibrotic and contain aggregates of proliferating vessels characteristic of stasis change.

others are associated with marked overlying epidermal hyperplasia and hyperkeratosis (Fig. 4–10A). This, coupled with dermal swelling and induration, variable vascular patterns, and uneven deposition of melanin and hemosiderin, may result in a polymorphous clinical appearance that mimics a number of dermatitides and neoplasms that affect the surface epidermis.

The critical histologic clue to stasis dermatitis is elaborate proliferation of superficial dermal vessels within a fibrotic papillary dermis, which often contains hemosiderin and recent hemorrhage (Fig. 4–10B). Care must be taken not to confuse these vascular changes with those of psoriasis, which also occur in the setting of relatively nonspongiotic overlying epidermal hyperplasia. Noteworthy in this regard is the presence of diffuse, randomly oriented papillary dermal fibrosis in association with the prominent vessels in stasis dermatitis, a feature not observed in psoriasis. Occasionally, chronically excoriated psoriasis will be associated with superimposed lichen simplex chronicus; however, the fibrosis in such lesions consists of vertically oriented streaking within dermal papillae rather than diffuse, randomly oriented collagen deposition.

Occasional lesions of stasis dermatitis are not predominated by epidermal alterations but rather by extensive vascular changes that result in histologic confusion with angioproliferative neoplasms. The term *acroangiodermatitis* has been applied to these variants of stasis dermatitis.

Psoriasiform Change Induced by Tumors[16]

- VARIABLE, OFTEN PSEUDOEPITHELIOMATOUS HYPERPLASIA
- ASSOCIATED WITH DERMATOFIBROMA, GRANULAR CELL TUMOR

Any discussion of commonly encountered forms of psoriasiform epidermal hyperplasia would be incomplete if inductive influences of underlying tumors were not considered. The two best examples of this phenomenon are dermatofibroma and granular cell tumor. Although the underlying mechanisms of this fascinating phenomenon remain poorly understood, the common occurrence of this finding, particularly in shave biopsy specimens, warrants consideration of the histopathologic alterations that may be produced. In the setting of dermatofibroma, there is generally some degree of overlying epidermal hyperplasia (Fig. 4–11). Usually this hyperplasia is composed of squamoid cells with abundant cytoplasm and polyhedral contours, but sometimes it is comprised of basaloid cells that closely resemble hair matrix epithelium or basal cell carcinoma. In fact, superficial biopsies of dermatofibromas have been diagnosed as basal cell carcinomas based upon these inductive changes. Often, however, there is slight hypercellularity at the base of such tissue fragments suggestive of an underlying proliferation of fibroblasts (Fig. 4–11C). Other tumors may show superficial alterations that resemble psoriasis (Fig. 4–11B). Granular cell tumors, particularly when they occur on the tongue, may result in such exuberant epidermal alteration that superficial biopsy specimens have been mistaken for invasive squamous cell carcinoma.

Psoriasiform Change Induced by Infection and Chemicals[17, 18]

- TUMOR-LIKE VERRUCOUS PROLIFERATIONS (PAPILLOMAVIRUS)
- IRREGULAR EPIDERMAL HYPERPLASIA (BLASTOMYCOSIS; HALOGENODERMA)

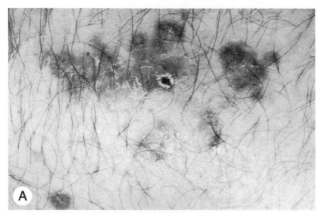

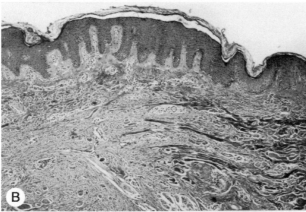

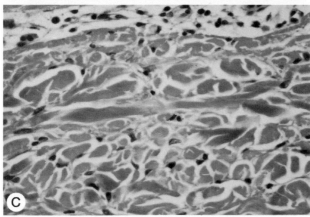

Figure 4–11. Psoriasiform epidermal hyperplasia overlying dermal tumors: dermatofibroma. **(A)** Multiple eruptive benign fibrous histiocytomas (i.e., dermatofibromas) on the thigh producing a scale-covered plaque. **(B)** Psoriasis-like epidermal hyperplasia is obvious at scanning magnification; this lesion is too subtle at this level of magnification to reveal itself as a dermatofibroma. Note, however, the hypercellular, altered dermis in the lower left portion of this field. **(C)** Inspection of the underlying dermis at a higher magnification shows proliferation of small fibroblasts within abnormal collagen bundles forming a symmetrical dermal nodule. Review of **B** reveals the lesion *(left),* bordered by normal reticular dermal collagen *(right).*

- PSORIASIFORM CHANGE WITH NEUTROPHILS (RUPIAL SECONDARY SYPHILIS)

This category pertains predominantly to marked pseudoepitheliomatous hyperplasia in the absence of an obvious underlying cause. In such instances, it is important to examine the underlying dermis carefully for evidence of inductive neoplasia (discussed previously) or marked or unusual inflammation, which could indicate a specific cause of the epithelial hyperplastic response. For example, many examples of verrucous epidermal hyperplasia or giant or unusual condyloma-like proliferations may upon close scrutiny have focal evidence of human papillomavirus (HPV) effect. Demonstration of viral protein by immunohistochemistry or DNA by in situ hybridization may enhance sensitivity for HPV detection in problematic lesions. Underlying inflammation containing neutrophils, especially when arranged in microabscesses or associated with necrosis, or granulomatous areas, should be evaluated for the presence of fungi, because certain deep mycotic infections (e.g., blastomycosis) are known to induce florid epithelial proliferation (Fig. 4–12). Also, a careful history for exposure to halogenated hydrocarbons (e.g., bromoderma, iododerma) should be sought in order to exclude these factors as environmental causes of the pseudoepitheliomatous hyperplastic response. Finally, it should be kept in mind that rupial secondary syphilis may produce a cutaneous lesion characterized by psoriasiform epidermal hyperplasia and neutrophilic infiltration. The presence of plasma cells and swollen endothelial cells, as well as a lichenoid and sometimes deep perivascular component to the inflammatory infiltrate, provides clues that the lesion is not ordinary psoriasis, prompting appropriate stains and serologic evaluation.

Rare Disorders That May Show Psoriasiform Hyperplasia

- PSORIASIFORM VARIANT CUTANEOUS T-CELL LYMPHOMA
- INCONTINENTIA PIGMENTI, VERRUCOUS STAGE[19]
- ACRODERMATITIS ENTEROPATHICA[20]
- PELLAGRA[21]
- NECROLYTIC MIGRATORY ERYTHEMA[22]
- ICHTHYOSIS (LAMELLAR)[23]
- PSORIASIFORM (HYPERTROPHIC) LUPUS ERYTHEMATOSUS[24]

Detailed discussion of the numerous rare disorders that may show psoriasiform epidermal hyperplasia is beyond the scope of this text, which focuses on more common conditions and variants. However, the previous list underscores the fact that certain examples of epidermal hyperplasia may provide important diagnostic clues to systemic disorders. Table 4–4 summarizes several of the salient comparative characteristics of these rare conditions, and the reader is referred to the suggested references for further details.

DIFFERENTIAL DIAGNOSIS

The histologic feature common to all forms of psoriasiform dermatitis is epidermal hyperplasia with or without a

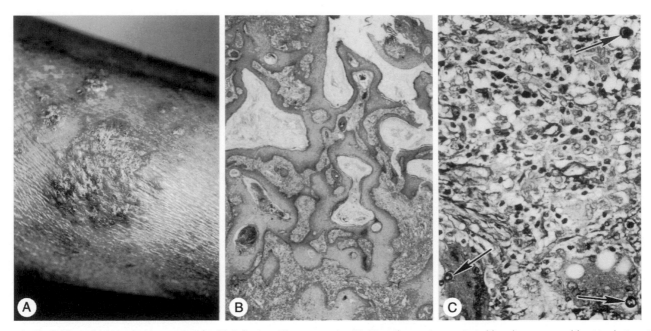

Figure 4–12. Epidermal hyperplasia associated with infection: Blastomycosis. **(A)** Hyperkeratotic, psoriasis-like plaque caused by North American blastomycosis (i.e., *Blastomyces dermatitides*). **(B)** On initial inspection, pseudoepitheliomatous epidermal hyperplasia predominates. **(C)** The inflammatory infiltrate is composed of mononuclear cells, including multinucleated giant cells, and admixed neutrophils; using the periodic acid–Schiff stain, typical yeast forms *(arrows)* are observed within giant cells.

Table 4–4. RARE DISORDERS ASSOCIATED WITH EPIDERMAL HYPERPLASIA

DISORDER	CLINICAL CHARACTERISTICS	HISTOLOGY
Psoriasiform cutaneous T-cell lymphoma (CTCL)	Verrucous, erythematous plaques	Pautrier microabscesses
Verrucous incontinentia pigmenti	Linear verrucous plaques following erythema and bullae; X-linked dominant inheritance	Verrucous acanthosis with whirling zones of dyskeratosis; persistent eosinophils
Acrodermatitis enteropathica	Zinc deficiency; hair loss, gastrointestinal complaints, bullous to verrucous skin lesions in infancy	Verrucous acanthosis with dyskeratotic epidermal cells; perivascular lymphocytes
Pellagra	Niacin deficiency; erythema, vesicles, and thickened plaques in photodistribution	Psoriasiform acanthosis, confluent parakeratosis, pallor to superficial keratinocytes
Necrolytic migratory erythema	Weight loss, diabetes mellitus, anemia, and vesicular to psoriasiform skin lesions (glucagonoma syndrome)	Psoriasiform acanthosis, pyknosis and necrosis of keratinocytes in uppermost epidermis
Lamellar ichthyosis	Ichthyosiform scales at birth, flexural skin may be more severely affected	Normal or thickened granular layer; compact, lamellar hyperorthokeratosis
Psoriasiform (hypertrophic) lupus erythematosus	Verrucous plaques in patients with chronic cutaneous lupus erythematosus	Hyperkeratosis, acanthosis, pseudoepitheliomatous hyperplasia associated with interface dermatitis

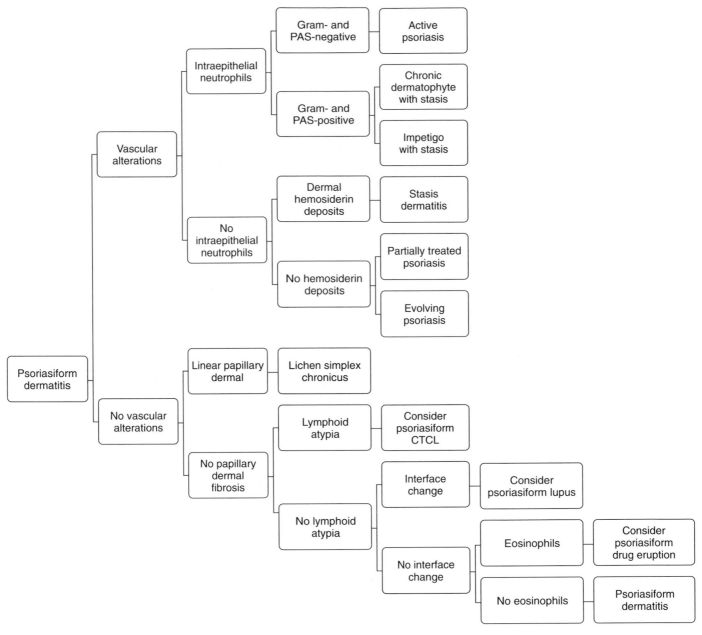

Figure 4–13. Algorithm for the diagnosis of psoriasiform dermatitis. The schematic is presented for conceptual purposes and is one of many diagnostic approaches. It also represents an oversimplification of a complicated diagnostic area. It may be modified by the reader to conform to other diagnostic criteria and "branch points" that may have been omitted or that may be of individual value.

characteristic inflammatory component. This hyperplasia is so characteristic that many diagnoses may be made based on the nature of the proliferative response within the four epidermal strata (i.e., basalis, spinosum, granulosum, and corneum). Table 4–2 emphasizes some of these simple differential features.

It is important when confronted with psoriasiform epidermal hyperplasia to remember the diversity of conditions that may give rise to this pattern. These vary from systemic disorders, such as Reiter syndrome, to infections, to genetically inherited conditions. It is therefore useful to approach lesions of psoriasiform dermatitis in a step-wise algorithmic approach, as outlined in Figure 4–13. The importance of

clinicopathologic correlation in the accurate diagnostic assessment of psoriasiform epidermal alterations cannot be overstated.

SELECTED REFERENCES

1. Soltani K, Van Scott EJ. Patterns and sequence of tissue changes in incipient and evolving lesions of psoriasis. Arch Dermatol 1972; 106:484.
2. Adler DJ, Rower JM, Hashimoto K. Annular pustular psoriasis. Arch Dermatol 1981; 117:313.
3. Brain S, Camp R, Dowd P, et al. Psoriasis and leukotriene B$_4$. Lancet 1982;2:762.

4. Braun-Falco O, Christophers E. Structural aspects of initial psoriatic lesions. Arch Dermatol Forsch 1974;251:95.
5. Cox AJ, Watson W. Histologic variations in lesions of psoriasis. Arch Dermatol 1972:106:503.
6. Gelfant S. The cell cycle in psoriasis: A reappraisal. Br J Dermatol 1976;95:577.
7. Harrist TJ, Mihm MC. Cutaneous immunopathology. Hum Pathol 1979;10:625.
8. Weinberger HW, Ropes MW, Kulka JP, et al. Reiter's syndrome, clinical and pathological observations. Medicine 1962;41:35.
9. Rowland Payne CME, Wilkinson JD, McKee PH, et al. Nodular prurigo—a clinicopathological study of 46 patients. Br J Dermatol 1985;113:431.
10. Wagner RF Jr, Grande DJ. Pseudoepitheliomatous hyperplasia vs squamous cell carcinoma. J Dermatol Surg Oncol 1986;12:632.
11. Braun-Falco O, Ryckmanns F, Schmoekel C, et al. Pityriasis rubra pilaris: A clinicopathological and therapeutic study. Arch Dermatol Res 1983;275:287.
12. Soeprono FF. Histologic criteria for the diagnosis of pityriasis rubra pilaris. Am J Dermatopathol 1986;8:277.
13. Wade TR, Finan MC. Psoriasiform dermatitis. In: Farmer ER, Hood AF, eds. Pathology of the Skin. Norwalk, CT: Appleton & Lange, 1990:94.
14. Bunch LW, Tilley JC. Pityriasis rosea. Arch Dermatol 1961;84:79.
15. Hood AF. Superficial and deep infiltrates of the skin. In: Farmer ER, Hood AF, eds. Pathology of the Skin. Norwalk, CT: Appleton & Lange, 1990:205.
16. Murphy GF, Elder DE. Non-Melanocytic Tumors of the Skin. Armed Forces Institute of Pathology Fascicle Series, monograph 1, series 3. Washington, DC: AFIP Press, 1991:223.
17. Schwartz J, Salfelder K. Blastomycosis: A review of 152 cases. Curr Top Pathol 1977;65:165.
18. Lauret P, Godin M, Bravard P. Vegetating iodides after an intravenous pyelogram. Dermatologica 1985;171:463.
19. Guerrier LJW, Wong CK. Ultrastructural evolution of the skin in incontinentia pigmenti (Bloch-Sulzberger). Dermatologica 1974;149:10.
20. Gonzalez JR, Botet MV, Sanchez JL. The histopathology of acrodermatitis enteropathica. Am J Dermatopathol 1982;4:303.
21. Stratigos JD, Katsambas A. Pellagra: A still existing disease. Br J Dermatol 1977;96:99.
22. Kahan RS, Perez-Figaredo RA, Neimans A. Necrolytic migratory erythema. Arch Dermatol 1977;113:792.
23. Williams ML, Elias PM. Heterogeneity in autosomal recessive ichthyosis. Arch Dermatol 1985;121:477.
24. Spann CR, Callen JP, Klein JB, et al. Clinical, serologic and immunogenetic studies in patients with chronic cutaneous (discoid) lupus erythematosus who have verrucous and/or hypertrophic skin lesions. J Rheum 1988;15:256.

5

Vesiculobullous Dermatitis

DEFINITIONS AND GENERAL CONSIDERATIONS

One of the most important and misunderstood areas of dermatopathology is vesiculobullous disease. This divergent group of disorders may be life-threatening, and accurate diagnosis and implementation of correct therapy may have profound therapeutic implications. The ability to make an accurate diagnosis, however, is often confounded by the histologic subtleties inherent in stage of lesion evolution, slight nuances in architecture and inflammatory cytology that separate certain disorders, and the plethora of divergent stimuli that may eventuate in the common theme of an intraepidermal or subepidermal blister (e.g., antibody attack, cellular attack, ischemia, viral cytopathologic changes).

The nomenclature of blistering diseases is relatively simple. The term *vesicles*, from the Latin word vesicula, meaning small blister, generally implies lesions ranging up to 0.5 cm in diameter. The term *bullae*, from the Latin word bulla, meaning bubble-like, connotes larger blisters. Blisters may form from spongiosis, reticular degeneration, vacuolar degeneration, acantholysis, and lysis of the dermal matrix (i.e., dermolysis).

This chapter concentrates on those disorders that commonly manifest as blisters at the most classic stage of their clinical evolution. Diseases that may form blisters but are better known for changes inherent in nonvesicular stages (e.g., erythema multiforme) or disorders that occasionally, but not ordinarily, give rise to blisters and erosions (e.g., lupus erythematosus, fixed drug eruption, lichen sclerosus) are discussed in other chapters.

GROSS PATHOLOGY

Appreciation of the gross pathology of blistering diseases is of critical importance in evaluation of a skin biopsy specimen. Early blisters may not appear as such, and the accompanying history may describe urticaria, erythema, induration, or simply pruritic, normal-appearing skin. Some blisters may be so fulminant and rapid that the predominant lesion is a shallow erosion. Later in the course of blistering disease, lesions may be appreciated primarily as pustules (due to superinfection), eschars, or zones of re-epithelialization. It is imperative to ascertain the type of lesion that was biopsied in evaluating the possibility of a blistering disorder. Ideally, a relatively recent, fluid-filled blister will be sampled. However, biopsy of the midportion of the lesion jeopardizes dermal-epidermal integrity and minimizes the possibility of gaining insight into the evolutionary histology of the process. Samples should ideally be obtained from the blister edge, with no more than two thirds of the biopsy diameter representing the blister and at least one third representing the presumably intact perilesional skin. Often, histologically, this clinically normal skin will be inflamed, and early blister formation will be seen. Biopsy specimens obtained in this manner will generally include a spectrum of histologic changes ranging from early stages of the formation of the blister at one edge or in the middle, and frank vesicle formation at the other edge. Such specimens are also optimal for direct immunofluorescence examination if triaged in appropriate transport medium (see Chap. 2).

GENERAL HISTOLOGY AND TEMPORAL EVOLUTION

The reaction patterns that may give rise to blisters are described in detail in Chapter 1. Regardless of whether a blister arises as a result of spongiosis, cell injury or death, acantholysis, or defective cell-matrix interactions, a common denominator is a fluid-filled cavity within the epidermis or superficial dermis. Most acute blisters contain proteinaceous serum transudate, and therefore are filled with homogeneous pink material histologically. Traumatized blisters may contain numerous erythrocytes, and superinfected blisters may be infiltrated by neutrophils and mimic primary neutrophilic

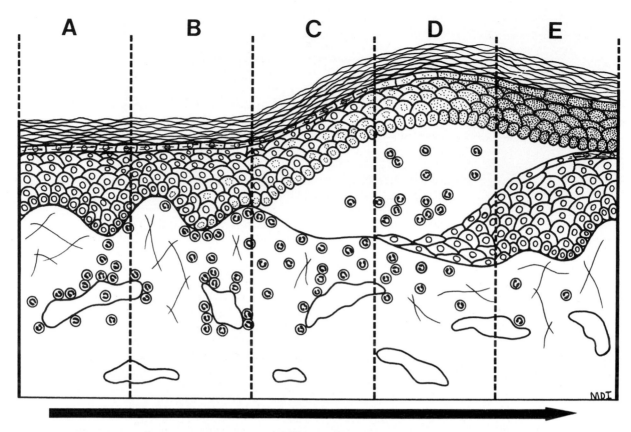

Time

Figure 5–1. Temporal evolution of subepidermal inflammatory blister. **(A)** The earliest phase of blister formation involves the local recruitment of inflammatory cells. Release of mediators by these cells, often in concert with concentration of these cells along with antibody and complement deposition along the dermal-epidermal junction **(B)**, results in separation of the dermal and the epidermal layer **(C)**. Initially, serum fills the forming cavity. **(D)** Eventually, inflammatory cells infiltrate the cavity, and squamous epithelial cells begin to cover the blister base. **(E)** Upon reaching confluence, these re-epithelializing cells begin to stratify, forming a new viable epidermal layer as the blister roof becomes progressively necrotic and eventually is sloughed. Biopsy of the edge of a blister may reveal several of these sequential steps and facilitate diagnosis. Biopsy of the center of the blister may confuse the diagnosis, because these sites frequently contain more chronic alterations.

and pustular dermatoses (see Chap. 8). Early stages of blister formation, however, are generally more subtle. Because most vesiculobullous disorders are inflammatory, their early counterparts usually show a superficial perivascular infiltrate, occasionally with leukocytes in association with epidermal cells in a pattern that may be very helpful diagnostically (e.g., degranulating eosinophils along the dermal-epidermal interface in early bullous pemphigoid). Subtle early cellular alterations also may be extremely helpful in discerning the cause of the blister (e.g., differentiating between spongiosis and acantholysis).

Whereas early evolutionary phases of blisters may provide important diagnostic clues, late stages are usually confusing and problematic. Dermatitis herpetiformis, for example, which during active stages is predominated by neutrophils, may contain eosinophils in later stages, resulting in confusion with active bullous pemphigoid. Resolving lesions of the subepidermal blistering disorder bullous pemphigoid, on the other hand, may show significant re-epithelialization along the blister base, giving the false impression in some samples that the blister cavity is really intraepidermal. Again, precise understanding of the evolutionary patterns of how blisters form and how they heal is integral to accurate histologic interpretation. Close clinicopathologic correlation is re-

quired in the evaluation of most forms of vesiculobullous dermatitis. Figure 5–1 provides a schematic representation of various evolutionary stages of a generic subepidermal blister to illustrate some of these conceptual and practical points.

HISTOLOGY OF SPECIFIC DISORDERS

Bullous Pemphigoid[1-3]

- SUBEPIDERMAL BLISTER
- EOSINOPHILS ALONG DERMAL-EPIDERMAL JUNCTION IN EARLY LESIONS
- LYMPHOCYTES AND EOSINOPHILS AROUND SUPERFICIAL VESSELS
- RE-EPITHELIALIZATION MAY GIVE APPEARANCE OF INTRAEPIDERMAL BLISTER
- DIRECT IMMUNOFLUORESCENCE USUALLY POSITIVE FOR LINEAR C3 ALONG DERMAL-EPIDERMAL JUNCTION

Bullous pemphigoid is characterized by subepidermal bullae and a chronic, relatively self-limited course. Although relatively rare among dermatitides in general, this disorder is more common than pemphigus or dermatitis herpetiformis. In the immunofluorescence laboratory at the University of Pennsylvania, for example, bullous pemphigoid accounts for more than 40% of all specimens of blistering diseases received for diagnostic evaluation. Bullous pemphigoid usually occurs after the age of 60 years and is very rare before the age of 40 years. Lesions of bullous pemphigoid may occur anywhere on the skin, but there is a predilection for the lower abdomen, groin, inner aspects of the thighs, and flexor surfaces of the forearms. In one third of patients, the mouth is involved, but these lesions are small, heal quickly, and are much less significant than oral lesions of pemphigus. The development of typical lesions of bullous pemphigoid may be heralded by one or more areas of localized pruritus in certain individuals. These lesions are often urticarial, and in some patients, urticarial lesions may predominate or persist in the relative absence of overt blisters. Cicatricial pemphigoid is an erosive, scarring variant with a predilection for involvement of conjunctival and mucosal epithelium.

Lesions generally consist of tense bullae filled with clear fluid upon variably erythematous bases (Fig. 5–2A). In any one patient with active disease, transitions between urticarial erythematous plaques, small vesicles, and frank bullae may be observed. Biopsy of early evolutionary stages or the edges of an established lesion is often most diagnostically informative (Fig. 5–3A).

At scanning magnification, bullous pemphigoid is easily recognized as a subepidermal, inflammatory blistering disorder. Early changes, often appreciated at the blister edge, consist of vacuolization at the dermal-epidermal junction and small collections of degranulating eosinophils and mast cells within the most superficial stratum of the papillary dermis, directly beneath the basement membrane zone (Fig. 5–2B, C). Vacuoles within basal keratinocytes coalesce to form a subepidermal bulla; within and below the bulla, there is an infiltrate composed of eosinophils, mast cells, lymphocytes, histiocytes, and rare neutrophils (Figs. 5–2D and 5–3B, C). Pulses of eosinophils in regions of spongiosis may occur (i.e., eosinophilic spongiosis). Epidermal regeneration, or re-epithelialization of the blister base, begins within 2 days of blister formation at the edges of the bulla and gradually extends centripetally toward the center of the bulla. Acantholysis is not observed, and neutrophilic papillary dermal microabscesses, a requisite feature for the diagnosis of dermatitis herpetiformis, are never seen. In urticarial lesions, the dermal infiltrate may predominate, with the epidermis showing only subtle basal layer vacuolization.

There are a number of disorders that may mimic bullous

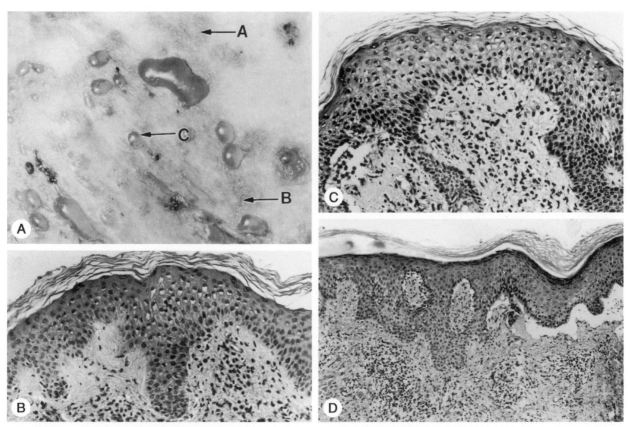

Figure 5–2. Bullous pemphigoid. **(A)** Numerous tense bullae are present on erythematous bases. Occasionally, lesions begin and persist as pruritic, urticarial plaques. Erythematous, often urticarial plaques (A, *arrow*) evolve into zones of microvesiculation (B, *arrow*) and eventually form overt, fluid-filled bullae (C, *arrow*). **(B)** The earliest evolutionary phase of bullous pemphigoid consists of superficial perivascular infiltration by lymphocytes and eosinophils, with occasional eosinophils in close proximity to the dermal-epidermal junction. This pattern could represent a drug eruption or insect-bite reaction, but there is no spongiosis, and the presence of eosinophils along the basement membrane zone is unusual. **(C)** The apposition of degranulating eosinophils along the dermal-epidermal junction is followed by basal layer vacuolization and microvesicle formation *(lower left).* **(D)** In time, a subepidermal blister forms, although at the edge *(left side of this panel),* most of the changes seen in **B** and **C** may be observed.

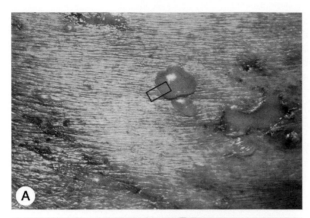

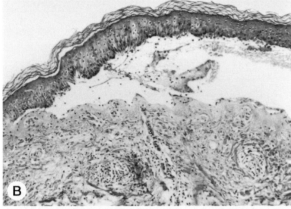

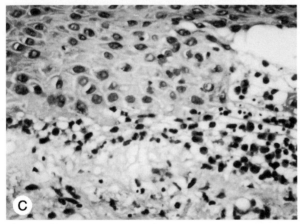

Figure 5–3. Bullous pemphigoid. **(A)** A biopsy specimen that includes perilesional skin of an established blister *(enclosed by rectangle)* will not only yield **(B)** an intact blister base and roof, but also **(C)** early alterations at the lesion edge, which facilitate accurate diagnosis. In **C**, note the intimate association between eosinophils containing bilobed nuclei and the finely vacuolated epidermal basal cell layer.

pemphigoid histologically. These include herpes gestationis, epidermolysis bullosa acquisita, insect-bite reactions, drug eruptions, old lesions of dermatitis herpetiformis, and rarely, certain stages of drug-induced erythema multiforme. Accordingly, direct immunofluorescence of a perilesional specimen including the edge of lesional skin is generally recommended as a confirmatory test when bullous pemphigoid is suspected by conventional histology. Immunofluorescence microscopy discloses deposition of C3, usually with IgG, in a linear pattern at the dermal-epidermal junction. C3 usually predom-

inates over IgG in intensity. Immunoelectron microscopy reveals that the bullous pemphigoid antigen to which these immune reactants bind is associated with the lamina lucida of the basement membrane and is present in the portion of basal keratinocyte cytoplasm that apposes the basement membrane. Circulating antibody directed against the dermal-epidermal junction is detected in 70% of patients. A proposed sequence of events in the pathogenesis of bullous pemphigoid is the deposition of immunoglobulin and complement at the dermal-epidermal junction, followed by degranulation of mast cells resulting in eosinophil recruitment and degranulation. The proteolytic enzymes released by eosinophils may then result in damage to the basement membrane zone, with subsequent blister formation.

The pathogenesis of bullous pemphigoid is now partially understood. Figure 5–4 depicts a schematic of the proposed pathogenesis of bullous pemphigoid.

Herpes Gestationis[4]

- PRURITIC ERUPTION DURING PREGNANCY
- FINDINGS MAY BE SIMILAR TO BULLOUS PEMPHIGOID
- SPONGIOSIS WITH INTRAEPIDERMAL EOSINOPHILS
- DYSKERATOTIC RATHER THAN VACUOLAR DEGENERATION OF BASAL CELLS
- INDIRECT IMMUNOFLUORESCENCE USUALLY NEGATIVE

Eruptions during pregnancy frequently generate the request that the dermatopathologist consider herpes gestationis in biopsy interpretation. Because herpes gestationis is very similar to bullous pemphigoid histologically, clinical parameters are very important in establishing a definitive diagnosis.

There are subtle yet important differences between the histology of herpes gestationis and bullous pemphigoid. Both are subepidermal blistering disorders. In herpes gestationis, however, there is often marked papillary dermal edema which expands dermal papillae and which, in tangential section, may appear to represent intraepidermal vesicles. The epidermis may show focal spongiosis and infiltration of eosinophils (i.e., eosinophilic spongiosis). Whereas bullous pemphigoid is associated with vacuolization of the basal cell layer, herpes gestationis often demonstrates dyskeratosis and colloid body formation, similar to that seen in lichen planus. Herpes gestationis must be differentiated from pruritic urticarial papules and plaques of pregnancy (PUPPP). PUPPP, an itchy papular eruption, generally does not vesiculate, shows no evidence of cytolytic or dyskeratotic injury along the dermal-epidermal junction, and is negative by routine direct immunofluorescence testing.

Immunofluorescence testing of lesional or nonlesional skin in herpes gestationis reveals findings identical to bullous pemphigoid. It has been hypothesized that herpes gestationis is a hormonally modulated autoimmune disease directed against chorioallantoic and trophoblastic (paternally derived) antigens that cross-react with basement membrane zone antigens. Circulating anti–basement membrane zone antibodies are less frequently detected in herpes gestationis than in bullous pemphigoid.

Figure 5–4. Pathogenesis of bullous pemphigoid. Circulating antibody to bullous pemphigoid antigen, a protein normally located in the lamina lucida of the dermal-epidermal basement membrane directly above the lamina densa and in basal keratinocyte cytoplasm in association with hemidesmosomes, binds to this antigen within lesional and perilesional skin. Antigen-antibody complex leads to recruitment and fixation of complement (C, C3a, C5a), resulting in activation and degranulation of dermal mast cells. This triggers release of eosinophil chemotactic factors (ECF-A) which result in the recruitment and degranulation of eosinophils. The resultant liberation of potent proteolytic enzymes causes basal cell layer cytolysis and degradation of adhesive bonds between basal lamina and epidermal cells, resulting in a forming subepidermal blister.

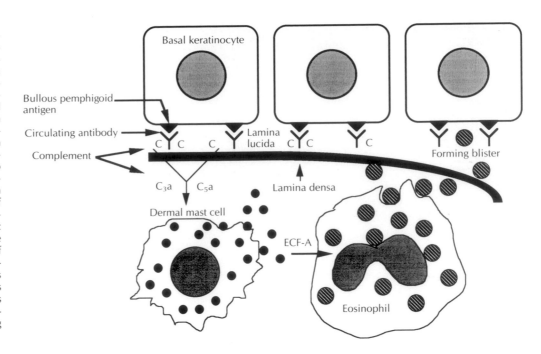

Epidermolysis Bullosa Acquisita[5]

- BLISTERS PROVOKED BY TRAUMA
- HISTOLOGY IDENTICAL TO BULLOUS PEMPHIGOID
- LINEAR IgG BY DIRECT IMMUNOFLUORESCENCE

True epidermolysis bullosa is rare, noninflammatory, and should not be confused with epidermolysis bullosa acquisita (EBA). EBA presents in adult life and involves skin over joint surfaces, particularly the hands and feet. Trauma may induce blisters, and healing involves scar and milia formation. The histology may be identical to that of bullous pemphigoid. Direct immunofluorescence, although often negative, may show a linear pattern for IgG that predominates over that of C3. Indirect immunofluorescence of split skin preparations, immunocytochemical mapping of basement membrane zone components of lesional skin, or immunoelectron microscopy of lesional skin may be required to definitively differentiate EBA from bullous pemphigoid (see Chap. 2). It is presently believed that EBA is caused by autoantibody formation and deposition below the lamina densa to the carboxyl terminus of type VII collagen.

Dermatitis Herpetiformis[6–8]

- SUBEPIDERMAL INFLAMMATORY BLISTERS
- NEUTROPHILIC MICROABSCESSES IN DERMAL PAPILLAE
- VACUOLAR DEGENERATION IN INTER-RETE BASAL CELLS
- IgA AND FIBRIN IN GRANULAR ARRAY IN DERMAL PAPILLAE

This relatively rare blistering disorder is characterized by itchy papulovesicular lesions, neutrophilic microabscesses within dermal papillae, and the presence of granular deposits of IgA at the dermal-epidermal junction. Adults 25 to 50 years old are the most commonly affected group. Lesions are characterized by symmetrical distribution of grouped (therefore, herpetiform) vesicles (Fig. 5–5A, B). The earliest sign of incipient eruption is marked pruritus and burning, followed 24 to 48 hours later by erythematous urticarial lesions. Close inspection with a hand lens allows the physician to see clusters of small vesicles surmounting the erythematous, urticarial areas. Fully developed lesions are characterized by bilateral, symmetrical, intensely pruritic grouped vesicles involving the shoulders, buttocks, and extensor surfaces of the extremities. Because lesions are grouped or localized and pruritic, the clinical differential diagnosis that accompanies a biopsy specimen may include insect-bite reaction, scabies, contact dermatitis, or pruritic variant of bullous pemphigoid.

Histologically, scanning magnification reveals a forming or established subepidermal blister associated with concentration of inflammatory cells within the tips of dermal papillae (Figs. 5–6 and 5–7). Early changes include deposition of fibrin in dermal papillae, nuclear dust (i.e., fragments) beneath a vacuolated basal cell layer overlying dermal papillae, and the notable absence of spongiosis or eosinophils (Figs. 5–6A and 5–7A). Importantly, neutrophils are not concentrated at rete tips, a common site of inflammatory involvement in linear IgA disease (discussed later). Old lesions may show influx of eosinophils, re-epithelialization, and impetiginization, which may confuse the diagnostic picture.

The pathogenesis of dermatitis herpetiformis is intriguing. Studies have shown that IgA and IgG antibodies that cross-react with gluten proteins are present in many patients with this condition. Moreover, patients may show evidence clinically or histologically of a sprue-like, gluten-sensitive enteropathy. These antibodies react with reticulin fibrils directly beneath the basement membrane of the skin or may be deposited there as circulating immune complexes. Genetic factors may play a role in prolonged formation or circulation of immune complexes in these patients. Therapy with a glu-

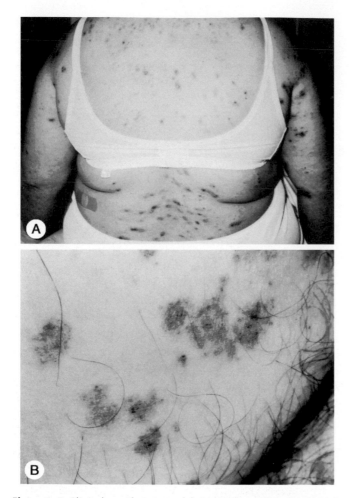

Figure 5–5. Clinical manifestations of dermatitis herpetiformis. **(A)** Multiple erythematous vesicles and erosions are present on the back of a patient. **(B)** Closer inspection reveals the clustered, herpetiform arrangement of lesions. Often, vesicles have a predilection for the extensor surfaces of the extremities, and lesions are almost always intensely pruritic. The clinical differential diagnosis that accompanies a biopsy specimen will often include contact dermatitis and pruritic forms of pemphigoid.

ten-free diet, although difficult to enforce, may cause remission of skin lesions. As is the case in many cutaneous disorders, diet and environmental stress may be major complicating issues in this debilitating disease. Figure 5–8 summarizes an overview of the presently proposed pathogenesis for this disorder.

Linear IgA Disease[9, 10]

- SUBEPIDERMAL INFLAMMATORY BLISTERS
- NEUTROPHILS IN DERMAL PAPILLAE AND AT RETE TIPS
- VACUOLAR DEGENERATION IN INTER-RETE AND RETE TIP BASAL CELLS
- IgA (AND FIBRIN) IN LINEAR ARRAY ALONG THE DERMAL-EPIDERMAL INTERFACE

Linear IgA dermatosis is not a variant of dermatitis herpetiformis. Clinically, linear IgA dermatosis is characterized by a vesiculobullous eruption that may occur in child-

hood or after puberty. Lesions often form large bullae, may be annular in configuration, and occur randomly. In contrast to dermatitis herpetiformis, intestinal lesions or association with gluten-induced autoimmunity are not typical. Clinical presentation may mimic bullous pemphigoid.

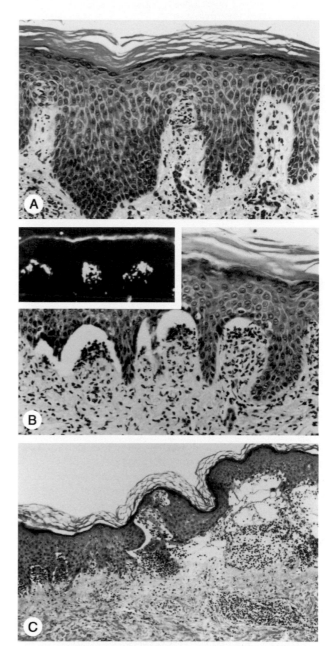

Figure 5–6. Histologic manifestations of dermatitis herpetiformis. **(A)** An early lesion shows subtle accumulation of neutrophils, nuclear dust, and fibrin within the tips of dermal papillae. Because the epidermis in this biopsy specimen appears slightly hyperplastic and spongiotic, possibly due to a primary irritant effect, the dermal changes could be overlooked in favor of an erroneous diagnosis of low-grade subacute spongiotic dermatitis. **(B)** A better-developed lesion shows neutrophilic microabscesses at the tips of the dermal papillae, producing cleft-like zones of dermal-epidermal separation overlying each papilla. Eosinophils are notably absent. Inset depicts low-power direct immunofluorescence of lesion shown in **B**. There are granular aggregates of IgA outlining each of four dermal papillae (see Chap. 2). **(C)** A fully evolved lesion shows a subepidermal blister *(right)* formed by confluence of suprapapillary microvesicles *(left)* associated with microabscesses similar to those depicted in **B**.

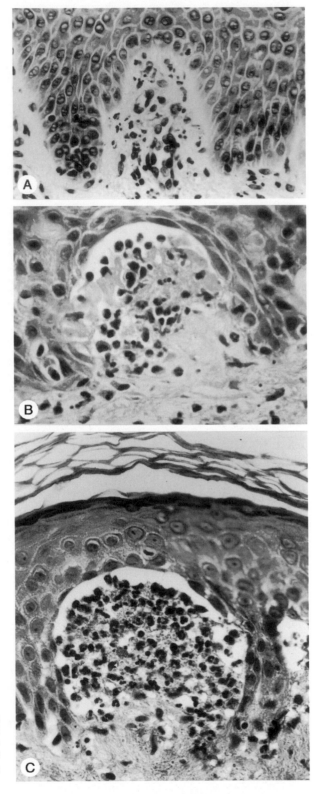

Figure 5–7. Sequential evolution of dermal papillary microabscess in dermatitis herpetiformis. **(A)** Scant numbers of fragmented neutrophils and fibrin in dermal papillae lead to **(B)** more overt aggregates of clumped fibin and neutrophils associated with early microvesicle formation directly over the papilla. **(C)** A fully formed microabscess is rounded in contour, composed exclusively of neutrophils, and associated with a crescentic microvesicle that surrounds the entire papilla.

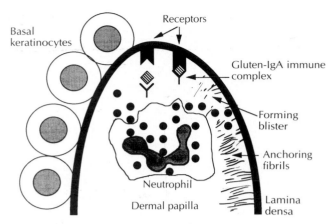

Figure 5–8. Pathogenesis of dermatitis herpetiformis. Circulating antibody of the IgA type formed in the intestinal lamina propria to dietary gluten and gluten-like proteins cross-reacts with similar antigens within anchoring filaments at the tips of dermal papillae. Alternatively, gluten-IgA immune complexes bind to receptors at this site. The formation of immune complexes evokes the recruitment of neutrophils, which become activated, degranulate, and release destructive proteolytic enzymes in the vicinity of the basal cells that overlie each dermal papilla. Basal cell layer cytolysis results in dermal papillary microvesicles that coalesce to form clinical blisters. The reason for the intense itching remains enigmatic, but it is possible that the release of inflammatory mediators within the superficial portion of the dermal papillae may have implications regarding afferent neural impulses.

Although the histologic appearance superficially may mimic dermatitis herpetiformis, important differences exist. Most critical of these is the localization of neutrophils evenly along the dermal-epidermal interface to include the tips of rete ridges (Fig. 5–9). Confirmation of this diagnosis requires direct immunofluorescence (see Chap. 2), which will reliably show a linear pattern of IgA deposition along the dermal-epidermal interface in contrast to the localized granular IgA deposits in dermatitis herpetiformis.

Pemphigus[11-13]

- INTRAEPIDERMAL ACANTHOLYTIC BLISTER
- SUPERFICIAL MIXED MONONUCLEAR INFILTRATE WITH EOSINOPHILS
- EVIDENCE OF INTERCELLULAR IMMUNE REACTANT DEPOSITION

Pemphigus refers to a group of uncommon diseases of the skin characterized clinically by vesicles and bullae and histologically by acantholysis. These disorders are associated with serum autoantibodies directed against antigens in the intercellular domains of the epidermis. There are four variant forms of pemphigus: pemphigus vulgaris (suprabasal acantholytic blister); pemphigus foliaceus (subcorneal acantholytic blister); pemphigus vegetans (suprabasal with epithelial hyperplasia); and pemphigus erythematosus (a cross-over disorder with features of lupus erythematosus and pemphigus vulgaris). The latter two variants are seen with a frequency that suggests that they practically do not exist.

Pemphigus vulgaris, by far the most common manifestation of this rare disorder, affects individuals of middle to old age and begins as a vesiculobullous eruption, often ini-

tially involving traumatized regions of skin. Scalp and oral mucosa are frequently involved. Bullae are characteristically flaccid, with a tendency to enlarge. Because of their superficial location within the epidermal layer, these bullae often rupture, producing new and healing surface erosions (Fig. 5–10A). Pemphigus foliaceus, a more benign and more superficial acantholytic process than pemphigus vulgaris, results in the formation of weeping surface erosions in a seborrheic distribution (i.e., face, midline chest, and back; Fig. 5–11A). It is not unusual to fail to detect evidence of intact, fluid-filled blisters in pemphigus vulgaris and especially in pemphigus foliaceus. However, when an intact blister is located, pressure on the blister roof readily results in centrifugal expansion (i.e., Nikolsky sign) and is an indication of the intraepidermal acantholytic nature of this disorder.

Histologically, the common denominator of the pemphigus group of disorders is acantholysis. This term implies dissolution, or lysis, of the intercellular adhesion sites within

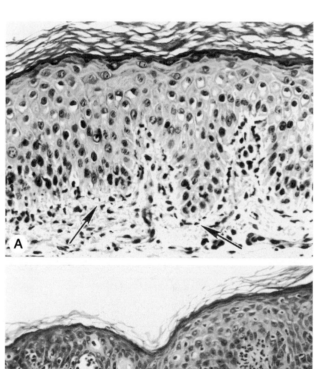

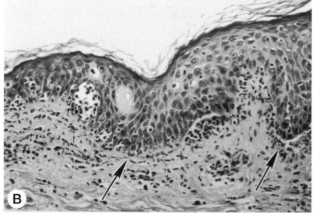

Figure 5–9. Linear IgA disease. **(A, B)** In this biopsy specimen, neutrophils are both aggregated within dermal papillae as well as aligned along the entire dermal-epidermal junction, including rete tips *(arrows)*. Direct immunofluorescence reveals linear, not granular, deposits of IgA in a pattern that resembles C_3 and IgG deposition in pemphigoid. Linear IgA dermatosis is not a variant of dermatitis herpetiformis. Clinically, linear IgA dermatosis is characterized by a vesiculobullous eruption that may occur in childhood or after puberty. Lesions often form large bullae, may be annular in configuration, and occur randomly. In contrast to dermatitis herpetiformis, intestinal lesions and association with gluten-induced autoimmunity are the exception. Clinical presentation may mimic bullous pemphigoid.

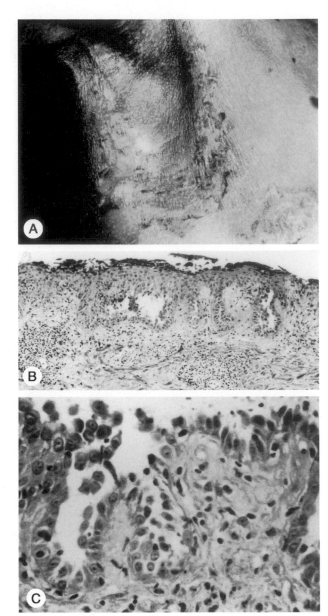

Figure 5–10. Pemphigus vulgaris. **(A)** Eroded plaques are formed by confluent, thin-roofed bullae on intertriginous skin. **(B)** At scanning magnification, there are discrete foci of suprabasal acantholysis resulting in early microvesiculation. **(C)** Rounded, acantholytic keratinocytes detached from neighboring cells are visible along the surface of the blister base. The relatively rigid dermal papillae covered with a single row of adherent basal cells produce a characteristic tombstone pattern. The underlying inflammatory infiltrate is superficial, perivascular, and composed primarily of lymphocytes and eosinophils.

a squamous epithelial surface. Acantholytic cells that are no longer attached to other epithelial cells lose their polyhedral shape and characteristically become rounded. In pemphigus vulgaris and pemphigus vegetans, acantholysis selectively involves the layer of cells immediately above the basal cell layer (Fig. 5–10B, C). The vegetans variant also shows considerable epidermal hyperplasia. In pemphigus foliaceus, a blister forms by similar mechanisms, but unlike pemphigus vulgaris, it selectively involves the superficial epidermis at the level of the stratum granulosum (Fig. 5–11B–D). Variable superficial dermal infiltration by lymphocytes, histiocytes, and eosinophils accompanies all forms of pemphigus.

Sera from patients with pemphigus vulgaris contain antibodies of the IgG type, which react with the intercellular cement substance of skin and mucous membranes. This phenomenon is the basis for direct and indirect diagnostic immunofluorescence testing of skin and serum, respectively. Lesional skin shows a net-like pattern of intercellular IgG

deposition localized to sites of developed or incipient acantholysis. Although cultured skin exposed to pemphigus antiserum develops acantholysis, it now appears that at least some of the acantholytic process is not the direct result of antibody-induced damage but rather is the consequence of synthesis and liberation of a proteinase, plasminogen activator, by epidermal cells, an event that is triggered by the pemphigus antibody. Figure 5–12 illustrates the proposed mechanism for acantholysis characteristic of pemphigus vulgaris.

Porphyria Cutanea Tarda[14]

- BLISTERS ON ACRAL, SUN-EXPOSED SKIN
- ABSENCE OF DERMAL INFLAMMATION
- DERMAL-EPIDERMAL CLEAVAGE PLANE
- THICKENED, HYALINIZED VESSEL WALLS WITHIN DERMAL PAPILLAE

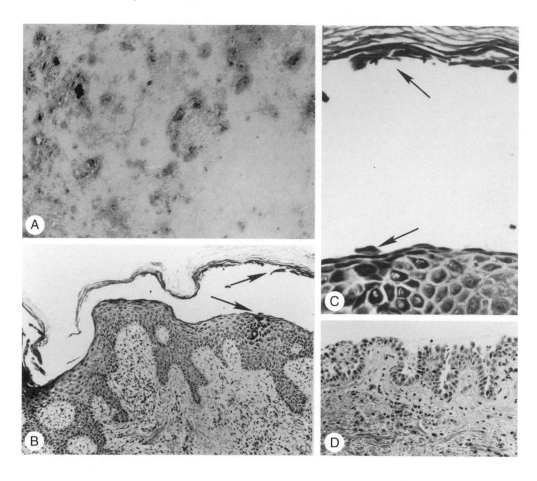

Figure 5-11. Pemphigus foliaceus (i.e., superficial pemphigus). **(A)** The clinical picture consists predominantly of superficial erosions with crust superimposed upon erythematous plaques. Intact blisters may not be observed. **(B)** Biopsy specimens of these lesions frequently reveals the base and a detached stratum corneum, which at scanning magnification may appear to represent normal skin. **(C)** Closer inspection reveals that the stratum corneum and stratum granulosum have been sloughed as the roof of a very superficial acantholytic blister. Residual acantholytic cells are easily detected by their rounded, partially detached contours *(arrows)*. The blister base in pemphigus foliaceus is therefore composed of an epidermal layer that is almost entirely intact. **(D)** This is in contrast to the blister base in pemphigus vulgaris, which is composed of an intact layer of basal cells adherent to a dermal layer exhibiting prominent, rigid dermal papillae (i.e., "tombstones").

Porphyria refers to a group of uncommon inborn or acquired disturbances of porphyrin metabolism. Porphyrins are pigments normally present in hemoglobin, myoglobin, and cytochromes. The classification of porphyrias is based on both clinical and biochemical features. The five major types are: (1) congenital erythropoietic porphyria; (2) erythrohepatic protoporphyria; (3) acute intermittent porphyria; (4) porphyria cutanea tarda; and (5) mixed porphyria. Cutaneous manifestations consist of urticaria and subepidermal

relatively noninflammatory vesicles that heal with scarring and are exacerbated by exposure to sunlight. The primary alterations seen by light microscopy are a subepidermal vesicle with associated marked thickening of vessel walls of microvessels within the superficial dermis (Fig. 5-13). The differential diagnosis includes other causes of noninflammatory subepidermal blisters (e.g., true forms of epidermolysis bullosa). These are generally easy to exclude based on clinical information.

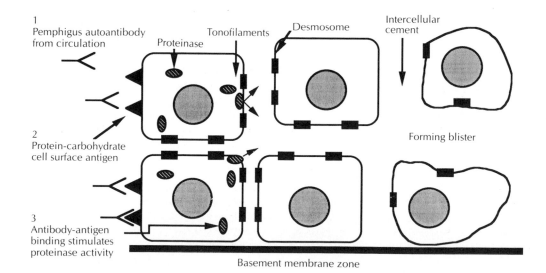

Figure 5-12. Pathogenesis of pemphigus vulgaris. Circulating antibody to intercellular cement proteins binds with relevant protein-carbohydrate cell surface antigens in the epidermal intercellular spaces (i.e., the sites where circulating IgG autoantibody is detected in lesional skin by direct immunofluorescence). This binding stimulates the synthesis of keratinocyte proteinases (e.g., plasminogen activator), resulting in gradual loosening of cell-cell adhesive bonds mediated by intercellular cement (e.g., cadherens, desmoplakin). Acantholytic cells that result are free of cell-cell attachments, and characteristically assume a rounded rather than polyhedral shape.

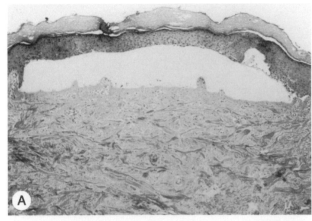

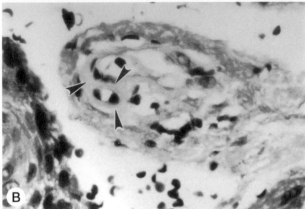

Figure 5–13. Porphyria cutanea tarda. **(A)** At scanning magnification, there is a noninflammatory subepidermal blister. Forms of epidermolysis bullosa also produce noninflammatory blisters. Toxic epidermal necrolysis, a type of cytotoxic dermatitis (see Chap. 6), is also described erroneously as another example of noninflammatory subepidermal blister formation. **(B)** The vessels in each dermal papilla have thickened, hyalinized walls *(arrowheads)* that are accentuated further by PAS stain.

Bullous Delayed Hypersensitivity Reaction

- SPONGIOSIS AT PERIPHERY OF INTRAEPIDERMAL BLISTER
- DERMAL ANGIOCENTRIC MONONUCLEAR CELL INFILTRATE
- EOSINOPHILS COMMON IN INFILTRATE
- VARIABLE DERMAL EDEMA AND FIBRIN DEPOSITION

The alterations and mechanisms responsible for the formation of intraepidermal spongiotic blisters have been discussed comprehensively in Chapter 3. In brief, one cause of intraepidermal blisters is spongiosis, in contrast to acantholysis or ballooning or reticular degeneration. Spongiosis results in mechanical lysis of intercellular adhesive connections as a result of increasing accumulation of intercellular edema. A prototypical disorder that results in spongiotic intraepidermal vesicle formation is *Rhus* contact dermatitis (i.e., poison ivy). The diagnosis of spongiotic intraepidermal vesicle formation relies on inspection of the edges of blisters at high magnification to detect widening of the intercellular space as a result of intercellular edema.

Bullous Manifestations of Ischemic Change

- SUBEPIDERMAL BLISTER WITH VARIABLE NECROSIS OF ROOF
- NONINFLAMMATORY: PRESSURE OR COMA BLISTER
    Adnexal necrosis
- INFLAMMATORY: BULLOUS VASCULITIS
    Fibrinoid necrosis of dermal vessels
    Nuclear karyorrhexis ("nuclear dust")
    Dermal hemorrhage

Blister formation may result from ischemic insult to the superficial dermis and, more commonly, to the epidermis. Injury to large vessels, which potentially may not be included in the biopsy specimen, will result in noninflammatory cytolytic injury to the basal cell layer, leading to sites of dermal-epidermal separation. Blisters caused by prolonged pressure necrosis, commonly as a result of coma due to drug ingestion or unconsciousness, will demonstrate, in addition to the more acute change of basal cell cytolysis, variable necrosis of the surface epidermal layer and notably of the epithelium of follicular and eccrine adnexae. Bullous vasculitis (Fig. 5–14) is one of the more common forms of ischemic bullae formation. In this condition, clinical bullae result from necrotizing vasculitis (see Chap. 7), involving leucocytoclasis, fibrinoid necrosis, and intralumenal thrombus formation, presumably leading to nutrient deficiency to the overlying epidermal layer.

Bullous Manifestations of Interface Change

- DERMAL-EPIDERMAL SEPARATION
- INFLAMMATORY CELLS ALIGNED ALONG THE DERMAL-EPIDERMAL INTERFACE AT BLISTER EDGE
- DYSKERATOTIC OR VACUOLATED KERATINOCYTES WITHIN THE LOWEST EPIDERMAL LAYERS

Chapter 6 contains an overview of the relevant disorders relating to bullous manifestations of interface change. These include erythema multiforme, toxic epidermal necrolysis, bullous lupus erythematosus, bullous/erosive lichen planus, and bullous fixed drug eruption. It is important to realize that just as vascular ischemia may produce blisters, so may interface dermatitis. Interface dermatitis generally results only in a band-like lymphocytic infiltrate along the dermal-epidermal interface and chronic alterations to basal cells (i.e., dyskeratosis, squamatization) that do not eventuate in dermal-epidermal separation. This observation implies that neutrophils and eosinophils may be far more potent than lymphocytes in producing the degree of acute epidermal injury that results in the formation of a subepidermal vesicle. However, in rare instances, interface dermatitis mediated by lymphocytes may produce erosive and bullous lesions due to the degree of basal cell layer and basement membrane zone destruction. The more common disorders that produce such alterations include erythema multiforme, lichen planus, and fixed drug

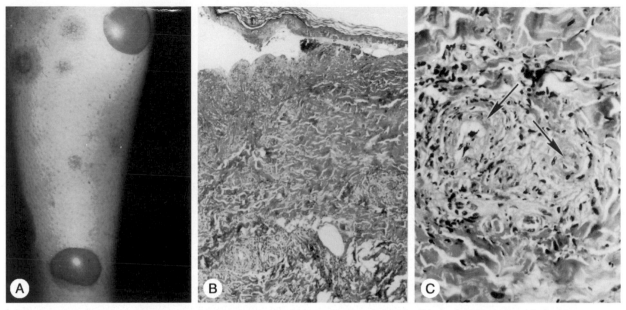

Figure 5–14. Bullous vasculitis. **(A)** Hemorrhagic blisters on purpuric bases. **(B)** Edge of vasculitis blister revealing subepidermal separation, necrotic blister roof, and basophilic inflammatory cells aggregated around superficial and mid-dermal vessels. **(C)** Higher magnification of involved dermal venules showing fibrinoid necrosis of vessel walls *(arrows)*, nuclear dust, and luminal obliteration due to endothelial necrosis and microthrombus formation.

eruption. Pityriasis lichenoides et varioliformis acuta may also result in bullous lesions due to lymphocyte-mediated dermal-epidermal separation. Bullous lupus erythematosus involves an admixture of neutrophils and lymphocytes along the basement membrane zone of a forming dermal-epidermal separation. Such lesions may mimic linear IgA disease, and direct immunofluorescence to exclude linear IgA deposits may be helpful.

Vesicles Due to Viral Infection[15, 16]

- CLUSTERED BLISTERS OR ERODED PLAQUES
- INTRAEPIDERMAL ACANTHOLYTIC BLISTER
- MULTINUCLEATED GIANT CELLS
- NUCLEAR MOLDING AND INTRANUCLEAR INCLUSIONS
- MIXED MONONUCLEAR OR NEUTROPHILIC INFLAMMATORY INFILTRATE

The most commonly encountered vesicular eruption resulting from viral infection is that of herpes simplex virus. Both the simplex and zoster variants produce grouped erythematous papules that rapidly develop central vesiculation (i.e., "dewdrops on rose petals"), although the latter occurs along a dermatomal distribution. Early vesicular lesions may be mistaken for other forms of vesicular dermatitis (e.g., acute spongiotic dermatitis, dermatitis herpetiformis; Fig. 5–15A). Older lesions may become superinfected, resulting in grouped pustules (Fig. 5–15B).

Histologically, acute early lesions of herpesvirus infection may disclose only a mixed superficial and periadnexal inflammatory infiltrate predominated by neutrophils and lymphocytes associated with disordered overlying epidermal maturation and slight cytoplasmic ballooning. Clues to the diagnosis are the presence of the mixed neutrophilic and lymphocytic (i.e., dirty) infiltrate and associated subtle epidermal changes. These changes may take the form of cytoplasmic pallor and disordered maturation, both nonspecific findings. Eventually, an intraepidermal acantholytic blister forms, which is easily detected at scanning magnification (Fig. 5–15C). Although acantholytic cells are present within the blister fluid, dyskeratotic cells are not observed. The acantholysis is not exclusively between the basal cell layer and suprabasal cells, as is the case in pemphigus vulgaris. At least some of the acantholytic cells will be multinucleated and show pallor and homogeneous clearing of nuclear chromatin, a characteristic cytopathic change of herpesvirus which correlates with the presence of intranuclear inclusions (Fig. 5–15D). The contours of the individual nuclei within the multinucleated cells mold to one another, an additional feature of diagnostic significance. As is emphasized in Figure 5–15D, these virally infected acantholytic cells may account for only a small minority of the cells within the blister cavity and therefore are easy to overlook.

Varicella-zoster has identical features to those described for herpes simplex infection, as does the exanthem of chicken pox. However, varicella-zoster often shows associated vasculitis within the superficial dermis, whereas herpes simplex does not. This vasculitis consists of a perivascular infiltrate of neutrophils and mononuclear cells with associated nuclear dust formation, fibrinoid necrosis of vessel walls, and perivascular hemorrhage. It therefore is indistinguishable from necrotizing cutaneous vasculitis. Herpesvirus infections may also at times preferentially involve the hair follicle. Therefore, follicular epithelium should also be carefully scrutinized for evidence of viral changes, particularly in biopsy specimens of vesicular dermatoses from facial or scalp skin (see Chap. 20).

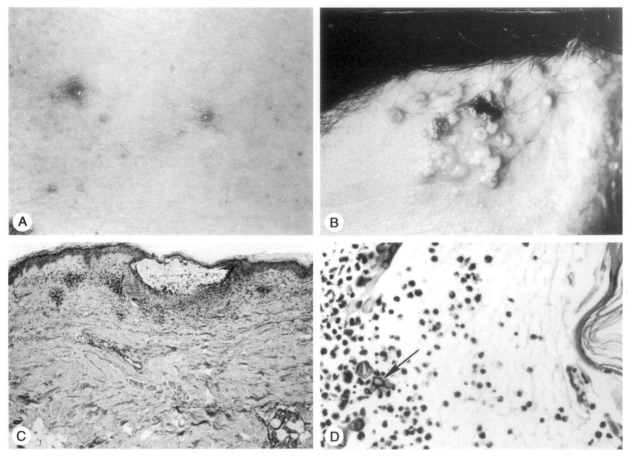

Figure 5–15. Herpesvirus infection with blister formation. **(A)** Varicella (chicken pox), showing drop-like vesicles on erythematous bases ("dew drops on rose petals"). **(B)** Herpes simplex, superinfected and presenting as grouped vesiculopustules. **(C)** Intraepidermal acantholytic vesicle with underlying dermal perivascular inflammatory infiltrate. **(D)** Vesicle cavity containing mixed inflammatory cells and rare, inconspicuous multinucleated giant cells *(arrow)* exhibiting nuclear molding and characteristic pale grey viral inclusions.

Bullae Due to Physical Factors

• NONSPONGIOTIC, NONACANTHOLYTIC INTRAEPIDERMAL BLISTER CONTAINING ERYTHROCYTES: FRICTION INJURY
• SUBEPIDERMAL BLISTER WITH KERATINOCYTE NECROSIS: THERMAL INJURY
• SUBEPIDERMAL BLISTER WITH KERATINOCYTE SHRINKAGE, DISTORTION, AND VASCULAR THROMBOSIS: FREEZE INJURY
• SUBEPIDERMAL BLISTER WITH KERATINOCYTE NUCLEAR ELONGATION AND PARALLEL ALIGNMENT: ELECTRICAL INJURY

There are a number of physical agents that may produce epidermal or dermal blisters. Unfortunately, most of these lack specific histologic alterations. Therefore, when a biopsy of a blister is encountered that does not fit well into the conventional diagnostic categories for primary immunologic or infectious vesicular disorders, it is prudent to consider external causes and to scrutinize the clinical history accordingly. *Friction blisters* are occasionally biopsied, particularly when they are associated with hemorrhage into the blister cavity which, with time, acquires a blue-black clinical appearance that may be confused with acral melanoma. Generally, biopsy reveals only an intraepidermal or subcorneal vesicle without evidence of active acantholysis or spongiosis. Inflammation is minimal. The blister cavity contains serum and erythrocytes undergoing cytolysis and coagulation necrosis. *Thermal burns* (i.e., infrared) and ultraviolet light B–induced injury (i.e., sunburn) usually produce subepidermal blisters as a result of individual cell or widespread keratinocyte necrosis. Inflammation may be minimal in comparison to the extent of epidermal injury. First-degree thermal burns differ from sunburn in that the former shows necrosis of the more superficial epidermal layers, whereas the latter shows individual cell necrosis (i.e., sunburn cells) of the basal cell layer. Second-degree thermal burns are characterized by full-thickness epidermal necrosis, usually dermal-epidermal separation and blister formation, and sometimes superficial dermal necrosis; adnexae, however, remain viable. Third-degree thermal burns involve adnexal necrosis as well as extensive dermal necrosis. It is important for the dermatopathologist to make these distinctions, because the presence of third-degree changes mandates skin grafting.

Freeze injury to viable skin produces diffuse nuclear and cytoplasmic shrinkage and distortion similar to that observed in routinely stained frozen sections. In addition, there may be evidence of widespread vascular thrombosis and subepidermal blister formation, which are probably the result of both direct epidermal injury and vascular ischemia. During the winter months in colder climates, freezing artifact may be seen in formalin-fixed tissue after transportation in fixative that was not pretreated with an antifreeze reagent. Fixed frozen tissue undergoes striking ballooning artifact to individual cells throughout the biopsy specimen that may render accurate interpretation impossible. Finally, *electrical injury* may produce dermal-epidermal separation as a result of direct epithelial necrosis, which is characterized by nuclear thinning, elongation, and alignment of each nucleus in par-

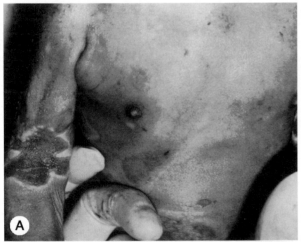

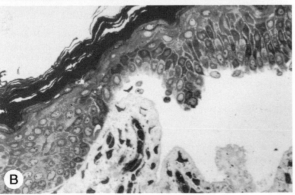

Figure 5–16. Epidermolysis bullosa. **(A)** Junctional epidermolysis bullosa showing typical erosions in flexural creases. **(B)** Dermal-epidermal blister cavity defined by 1-μm section.

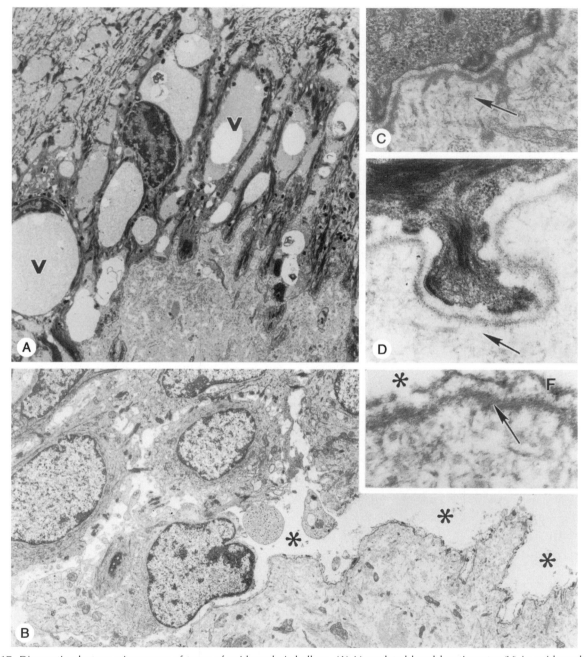

Figure 5–17. Diagnostic electron microscopy of types of epidermolysis bullosa. **(A)** Vacuolated basal keratinocytes (V) in epidermolysis bullosa simplex. **(B)** Lamina lucida split (*) in junctional epidermolysis bullosa (*note inset,* where lamina densa *[arrow]* remains on blister base; F, fibrin coat on surface of base). **(C)** Normal dermal-epidermal junction with full complement of anchoring fibrils *(arrow)* beneath the lamina densa. **(D)** Markedly diminished anchoring fibrils *(arrow)* in dystrophic (dermolytic) form of epidermolysis bullosa, at site where separation occurs beneath the lamina densa.

allel to the next diffusely throughout the specimen. Similar alterations are routinely encountered at the edges of biopsy specimens exposed to electrocautery.

Rare Disorders

- BULLOUS MASTOCYTOSIS[17]
- STAPHYLOCOCCUS SCALDED SKIN SYNDROME[18]
- BULLOUS CONGENITAL ICHTHYOSIFORM ERYTHRODERM[19]
- EPIDERMOLYSIS BULLOSA[20]
- INCONTINENTIA PIGMENTI, VESICULAR STAGE[21]

There are a number of rare disorders that may manifest clinically with vesicles and bullae. A rare variant of *mastocytosis*, for example, produces bullous lesions, although the exact pathogenesis of this phenomenon is poorly understood. *Staphylococcal scalded skin syndrome*, which is also discussed in Chapter 8, results in the formation of subcorneal blisters due to acantholysis resulting from liberation of the epidermolytic toxin exfoliatin from a distant site of infection. *Bullous congenital ichthyosiform erythroderm* is a dominantly inherited disorder characterized by diffuse epidermolytic hyperkeratosis (see Chap. 18) and superficial epidermal vesiculation within the first several years of life.

Epidermolysis bullosa consists of a family of genetically inherited disorders that present as blistering and erosive lesions at birth or soon thereafter at sites of minor trauma (Fig. 5–16A). The characteristic light microscopic morphology of epidermolysis bullosa is a subepidermal blister in the absence of inflammation (Fig. 5–16B). In addition to clinical characteristics that help to sort out the different forms of the disease, there are ultrastructural features that are also of diagnostic assistance (Fig. 5–17). For example, whereas *epidermolysis bullosa simplex* is characterized by basal cell layer cytolysis (Fig. 5–17A), *junctional epidermolysis bullosa* shows dermal-epidermal separation at the level of the lamina lucida (Fig. 5–17B). *Dystrophic or scarring variants*, on the other hand, are characterized by defective anchoring fibrils beneath the lamina densa (Fig. 5–17D), resulting in dermolytic blisters.

Finally, the *vesicular stage of incontinentia pigmenti* (also briefly discussed and illustrated in Chapter 3) is a rare bullous eruption of the newborn. It is an X-linked dominantly inherited disease characterized by an initial stage of linear erythema and bullae predominantly affecting the extremities (Fig. 5–18A). This is followed by development of verrucous and hyperpigmented lesions (see Chap. 4). The vesicles are caused by intraepidermal spongiosis (Fig. 5–18B) with associated infiltration of eosinophils and mononuclear cells. The finding of clustered dyskeratosis in association with spongiosis may be diagnostically helpful in differentiating this disorder from other forms of spongiotic dermatitis containing eosinophils.

DIFFERENTIAL DIAGNOSIS

Figure 5–19 presents an overview of some of the important branch points in the diagnostic decision making neces-

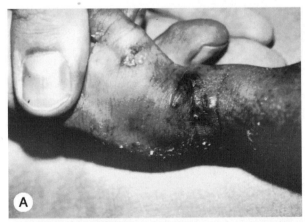

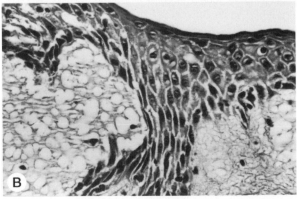

Figure 5–18. Incontinentia pigmenti, vesicular stage (see also Chap. 3). **(A)** Vesicular and pigmented lesions on distal extremity skin precede verrucous plaques that will supervene. **(B)** Histologic examination reveals the formation of large intraepidermal blisters resulting from spongiosis.

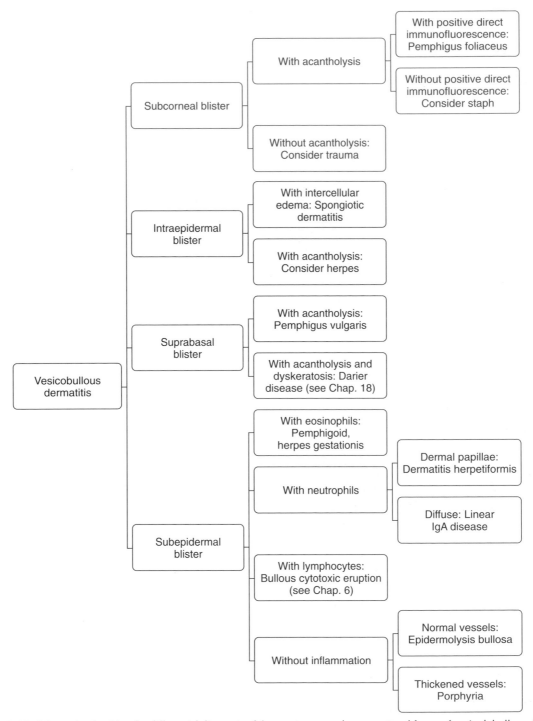

Figure 5–19. Schematic algorithm for differential diagnosis of the most commonly encountered forms of vesiculobullous dermatitis.

sary to systematically evaluate common forms of vesiculo-bullous disease. As with other similar approaches in this text, there are numerous exceptions to these rules, and oversimplification is inherent in such an approach. It provides, however, an initial approach for understanding the many potentially confusing similarities and differences among the numerous disorders that comprise the category of vesiculobullous dermatitis.

SELECTED REFERENCES

1. Farmer ER. Subepidermal bullous diseases. J Cutan Pathol 1985;12:316.
2. Nishioka K, Hashimoto K, Katayama I, et al. Eosinophilic spongiosis in bullous pemphigoid. Arch Dermatol 1984;120:1166.
3. Dvorak AM, Mihm MC Jr, Osage JE, et al. Bullous pemphigoid, an ultrastructural study of the inflammatory response. J Invest Dermatol 1982;78:91.
4. Holmes RC, Black MM. Herpes gestationis. Dermatol Clin 1983;1:195.
5. Gammon WR, Briggaman RA, Woodly DT, et al. Epidermolysis bullosa acquisita—a pemphigoid-like disease. J Am Acad Dermatol 1984;11:820.
6. Lawley TJ, Yancey KB. Dermatitis herpetiformis. Dermatol Clin 1983;1:187.
7. Braun-Falco O. Pathology of blister formation. In: Kopf AW, Andrade R, eds. Year Book of Dermatology. Chicago: Year Book Medical Publishers, 1969:16.
8. Katz SI, Hall RH, Lawley TJ, et al. Dermatitis herpetiformis: The skin and the gut. Ann Intern Med 1980;93:857.
9. Ackerman AB. Histologic Diagnosis of Inflammatory Skin Diseases: A Method of Pattern Analysis. Philadelphia: Lea & Febiger, 1978.
10. Smith SB, Harrist TJ, Murphy GF. Linear IgA bullous dermatosis vs dermatitis herpetiformis. Arch Dermatol 1984;120:324.
11. Bhogal B, Wojnarowska F, Black MM, et al. The distribution of immunoglobulins and the C3 component of complement in multiple biopsies from uninvolved and perilesional skin in pemphigus. Clin Exp Dermatol 1986;11:49.
12. Katz SJ. Blistering diseases of the skin, new insights. N Engl J Med 1985;313:1657.
13. Lever WF, Hashimoto K. The etiology and treatment of pemphigus and pemphigoid. J Invest Dermatol 1969;53:373.
14. Harber LC, Poh-Fitzpatrick MB, Walther RR. Cutaneous aspects of the porphyrias. Acta Derm Venereol (Suppl) 1982;100:9.
15. McSorsley J, Shapiro L, Brownstein MH, et al. Herpes simplex and varicella-zoster: Comparative histopathology of 77 cases. Int J Dermatol 1974;13:69.
16. Cohen C, Trapuck S. Leukocytoclastic vasculitis associated with cutaneous infections by herpesvirus. Am J Dermatopathol 1984;6:561.
17. Mihm MC, Clark WH, Reed RJ, et al. Mast cell infiltrates of the skin and the mastocytosis syndrome. Hum Pathol 1973;4:231.
18. Dimond RL, Wolff HH, Braun-Falco O. The staphylococcal scalded skin syndrome. Br J Dermatol 1977;28:483.
19. Ackerman AB. Histopathologic concept of epidermolytic hyperkeratosis. Arch Dermatol 1970;102:253.
20. Fine JD. Changing clinical and laboratory concepts in inherited epidermolysis bullosa. Arch Dermatol 1988;124:523.
21. Takematsu H, Terui T, Torinuki W, et al. Incontinentia pigmenti: Eosinophil chemotactic activity of the crusted scales in the vesiculobullous stage. Br J Dermatol 1986;115:61.

6

Cytotoxic Dermatitis

DEFINITIONS AND GENERAL CONSIDERATIONS

There are only a finite number of reaction patterns that may occur in human skin consequent to infiltration by reactive T lymphocytes. One pattern, discussed in Chapter 3, involves intercellular epidermal edema, or spongiosis. Spongiosis may occur when antigen-specific T cells of the helper subtype infiltrate at sites of antigen challenge. Other subtypes of effector lymphocytes, however, may produce very different alterations within the epidermal layer. For example, experimentally, when autosensitized cytotoxic T cells enter the skin, the pattern consistently involves degeneration and death of keratinocytes (i.e., cytotoxicity), particularly those of the lower epidermal layers. Acute cytotoxicity may take the form of basal cell layer vacuolization, an accelerated rate of programmed cell death (i.e., apoptosis), or direct cell-cell killing via effector-target cell apposition (i.e., satellitosis). Chronic cytotoxicity is manifested by abnormal keratinization (i.e., dyskeratosis), cell death with mummification of cytoplasmic contents (i.e., colloid body formation), or altered cellular maturation for a specific epidermal stratum (i.e., squamatization of the basal cell layer). These acute and chronic alterations, usually concentrated at the dermal-epidermal junction, coupled with lymphocyte infiltration along this interface, have earned for cytotoxic dermatitis the alternative designation of *interface dermatitis*.

The underlying causes of most forms of cytotoxic dermatitis are protean, although it is generally assumed that autoantigens within the epidermal layer provoke an autoimmune reaction directed against keratinocytes. In connective tissue disorders such as lupus erythematosus, the primary abnormality appears to reside in the effector pathway, with immune recognition and attack directed against epitopes that normally are exempt from host surveillance. In other settings such as erythema multiforme, infectious agents and ingested drugs are likely to alter epidermal antigens in a manner that provokes reactivity of an otherwise normal T-cell axis. In situations such as lichen planus, it remains unclear whether target or effector pathways are the primary stimulants for lesion formation.

Special note should be made regarding the meaning and significance of the term apoptosis. Although some contemporary dermatopathology authorities contend that the term should be pronounced with a silent second "p," as is the case in the term ptosis, medical dictionaries and Greek academicians agree that the preferred pronunciation is dictated by the phonetic interpretation of the spelling. Strictly speaking, the term apoptosis connotes programmed cell death. By programmed, it is implied that the cell is not simply starved as a result of nutrient depletion or ripped apart as in a traumatic wound. Rather, there are precise events determined at the genomic or receptor-mediated level that initiate nuclear degeneration involving chromosomal nicking by intrinsic endonucleases. Accordingly, apoptosis is both an event that occurs normally in the epidermis and as an essential component of follicular cycling, and an event that occurs as a result of cytotoxicity as a consequence of mediators such as tumor necrosis factor (TNF) binding to the TNF receptor, which stimulates an identical degenerative process. Apoptotic cells show progressive nuclear pyknosis as well as eventual nuclear fragmentation and cytoplasmic shrinkage such that intermediate filaments become increasingly prominent with routine histologic stains. Accordingly, such cells may appear to be dyskeratotic. Only refined stains that permit detection of chromosomal fragmentation within intact nuclei permit absolute distinction between early apoptotic cells and cells with an accelerated or abnormal program for cytoplasmic keratinization.

GROSS PATHOLOGY

The clinical appearance of cytotoxic dermatitis is very different in acute and chronic forms of disease. Because early lesions often involve abrupt destruction of the basal cell layer, there may be blister formation or erosion of the epidermal surface. Accordingly, acute forms of cytotoxic dermatitis

Table 6–1. CLINICAL APPEARANCE OF VARIOUS FORMS OF CYTOTOXIC DERMATITIS

GROSS PATHOLOGY	HISTOLOGY	REPRESENTATIVE DISORDERS
Urticarial	Dermal edema, angiocentric lymphocytic infiltrate with mild basal cell layer injury	Erythema multiforme, early
Vesiculobullous	Marked basal cell layer injury	Erythema multiforme, advanced
Erythematous plaque	Marked dermal inflammation, focal epidermal injury	Fixed drug eruption, active
Pigmented macule	Dermal melanin incontinence	Fixed drug eruption, inactive
Hyperkeratotic plaque	Epidermal hyperplasia with hyperkeratosis, focal basal layer injury	Lichen planus
Erosion	Epidermal slough after diffuse, severe, basal layer injury	Lichen planus, erosive
Translucent, scaling plaque with telangiectasia	Epidermal atrophy, hyperkeratosis, vessel ectasia	Lupus erythematosus

may be considered in the clinical differential diagnosis of primary vesiculobullous disorders of the skin (see Chap. 5). Certain chronic forms of cytotoxic dermatitis may produce lichenoid plaques as a result of inflammation and associated epidermal hyperplasia and therefore be confused with forms of psoriasiform dermatitis. Other types of chronic cytotoxic dermatitis result in epidermal atrophy, vascular ectasia, and loss of melanin pigment into the underlying dermis and therefore may be confused with variants of cutaneous T-cell lymphoma, superficial basal cell carcinomas, or even primary abnormalities of skin pigmentation. Table 6–1 describes representative examples of each clinical type of cytotoxic dermatitis.

GENERAL HISTOLOGY AND TEMPORAL EVOLUTION

The generic forms of cytotoxic dermatitis share the following common features: (1) a superficial perivascular and interstitial papillary dermal infiltrate; (2) apposition of lymphocytes along a focally damaged basal cell layer characterized by either vacuolization, dyskeratosis, or squamatization; (3) epidermotropic migration of lymphocytes associated with necrosis of epidermal cells in direct contact; and (4) epidermal pigment incontinence and dermal fibrosis or basement membrane thickening with chronicity. The evolutionary stages of cytotoxic dermatitis are diagrammed in Figure 6–1, although most disorders are routinely encountered histologically in only one or two of the multiple steps implied in this conceptual schematic. Early in the course of the disease, only a sparse superficial dermal perivascular lymphocytic infiltrate with hints of lymphoid migration into the papillary dermis may be seen. Somewhat later, lymphocytes become aligned along the dermal-epidermal interface in association with subtle evidence of basal cell layer destruction. This tagging of lymphocytes is typical of early stages of erythema multiforme, although it also may be encountered in acute and subacute forms of lupus erythematosus. Generally, the stratum corneum maintains a basket-weave configuration at this juncture, because adequate time has not elapsed for transmission of evidence of full-thickness epidermal injury. Eventually, the interstitial component of the papillary dermal infiltrate begins to fill and expand this stratum, resulting in a band-like architecture.

With chronicity, there is progressive squamatization and dyskeratosis of the basal cell layer, dyskeratosis (possibly apoptosis), melanin pigment incontinence, epidermotropism of lymphocytes with apposition to degenerating keratinocytes (when lymphocytes predominate about a single target keratinocyte, a phenomenon termed satellitosis) and abnormalities of the stratum corneum (hyperkeratosis and/or parakeratosis). In certain lesions, the dermal-epidermal interface may be so compromised that microscopic zones of cleft-like separation or even clinical bullae are formed (Fig. 6–1).

HISTOLOGY OF SPECIFIC DISORDERS

Erythema Multiforme[1, 2]

- SUPERFICIAL PERIVASCULAR LYMPHOCYTIC INFILTRATE
- LYMPHOCYTIC VASCULITIS
- TAGGING OF LYMPHOCYTES ALONG DERMAL-EPIDERMAL INTERFACE (EARLY OR AT EDGE)
- BASAL CELL VACUOLIZATION WITH BLISTER FORMATION (LATE OR AT CENTER)
- ZONAL EPIDERMAL NECROSIS

Erythema multiforme is an uncommon but not rare, self-limiting disorder that appears to be an acute cytotoxic manifestation of cell-mediated hypersensitivity to certain infections and drugs. Unlike contact allergy, which is a form of spongiotic dermatitis (see Chap. 3), erythema multiforme is a prototype of an acute cytotoxic reaction pattern. This disorder may affect individuals of any age and is associated with the following conditions: (1) infections such as herpes simplex, mycoplasma, histoplasmosis, coccidioidomycosis, typhoid, and leprosy; (2) administration of certain drugs, such as sulfonamides, penicillin, barbiturates, salicylates, hydantoins, and antimalarials; (3) malignancy (i.e., carcinomas and lymphomas); and (4) collagen-vascular (i.e., connective tissue) diseases, such as lupus erythematosus, dermatomyositis, and polyarteritis nodosa.

Clinically, affected individuals present with an array of "multiform" lesions, including macules, papules, vesicles, and bullae, as well as the characteristic target lesion, consisting of a red macule or papule with a pale, vesicular or eroded center (Figs. 6–2A and 6–3A). Although lesions may be widely distributed, symmetric involvement of the extremities frequently occurs. An extensive and symptomatic febrile form of the disease, which is more common in children, is called the *Stevens-Johnson syndrome*. In this disorder, erosions and hemorrhagic crusts involve the lips and oral mucosa. In addition, the conjunctiva, urethra, and anogenital regions may also be involved. Life-threatening sepsis may

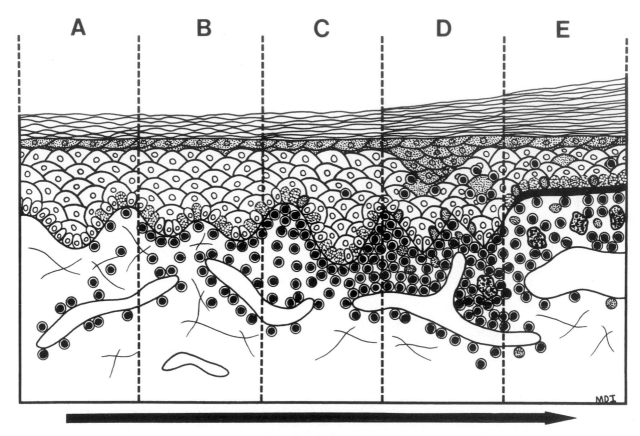

Figure 6–1. Temporal evolution of acute and chronic phases of cytotoxic dermatitis. **(A–C)** The temporal evolution of prototypical cytotoxic dermatitis commences with a dermal angiocentric infiltrate with progressive alignment or tagging of lymphocytes along the dermal-epidermal interface. This is associated with degenerative alterations in basal keratinocytes. Note that by **C**, the infiltrate has begun to fill the papillary dermis, producing a band-like interstitial pattern as well as an angiocentric pattern. **(D)** In certain disorders, such as lichen planus, chronicity takes the form of hyperkeratosis, hypergranulosis, and redefinition of the rete ridge pattern to form jagged ''teeth.'' Note satellitosis of lymphocytes about midepidermal keratinocytes undergoing degenerative changes. **(E)** In other conditions, such as discoid lupus erythematosus, chronicity produces hyperkeratosis and epidermal atrophy, with complete loss of the rete ridge pattern. Thickening of the basement membrane characteristically occurs in this disorder. Chronic destruction of basal cells containing melanin also results in accumulation of melanophages within the papillary dermis (**D, E:** *melanophages, larger cells amidst lymphocytes*).

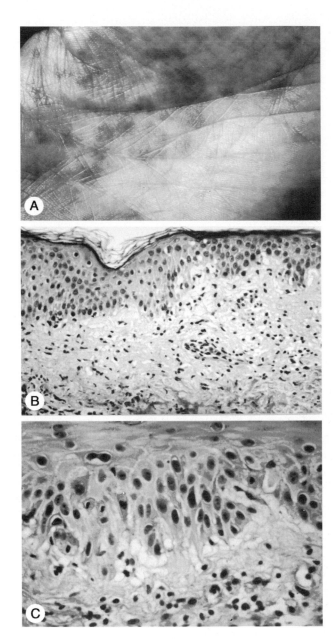

Figure 6–2. Erythema multiforme, early lesion. **(A)** Erythematous macules and dermal plaques on the palm are the result of **(B)** superficial perivascular lymphocytic infiltration with associated papillary dermal edema. **(C)** Higher magnification discloses characteristic early tagging of occasional lymphocytes along the dermal-epidermal interface, with early vacuolization of basal keratinocytes.

result due to infection of involved areas in Stevens-Johnson syndrome. Another variant of erythema multiforme, termed *toxic epidermal necrolysis*, is characterized by diffuse necrosis and sloughing of cutaneous and mucosal epithelial surfaces. This produces a clinical picture similar to that of an extensive thermal burn.

Histologically, the earliest phases of erythema multiforme are characterized by alignment or tagging of lymphocytes along a focally vacuolated dermal-epidermal interface (Fig. 6–2B, C). At this juncture, there is an associated superficial perivascular lymphocytic infiltrate, often containing eosinophils, and papillary dermal edema. As lymphocytes migrate into the epidermis, they appear to provoke single-cell and focally clustered epidermal necrosis. With progressive accumulation of lymphocytes along a damaged dermal-epidermal interface (Fig. 6–3B, C), subepidermal blister formation eventually ensues (Fig. 6–3D). The roof of the blister often shows extensive necrosis (Fig. 6–3D), and in healing

lesions, the roof may cover a blister base lined with a new, re-epithelializing layer of flattened keratinocytes (Fig. 6–3E).

Some observers have categorized erythema multiforme as a type of lymphocytic vasculitis. Although the degree of vascular injury is not akin to that observed in necrotizing cutaneous vasculitis mediated by neutrophils, there indeed is endothelial enlargement, subtle degenerative alterations, and perivascular hemorrhage in erythema multiforme. These features may be useful in diagnosing early lesions, when predominantly dermal alterations are present.

Acute Graft-Versus-Host Disease[3, 4]

- SPARSE SUPERFICIAL PERIVASCULAR LYMPHOCYTIC INFILTRATE
- SATELLITE CELL NECROSIS WITHIN EPIDERMIS
- DISORDERED EPIDERMAL MATURATION

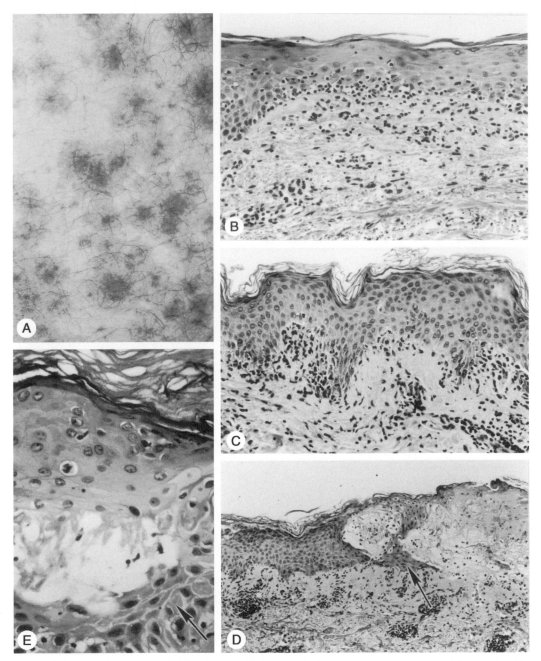

Figure 6–3. Erythema multiforme, advanced and healing lesions. **(A)** Targetoid plaques are formed by central zones of epidermal necrosis and incipient vesiculation surrounded by a peripheral, advancing, erythematous rim. **(B, C)** The rim shows well-developed alterations, which are depicted in Figure 6–2B, C. Note the extensive lymphocyte tagging and basal cell layer vacuolization. **(D)** The center of the lesion *(right)* shows full-thickness epidermal necrosis with early detachment of the epidermal layer. The underlying dermis has already been partially recovered by re-epithelialization *(arrows)*. **(E)** The basal cells of the former blister roof are ragged and necrotic. The basal cells of the re-epithelialized layer *(arrow)* are infiltrated by lymphocytes, indicating that complete resolution of the inflammatory component has not yet occurred.

Acute graft-versus-host disease (GVHD) is a major complication of allogeneic bone marrow transplantation. It is perhaps more common than is generally realized, because it also may be provoked by transfusion of nonirradiated blood products. GVHD is divided into two phases: acute disease, with an onset within 100 days of bone marrow transplantation, and chronic disease, which occurs after the first 100 days. This definition is somewhat arbitrary, however, and variations to this time frame exist. Although acute GVHD is predominated by epidermal alterations, chronic GVHD is characterized by dermal sclerosis that clinically and histolog-

ically is virtually indistinguishable from scleroderma. Biopsy of acute GVHD is generally performed to exclude drug eruption and viral exanthem. Acute GVHD is characterized clinically by an ill-defined maculopapular eruption that frequently involves the skin of the palms and soles (Fig. 6–4A). Suspicion of acute GVHD is heightened when abnormal liver function tests or diarrhea exist, because the liver and gut are also main targets of the cytotoxic attack.

Histologically, a helpful diagnostic feature of acute GVHD is the presence of significant epidermal injury (i.e., basal cell layer vacuolization and single cell necrosis) that is

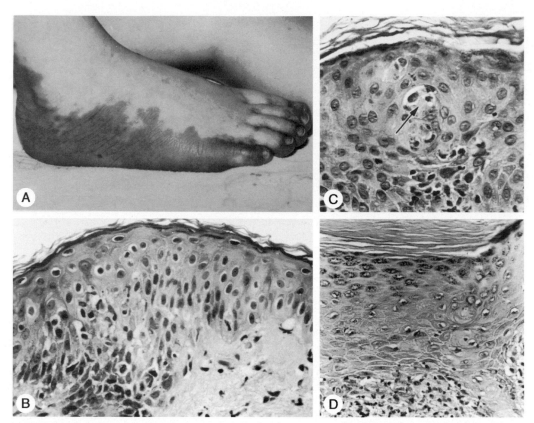

Figure 6–4. Acute and chronic graft-versus-host disease. **(A)** There is confluent erythema of the palms and soles; elsewhere on the body surface there may be a maculopapular exanthem. **(B)** The histology is characterized by a relatively sparse infiltrate of lymphocytes within the papillary dermis, with migration of these cells into the overlying epidermal layer. **(C)** Both basal cell layer vacuolization and satellitosis may occur; the latter is characterized by aggregation of intraepidermal lymphocytes about a target keratinocyte undergoing necrosis *(arrow).* **(D)** Lesions depicted in **A–C** above may become chronic, with progressive epidermal hyperplasia, hypergranulosis, and hyperkeratosis as well as development of a jagged dermal-epidermal interface infiltrated by lymphocytes in apposition to necrotic keratinocytes. These alterations resemble those of classic lichen planus, although the clinical setting in which they occur is very different. Acute graft-versus-host disease may also produce dermal sclerosis that is indistinguishable from scleroderma in certain individuals (i.e., dermal or sclerodermoid type).

out of proportion to a relatively sparse superficial dermal perivascular lymphocytic infiltrate (Fig. 6–4*B*). A characteristic finding is satellite cell necrosis, or satellitosis, a reaction pattern whereby a necrotic keratinocyte, commonly referred to as an apoptotic cell, is surrounded by several lymphocytes in direct apposition (Fig. 6–4*C*). Although originally described in experimental acute GVHD, this finding is not entirely specific and also may be observed in other forms of cytotoxic dermatitis, such as lichen planus and erythema multiforme. Because the term apoptosis, when rigidly defined, implies programmed cell death, it remains to be determined whether many of the necrotic cells in certain forms of cytotoxic dermatitis represent true apoptotic cells. Other features that may be seen in acute GVHD include increased mitotic activity and abnormal or disordered epidermal maturation. Early acute GVHD may have extraordinarily subtle findings, necessitating serial biopsies at 7- to 10-day intervals to assess disease progression, which is generally expected to occur in this disorder, as opposed to viral exanthems. One helpful site to examine at early time points (e.g., 2 to 3 weeks after transplantation or transfusion) is the infundibulum of hair follicles, which in both experimental and human disease has proven to be a very early site of target cell injury. The histology of chronic GVHD may resemble lichen planus

(Fig. 6–4*D*) or may be indistinguishable from scleroderma (see Chap. 19).

Pityriasis Lichenoides et Varioliformis Acuta[5]

- SUPERFICIAL AND DEEP PERIVASCULAR LYMPHOCYTIC INFILTRATE
- LYMPHOCYTIC VASCULITIS WITH PAPILLARY DERMAL AND INTRAEPIDERMAL HEMORRHAGE
- BASAL CELL LAYER VACUOLIZATION AND ZONAL EPIDERMAL NECROSIS
- FOCAL PARAKERATOSIS CONTAINING NEUTROPHILS

Pityriasis lichenoides et varioliformis acuta (PLEVA) is a disorder characterized by successive crops of erythematous papules and nodules, predominantly involving the skin of the trunk. Individual lesions last for several weeks and are characterized by juicy red papules that may undergo central necrosis (Fig. 6–5*A*). New crops of lesions frequently develop

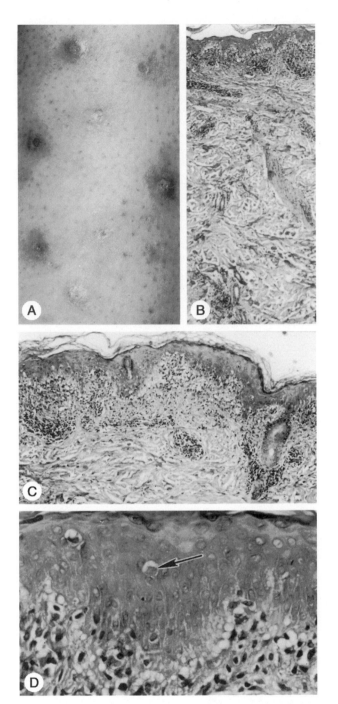

Figure 6–5. Pityriasis lichenoides et varioliformis acuta. (**A**) Biopsy specimens of erythematous, indurated nodules generally reveal (**B**) a superficial and deep angiocentric dermal infiltrate with an interface component at scanning magnification. Upon closer inspection, early focal parakeratosis, basal cell layer vacuolization (**C, D**), and hemorrhage into the papillary dermis are observed. In more advanced lesions, individual and zonal epidermal necrosis (**D,** *arrow*) and infiltration of parakeratotic scale by neutrophils are generally detected.

before old ones have completely resolved; therefore, the entire clinical course may last for several to many months. The clinical appearance of the lesions may prompt a differential diagnosis that includes insect-bite reaction, lymphomatoid papulosis or other lymphohematopoietic disorders, or pityriasis lichenoides chronica (PLC). PLC is regarded as a mild, superficial, more persistent variant of PLEVA.

At scanning magnification, the inflammatory infiltrate in PLEVA shows a superficial and deep angiocentric pattern as well as a cytotoxic (i.e., lichenoid) pattern of infiltration along the dermal-epidermal junction (Fig. 6–5B). At higher magnification, the lichenoid portion of the infiltrate is associated with basal cell layer vacuolization and epidermotropism with associated satellitosis (Fig. 6–5C, D). Often, single-cell and zonal necrosis involving clusters of keratinocytes independent of infiltrating lymphocytes are also observed. The stratum corneum may show foci of parakeratosis infiltrated by neutrophils. Perivascular extravasation of erythrocytes is frequently present about superficial vessels, an indicator that in addition to erythema multiforme, PLEVA may represent yet another example of lymphocytic vasculitis. PLC demonstrates many of the features of PLEVA, but in PLC, the dermal infiltrate spares the deep vessels, and dermal pigment incontinence is also apparent.

Table 6–2 summarizes some of the salient differential diagnostic features of PLEVA and conditions with which it may be clinically and histologically confused.

Lupus Erythematosus and Dermatomyositis[6–8]

- LYMPHOCYTIC INFILTRATE WITHIN PAPILLARY DERMIS AND PERIADNEXAL ADVENTITIA
- BASAL CELL LAYER VACUOLIZATION WITH VARIABLE COLLOID BODY FORMATION
- EPIDERMAL ATROPHY WITH HYPERKERATOSIS
- DERMAL MUCIN DEPOSITION

The cutaneous manifestations of lupus erythematosus are many and varied, and include: (1) classic discoid lupus erythematosus; (2) acute and subacute forms of discoid lupus erythematosus, characterized by subtle histologic changes and neutrophils along the dermal-epidermal interface; (3) predominantly dermal forms of lupus, including lupus panniculitis (see Chap. 10); and (4) necrotizing vasculitic lesions (see Chap. 7). In addition, the malar erythema of systemic lupus erythematosus is a distinctive clinical lesion but is not characterized by specific diagnostic findings in biopsy specimens. Clinically, discoid plaques of lupus erythematosus, which predominate in disease localized just to the skin but may also occur in the setting of systemic disease, are well-defined lesions characterized by erythema, telangiectasia, epidermal atrophy with occasional slight scale, and variability in pigmentation (Fig. 6–6A). Lesions may contain patulous follicular infundibula filled with cornified plugs. As a rule, discoid plaques are asymptomatic and preferentially affect the scalp, face, upper trunk, and upper extremities. Scalp lesions are frequently associated with alopecia (Fig. 6–6B), and therefore must be considered in the differential diagnosis of inflammatory alopecia (see Chap. 20).

The histologic alterations of discoid lupus erythematosus are characteristic. At scanning magnification, there is diffuse epidermal atrophy with loss of rete ridges (Fig. 6–6C). Appendages are either diminished due to local destruction, or atrophic, with thinned epithelium forming follicular infundibula. The surface scale is composed of increased amounts of compacted orthokeratin, and ectatic follicles are plugged with similarly abnormal keratin. The inflammatory

Table 6–2. DIFFERENTIAL DIAGNOSTIC FEATURES OF PLEVA

	PLEVA	PLC	LYMPHOMATOID* PAPULOSIS	INSECT-BITE REACTION
Infiltrate				
Depth	Superficial and deep	Superficial	Superficial and deep	Superficial and deep
Location	Angiocentric and lichenoid	Angiocentric and lichenoid	Angiocentric and interstitial	Angiocentric and interstitial
Composition	Lymphocytes	Lymphocytes	Lymphocytes and atypical Reed-Sternberg–like cells	Lymphocytes and eosinophils
Spongiosis	Absent	Absent	Absent	Often present
Dyskeratosis	Present	Present	Absent	Usually absent
Vascular injury	Variable	Absent	Prominent	Variable

*See Chapter 14 for further information.

infiltrate is perivascular and periadnexal, and involves the superficial and deep dermis. There is also a variably dense lichenoid infiltrate along the dermal-epidermal interface, which shows coarse vacuolization of the stratum basalis (Fig. 6–6D) and, with PAS staining, variable thickening of the basement membrane. Occasional dyskeratotic cells, sites of satellitosis, and superficial dermal colloid bodies may also be observed. A helpful feature in making the diagnosis is the presence of diffuse mucin deposition within the superficial and deep dermis, recognized as finely granular strands of pale, grey-blue material dispersed within the slightly widened spaces separating collagen bundles. The use of a combined alcian blue–PAS stain permits visualization of dermal mucin and the widened basement membrane in a single section.

Certain lesions of lupus erythematosus show a predominance of dermal alterations with only minor or subtle alterations of the surface epidermis. For diagnostic purposes, such lesions are referred to as lupus erythematosus of predominantly dermal type. Lupus erythematosus of the face may show predominantly follicular involvement. As mentioned previously, acute, subacute, and bullous variants of lupus are characterized by very subtle interface change, often without significant atrophy. A clue to the diagnosis is the presence of neutrophils along the dermal-epidermal junction, a feature that may cause confusion with linear IgA disease. A rare and fascinating histologic variant of lupus erythematosus produces hypertrophic lesions exhibiting verrucous epidermal hyperplasia in the presence of cytotoxic alterations along the dermal-epidermal interface. The histology of dermatomyositis is generally indistinguishable from that of lupus erythematosus; immunofluorescence, serologic, and clinical findings are therefore critical to differentiating between the cutaneous lesions of these two disorders.

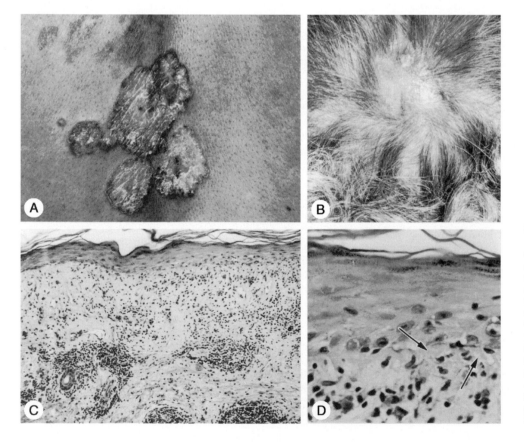

Figure 6–6. Lupus erythematosus. **(A)** Discoid plaques of lupus erythematosus clinically show erythema, central atrophy and hyperkeratosis, and peripheral hyperpigmentation. **(B)** When hair-bearing surfaces are affected, hair loss often occurs. **(C, D)** Histologically, there is a superficial, deep, perivascular and periadnexal infiltrate of lymphocytes; dermal pallor resulting from infiltration of pale-staining, particulate mucin; and diffuse epidermal atrophy with associated basal cell layer vacuolization and hyperkeratosis. Note the association of subepidermal lymphocytes with degenerating basal cells in **D** (arrows).

Lichen Planus[9, 10]

- BAND-LIKE INFILTRATE OF LYMPHOCYTES IN PAPILLARY DERMIS
- EPIDERMAL HYPERPLASIA WITH ZONAL HYPERGRANULOSIS AND HYPERKERATOSIS
- SQUAMATIZATION AND DYSKERATOSIS OF BASAL CELL LAYER
- OCCASIONAL CLEFTS BETWEEN EPIDERMIS AND DERMIS DUE TO BASAL CELL LAYER DESTRUCTION
- PAPILLARY DERMAL COLLOID BODY FORMATION
- "SAW-TOOTH" DERMAL-EPIDERMAL INTERFACE
- PAPILLARY DERMAL FIBROSIS (OLD LESIONS)

The clinical signs and symptoms of lichen planus account for their description as pruritic, pink, polygonal papules. This common disorder presents as crops of flat-topped papules, often arranged in linear configuration, presumably elicited at sites of trauma (i.e., Koebner phenomenon; Fig. 6–7A). The surface of individual lesions show delicate white lines known as Wickham striae. These appear to correlate with hyperplastic rete ridges, which intimately interdigitate with dermal papillae replete with lymphocytes. Coalescence of individual papules may result in plaques that mimic psoriasis or other forms of chronic dermatitis. Lichen planus–like drug eruptions also occur commonly; therefore, the clinical differential diagnosis may also include iatrogenic causes. The pathogenesis of lichen planus remains obscure; leading hypotheses implicate cell-mediated autoimmune mechanisms. The fact that chronic epidermal injury in lichenoid variants of GVHD may be indistinguishable histologically from ordinary lichen planus supports this hypothesis.

At scanning magnification, the histologic alterations of lichen planus are characteristic. There is epidermal hyperplasia with hyperkeratosis and acanthosis associated with an epidermal-dermal junction that resembles the teeth of a saw (Fig. 6–7B) rather than the normally smooth, undulant interface between rete redges and dermal papillae. At higher magnification, the basal cell layer shows variable vacuolization, dyskeratosis, and prominent squamatization (Fig. 6–7C) in association with a lymphocytic infiltrate that is intimately associated with these epidermal alterations. With chronicity and resolution, this lymphocytic infiltrate becomes less pronounced, and the papillary dermis may acquire deposits of thickened collagen bundles. Moreover, the mid- and lower epidermis, as well as the papillary dermis, may contain individual and clustered dyskeratotic cells (Fig. 6–7D). These presumed targets of cytotoxic attack are the colloid bodies that contain IgM on inspection by direct immunofluorescence (see Chap. 2).

Lichen planus may preferentially involve follicular infundibular epithelium as well as interfollicular epithelium in a diffuse manner, leading to localized follicular papules (Fig. 6–8A) or clinical erythroderma, respectively (see Chap. 20). This condition, known as *lichen planopilaris*, is characterized by peri-infundibular lymphocytic infiltrates (Fig. 6–8B), which induce many of the alterations in infundibular epithelium that are produced in interfollicular epithelium in ordinary lichen planus. These alterations include follicular infun-

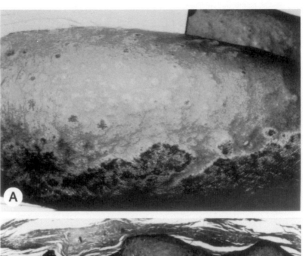
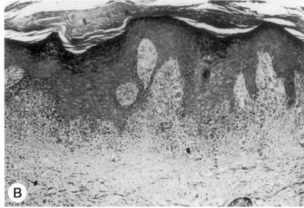
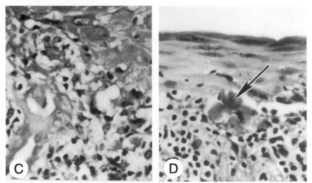

Figure 6–7. Lichen planus. **(A)** Clinically, lichen planus is characterized by numerous flat, pruritic papules which may coalesce to form hyperkeratotic plaques. Marked associated hyperpigmentation, resulting from chronic dermal pigment incontinence, is also present in this individual. **(B)** The characteristic histology of lichen planus at scanning magnification involves a band-like infiltrate of lymphocytes within the papillary dermis that is intimately associated with a jagged dermal-epidermal interface. The epidermal layer is hyperplastic, with hypergranulosis and hyperkeratosis. **(C, D)** At higher magnification, lymphocytes infiltrating the dermal-epidermal interface are associated with basal cells with a polyhedral contour (i.e., squamatized cells) (*upper right corner of* **C**) and small eosinophilic bodies (i.e., colloid bodies, *arrow*) representing necrotic, anucleate epidermal cells.

dibular acanthosis, hypergranulosis, hyperkeratosis, and infundibular basal cell layer dyskeratosis and squamatization (Fig. 6–8C).

The histologic differential diagnosis of lichen planus includes lichen planus–like drug eruption, benign lichen planus–like keratoses, lichenoid actinic keratosis, lichenoid secondary syphilis, and lichenoid GVHD. Table 6–3 sum-

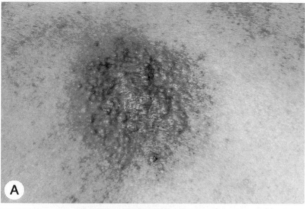

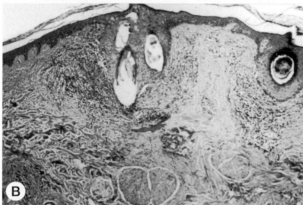

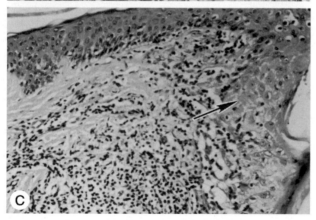

Figure 6–8. Lichen planus, follicular involvement (i.e., lichen plano-pilaris). **(A)** A cluster of follicular papules is associated with hyperpigmentation indicative of chronic destruction of pigment-containing epithelial cells. **(B)** At scanning magnification, there is an interface infiltrate of lymphocytes about the dilated and plugged follicular infundibula. **(C)** The infiltrate does not extend as deeply as in follicular lupus erythematosus, and the follicular epithelium is hyperplastic, not atrophic *(arrow).* As is the case in interfollicular lichen planus, the infundibular epithelium may also show hyperkeratosis and hypergranulosis, and the basal cells infiltrated by lymphocytes may demonstrate squamatization and colloid body formation.

marizes the salient differences and similarities among these diagnostic considerations.

Lichen Nitidus[11]

- FOCAL MICRONODULE OF HISTIOCYTES IN PAPILLARY DERMIS
- EPIDERMAL COLLARETTE ABOUT HISTIOCYTIC NODULE
- BASAL CELL VACUOLIZATION AND DYSKERATOSIS OVERLYING HISTIOCYTES

The clinical picture of lichen nitidus is predominated by multiple, often grouped, nonfollicular, asymptomatic, flesh-colored papules (Fig. 6–9A). Unlike lichen planus, lesions are quite small (i.e., 1 to 3 mm), do not coalesce, and do not itch. Skin of the upper extremities, abdomen, and penis are most frequently involved.

Histologically, lichen nitidus demonstrates a rounded aggregate of mononuclear cells within the superficial dermis, beneath a thinned epidermal layer and often surrounded by a peripheral epithelial collarette (Fig. 6–9B). The overlying stratum corneum may show parakeratosis, and the basal cell layer overlying the inflammatory infiltrate may be vacuolated or squamatized. Occasional colloid bodies, as seen in lichen planus, may also be observed at the dermal-epidermal interface. At higher magnification, the inflammatory dermal component is predominantly composed of histiocytes (Fig. 6–9C) admixed with lymphocytes. In contrast to lymphocytes, the histiocytic component is characterized by mononuclear cells with larger, paler nuclei and abundant pink cytoplasm. The primary diagnostic differences between lichen nitidus and lichen planus are detailed in Table 6–3.

Lichenoid Reaction Patterns[12, 13]

- MIXED PAPILLARY DERMAL INFILTRATE (PLASMA CELLS, EOSINOPHILS)
- PARAKERATOTIC SCALE
- POSSIBLE KERATINOCYTE DYSPLASIA (LICHENOID ACTINIC KERATOSIS)

There are a number of commonly encountered disorders that may mimic primary lichen planus or lichen nitidus as a result of the presence of a lichenoid reaction pattern. Common to all of these disorders is a band-like infiltrate of lymphocytes, often admixed with other cell types, within the papillary dermis. As in lichen planus and lichen nitidus, the basal cell layer may show evidence of chronic cytotoxic destruction, with vacuolization, squamatization, and colloid body formation. The reason for the development of lichenoid reaction patterns is unclear, although it most probably relates

Table 6–3. DIFFERENTIAL DIAGNOSIS OF LICHEN NITIDUS AND LICHEN PLANUS

	LICHEN NITIDUS	**LICHEN PLANUS**
Size	0.1–0.3 cm	0.5–1 cm
Pruritus	Usually absent	Usually present
Coalescence	Unusual	Frequently occurs
Collarette	Present	Absent
Epidermal hyperplasia	Absent	Present
Epidermal atrophy	Present	Usually absent
Parakeratosis	Present	Absent
Lymphocytes	Minor population	Predominant population
Histiocytes	Predominant population	Minor population

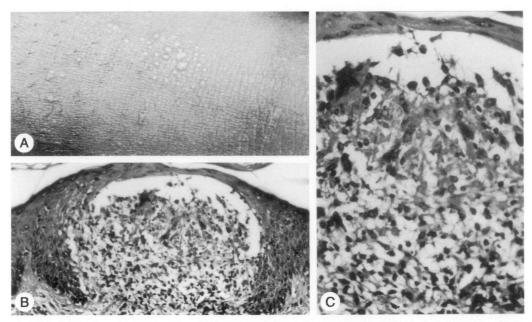

Figure 6–9. Lichen nitidus. **(A)** Multiple nonfollicular papules, smaller than the flat-topped papules of lichen planus, are observed clinically. **(B)** Histologically, there is a micronodule of inflammatory cells (i.e., histiocytes and lymphocytes) embraced by an epidermal collarette. Interface changes similar to those observed in lichen planus are observed in the basal cell layer of the overlying epidermis. **(C)** At high magnification, the majority of inflammatory cells are histiocytic. The overlying epidermis is separated from the infiltrate by a cleft-like space resulting from destruction of basal cells and associated dermal-epidermal integrity.

to the local or systemic sensitization of cytotoxic cells to autoantigens within the epidermis.

Common causes of lichenoid reaction patterns include lichenoid actinic keratoses, solitary lichenoid keratoses, and lichen planus–like drug eruptions. Lichenoid keratoses are discussed in greater depth in Chapter 11. Generally, the presence of true keratinocyte dysplasia within the lower epidermal layers distinguishes lichenoid actinic keratoses from all other forms of lichenoid reaction. The presence of parakeratosis is also helpful in differentiating lichenoid reactions from lichen planus, which shows only hyperkeratosis. When lymphocytes predominate in the inflammatory infiltrate, detection of rare plasma cells and/or eosinophils is also of assistance in making the diagnosis, because in true lichen planus, there is a relatively pure infiltrate of small lymphocytes. Lichen planus–like drug eruptions may closely mimic lichen planus, except for the presence of easily observed eosinophils within the band-like inflammatory component of the former (Fig. 6–10).

Fixed Drug Eruption[14, 15]

- SUPERFICIAL PERIVASCULAR AND PAPILLARY DERMAL LYMPHOCYTIC INFILTRATE
- DEEP PERIVASCULAR COMPONENT AND/OR EOSINOPHILS SOMETIMES PRESENT
- BASAL CELL LAYER VACUOLIZATION
- MELANIN WITHIN PAPILLARY DERMAL MACROPHAGES (PIGMENT INCONTINENCE)

Fixed drug eruption is both clinically and histologically distinctive. As the name implies, the lesion occurs repeatedly at the same site after drug ingestion. Common offenders include trimethoprim-sulfamethoxazole, aspirin, tetracycline, phenolphthalein, phenylbutazone, and an extensive list of other pharmaceutical agents, including oral contraceptives. The active lesion consists of an erythematous, edematous plaque (Fig. 6–11A). As the plaque flares up and subsides, melanin pigment is deposited, imparting a gray-brown hue. Inactive phases are characterized by macular zones of hyperpigmentation demarcating the site of the preceding plaque. With repeated eruptions followed by quiescent periods at a single site, progressive macular darkening occurs. Any cutaneous site may be affected, although the glans penis is a frequent region of involvement.

Histologically, fixed drug eruptions demonstrate a lichenoid (i.e., cytotoxic) pattern of lymphocytic infiltration within the papillary dermis, along with a superficial and at least mid-dermal perivascular lymphocytic infiltrate (Fig. 6–11B). Occasional eosinophils and activated histiocytes may also be admixed within the infiltrate. At higher magnification, lymphocytes are present along a vacuolated dermal-epidermal junction, which may show colloid body formation (Fig. 6–11C). Lymphocytes also migrate into the epidermis, where they are associated with zones or clusters of necrotic keratinocytes, a finding similar to that seen in erythema multiforme. In active as well as inactive lesions, there is often striking melanin pigment incontinence within the underlying papillary dermis (Fig. 6–11D). It should be remembered, however, that any cytotoxic dermatitis may result in marked papillary dermal deposition of melanin pigment in black skin; therefore, the finding of pigment incontinence need not indicate repeated insult or chronicity in that setting.

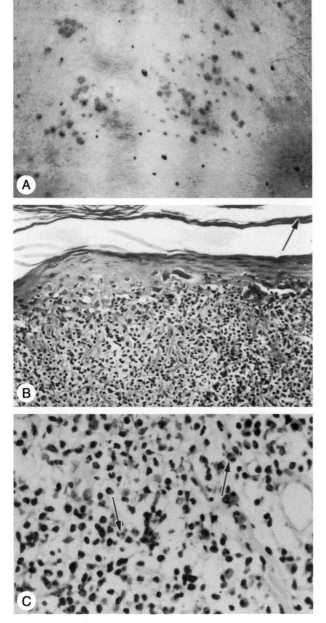

Figure 6–10. Lichenoid drug eruption. **(A)** Multiple flat, erythematous papules are observed clinically (smaller, darker papules are incidental hemangiomas). **(B)** At medium magnification, there is a band-like inflammatory infiltrate associated with chronic interface changes with prominent single-cell epidermal necrosis with colloid body formation. The scale shows focal compact hyperkeratosis *(arrow)* and parakeratosis. **(C)** Eosinophils *(arrows)* as well as lymphocytes are observed in the infiltrate, in contrast to true lichen planus, which contains only lymphocytes.

Secondary Syphilis[16]

- BAND-LIKE PAPILLARY DERMAL LYMPHOCYTIC INFILTRATE WITH PLASMA CELLS AND POORLY FORMED GRANULOMAS
- SUPERFICIAL DERMAL VESSEL LUMENS INCONSPICUOUS DUE TO ENDOTHELIAL SWELLING
- BASAL CELL LAYER VACUOLIZATION
- VARIABLE EPIDERMAL ATROPHY OR HYPERPLASIA

Secondary syphilis is recognized both clinically and histologically as the mimic of a number of unrelated conditions. With regard to clinical appearance, secondary syphilis frequently presents as small, erythematous plaques that resemble pityriasis rosea or small-plaque parapsoriasis. It may also present with lichenoid or psoriasiform lesions; the latter are often referred to as rupial secondary syphilis. Involvement of the palms, soles, and mucosal surfaces may be a helpful clue to alert the clinician to the possibility of secondary syphilis (Fig. 6–12A).

Histologically, lichenoid secondary syphilis demonstrates a band-like infiltrate of lymphocytes and histiocytes within the papillary dermis. The epidermis shows a variable degree of injury to the basal cell layer (Fig. 6–12B). The epidermis is usually not acanthotic with a jagged dermal-epidermal interface, as is seen in lichen planus; rather, the epidermal rete may be lost and the epidermal layer thinned, or the rete may demonstrate psoriasiform hyperplasia, with the epidermal layer thickened. A diagnostic clue may be the presence of unusual numbers of activated histiocytes, often associated with vague foci of granuloma formation. Another helpful clue is the detection of plasma cells and enlarged or

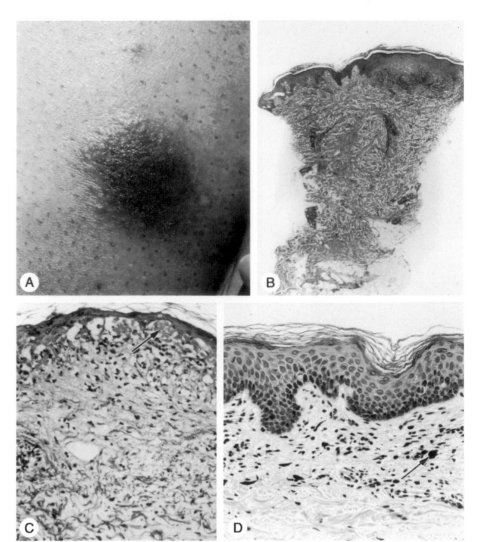

Figure 6–11. Fixed drug eruption. **(A)** A chronic zone of macular hyperpigmentation has become indurated and peripherally erythematous. This is indicative of recrudescence of this fixed form of cytotoxic dermatitis. **(B, C)** Histologically, there is a superficial and mid-dermal angiocentric infiltrate, as well as a prominent lichenoid component within the papillary dermis. Zonal necrosis of keratinocytes *(arrow)* may also be observed. Inflammatory destruction of basal cells with associated dermal melanophage formation is the hallmark of fixed drug eruption. **(D)** Inactive phases may only demonstrate persistent melanophages within the papillary dermis *(arrow)*.

activated endothelial cells within the papillary dermis (Fig. 6–12*C*). At times, the degree of endothelial swelling is so pronounced that vascular lumens are no longer detectable. Silver stains (i.e., Warthin-Starry or Dieterle) may disclose thin, spiraling spirochetes amidst the dermal infiltrate and within the epidermal layer or follicular structures. Special stains are often negative, however, with the exception of the hyperplastic variant of secondary syphilis that affects mucosal surfaces, condyloma lata. In the setting of lichenoid dermatitis that contains plasma cells, vague granulomatous foci, or marked occusive endothelial activation, or that presents clinically as a nonlichenoid dermatitis (e.g., pityriasis rosea, guttate parapsoriasis, psoriasis), it is often prudent to raise the possibility of syphilis and recommend appropriate serologic testing. Special stains should also be performed, because a small number will yield positive results, and because seronegative lesions may occur in the setting of immunodeficiency.

Lichenoid Eruption of AIDS[17]

- SPARSE SUPERFICIAL PERIVASCULAR AND INTERSTITIAL LYMPHOCYTIC INFILTRATE
- OCCASIONAL PLASMA CELLS
- SATELLITE CELL KERATINOCYTE NECROSIS
- DISORDERED EPIDERMAL MATURATION

Patients with acquired immunodeficiency syndrome (AIDS) or AIDS-related complex (ARC) may develop generalized maculopapular exanthems that resemble morbilliform drug eruptions and viral exanthems (Fig. 6–13*A*). Unlike drug eruptions or viral rashes occurring in immunologically intact individuals, the histology of many of these lesions closely resembles the alterations characteristic of acute GVHD. Interestingly, there are a number of immunologic similarities between bone marrow recipients experiencing acute GVHD and patients with AIDS.

Histologically, there is a sparse papillary dermal infiltrate of lymphocytes and often occasional plasma cells associated with basal cell layer vacuolization and keratinocyte necrosis (Fig. 6–13*B*). Satellitosis, in which epidermotropic lymphocytes surround necrotic keratinocytes, is frequently encountered. The epidermal layer may show focal parakeratosis and evidence of disordered maturation (i.e., irregularity in maturation from the vertically oriented cells of the stratum basalis to the horizontally oriented cells of the uppermost stratum corneum).

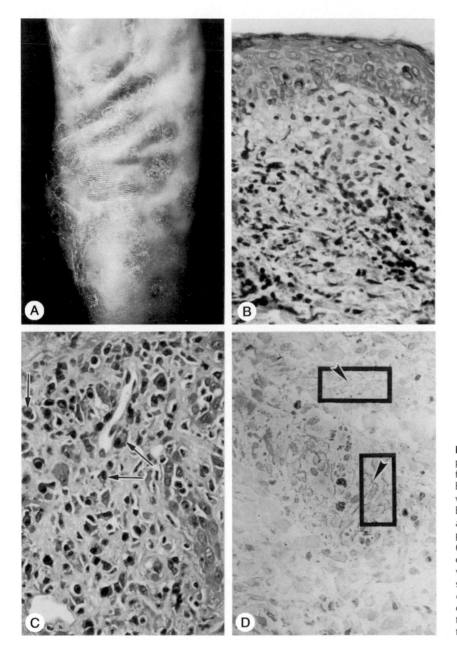

Figure 6–12. Lichenoid secondary syphilis. **(A)** Hyperpigmented, scaling plaques on the palms and soles are frequently observed. **(B)** A biopsy specimen reveals a band-like interstitial infiltrate of mononuclear cells within the papillary dermis, associated with variable basal cell layer vacuolization. Granulomatous foci also are often observed (note the vague collection of pale histiocytes centrally beneath the epidermal layer). **(C)** At higher magnification, plasma cells *(arrows)* and enlarged endothelial cells that focally occlude microvascular lumens are usually detected. **(D)** Dieterle stain may reveal slender, spiraling organisms *(enclosed in rectangles, arrowheads)* within perivascular connective tissue or within the epidermal layer, although serologic confirmation often is more sensitive than tissue stains in establishing a definitive diagnosis.

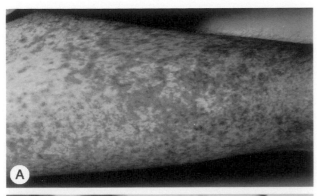

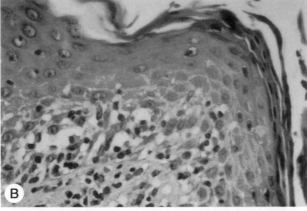

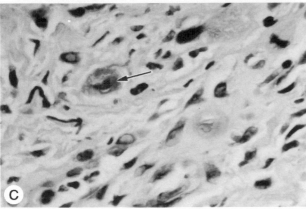

Figure 6–13. Lichenoid eruption in patients with acquired immunodeficiency syndrome. **(A)** Clinically, there may be a maculopapular exanthem, raising the possibilities of viral rash or drug eruption. **(B)** Interface change may resemble that seen in acute graft-versus-host disease, although epidermal alterations, such as parakeratosis and hyperplasia, may also be present. **(C)** The inflammatory component should be inspected closely for evidence of associated pathology or infection; in this case, inclusions of cytomegalovirus *(arrow)* were observed in some cells.

The differential diagnosis of lichenoid dermatitis of AIDS should include GVHD, especially if the patient has received nonirradiated blood products within 100 days of onset; lichenoid secondary syphilis; drug eruption; viral exanthem; and erythema multiforme. Lesional skin biopsies in GVHD generally do not contain plasma cells. Although secondary syphilis biopsies may contain plasma cells, occlusive endothelial activation is not typical of the lichenoid dermatitis of AIDS. This latter condition may be problematic to differentiate from syphilis, however, particularly because

AIDS patients may have seronegative syphilis. Although certain drug eruptions may have a lichenoid pattern, they generally contain eosinophils, a finding not observed in lichenoid dermatitis of AIDS. Nonspecific viral exanthems often show a sparse superficial perivascular lymphocytic infiltrate with foci of perivascular hemorrhage, and cytotoxic alterations within the epidermal layer are usually not observed. Targetoid lesions of erythema multiforme are not typical of the clinical presentation of the lichenoid dermatitis of AIDS.

Biopsy specimens of dermatitis from patients with known or suspected immunodeficiency may harbor other alterations indicative of contemporaneous infections or infestations within epidermal and dermal components. For example, alterations of cytomegalovirus infection (Fig. 6–13C) and atypical mycobacteria in association with unrelated cutaneous pathology in skin lesions may occur. Therefore, biopsy specimens from this patient population must be scrutinized with great care, both at scanning magnification and at higher-power magnification.

Rare Disorders

The category of lichenoid dermatitis contains a number of uncommonly encountered disorders, many of which have already been discussed in this chapter. This is because it is helpful to compare and contrast the findings in these conditions with the often subtle variations that are seen in more common forms of cytotoxic dermatitis. In addition, some of the less commonly encountered disorders, if diagnostically overlooked, may result in treatment omission or mistreatment, which could significantly influence patient morbidity and mortality. Such relatively rare disorders in general dermatologic practice include acute GVHD, lichenoid secondary syphilis, and lichenoid dermatitis as a presenting sign of ARC or AIDS.

DIFFERENTIAL DIAGNOSIS

When confronted with cytotoxic dermatitis, it is first important to determine histologically whether the lesion is acute or subacute to chronic. Generally, acute lesions retain a normal basket-weave stratum corneum, whereas more chronic lesions show scale abnormalities, colloid body formation, and pigment incontinence. Epidermal hyperplasia or atrophy also indicate chronicity. In the setting of acute cytotoxic dermatitis, diagnostic possibilities of erythema multiforme, acute GVHD, and lichenoid drug eruptions must be considered and correlated with the gross appearance of lesions and related clinical parameters. Chronic cytotoxic dermatitis with lichen planus–like features raises the possibilities of true lichen planus, lichen planus–like drug eruption, lichenoid chronic GVHD, and lichenoid forms of keratoses. Both histologic and clinical features of such lesions generally permit accurate diagnosis. Cytotoxic dermatitis with epidermal atrophy raises the possibility of lupus erythematosus and dermatomyositis, and scrutiny for basal lamina thickening, mucin deposition, and correlation with serologic parameters is often indicated. Cytotoxic involvement of hair follicles raises the possibility of lichen planopilaris when infundibular hyperplasia is present and follicular lupus erythematosus when infundibular atrophy is observed. Cytotoxic dermatitis with a deep angiocentric component may occur in lupus erythematosus, PLEVA, and in certain lichenoid drug eruptions. Fortunately, each of these disorders has characteristic histologic alterations that permit accurate diagnosis. It is always important to keep lichenoid secondary syphilis and lichenoid eruption of AIDS in mind when evaluating cytotoxic dermatitis.

SELECTED REFERENCES

1. Huff JC, Weston WL, Tonneson MG. Erythema multiforme: A critical review of characteristics, diagnostic criteria, and causes. J Am Acad Dermatol 1983;18:763.
2. Bedi TR, Pinkus H. Histological spectrum of erythema multiforme. Br J Dermatol 1971;95:243.
3. Weedon D, Searle J, Kerr JFR. Apoptosis: Its nature and implications for dermatopathology. Am J Dermatopathol 1979;1:133.
4. Lever R, Turbitt A, Mackie R, et al. A prospective study of the histological changes in the skin in patients receiving bone marrow transplants. Br J Dermatol 1986;114:161.
5. Hood AF, Mark EJ. Histopathologic diagnosis of pityriasis lichenoides et varioliformis acuta and its clinical correlation. Arch Dermatol 1982;118:478.
6. Hood AF. Pathology of cutaneous lupus erythematosus. Adv Dermatol 1988;3:153.
7. Clark WH Jr, Reed RJ, Mihm MC. Lupus erythematosus. Histopathology of cutaneous lesions. Hum Pathol 1973;4:157.
8. Janis JF, Winkelmann RK. Histopathology of the skin in dermatomyositis. Arch Dermatol 1968;97:640.
9. Grubauer G, Romani N, Kofler H et al. Apoptotic keratin bodies as autoantigen causing the production of IgM-anti-keratin intermediate filament autoantibodies. J Invest Dermatol 1986; 87:466.
10. Ragaz A, Ackerman AB. Evolution, maturation, and regression of lesions of lichen planus. Am J Dermatopathol 1981;3:5.
11. Ellis FA, Hill WF. Is lichen nitidus a variety of lichen planus? Arch Dermatol Syphilol 1938;38:568.
12. Shiohara T. The lichenoid tissue reaction: An immunological perspective. Am J Dermatopathol 1988;10:252.
13. Weedon D. The lichenoid tissue reaction. J Cutan Pathol 1985;12:279.
14. Korkij WK, Soltani K. Fixed drug eruption. A brief review. Arch Dermatol 1984;120:520.
15. Hindsen M, Christensen OB, Gruic V, et al. Fixed drug eruption: An immunohistochemical investigation of the acute and healing phase. Br J Dermatol 1987;116:351.
16. Abell E, Marks R, Wilson Jones E. Secondary syphilis: A clinicopathological review. Br J Dermatol 1975;93:53.
17. Rico MJ, Kory WP, Gould EW, et al. Interface dermatitis in patients with the acquired immunodeficiency syndrome. J Am Acad Dermatol 1987;16:1209.

7
Angiocentric Dermatitis

DEFINITIONS AND GENERAL CONSIDERATIONS

The term angiocentric dermatitis is used here to define those disorders characterized throughout their course primarily by perivascular inflammatory infiltrates, with or without vasculitis. Although all forms of dermatitis are, per force, angiocentric from the outset, some are distinguished by subsequent localization of immune cells in nonangiocentric tissue compartments (e.g., the epidermis in the case of spongiotic and cytotoxic dermatitis; the subcutaneous fat in the case of panniculitis). Because the epidermis is relatively unaltered in angiocentric dermatitis, these conditions are often diagnosed at scanning magnification after the normal overlying epidermal layer is appreciated. Vasculitis, an unfortunate term that merely implies inflammation of the vessel, is used to describe vessel injury manifested by varying degrees of endothelial degeneration and necrosis. Accordingly, vasculitis is present when endothelial cells exhibit little more than degenerative cytoplasmic vacuolization and hypereosinophilia. Classical fibrinoid necrosis defines a condition in which injury has progressed so far as to render the vessel wall permissive to the leakage of blood cells and serum components, including fibrin.

The term lymphocytic vasculitis implies damage to the vessel wall provoked primarily by lymphocytes. It is generally characterized by a perivascular angiocentric pattern with associated hemorrhage but without classic fibrinoid necrosis of the vessel wall. Lymphocytic vasculitis is a reaction pattern that may be seen in a diverse array of conditions, including erythema multiforme, pityriasis lichenoides et varioliformis acuta, and pigmentary purpura, and in dysplastic and malignant cutaneous lymphocytic infiltrates. In the setting of pure angiocentric dermatitis without evidence of epidermal alterations or chronicity, lymphocytic vasculitis may suggest the exanthem of systemic viral infection.

GROSS PATHOLOGY

In general, angiocentric dermatitis typically produces a zone of dermal induration when dermal edema collects in the setting of minimal inflammation. With progressive increase in the severity of the inflammatory response, such zones of induration become progressively erythematous. Erythema may be more pronounced at the perimeter than in the center of the lesion, a pattern indicative of centrifugal lesion propagation as concentric waves, which is suggestive of a primary angiocentric process. Extravasation of erythrocytes results in nonblanching purpura, which may be palpable. Epidermal change is generally absent, although sudden blister formation or necrosis in purpuric lesions may indicate the onset of secondary ischemic necrosis.

As might be expected in a primarily dermal inflammatory process, scaling, crust formation, irregular epidermal topography, or variability in epidermally derived pigmentation are not typical features, because the epidermal layer is not appreciably affected. Rather, the character of clinical lesions relates primarily to the nature of the dermal inflammatory component. When perivascular and interstitial edema predominate, lesions are generally edematous plaques (i.e., hives or urticaria) that have blanchable erythema and are evanescent in time course. Persistence of such lesions beyond 24 hours often indicates a component of vascular injury (i.e., urticarial vasculitis). Angiocentric infiltrates that involve inflammatory cells that remain intimately associated with vessel walls may enlarge to become well-circumscribed, erythematous plaques with slightly elevated borders, producing gyrate or polycyclic formations on the skin surface. Erythematous papules and plaques caused by angiocentric lymphocytic infiltrates may occasionally appear vesicular and polymorphous when accompanied by marked superficial dermal edema. Although all of these examples involve blanchable erythema (i.e., redness that disappears on compression), the presence of perivascular hemorrhage caused by injury to vessel walls results in deep red-purple erythema (i.e., purpura), which does not blanch. Moreover, when perivascular hemorrhage is appreciable, lesions are not only observed, but may be palpated (i.e., palpable purpura). Repeated hemorrhage to skin may result in transient (i.e., acute purpura), as well as persistent (e.g., hemosiderin deposition) pigmentation (e.g., pigmentary purpura). Whereas necrotizing angiocentric injury to superficial dermal vessels produces acute and chronic clinical manifestations of perivascular hemorrhage, similar damage to larger, subcutaneous vessels results in gross pathology dominated by secondary ischemia and necrosis to the subcutis, dermis, and epidermis. Because such infarctive lesions often occur at multiple foci along the course of deep vessels, the clinical nodules they produce may be linear in configuration or result in indurated, painful plaques that mimic panniculitis.

GENERAL HISTOLOGY AND TEMPORAL EVOLUTION

The earliest phases of angiocentric dermatitis show both intraluminal and perivascular accumulation of inflammatory cells. An example of this phenomenon is urticaria, which is often only several hours old at the time of biopsy. In urticaria, there characteristically are intraluminal neutrophils as well as scant perivascular collections of lymphocytes, neutrophils, and sometimes eosinophils. Established lesions of angiocentric dermatitis generally show a predominance of perivascular inflammatory cells, as in erythema annulare centrifugum, in which lymphocytes within the perivascular adventitia are tightly apposed to vessel walls. In some but not all forms of angiocentric dermatitis, late lesions demonstrate both perivascular and interstitial infiltrates of inflammatory cells. Established or chronic dermal delayed hypersensitivity responses to injected antigens, such as in arthropod bites and stings, commonly result in this interstitial pattern. Figure 7–1 summarizes the temporal evolution of angiocentric dermatitis. Although this figure provides a theoretical schema for the evolution of certain conditions in this category, it is important to remember that not all types of angiocentric dermatitis evolve through all three phases,

and many are characterized by only one or two of the phases throughout their natural progression.

Because the general histology of angiocentric dermatitis is subtle, especially in the absence of overt vasculitis, care must be taken not to confuse the general histology of this group of disorders with nonspecific chronic inflammation. Such diagnoses do not add to the understanding of the clinical inflammation that prompted the biopsy and commonly overlook essential, albeit covert, clues to accurate diagnosis. Each of the conditions discussed in the following sections has characteristic findings that facilitate its recognition. Coupled with understanding of the gross pathology and clinical characteristics of individual lesions, precise clinicopathological diagnoses are often possible. For example, whereas individual lesions of ordinary urticaria generally occur and regress within 24 hours, urticarial vasculitis commonly persists for several days. Association of polymorphous light eruption with exposure to ultraviolet light, erythema chronicum migrans with tick-bite exposure, and urticarial papular eruptions with pregnancy are other examples of how even rudimentary knowledge of clinical parameters may facilitate diagnosis of this group of histologically protean disorders.

HISTOLOGY OF SPECIFIC DISORDERS

Angiocentric, without Vascular Injury

Urticaria[1-3]

- SPARSE, SUPERFICIAL, PERIVASCULAR INFILTRATE OF LYMPHOCYTES AND NEUTROPHILS
- INTRALUMINAL NEUTROPHILS ADHERENT TO ENDOTHELIAL MEMBRANES
- SUPERFICIAL DERMAL EDEMA WITH LYMPHATIC ECTASIA
- INTERSTITIAL NEUTROPHILS AND NUCLEAR FRAGMENTS IN SOME LESIONS

Urticaria, or hives, refers to a common disorder of the skin resulting in pruritic, pink-white wheals. These wheals are localized zones of dermal edema that produce isolated, polycyclic, and often coalescent plaques surmounted by a

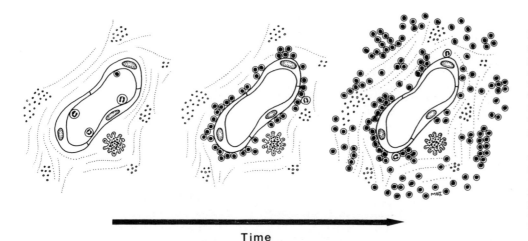

Figure 7–1. Temporal evolution of angiocentric dermatitis. The earliest phases of angiocentric dermatitis *(left)* are often characterized by little more than margination of leukocytes along the endothelial lumen. In time, transmural diapedesis results in accumulation of leukocytes in the immediate perivascular space *(center)*. Depending on the nature of the provocative agent or antigen and the adhesion pathways that are set into motion, leukocytes may migrate away from the vessel wall, producing an interstitial pattern as well as an angiocentric pattern *(right)*. The latter phenomenon often occurs in insect-bite reactions to injected antigen.

Time

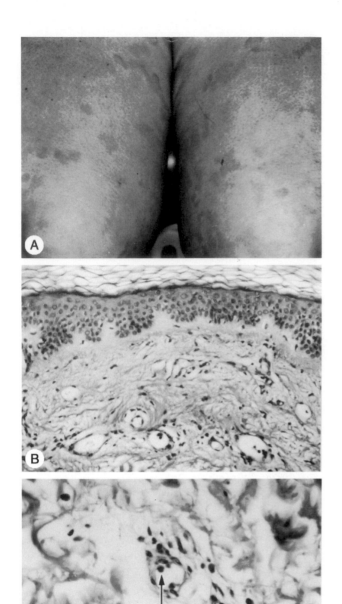

Figure 7–2. Urticaria. **(A)** Clinically, there are erythematous, edematous, often circinate or polycyclic plaques covered by a normal epidermal surface. Individual lesions generally last for less than 24 hours. **(B)** At scanning magnification, there is superficial dermal edema and dilated lymphatic channels. The edema is manifested as a widening of spaces that separate adjacent collagen bundles. **(C)** At higher magnification, there is a scant inflammatory infiltrate composed of lymphocytes and occasional neutrophils within an edematous perivascular space. The finding of intraluminal neutrophils *(arrow)* adherent to the endothelial luminal membrane is characteristic.

smooth, normal-appearing epidermal surface (Figs. 7–2A and 7–3A). About 20% of the general population will experience at least one episode of urticaria during their lifetime. Clinically, most forms of urticaria can be divided into acute and chronic forms. Acute urticaria consists of a single, self-limiting episode involving lesions that last for less than 24 hours. Chronic urticaria involves repeated episodes of eva-

nescent wheals or persistent lesions that last more than 24 hours (i.e., urticarial vasculitis). Although the cause of many instances of urticaria remains unknown, there are a number of well-defined clinical forms. These include immunologic urticaria, which is presumably mediated by IgE or complement, and nonimmunologic urticaria, which is due to the direct effects of drugs or physical agents. Angioedema is a form of clinical urticaria in which edema of both the dermis and subcutaneous fat may produce life-threatening swelling of skin and mucosa, leading to airway obstruction.

The link between the clinical presentation of urticaria (i.e., localized or diffuse cutaneous swelling) and the histopathology is mast cell degranulation. Mast cells are normally situated about small cutaneous venules. When these cells are triggered to degranulate, histamine is liberated, resulting in interendothelial gaps and increased microvascular permeability. This results in progressive accumulation of edema fluid within the intervascular interstitium. Because mast cells also contain other proinflammatory mediators, such as certain cytokines, affected endothelial cells also attract circulating leukocytes, resulting in an angiocentric inflammatory pattern.

Histologically, the findings may be extraordinarily subtle, leading to confusion with normal skin. However, there is always at least superficial dermal edema, manifested by increased spacing between adjacent bundles of collagen (Fig. 7–2B, C). This edema may be readily appreciated as a diffuse zone of papillary dermal pallor at scanning magnification. A frequently overlooked finding that invariably occurs coincident with even subtle dermal edema is dilation of lymphatic channels (Fig. 7–2B). At higher magnification, the subtle pattern of angiocentric inflammation consists of a sparse cuff of lymphocytes and sometimes eosinophils about affected venules; a helpful feature is the presence of intraluminal neutrophils adherent to luminal endothelial cells (Fig. 7–2C). Certain forms of urticaria are described as neutrophil-rich. These lesions usually show a diffuse dermal edema with associated interstitial permeation of intervenular collagen by neutrophils, a superficial and often deep sparse angiocentric infiltrate of lymphocytes and occasional neutrophils, and intraluminal adherent neutrophils (Fig. 7–3C, D).

It is difficult to determine the cause of urticaria from the associated histology. Certain insect-bite reactions (i.e., papular urticaria), drug eruptions, viral exanthems, and food allergies may all show the histology of urticaria. It is also important to recognize that certain nonurticarial disorders may have urticarial evolutionary phases, such as bullous pemphigoid (see Chap. 5) and very early lesions of allergic contact dermatitis (see Chap. 3).

Urticarial Papules of Pregnancy[4, 5]

- SUPERFICIAL AND MID-DERMAL MIXED INFLAMMATORY INFILTRATE COMPOSED OF LYMPHOCYTES, EOSINOPHILS, AND RARE NEUTROPHILS
- SUPERFICIAL DERMAL EDEMA
- ABSENCE OF EPIDERMAL BASAL CELL LAYER VACUOLIZATION
- SUPERFICIAL PAPILLARY DERMIS FREE OF EOSINOPHILS

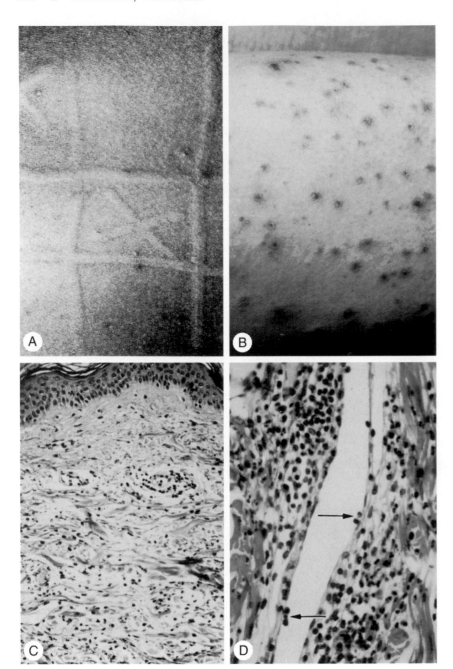

Figure 7–3. Various forms of urticaria. **(A)** Dermatographism, or urtication, at sites of trauma or stroking is a form of physically induced urticaria. **(B)** Pruritic urticaria papules and plaques of pregnancy (PUPPP) is characterized by often excoriated, discrete, erythematous papules. **(C)** Neutrophil-rich urticaria. Note the interstitial as well as angiocentric pattern of neutrophil infiltration within an edematous superficial dermis. **(D)** Higher magnification of an involved vessel demonstrates an angiocentric infiltrate of lymphocytes and neutrophils with adherent neutrophils within the vessel lumen *(arrows).*

Pruritic urticarial papules and plaques of pregnancy (PUPPP) is a characteristic urticarial eruption that occurs in the third trimester of pregnancy. Lesions begin as small urticarial papules that coalesce to form plaques (Fig. 7–3*B*). Skin of the abdomen surrounding the umbilicus and in association with striae is most commonly affected. Histologically, the findings resemble urticaria, as described previously. Eosinophils are generally present within the inflammatory infiltrate, although unlike bullous pemphigoid or herpes gestationis, basal cell layer vacuolization and degranulation of eosinophils along the dermal-epidermal interface are not observed. In addition, in contrast to herpes gestationis, direct immunofluorescence of perilesional skin is negative in PUPPP (see Chap. 2).

Erythema Marginatum[6]

- ANGIOCENTRIC AND INTERSTITIAL DERMAL INFILTRATE OF NEUTROPHILS
- NUCLEAR DUST WITHOUT VASCULITIS OR HEMORRHAGE
- OCCASIONAL NEUTROPHILS IN DERMAL PAPILLAE

Erythema marginatum, along with subcutaneous nodules, polyarthritis, carditis, and chorea, is one of the five major criteria for the diagnosis of rheumatic fever. The gross pathology consists of dull red, often polycyclic, coalescent, relatively flat plaques, most frequently involving abdominal

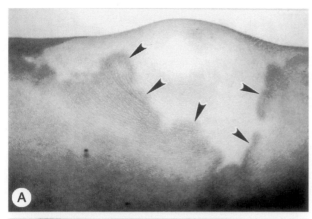

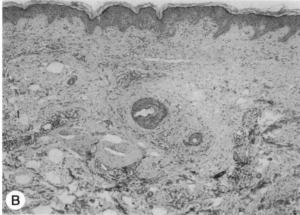

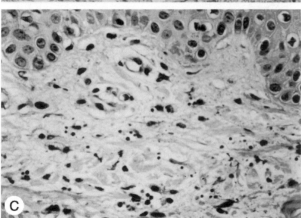

Figure 7–4. Erythema marginatum. **(A)** Clinically, there are confluent zones of erythema and edema with a characteristically sharply demarcated advancing border *(arrowheads)*. **(B)** At scanning magnification, there is an angiocentric and interstitial inflammatory infiltrate within the superficial and mid-dermis, beneath a normal overlying epidermal layer. **(C)** The urticarial quality of erythema marginatum is appreciated in this field, showing superficial dermal edema and an interstitial infiltrate of neutrophils similar to the histologic picture of neutrophil-rich urticaria. In both, however, lymphocytes also participate, and accordingly, these lesions are not considered primarily under the category of granulocytic dermatitis.

skin (Fig. 7–4A). At scanning magnification, there is a sparse superficial and deep angiocentric infiltrate, as well as a less well developed interstitial inflammatory component (Fig. 7–4B). At higher magnification, it is seen that the infiltrate is composed predominantly of neutrophils with associated nuclear dust (Fig. 7–4C), but it occurs in the absence of fibrin-

oid necrosis of vessel walls or evidence of erythrocyte extravasation. Occasional neutrophils may collect in dermal papillae; these must not be confused with the forming, neutrophilic microabscesses seen in early dermatitis herpetiformis.

Erythema marginatum has a subtle histologic picture that may be confused with a number of entities, including neutrophil-rich urticaria, neutrophilic dermatitis of rheumatoid arthritis, and early evolutionary stages of Sweet syndrome. Generally, neutrophil-rich urticaria will show more dermal edema than is characteristic of erythema marginatum. Differentiation from other forms of neutrophilic dermatitis in early evolutionary stages and without associated vasculitis may be problematic and will rely on recognition of the more angiocentric pattern observed in erythema marginatum and the patient's correlative clinical history.

Erythema Annulare Centrifugum[7, 8]

- SUPERFICIAL PERIVASCULAR LYMPHOCYTIC INFILTRATE
- LYMPHOCYTES TIGHTLY AGGREGATED ABOUT VESSEL WALLS (COAT-SLEEVE PATTERN)
- MILD, FOCAL SPONGIOSIS AND PARAKERATOSIS IN SOME LESIONS

This common but poorly understood disorder typically begins as an erythematous papule that rapidly enlarges to form an erythematous plaque with prominent central clearing (Fig. 7–5A). The advancing edge of the lesion is slightly elevated and often retains an adherent zone of scale along the inner aspect of the border (i.e., trailing scale). Lesions are generally asymptomatic or slightly pruritic, and affected individuals usually do not have an underlying or predisposing condition. The clinical differential diagnosis often includes dermatophyte infection, eczematous dermatitis, or deeper forms of gyrate erythema.

Histologically, scanning magnification reveals a well-defined, perivascular inflammatory infiltrate composed of lymphocytes tightly clustered about superficial and mid-dermal vessels (Fig. 7–5B). Often, the apposition of inflammatory cells to affected vessels is so discrete that vascular channels so outlined resemble Chinese figure writing, a finding of assistance in remembering the pattern of figurate erythema. At higher magnification, the tight perivascular cuff of lymphocytes may be even better appreciated (Fig. 7–5C). The overlying epidermis is generally unaffected, although if the region of the clinical lesion showing the trailing scale is biopsied, focal parakeratosis and mild epidermal hyperplasia may be observed in the specimen.

Erythema Chronicum Migrans[9, 10]

- SUPERFICIAL AND DEEP, TIGHTLY AGGREGATED PERIVASCULAR INFLAMMATORY INFILTRATE
- INFLAMMATORY INFILTRATE COMPOSED PREDOMINANTLY OF LYMPHOCYTES, WITH OCCASIONAL EOSINOPHILS AND PLASMA CELLS
- EPIDERMAL HYPERPLASIA WITH CHRONICITY AND IN CENTER OF LESIONS

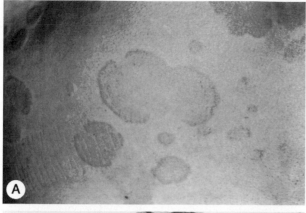

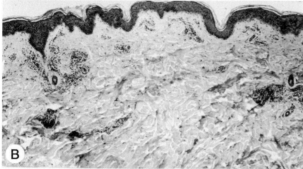

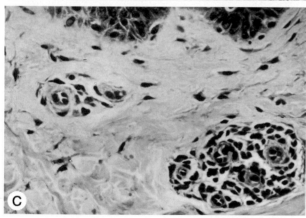

Figure 7–5. Erythema annulare centrifugum. **(A)** The gross pathology is characterized by annular, erythematous plaques, often with a fine, adherent collarette of scale that trails just behind the advancing edge of each lesion. **(B, C)** Histologically, there is a superficial and sometimes mid-dermal angiocentric infiltrate of lymphocytes, which are tightly aggregated in the perivascular space (i.e., coat-sleeve pattern). When the biopsy specimen includes the edge of a lesion, foci of mild epidermal hyperplasia and parakeratosis may be detected in the overlying epidermal layer.

Erythema chronicum migrans represents a local hypersensitivity reaction to local injection of the spirochete *Borrelia burgdorferi* by tick bite inoculation. As such, this condition represents an important potential marker for the development of Lyme disease. Indeed, erythema chronicum migrans may coexist with the symptom complex of Lyme disease, which includes myalgias, malaise, and arthralgias, and which may eventuate in overt cardiac, neurologic, and arthritic lesions. The clinical appearance of erythema chronicum migrans is that of a papule which enlarges to form an erythematous plaque with a smooth, indurated border, and a

variable degree of central clearing (Fig. 7–6A). A persistent zone of central erythema or hemorrhage indicative of the bite punctum may be apparent in some lesions.

Histologically, erythema chronicum migrans, unlike erythema annulare centrifugum, demonstrates a superficial and deep angiocentric inflammatory infiltrate composed predominantly of lymphocytes with occasional admixed eosinophils and plasma cells (Fig. 7–6B). The depth of angiogenic extension into the reticular dermis of erythema chronicum migrans is an important diagnostic feature of this disorder. The overlying epidermis is relatively unaffected, although biopsy specimens from the central punctum may show epidermal hyperplasia and occasionally granulomatous inflammation in sites of retained mouth parts of the offending tick.

Polymorphous Light Eruption[11–13]

- SUPERFICIAL AND DEEP PERIVASCULAR LYMPHOCYTIC INFILTRATE
- INFILTRATE GRADUALLY DIMINISHES WITH DERMAL DEPTH
- VARIABLE PAPILLARY DERMAL EDEMA
- ABSENCE OF ADNEXAL INFLAMMATION

The histology of polymorphous light eruption, when correlated closely with the clinical appearance and setting in which lesions occur, is characteristic. The eruption, as the name implies, involves multiple erythematous papules and plaques that develop in sun-exposed skin (Fig. 7–7A). Because photosensitivity is a cause of exacerbated lupus erythematosus, lupus is commonly cited in the clinical differential diagnosis. In addition, photoeczematous eruptions (see Chap. 3) and phototoxic eruptions (i.e., exaggerated sunburn reaction) are also frequently listed among the clinical diagnostic considerations.

Histologically, polymorphous light eruption may initially mimic lupus erythematosus, and I have seen a number of examples of the former that have proven to be erroneously diagnosed as the latter. At scanning magnification, there is a superficial and deep dermal angiocentric infiltrate of lymphocytes that gradually fades in severity from the superficial to deep dermis. In addition, there is often marked papillary dermal edema (Fig. 7–7B, C). In contrast to lupus erythematosus, there is absent or minimal basement membrane thickening, dermal mucinosis, or cytotoxic alteration of the basal cell layer or follicular epithelium. Table 7–1 summarizes the salient diagnostic differences between polymorphous light eruption and photoexacerbated lupus erythematosus.

Table 7–1. DIFFERENTIAL DIAGNOSIS OF POLYMORPHOUS LIGHT ERUPTION AND CUTANEOUS LUPUS ERYTHEMATOSUS

	POLYMORPHOUS LIGHT ERUPTION	CUTANEOUS LUPUS ERYTHEMATOSUS
Epidermal atrophy	Absent	Present
Basement membrane thickening	Absent	Present
Degree of deep infiltrate	Grades off	Prominent
Adnexal involvement	Absent	Present
Dermal mucinosis	Minimal	Present

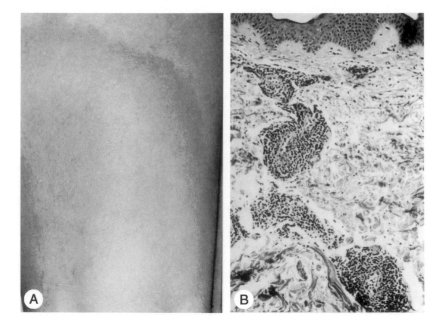

Figure 7–6. Erythema chronicum migrans. **(A)** An expanding, indurated, erythematous plaque developed at the site of a previous tick bite. There is no epidermal change at the advancing border of this annular lesion, in contrast to erythema annulare centrifugum. **(B)** The tight, perivascular lymphocytic infiltrate appreciated in erythema annulare centrifugum is even more prominent and extends more deeply into the dermis in erythema chronicum migrans.

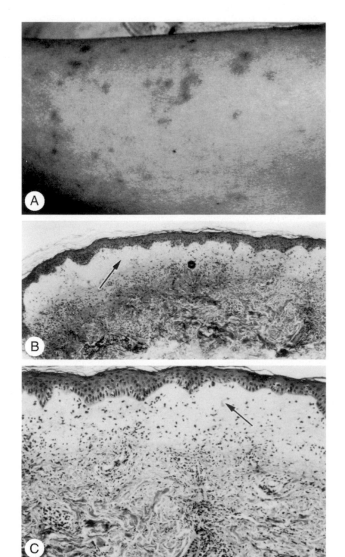

Figure 7–7. Polymorphous light eruption. **(A)** Clinical lesions vary from papules to plaques to vesicles at sites of sun exposure. **(B)** Scanning and **(C)** high magnification of a representative biopsy specimen of an early lesion reveals a brisk, superficial and mid-dermal, angiocentric, lymphocytic infiltrate associated with marked papillary dermal edema (*arrows*). Unlike phototoxic and photoeczematous eruptions, where epidermal dyskeratosis and spongiosis occur, respectively, the epidermal layer is relatively unaffected in a polymorphous light eruption.

Jessner Lymphocytic Infiltrate[14]

- SUPERFICIAL AND DEEP ANGIOCENTRIC INFILTRATE WITH HISTIOCYTES
- PERIFOLLICULAR EXTENSION ABOUT ADVENTITIAL VESSELS
- NO INTERFACE CHANGE
- PREDOMINANTLY LYMPHOCYTES ADMIXED WITH HISTIOCYTES
- MILD DERMAL MUCINOSIS

Jessner lymphocytic infiltrate is as poorly understood as the name implies. It generally involves facial skin as a well-defined erythematous, boggy plaque that may persist for many months to years. Typically, there is little or no evidence of follicular involvement, such as the presence of keratotic infundibular plugs or alopecia. Although exposure to sunlight may exacerbate some lesions, this association is far from constant. Clinically, there is a well-defined, indurated, erythematous plaque lacking follicular infundibular ectasia or keratotic plugging, as is typical of lupus erythematosus (Fig. 7–8A).

Histologically, there is a superficial and deep perivascular mononuclear cell infiltrate containing an admixture of small lymphocytes and large, pale histiocytes (Fig. 7–8B, C). Although perifollicular adventitia may appear to be involved at scanning magnification, inspection at higher power will reveal extension only about periadnexal vessels and the absence of true interface changes. Epidermotropism into the overlying epidermis is not present, and dermal mucin deposition is minimal.

Dermal Delayed Hypersensitivity[15]

- SUPERFICIAL AND OFTEN DEEP DERMAL ANGIOCENTRIC INFILTRATE
- FREQUENTLY PERIVENULAR INFILTRATION OF INTERSTITIAL CONNECTIVE TISSUE
- LYMPHOCYTES, HISTIOCYTES, AND OFTEN EOSINOPHILS
- VARIABLE DERMAL EDEMA

Delayed hypersensitivity reactions, also discussed in Chapter 3 in the context of spongiotic dermatitis, all begin as angiocentric infiltrates. As lesions evolve, however, many develop acute, subacute, and chronic epidermal alterations ranging from spongiotic to hyperplastic reactions. These alterations are generally associated with epidermotropic lymphocyte migration from the dermis into the epidermal layer. Depending on the nature and route of delivery (topical versus systemic) of the antigenic stimulus, however, certain delayed hypersensitivity reactions may show little or no epidermal alteration during their clinical course. Clinically, such lesions generally appear as vague, indurated, erythematous plaques covered by a normal skin surface devoid of vesiculation or excessive scale (Fig. 7–9A).

The histology of dermal delayed hypersensitivity reactions discloses a superficial and sometimes deep angiocentric infiltrate of lymphocytes and occasional eosinophils beneath a normal epidermal layer (Fig. 7–9B). Dermal edema may be observed, as well as intraluminal neutrophils adherent to ad-

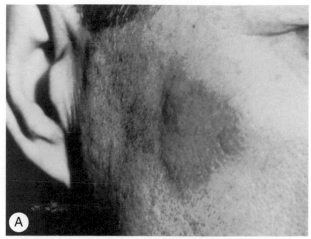

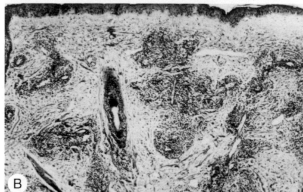

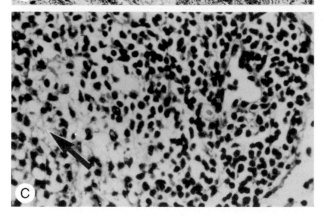

Figure 7–8. Jessner lymphocytic infiltrate. **(A)** A well-formed, boggy, erythematous plaque on the face with little or no evidence of epidermal or follicular involvement. **(B)** Low magnification of a biopsy specimen reveals a brisk, angiocentric, mononuclear cell infiltrate in the superficial and deep dermis. Although this clinical picture may raise the possibility of a predominantly dermal form of lupus erythematosus, note that hair follicles and other adnexal structures are not affected by the inflammatory infiltrate. **(C)** The mononuclear cells are composed of small lymphocytes admixed with larger, pale-staining histiocytes; foci of associated extracellular mucin *(arrow)* may also be observed.

jacent endothelial cells, a finding also encountered in urticaria. When the reaction is elicited by injected antigen, such as in certain arthropod bites and stings, an interstitial pattern of inflammatory cell migration involving intervenular connective tissue may also be observed.

Angiocentric, with Vascular Injury

Neutrophilic Venulitis (Leukocytoclastic Vasculitis)[16-19]

- MIXED SUPERFICIAL PERIVASCULAR INFLAMMATORY INFILTRATE COMPOSED OF NEUTROPHILS, LYMPHOCYTES, AND SOMETIMES EOSINOPHILS
- NUCLEAR FRAGMENTS (I.E., DUST) ABOUT VESSEL WALLS
- ENDOTHELIAL SWELLING AND DEPOSITION OF FIBRIN IN VESSEL WALLS (I.E., FIBRINOID NECROSIS)
- PERIVASCULAR HEMORRHAGE
- SECONDARY ISCHEMIC EPIDERMAL ALTERATIONS (I.E., BASAL CELL LAYER VACUOLIZATION AND NECROSIS) IN ADVANCED LESIONS

Necrotizing cutaneous vasculitis, or neutrophilic venulitis, is the cause of classic palpable purpura. Lesions occur at presumed sites of immune complex deposition, and therefore preferentially may involve dependent regions, such as lower extremities. Clinically, there are indurated, flat to slightly raised, red-purple plaques that may coalesce (Fig. 7–10A). Associated epidermal ischemia may result in central sloughing or bulla formation in certain instances (Fig. 7–10B). The causes of neutrophilic venulitis include drugs, infectious agents, and autoantigens, although the offending agent is never uncovered in a significant number of cases. The presence of necrotizing cutaneous vasculitis does not correlate with the coexistence of necrotizing vascular lesions in internal viscera.

Common to all variants of neutrophilic venulitis is variable infiltration of vessel walls by polymorphonuclear leukocytes associated with necrotizing vascular injury. In classic leukocytoclastic or hypersensitivity vasculitis, the superficial vascular plexus is preferentially involved, a feature that is best appreciated at scanning magnification (Fig. 7–10C). Continuation of the superficial vasculature within the adventitial sheath that surrounds hair follicles and sweat glands may produce the deceptive appearance of deep dermal involvement. At higher magnification, postcapillary venules show granular deposits of pink-purple, refractile fibrin within their walls, often best appreciated by racking down the substage condenser. This fibrinoid necrosis is associated with a permeative cuff of lymphocytes, neutrophils, and occasional eosinophils undergoing nuclear fragmentation and, in some lesions, with intraluminal fibrin thrombi (Fig. 7–10D, E). In biopsy specimens of very early lesions, multiple levels may be required to reveal fibrinoid necrosis. Perivascular hemorrhage and secondary ischemic epidermal necrosis or dermal-epidermal separation may also be encountered (Fig. 7–10E).

Care should be taken to distinguish ordinary necrotizing venulitis from vasculitis associated with locally formed immune complexes in infections such as gonococcemia and meningococcemia. In general, bacterial forms of vasculitis will have extensive fibrin thrombus formation, epidermal necrosis, and formation of intradermal and/or intraepidermal pustules. Such lesions should be stained for bacteria, although culture of fresh biopsied tissue is a more sensitive gauge of the presence or absence of bacteria.

Clinical variants of neutrophilic venulitis include cryoglobulinemia, erythema elevatum diutinum, and granuloma faciale. Cryoglobulinemia, caused by intravascular precipitation of abnormal circulating immunoglobulins that precipitate in the cold, is manifested as purpuric macules and sometimes ulcers of the distal extremities, where temperature regulation may be environmentally compromised (Fig. 7–11A). Erythema elevatum diutinum, a form of chronic neutrophil-mediated vasculitis, appears as persistent, red-brown to purple papules and nodules that become progressively indurated over time on the extensor surfaces of the extremities (Fig. 7–12A). Granuloma faciale presents as asymptomatic, soft, brown-red plaques involving facial skin (Fig. 7–13A). Granuloma faciale lesions characteristically contain dilated follicular ostia.

The histology of cryoglobulinemia is characterized by multiple, pale, pink, homogeneous, waxy, intraluminal thrombi associated with perivascular hemorrhage that is often out of proportion to the mild degree of inflammatory vasculitic injury (Fig. 7–11B). In contrast to fibrin thrombi, which stain with phosphotungstenic acid hematoxylin (PTAH) but not the periodic acid–Schiff (PAS) reagent, the intraluminal thrombi of cryoglobulinemia are PTAH-negative and PAS-

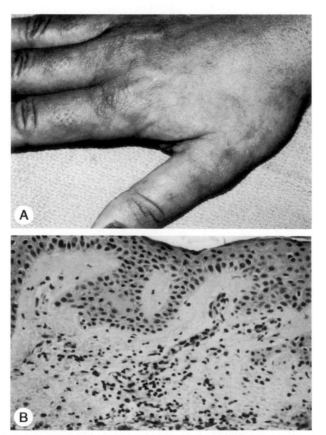

Figure 7–9. Dermal delayed hypersensitivity. **(A)** Clinical lesions may vary from vague zones of erythema to urticarial plaques; pruritus is common. **(B)** Biopsy specimens reveal superficial and sometimes deep perivascular lymphocytic infiltrate without significant epidermal alterations. Admixed eosinophils are often encountered.

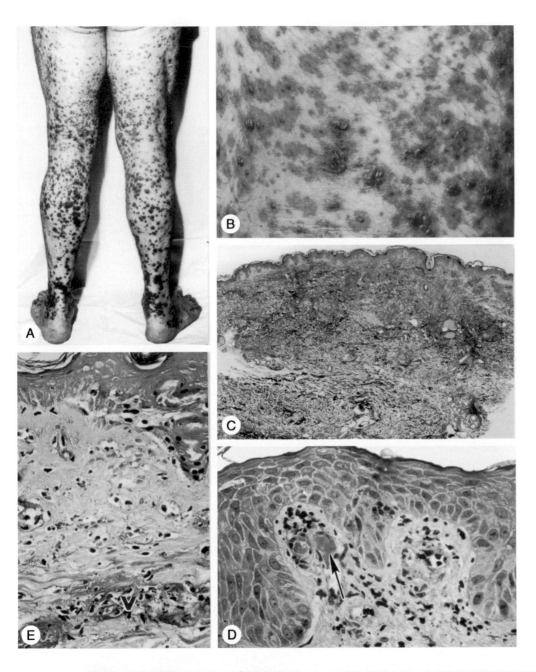

Figure 7–10. Necrotizing neutrophilic venulitis. **(A)** These palpable purpura characteristically involve the lower extremities. **(B)** Some lesions show early blister formation, the result of extensive epidermal necrosis (see **E**). **(C)** On scanning magnification, there is a superficial angiocentric infiltrate, often with a red-purple hue due to associated hemorrhage and fibrin deposition. **(D, E)** Individual venules (v) within the superficial vascular plexus show fibrinoid necrosis, fibrin thrombus formation *(arrow)*, and an angiocentric cuff of fragmented neutrophils (i.e., nuclear dust) and lymphocytes.

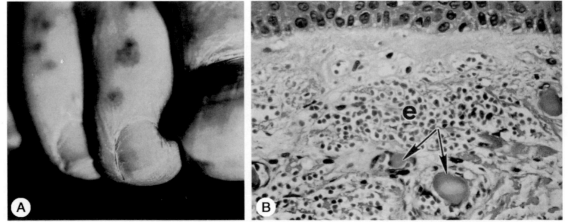

Figure 7–11. Necrotizing vasculitis: Cryoglobulinemia. **(A)** These purpuric lesions occur on distal extremities and digits that are prone to lower temperatures and thromboembolic events. **(B)** Glassy thrombi *(arrows)* within superficial vessels are surrounded by recently extravasated erythrocytes (e) and rare inflammatory cells. Compare these thrombi to the more granular fibrin thrombi that characterize neutrophilic venulitis (see Fig. 7–10D).

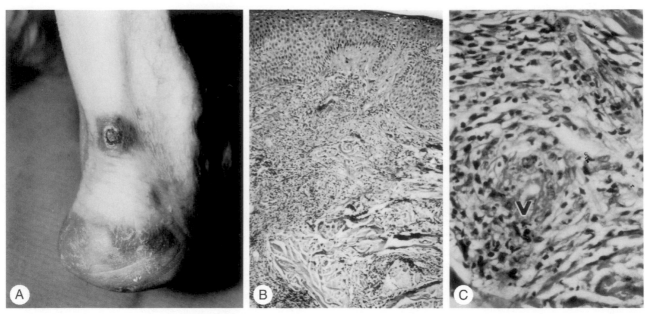

Figure 7–12. Erythema elevatum diutinum. **(A)** More chronic necrotizing vasculitis is manifested by long-standing hemorrhagic nodules with ulceration, typically on distal extremities. **(B, C)** Histologically, there is a brisk, superficial and mid-dermal, mixed inflammatory infiltrate composed of lymphocytes and neutrophils associated with necrotizing vascular injury **(C,** v). There is superficial dermal and perivascular fibrosis **(C,** *top*), a manifestation of chronic, repeated vascular insult.

positive. In erythema elevatum diutinum, there is a brisk superficial and mid-dermal mixed inflammatory perivascular infiltrate composed of lymphocytes and variably fragmented neutrophils associated with necrotizing vascular injury (Fig. 7–12*B, C*). Hemosiderin deposition and characteristic, vaguely concentric perivascular fibrosis are diagnostically helpful and provide testimony regarding the chronicity of the vascular injury (Fig. 7–12*C*). In granuloma faciale, scan-

ning magnification will reveal coalescent angiocentric infiltration by inflammatory cells within the superficial and deep dermis. The inflammatory component characteristically spares a thin mantle of dermis directly beneath the epidermal and adnexal basement membrane zones (i.e., Grenz zone or zone of sparing; Fig. 7–13*B*). Vessels may be nearly totally obliterated by fragmented neutrophils that demarcate their preexisting loci (Fig. 7–13*C*).

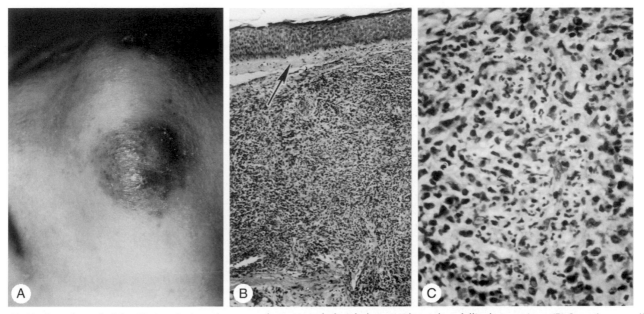

Figure 7–13. Granuloma faciale. **(A)** A typical, erythematous, brown-purple facial plaque with patulous follicular openings. **(B)** Scanning magnification reveals coalescent aggregates of inflammatory cells within the superficial and deep dermis; these begin as angiocentric foci. Note the characteristic sparing of the dermis directly beneath the epidermal layer *(arrow)* and around hair follicles (not shown); this area is known as the Grenz zone. **(C)** At higher magnification, foci of fragmented neutrophils demarcate sites of preexisting vessels that have been nearly totally obliterated.

Urticarial Vasculitis[20, 21]

- MIXED SUPERFICIAL PERIVASCULAR INFLAMMATORY INFILTRATE COMPOSED OF LYMPHOCYTES AND RARE NEUTROPHILS
- FOCAL PERIVASCULAR HEMORRHAGE WITH ENDOTHELIAL SWELLING AND VACUOLIZATION
- ABSENCE OF TRUE FIBRINOID NECROSIS
- CLINICAL PERSISTENCE OF INDIVIDUAL LESIONS >24 HOURS

Urticarial vasculitis, which may be associated with viral hepatitis and connective tissue diseases, consists of erythematous to slightly purpuric wheals that persist as individual lesions for longer than 24 hours. The histology of urticarial vasculitis may be indistinguishable from ordinary urticaria by light microscopy, because overt fibrinoid vessel necrosis does not occur. Direct immunofluorescence, examination of plastic-embedded 1-μ-thick sections, and most importantly, clinical correlation are critical to accurate diagnosis of urticarial vasculitis.

Lymphocytic Vasculitis[22]

- PERIVENULAR LYMPHOCYTIC INFILTRATE OFTEN CONFINED TO SUPERFICIAL DERMIS
- PERIVASCULAR HEMORRHAGE AND HEMOSIDERIN DEPOSITION WITH CHRONICITY
- VARIABLE ENDOTHELIAL INJURY AND FIBRINOID NECROSIS

The concept of lymphocytic vasculitis is useful in defining several disorders in which perivascular cuffs of lymphocytes are associated with vascular damage to a degree that perivascular hemorrhage may ensue. Accordingly, Table 7–2 lists all potential members of this group, although several have been discussed previously, because epidermal alterations predominated over the dermal patterns of angiogenic inflammation.

Two disorders that are discussed under the category of angiocentric dermatitis are progressive pigmentary purpura and vasculitic insect-bite reactions. Progressive pigmentary purpura, also known as Schamberg disease, presents grossly as multiple, often coalescent, asymptomatic, red-brown macules and shallow plaques (Fig. 7–14A). The angiocentric lymphocytic inflammation is sparse and characteristically centered about small vascular loops within dermal papillae (Fig. 7–14B). Overt vascular injury or fibrinoid necrosis is not encountered; it is therefore presumed that the lesion that permits chronic erythrocyte extravasation is too subtle to be appreciated by conventional microscopy. Within the perivas-

Table 7–2. DISORDERS SHOWING ANGIOCENTRIC LYMPHOID INFILTRATION AND ASSOCIATED ACUTE OR CHRONIC HEMORRHAGE

Erythema multiforme
Pityriasis rosea
Pityriasis lichenoides et varioliformis acuta
Pityriasis lichenoides chronica
Connective tissue diseases
Progressive pigmentary purpura
Vasculitic insect-bite reactions

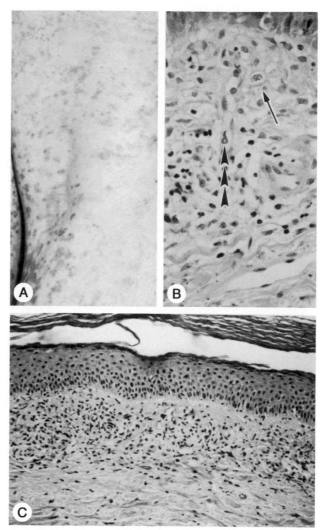

Figure 7–14. Lymphocytic vasculitis or pigmentary purpura. (A) Multiple asymptomatic, red-brown macules and shallow plaques. (B) Angiocentric lymphocytic inflammation in progressive pigmentary purpura is distinctively centered about capillary loops *(arrowheads)* within the most superficial regions of the papillary dermis. Recent perivascular hemorrhage and hemosiderin deposits *(arrow)* are testimony to this subtle form of vascular injury. (C) The angiocentric inflammatory component in some lesions is brisk, leading to a lichenoid pattern via confluence (i.e., lichenoid purpura).

cular space, there is recent hemorrhage as well as siderophages (i.e., macrophages containing hemosiderin). These latter cells may be best appreciated by the use of an iron stain. Lichenoid variants of pigmentary purpura show coalescence of the angiocentric pattern to form a band of lymphocytes within the superficial papillary dermis (Fig. 7–14C). True interface change (i.e., basal cell layer vacuolization, colloid body formation) is not observed.

Insect-bite reactions showing lymphocytic vasculitis may be markedly hemorrhagic clinically (Fig. 7–15A). Histologically, there is generally a superficial and deep perivascular infiltrate of activated lymphocytes and admixed eosinophils, often with a vaguely wedge-shaped architecture (Fig. 7–15B). Examination of involved vessels at higher magnification reveals vascular injury that is often striking in degree, with near-complete effacement of the preexisting vessel architecture by fibrin and inflammatory debris (Fig. 7–15C).

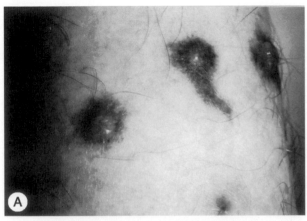

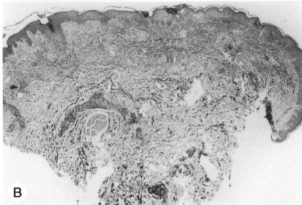

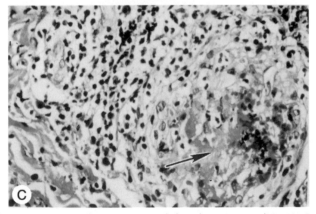

Figure 7–15. Insect-bite reaction with lymphocytic vasculitis. **(A)** Purpuric nodules occur at sites of arthropod stings. **(B)** Scanning magnification reveals a superficial and deep angiocentric inflammatory infiltrate beneath an essentially normal epidermal layer. **(C)** Extensive vascular injury and necrosis, with luminal obliteration by coagulated fibrin *(arrow)*, is associated with a perivascular lymphocytic infiltrate containing occasional eosinophils.

Cutaneous Polyarteritis Nodosa[23]

- INVOLVEMENT OF DEEP DERMAL AND SUBCUTANEOUS SMALL- TO MEDIUM-SIZED ARTERIES
- INFLAMMATORY INFILTRATION OF WALL, OFTEN SEGMENTAL
- MIXED INFILTRATE OF MONONUCLEAR CELLS, NEUTROPHILS, AND RARELY, EOSINOPHILS
- INTIMAL PROLIFERATION WITH CHRONICITY

Cutaneous polyarteritis nodosa of the benign variety, without systemic involvement, presents as painful, sometimes ulcerated nodules, often arranged in linear distribution, indicative of the course of the underlying artery. Lesions representing cutaneous involvement in systemic disease tend to resemble severe leukocytoclastic vasculitis with ulceration but without nodule formation. Both benign and systemic variants show a predilection for skin of the lower extremities, and both may be associated with a net-like pattern of erythema (i.e., livedo) involving the adjacent cutaneous surface (Fig. 7–16A).

Histologically, a deep biopsy specimen from a well-selected site of involvement is required for the evaluation of polyarteritis nodosa. At scanning magnification, there is an angiocentric inflammatory infiltrate involving small- to medium-sized arteries within the deep dermis and subcutis (Fig. 7–16B). At higher magnification, the walls of the involved arteries are infiltrated primarily by mononuclear cells and neutrophils with foci of nuclear dust formation (Fig. 7–16C, D). Eosinophils are rarely observed. The infiltration may be segmental, with regions of sparing in vessels sectioned longitudinally, and focally involve only part of the wall of vessels sectioned transversely. Occlusive intraluminal fibrin thrombi may be present in acute lesions, and with chronicity, these thrombi may organize and become associated with obliterative intimal proliferative lesions. The affected vessels may be differentiated from inflamed veins with thickened walls by detection of an internal elastic lamina in routinely stained sections. When the elastic lamina has been fragmented or partially destroyed, elastic tissue histochemistry may be necessary to identify residua of this structure. Secondary inflammatory changes may also be seen in the adjacent dermis as well as in the subcutaneous fat. The secondary panniculitis of polyarteritis nodosa may assume a lobular pattern and thus produce confusion with early lesions of nodular vasculitis or erythema induratum (see Chap. 10).

Migratory Thrombophlebitis[24]

- INVOLVEMENT OF DEEP DERMAL OR SUBCUTANEOUS VEINS
- LUMINAL THROMBOSIS
- INFILTRATION OF VEIN WALL BY MONONUCLEAR CELLS, OCCASIONALLY MULTINUCLEATED

The clinical appearance of superficial migratory thrombophlebitis consists of multiple coalescent tender nodules and indurated plaques occurring often but not invariably on the lower extremities (Fig. 7–17A). In addition to panniculitis, the differential diagnosis therefore often includes cutaneous polyarteritis nodosa. Histologically, medium-sized subcutaneous veins show expansion of their walls by edema fluid and inflammatory cell infiltration (Fig. 7–17B). The lumina of involved vessels are characteristically occluded by recent or organizing thrombi. Inflammation may spill over into the surrounding fat, producing a localized mantle of secondary panniculitis. At higher magnification, the inflammatory component within the vessel wall of established lesions consists of lymphocytes and histiocytes with occasional multinucleated macrophages (Fig. 7–17C). Neutrophils may

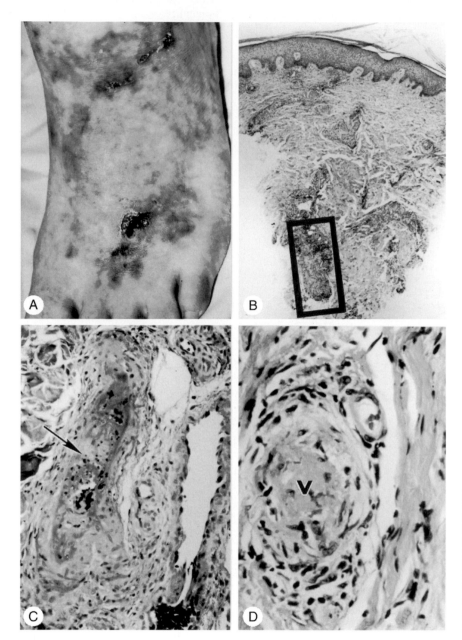

Figure 7–16. Cutaneous polyarteritis nodosa. **(A)** Painful, nodular lesions along the line of arteries underlying the skin of the dorsum of the foot. Note the livedo pattern of mottled erythema that accompanies the vascular insult. **(B)** A deep biopsy specimen includes a medium-sized cutaneous artery *(enclosed in rectangle)* infiltrated by inflammatory cells. **(C, D)** Higher magnifications of affected arteries reveal mixed inflammatory cells within the vessel wall **(C,** *arrow)* and luminal obliteration by fibrin and cellular debris **(D,** v). Obsolescent lesions demonstrate marked intimal fibrosis and luminal recanalization.

Table 7–3. RARE FORMS OF ANGIOCENTRIC DERMATITIS

DISORDER	VESSEL TYPE	INFLAMMATORY COMPONENT	CLINICAL FEATURES
Kawasaki disease	Superficial dermal venules	Lymphocytes	Fever, conjunctivitis, palm and sole redness, mucosal erythema, cervical adenopathy
Degos disease	Deep dermal venules	Lymphocytes	Porcelain white infarcts, gut and central nervous system lesions
Allergic granulomatosis	Small arteries and veins	Neutrophils and eosinophils; palisaded dermal granulomas	Asthma, eosinophilia, pulmonary infiltrates
Wegener granulomatosis	Small arteries and veins	Neutrophils; dermal necrotizing granulomas	Necrotizing upper airway granulomas, pulmonary vasculitis, glomerulonephritis
Giant cell arteritis	Temporal artery	Lymphocytes and macrophages	Lateral forehead pain, blindness

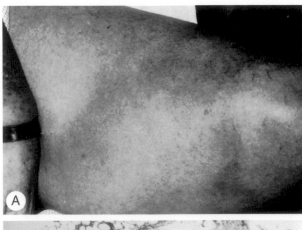

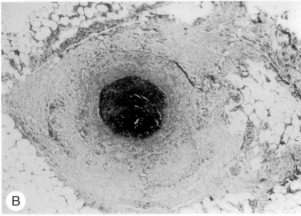

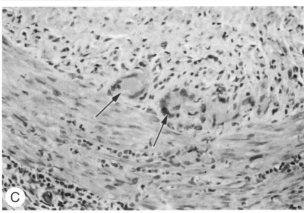

Figure 7–17. Superficial migratory thrombophlebitis. **(A)** Coalescent nodules form linear plaques that are exquisitely tender. **(B)** A subcutaneous vein is occluded by a thrombus and shows thickening of its wall due to edema and inflammatory infiltration. **(C)** The wall of the affected vein is infiltrated by mononuclear cells and occasional multinucleated giant cells *(arrows)*.

be detected in early evolutionary phases of this disorder. In healing lesions, in which organization of the luminal thrombus has occurred, multinucleated cells may persist, a finding of diagnostic value in reconstructing the earlier inflammatory phase.

Rare Disorders

- KAWASAKI DISEASE[25]
- DEGOS DISEASE[26] (Fig. 7–18)
- ALLERGIC GRANULOMATOSIS[27]

- WEGENER GRANULOMATOSIS[28]
- GIANT CELL ARTERITIS[29]

These disorders are rare and will not be discussed in depth. Table 7–3, however, summarizes some of the salient clinical and pathologic features of these entities.

DIFFERENTIAL DIAGNOSIS

The differential diagnostic approach to angiocentric dermatitis involves several obvious branch points. First, it should be determined whether or not the process involves vascular injury or necrosis. Next, the size and nature of the vessel (e.g., artery, arteriole, vein, venule, capillary) should be identified. The character, composition, and extent of the inflammatory component should then be considered. Whether or not extravascular alterations are present (e.g., granulomas, abscesses) should be ascertained. And perhaps most importantly, the gross pathology and clinical history should be carefully considered. With this approach, most common forms and presentations of angiogenic dermatitis can be sorted into diagnostic categories that will permit the generation of a limited and focused differential diagnosis. This approach should also avoid the all too common and unacceptable pitfall of designating various forms of angiogenic

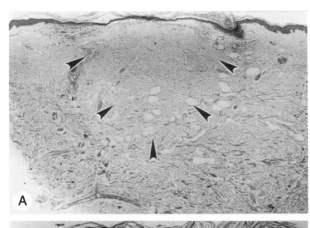

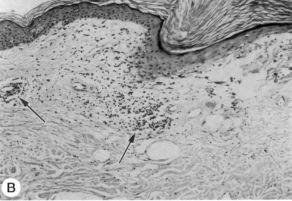

Figure 7–18. Rare forms of angiocentric dermatitis: Malignant atrophic papulosis. **(A)** At scanning magnification, there is a wedge-shaped dermal infarct *(arrowheads)* bordered by an angiocentric lymphocytic infiltrate and surmounted by epidermal atrophy and hyperkeratosis. **(B)** Higher magnification reveals cuffs of lymphocytes about small venules *(arrows)*; occasionally, necrotizing vascular injury is documented at the base of the zone of infarcted dermis.

dermatitis acute or chronic inflammation in lieu of a legitimate diagnosis.

SELECTED REFERENCES

1. Winkelmann RK, Reizner GT. Diffuse dermal neutrophilia in urticaria. Hum Pathol 1988;19:389.
2. Soter NA. Chronic urticaria as a manifestation of necrotizing venulitis. N Engl J Med 1977;296:1440.
3. Soter NA, Wasserman SI. Urticaria, angioedema. Int J Dermatol 1979;18:517.
4. Callen JP, Hanno R. Pruritic urticarial papules and plaques of pregnancy (PUPPP). J Am Acad Dermatol 1981;5:401.
5. Lawley TJ, Hertz HC, Wade TR, et al. Pruritic urticarial papules and plaques of pregnancy. J Am Med Assoc 1979;241:1696.
6. Troyer C, Grossman ME, Silvers DN. Erythema marginatum in rheumatic fever: Early diagnosis by skin biopsy. J Am Acad Dermatol 1983;8:724.
7. Bressler GS, Jones RE Jr. Erythema annulare centrifugum. J Am Acad Dermatol 1981;4:597.
8. Harrison PV. The annular erythemas. Int J Dermatol 1979;18:282.
9. Berger BW, Kaplan MH, Rothberg IR, Barbour AG. Isolation and characterization of the Lyme disease spirochete from the skin of patients with erythema chronicum migrans. J Am Acad Dermatol 1985;13:444.
10. Berger BW. Erythema chronicum migrans of Lyme disease. Arch Dermatol 1984;120:1017.
11. Hood AF, Elpern DJ, Morison WL. Histologic findings in papulovesicular light eruption. J Cutan Pathol 1986;13:13.
12. Muhlbauer JE, Bahn AK, Harrist TJ, et al. Papular polymorphic light eruption: An immunoperoxidase study using monoclonal antibodies. Br J Dermatol 1983;108:153.
13. Hozle E, Plewig G, Hofman C, et al. Polymorphous light eruption: Experimental reproduction of skin lesions. J Am Acad Dermatol 1982;7:111.
14. Jessner M, Kanof NB. Lymphocytic infiltration of the skin. Arch Dermatol Syphilol 1953;68:447.
15. Dvorak HF, Mihm MC, Dvorak AM. Morphology of delayed type hypersensitivity in man. J Invest Dermatol 1976;67:391.
16. Sams WM Jr. Necrotizing vasculitis. J Am Acad Dermatol 1980;3:1.
17. Sanchez NP, Van Hale HM, Su WPD. Clinical and histopathologic spectrum of necrotizing vasculitis. Arch Dermatol 1985;121:220.
18. Frost FA, Heenan PJ. Facial granuloma. Australas J Dermatol 1984;25:121.
19. Leboit PE, Ven TSB, Wintroub B. The evolution of lesions in erythema elevatum diutinum. Am J Dermatopathol 1986;8:392.
20. Gammon WR, Wheeler CE Jr. Urticarial vasculitis. Arch Dermatol 1979;115:76.
21. Fauci AS. The spectrum of vasculitis. Ann Intern Med 1978;89:660.
22. Massa MC, Su WPD. Lymphocytic vasculitis: Is it a specific clinicopathological entity? J Cutan Pathol 1984;11:132.
23. Diaz-Perez JL, Schroeter AL, Winkelmann RK. Cutaneous polyarteritis nodosa. Arch Dermatol 1980;116:56.
24. James WD. Trousseau's syndrome. Int J Dermatol 1984;23:205.
25. Bell DM, Brink EW, Nitzkin JL, et al. Kawasaki syndrome. N Engl J Med 1981;304:1568.
26. Soter N, Murphy GF, Mihm MC. Lymphocytes and necrosis of the cutaneous microvasculature in malignant atrophic papulosis. J Am Acad Dermatol 1982;7:620.
27. Strauss L, Churg J, Zak FG. Cutaneous lesions of allergic granulomatosis. A histopathologic study. J Invest Dermatol 1951;17:349.
28. Feinberg R. The protracted superficial phenomenon in pathergic (Wegener's) granulomatosis. Hum Pathol 1981;12:458.
29. Baum EW, Sams WM, Payne RR. Giant cell arteritis. A systemic disease with rare cutaneous manifestations. J Am Acad Dermatol 1982;6:1081.

8
Granulocytic Dermatitis

DEFINITIONS AND GENERAL CONSIDERATIONS

Granulocytes are defined for the purposes of this chapter as mature hematopoietic cells that display cytoplasmic granules visible by high-power light microscopy. Accordingly, granulocytes are segregated in the categories listed in Table 8–1.

There are a finite number of dermatoses that are dominated by granulocytes. The prototypical cause of granulocytic infiltration of the skin is bacterial infection. Neutrophils within scale-crust associated with superficial forms of bacterial infection (e.g., impetigo) produce a clinical and histologic picture often referred to as *impetiginization*. Clinical pustules are generally associated with *microabscesses,* which consist of small, tumor-like aggregates of granulocytes. Microabscesses may occur within or beneath the stratum corneum, within the epidermis or follicular epithelium, or within the dermis. *Pyoderma* is a term used to refer to diffuse, extensive, and permeative infiltration of the dermis by granulocytes.

GROSS PATHOLOGY

The clinical spectrum of granulocytic dermatitis is quite variable. Small lesions associated with microabscess formation often present as pinpoint pustules, whereas large, deep abscesses may appear as painful erythematous nodules. Considerable edema and fibrin extravasation often accompany less localized granulocytic infiltrates, producing indurated, erythematous plaques. The potent complement of proteolytic enzymes released by activated granulocytes frequently produces secondary injury to surrounding cells and structures, especially in chronic lesions. In these instances, it is not unusual for epidermal breakdown and frank ulceration to ensue. Tumoral aggregates of malignant granulocytes result in a clinical lesion termed chloroma, which characteristically appears as a nodule with a green hue.

GENERAL HISTOLOGY AND TEMPORAL EVOLUTION

As mentioned previously, the general histologic appearance of granulocytic dermatitis depends on the predominant cell type (e.g., neutrophil or eosinophil) and the architectural pattern produced on cutaneous infiltration (e.g., aggregated versus diffuse, association with preexisting structures such as hair follicles). Although acute lesions generally show only infiltrating granulocytes and edema, which is often extensive, chronic lesions will often demonstrate secondary tissue injury and fibrosis. The issue of secondary injury is an important one, because certain differential diagnoses may hinge on reconstruction of the chronology of events within a biopsy specimen. For example, similar patterns of neutrophilic infiltration may be produced in septic vasculitis and acute febrile neutrophilic dermatitis. The former, however, is characterized by primary vascular injury, which is present at very early stages of lesion formation and is often detected at the edge of a given lesion. The latter, conversely, may show foci of secondary vessel injury in established regions, but zones of early neutrophil infiltration, again at the margin of a lesion, are entirely devoid of vessel degeneration or necrosis.

Table 8–1. TYPES OF GRANULOCYTES IN HUMAN DERMATITIS

GRANULOCYTE TYPE	CHARACTERISTIC FEATURE	PROTOTYPICAL DISORDER
Neutrophil	Multilobed nucleus	Impetigo
Eosinophil	Bilobed nucleus, densely eosinophilic cytoplasmic granules	Well syndrome
Basophil	Bilobed nucleus, vague, amphophilic cytoplasmic granules	Rarely encountered in human skin*

*Described in rodent cutaneous basophil hypersensitivity and rarely documented in human dermatitis.

HISTOLOGY OF SPECIFIC DISORDERS

Impetigo[1-3]

- NEUTROPHILS WITHIN STRATUM CORNEUM
- SCALE-CRUST FORMATION
- SUBCORNEAL PUSTULES
- OCCASIONALLY, SUPERFICIAL ACANTHOLYTIC EPIDERMAL BLISTERS
- REACTIVE LYMPHOCYTIC INFILTRATE ABOUT SUPERFICIAL VESSELS

Impetigo is a common superficial infection of the skin, generally caused by staphylococci and streptococci. Impetigo is most often seen in infants, young children, and adults in poor health. Cultures most frequently grow coagulase-positive staphylococcus, group A β-hemolytic streptococci, or both. Nephritogenic strains of streptococcus cause impetigo, particularly in tropical areas and in the southern United States.

Impetigo usually involves exposed skin, particularly that of the face and hands. Initially, it is an erythematous macule, but multiple small pustules rapidly supervene. As pustules break, shallow erosions form and are covered with drying serum, which gives the characteristic clinical appearance of honey-colored crust (Fig. 8–1A). If the crust is not removed, new lesions form about the periphery, and extensive epidermal damage may ensue. Clinical variants of impetigo include impetigo contagiosa, an epidemic form of this disorder affecting preschool children, and bullous impetigo, which is characterized by rapidly progressive vesicles and bullae which may be confused with staphylococcal scalded-skin syndrome (SSSS).

The characteristic microscopic feature of impetigo is accumulation of neutrophils within and beneath the stratum corneum, often with the formation of a subcorneal pustule (Fig. 8–1C, D). Special stains reveal the presence of bacteria in these foci. Nonspecific, reactive epidermal alterations and superficial dermal inflammation accompany these findings. Rupture of pustules results in superficial layering of serum, neutrophils, and cellular debris to form the characteristic clinical crust. Bullous forms of impetigo are characterized by an acantholytic blister at or directly beneath the level of the granular cell layer. Bullae are fluid filled, and neutrophils are frequently scarce. Bullous impetigo may be differentiated from SSSS, which produces similar epidermal changes as a result of distant release of the phage group II staphylococcal toxin exfoliatin, by demonstration of bacteria in lesions by culture of tissue staining in the former, and by the tendency of bullous impetigo, but not SSSS, to show inflammatory

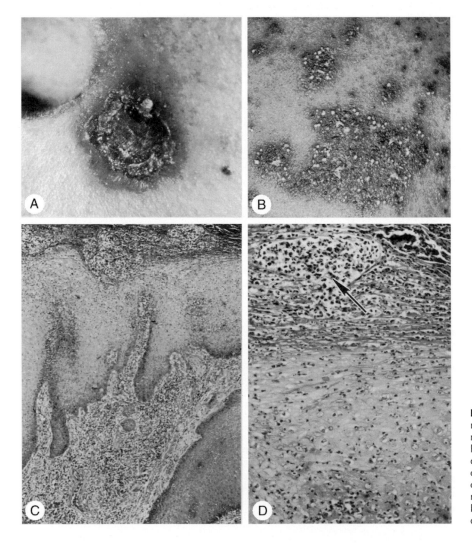

Figure 8–1. Impetigo. **(A)** Bacterial superinfection results in characteristic honey-colored crust surmounting this shallow facial erosion. **(B)** Impetigo herpetiformis, showing multiple grouped pustules covering an erythematous and focally eroded zone of intensive bacterial colonization. **(C, D)** The edge of an impetiginized ulcer shows pseudoepitheliomatous hyperplasia surmounted by scale crust heavily infiltrated by neutrophils (**D**, *arrow*) and colonized by bacteria.

infiltration of the superficial dermis that underlies the forming blister.

It should be remembered that these findings are of significance only in the context of the gross pathology. For example, these histologic findings, along with demonstration of bacteria by special stains or culture, result in a diagnosis when the biopsy specimen is obtained from a crusted or pustular lesion in a child. However, in adults, impetiginization may be a secondary phenomenon, as is frequently the case in actinic keratoses.

Subcorneal Pustular Dermatosis[4, 5]

- ANNULAR OR SERPIGINOUS PUSTULES CLINICALLY
- MICROPUSTULES DIRECTLY BENEATH STRATUM CORNEUM
- NEUTROPHILS PREDOMINATE WITHIN PUSTULES
- EPIDERMAL SPONGIOSIS
- MIXED SUPERFICIAL DERMAL INFLAMMATORY INFILTRATE

Subcorneal pustular dermatosis (SPD), also referred to as Sneddon-Wilkinson disease, is a chronic dermatitis characterized by aggregated pustules, often arranged in serpiginous arrays, most often involving abdominal skin and the skin of the axillary and inguinal folds (Fig. 8–2A, B). Early pustules may contain both clear serum and neutrophils, and pus may segregate within the lower half of larger pustules

(Fig. 8–2A). SPD is associated with monoclonal gammopathy, most commonly IgA paraproteinemia, and with the eventual development of IgA myeloma.

Histologically, scanning magnification reveals a well-formed subcorneal pustule filled with mature neutrophils and admixed serum (Fig. 8–2C, D). Adjacent to the blister, there may be spongiosis, and in advanced lesions, secondary acantholysis may be observed. There is a variable underlying dermal infiltrate composed of lymphocytes, neutrophils, and occasionally eosinophils.

Differentiation of lesions of SPD from those of bullous impetigo may be difficult by histology alone. Impetigo may show bacteria by special stains, but this is not invariable, and culture is a more sensitive means of detecting organisms. Correlation with the clinical setting in which the lesions arose (e.g., facial vesiculopustules in a child versus serpiginous truncal pustules in an adult) will generally assist in assigning the correct diagnosis.

Pustular Candidiasis[6, 7]

- SUBCORNEAL AND OCCASIONAL SPONGIFORM PUSTULES
- REACTIVE EPIDERMAL HYPERPLASIA AND FOCAL SPONGIOSIS
- BRANCHING MYCELIA AND SPORES WITHIN STRATUM CORNEUM

Acute mucocutaneous candidiasis is caused by *Candida albicans,* a dimorphous fungus producing both yeast and

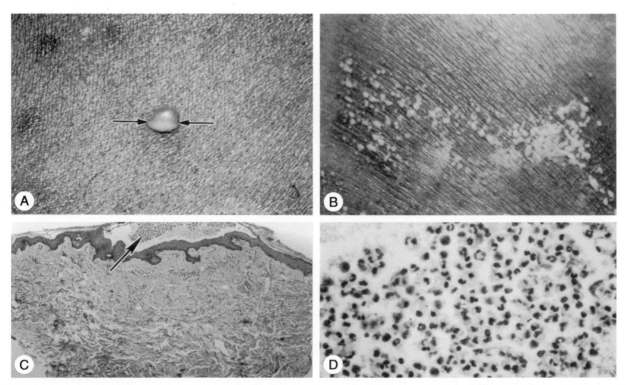

Figure 8–2. Subcorneal pustular dermatosis. **(A)** A solitary subcorneal vesiculo-pustule shows an interface *(arrows)* between serum *(upper half)* and purulent exudate *(lower half).* **(B)** An established plaque of subcorneal pustular dermatosis shows multiple coalescent pustules on an erythematous base. **(C)** Scanning magnification discloses a pure accumulation of neutrophils directly beneath the stratum corneum *(arrow).* **(D)** Higher magnification. In contrast to pustular psoriasis (see Chap. 4), changes of psoriasiform epidermal hyperplasia do not predominate, and neutrophils do not significantly accumulate in the epidermal layers (e.g., as in spongiform pustules).

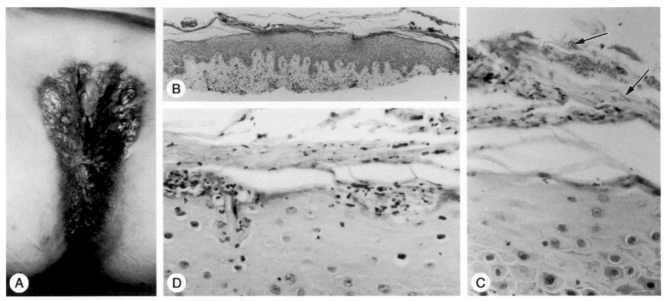

Figure 8–3. Pustular candidiasis. **(A)** Beefy red pustular eruption affecting genital skin in the diaper region of an infant. **(B)** Scanning magnification reveals dense aggregates of neutrophils within a stratum corneum overlying a diffusely hyperplastic epidermal layer. **(C, D)** Higher magnification of budding yeast forms *(arrows)*, stained by periodic acid–Schiff, within the affected stratum corneum.

filamentous growth in the superficial epidermal layers. It is a benign, self-limiting disease that occurs as a result of immunosuppression, changes in the topical cutaneous environment (e.g., excessive sweating), and overgrowth of this commensal organism in the setting of systemic antibiotic therapy. Intertriginous areas, the oral cavity, paronychial skin, and the vulva are preferentially affected (Fig. 8–3A). Generalized neonatal and congenital forms exist in which infection is acquired via passage through the birth canal or as a result of ascending intrauterine spread. Clinical lesions consist of beefy red plaques covered by small pustules.

Histologically, there are multiple foci of neutrophilic infiltration of the stratum corneum, which are best appreciated at scanning magnification (Fig. 8–3B). Well-formed foci are represented by subcorneal pustules, often associated with foci of neutrophilic infiltration and spongiosis involving the upper stratum spinosum (Fig. 8–3D; i.e., spongiform pustules similar to those observed in psoriasis). Mycelia and spores may be detected by PAS stain in the affected stratum corneum, although they are also often apparent in routinely stained sections as well (Fig. 8–3C). Mycelia are pseudoseptate and may show branching; spores are round to ovoid and range between 2 and 5 µm in diameter. Invasion of the epidermal layer by organisms raises the possibility of chronic mucocutaneous candidiasis, a form of infection associated with defective cell-mediated immunity.

Erythema Toxicum Neonatorum[8, 9]

- MACULES, PAPULES, AND PUSTULES WITHIN 48 HOURS AFTER BIRTH
- INTRAFOLLICULAR SUBCORNEAL PUSTULES
- EOSINOPHILS ABOUT VESSELS, WITHIN FOLLICULAR EPITHELIUM, AND COMPOSING PUSTULES

Erythema toxicum neonatorum is a benign, self-limiting eruption that affects newborns within the first several days of life. A relatively common and poorly understood disorder, it may produce enormous initial concern in parents and in physicians not familiar with its occurrence. Clinically, there are punctate macules, papules, and pustules with a follicular distribution involving the trunk and extremities (Fig. 8–4A). Generally, there is eosinophilia within the peripheral blood. An easy way to establish the diagnosis is by scraping a pustular lesion and examining a smear of the exudate, which characteristically will be dominated by eosinophils (Fig. 8–4D).

Biopsy specimens will reveal different alterations depending on the stage of lesional evolution. Early lesions will demonstrate only a perifollicular lymphocytic and eosinophilic infiltrate, often centered about hair follicles. With time, eosinophils progressively migrate into follicular epithelium, where small follicular infundibular abscesses form (Fig. 8–4B, C). It should be remembered that although incontinentia pigmenti may also produce subcorneal eosinophilic pustules, they are invariably interfollicular rather than follicular in location.

Pustular Folliculitis[10, 11]

- NEUTROPHILIC INFILTRATION OF FOLLICULAR INFUNDIBULUM
- MICROABSCESSES WITHIN AND AROUND FOLLICLES
- OCCASIONAL SITES OF FOLLICULAR PERFORATION
- REACTIVE DERMAL ALTERATIONS (E.G., CHRONIC INFLAMMATION, FIBROSIS)

Pustular folliculitis describes a family of acute inflammatory disorders of the superficial portion of the hair follicle

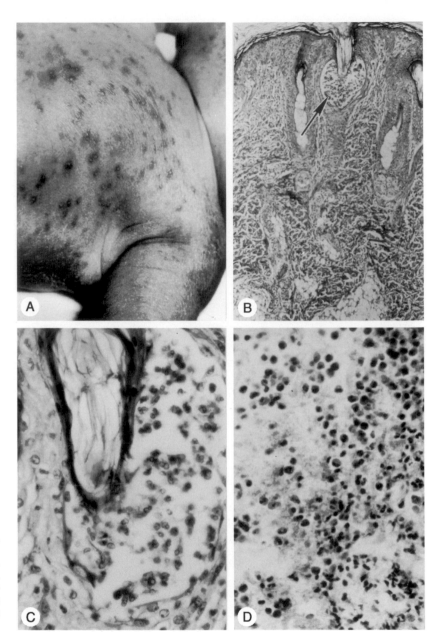

Figure 8–4. Erythema toxicum neonatorum. **(A)** Multiple erythematous pustules are present on the truncal skin of a newborn infant. **(B, C)** Histologically, there are follicular infundibular pustules *(arrow)* composed almost exclusively of eosinophils containing characteristically bilobed nuclei. **(D)** Scraping of superficial pustules permits examination of the inflammatory component as a smear. When eosinophils predominate in this clinical setting, this approach will obviate a skin biopsy.

characterized by neutrophilic infiltration and occasional follicular perforation and destruction. Acute folliculitis may refer to early pustular lesions of acne vulgaris, impetiginization of follicular eczema (acute superficial folliculitis of Bockhart), and deeper forms of abscess-forming folliculitis that may produce clinical furuncles. Eosinophilic pustular folliculitis is a form of superficial folliculitis dominated by eosinophils and associated with acquired immunodeficiency syndrome. Perforating folliculitis is a generic term applied to situations in which follicular epithelium is focally destroyed, leading to extrusion of purulent material and follicular contents into the adjacent dermis. Specific forms of perforating folliculitis (e.g., elastosis perforans serpiginosa) are discussed elsewhere in this text (see Chap. 18). Pustular folliculitis may also result from infection with organisms such as *Malassezia* (e.g., pityrosporum folliculitis) or bacteria other than *Staphylococcus* (e.g., *Pseudomonas* folliculitis).

The features common to all forms of pustular folliculitis

include early infiltration of follicular epithelium by neutrophils, often preferentially involving the infundibulum and region of origination of the sebaceous duct, eventuating in follicular infundibular microabscess formation (Fig. 8–5*B, C*). These early stages correlate with the formation of erythematous, often painful papules containing an enlarging, centrally located tan-yellow pustule (Fig. 8–5*A*). Persistence of neutrophils and their enzymes within the follicular epithelium may cause localized destruction of epithelium, resulting in extrusion of the abscess into the surrounding perifollicular adventitia (Fig. 8–5*C*). Extrusion of follicular contents and potentially of associated bacteria, fungi, and parasites into the dermis may provoke the formation of a larger abscess and increased pain and nodularity clinically (Fig. 8–6*A, B*). Perhaps the most common and painful cause of a large dermal abscess is the rupture of a follicular infundibular cyst, producing on a larger scale the tissue reaction that accompanies microperforations in the setting of purulent folliculitis

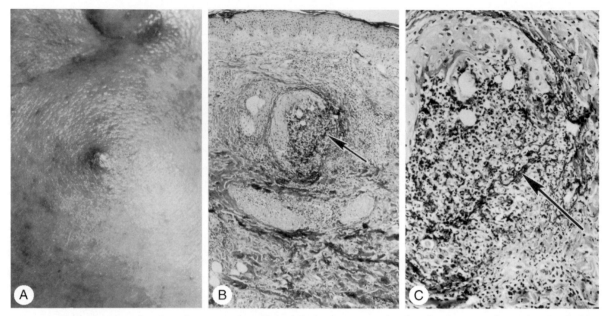

Figure 8–5. Pustular folliculitis. **(A)** The clinical appearance is that of erythematous papules that develop central pustules. **(B, C)** Biopsy reveals destructive follicular infundibular pustules composed of neutrophils. Follicular perforation *(arrows)* may result in secondary inflammation to follicular contents extruded into the dermis.

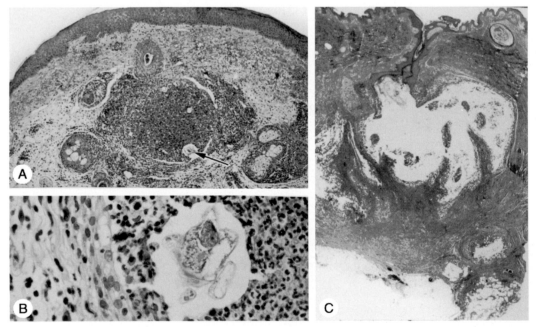

Figure 8–6. Dermal abscess secondary to perforating folliculitis. **(A)** A mid-dermal abscess composed of neutrophils contains a free *Demodex* mite *(arrow)*, evidence that follicular perforation was the cause of this lesion. **(B)** Higher magnification of a *Demodex* mite. **(C)** A large dermal abscess is secondary to rupture of a follicular cyst.

Table 8–2. DISTINGUISHING FEATURES OF COMMON FORMS OF PUSTULAR FOLLICULITIS

DISORDER	CLINICAL APPEARANCE	HISTOLOGY
Acute folliculitis	Tender, red pustules or tender nodules	Infundibular microabscess or dermal abscess with perforation
Eosinophilic pustular folliculitis	Often, annular arrangements of follicular papules and pustules; AIDS or AIDS-related complex (ARC)	Spongiosis about the sebaceous duct; mixed infiltrate with eosinophils; *Demodex* mite may be entrapped
Perforating folliculitis	Painful erythematous nodules; some may drain	Thinning and disruption of follicular epithelium; dermal abscess with foreign-body response
Pityrosporum folliculitis	Erythematous small papules and pustules, often on trunk; may also have lacrimal obstruction	Acute folliculitis with microperforations containing 2–4 μm budding yeast forms
Pseudomonas folliculitis	Pruritic pustules after exposure to water (e.g., hot tubs)	Pilar canal distended by neutrophils; gram-negative rods on Gram stain

(Fig. 8–6C). With time, foreign-body giant cell reaction may occur, as may perifollicular fibrosis. There are several types of pustular folliculitis that may be partially differentiated based on clinical and pathologic parameters. These types are summarized in Table 8–2.

Acute Febrile Neutrophilic Dermatosis[12, 13]

- TENDER, RAISED PLAQUES ASSOCIATED WITH FEVER AND LEUKOCYTOSIS
- COALESCENT NODULAR NEUTROPHILIC INFILTRATE IN SUPERFICIAL AND DEEP DERMIS
- NUCLEAR DUST WITHOUT PRIMARY VASCULAR INJURY
- MARKED SUPERFICIAL DERMAL EDEMA

Also referred to as Sweet syndrome, acute febrile neutrophilic dermatosis is characterized by tender plaques on the face and extremities (Fig. 8–7). Most lesions are erythematous and range in size from 0.5 cm to 2 cm. Onset may be sudden, and associated fever and leukocytosis are the rule. Women are preferentially affected over men, and multiple recurrences may be observed after regression of individual lesions. Vesicular and bullous forms may also develop. Although the pathogenesis is unclear, defective neutrophil chemotaxis or adhesion is probably responsible. There is an association of Sweet-like neutrophilic dermatitis, particularly bullous forms, with myeloproliferative disorders such as acute myelogenous and myelomonocytic leukemia.

The histopathology of acute febrile neutrophilic dermatosis is characterized by coalescent aggregates of neutrophils, some arranged in perivascular array, within the superficial and deep dermis (Fig. 8–8A). Closer inspection reveals nuclear fragmentation (i.e., dust) and occasional fibrin deposits but no evidence of true primary necrotizing vasculitis (Fig. 8–8B). Although the epidermis is generally spared, some lesions will show spongiosis and upward percolation of individual neutrophils between adjacent keratinocytes. The papillary dermis may be markedly edematous, accounting for the superficial dermal vesicles that occur in blistering variants.

Eosinophilic Cellulitis[14, 15]

- SUPERFICIAL AND DEEP DERMAL INFILTRATE OF EOSINOPHILS
- EOSINOPHIL DEGRANULATION
- FLAME FIGURES RIMMED BY EOSINOPHILS AND/OR PALISADES OF GIANT CELLS
- SUPERFICIAL DERMAL EDEMA WITH OCCASIONAL SUBEPIDERMAL BLISTERS

Eosinophilic cellulitis, or Well syndrome, is relatively rare, but is discussed here to contrast it with acute febrile neutrophilic dermatosis. Affected individuals develop recurrent painful or pruritic plaques that are often ill-defined and erythematous. Rapid spread over several days is the rule, followed by gradual resolution of indurated residua over 1 to 2 months. Some but not all patients develop peripheral blood eosinophilia.

Histologically, the superficial and deep dermis are infiltrated by diffuse to vaguely nodular collections of degranulating eosinophils (Fig. 8–8C). These cells are not associated with primary vasculitis, although marked superficial dermal edema and even dermal bulla formation may be observed. Degranulation is characterized by recognizable hypereosinophilic cytoplasmic granules within the extracellular matrix immediately adjacent to the eosinophil plasma membrane. As these cells persist within the dermis, characteristic flame figures become prominent. Flame figures are jagged clusters of degenerating, hypereosinophilic collagen rimmed by degranulating eosinophils and imparting the impression of a

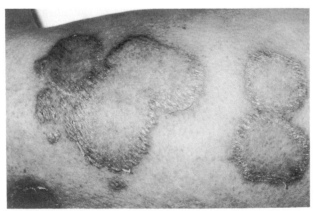

Figure 8–7. Acute febrile neutrophilic dermatosis (i.e., Sweet syndrome). The clinical appearance is characterized by raised, tender erythematous plaques.

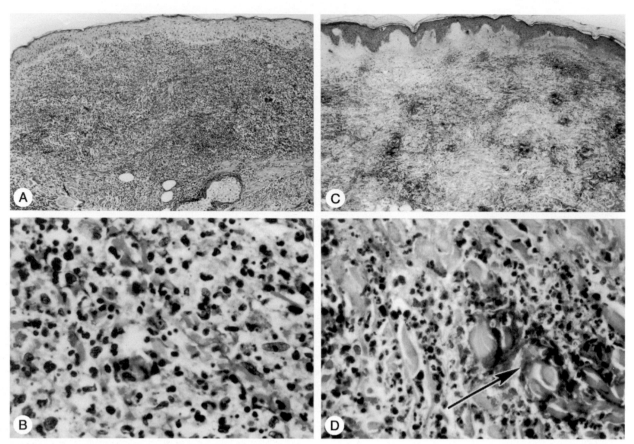

Figure 8–8. Comparison between acute febrile neutrophilic dermatosis and eosinophilic cellulitis. **(A, B)** Sweet syndrome is composed primarily of neutrophils and fibrin within the superficial and deep dermis. Pronounced lesions may be indistinguishable from early pyoderma gangrenosum. Primary vasculitis is not observed, although secondary injury to entrapped vessels may be documented. **(C, D)** Well syndrome is characterized by patchy superficial and deep infiltrates composed predominately of eosinophils. Eosinophilic degeneration of collagen bundles associated with degranulating eosinophils **(D,** *arrow)* is typical and is termed a flame figure.

burst of fire within the otherwise normal tinctorial quality of the background matrix (Fig. 8–8D). With chronicity, flame figures may eventually become surrounded by a palisade of giant cells. Flame figures are relatively specific for eosino-

philic cellulitis, although florid eosinophil-rich arthropod-bite reactions may occasionally show similar alterations. Comparative features of Sweet syndrome and Well syndrome are outlined in Table 8–3.

Table 8–3. COMPARISON OF CLINICOPATHOLOGIC FEATURES OF SWEET AND WELL SYNDROME

CLINICOPATHOLOGIC FEATURE	SWEET SYNDROME	WELL SYNDROME
Clinical features		
Symptoms	Painful plaques	Painful or pruritic plaques
Blisters	Occasionally present	Occasionally present
Fever	Often present	Unusual
Blood	Leukocytosis	Sometimes eosinophilia
Marrow	Leukemia-associated*	No leukemia association
Architecture	Nodular to diffuse, superficial and deep	Nodular to diffuse, superficial and deep
Cytology	Neutrophils	Eosinophils
Granules	Nuclear dust	Eosinophil degranulation
Vascular alterations	None	None
Dermal edema	Papillary	Papillary
Blister formation	Dermal	Dermal
Flame figures	Absent	Present

*Occasional cases, only.

Pyoderma Gangrenosum[16, 17]

- ULCERATED NODULES AND PLAQUES
- CHARACTERISTIC RED-PURPLE, UNDERMINED BORDERS
- DERMIS REPLACED BY DIFFUSE INFILTRATE OF NEUTROPHILS
- NEUTROPHILIC VASCULITIS ABSENT
- STERILE CULTURE

Pyoderma gangrenosum is a disorder that probably represents, along with acute febrile neutrophilic dermatosis, a point along a spectrum of disordered neutrophil chemotaxis. Like acute febrile neutrophilic dermatosis, pyoderma gangrenosum is associated with myeloproliferative disorders. It is also associated with ulcerative colitis, rheumatoid-like polyarthritis, and a primarily IgA-type monoclonal gammopathy, although about one half of cases fail to reveal associated pathology. The lesions of pyoderma gangrenosum are clinically characteristic, consisting of one or more well-defined ulcers bordered by dark-red to purple, undermined edges (Fig. 8–9A). Lesions may begin as fluctuant nodules that quickly break down to form shallow ulcers. Biopsy is often performed to exclude ulcerative lesions of vasculitis, infection, and factitia.

Early lesions and alterations at the edge of an ulcer will demonstrate a mixed inflammatory infiltrate, often with a pronounced perivascular cuff of lymphocytes. There is generally overlying epidermal hyperplasia, which grows downward into the well-defined edge of the ulcer base to produce the punched-out, undermined appearance appreciated clinically (Fig. 8–9B). The ulcer base consists of a sea of neutrophils which replace the dermal matrix but are not associated with primary neutrophilic vasculitis (Fig. 8–9C). Special stains for bacteria and fungi, as well as cultures, are consistently negative if deep lesional tissue is examined to exclude superficial contamination.

The diagnosis of ulcerative colitis is based on tight clinicopathologic correlation and exclusion of conditions that could mimic florid tissue infiltration by neutrophils, particularly infection. Lesions generally respond favorably to therapy with corticosteroids, making exclusion of infection mandatory before implementation of treatment.

Bacterial Pyoderma[18]

- MIXED INFLAMMATORY INFILTRATE COMPOSED PREDOMINANTLY OF NEUTROPHILS
- DIFFUSE TISSUE EDEMA
- SECONDARY VASCULAR INJURY COMMON
- VARIABLE EPIDERMAL HYPERPLASIA AND ULCERATION

The category of bacterial pyoderma is discussed here because it is common and may be misdiagnosed as disorders ranging from vasculitis to squamous cell carcinoma. In classic cases, there is a predisposing condition that favors bacterial invasion and growth within the dermis. Most commonly, there will be associated diabetes mellitus or ischemic changes due to peripheral vascular disease. Zones of cellulitis become painful, warm, and indurated due to cellular infiltration and edema (Fig. 8–10A). Epidermal bullae and sloughing may be

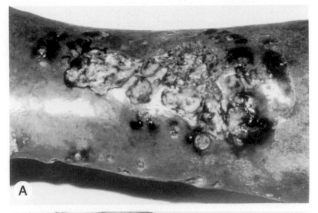

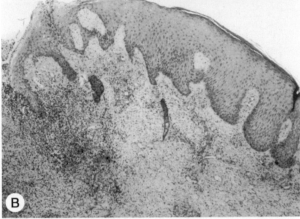

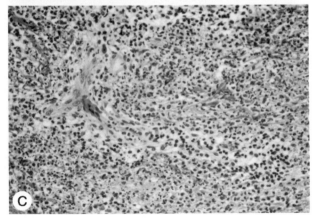

Figure 8–9. Pyoderma gangrenosum. **(A)** The clinical appearance of well-demarcated ulcers with undermined, red-purple borders is typical. **(B)** A biopsy specimen of the edge of an ulcer shows early pseudoepitheliomatous hyperplasia and a marked dermal inflammatory infiltrate. **(C)** Beneath the ulcer base, the dermis is entirely replaced by sheets of neutrophils.

seen in advanced lesions. A variant form, termed *blastomycosis-like pyoderma,* is associated with the development of vegetating, verrucous plaques and pustules bearing a superficial resemblance to cutaneous blastomycosis. Although most forms of pyoderma are associated with ordinary pathogenic bacteria, such as *Staphylococcus aureus,* others may result from more esoteric gram-positive forms, such as *Actinomyces israelii.* Cervicofacial actinomycosis results in indurated plaques containing abscesses and draining sinuses from which characteristic sulfur granules occasionally extrude (Fig. 8–11A).

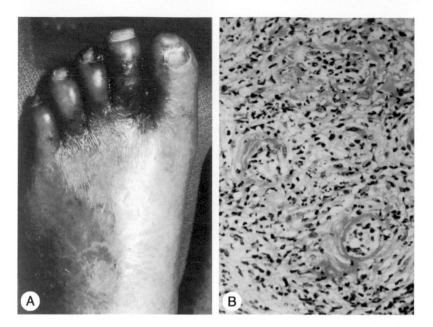

Figure 8–10. Bacterial pyoderma. **(A)** The ischemic foot of this diabetic patient has become superinfected by bacteria, producing increased erythema, edema, and local pain. **(B)** Biopsy specimens and culture reveal a mixed inflammatory infiltrate composed predominately of neutrophils; Gram stain revealed intracellular bacteria. Certain pyodermas may be characterized by marked epidermal hyperplasia (e.g., blastomycosis-like pyoderma).

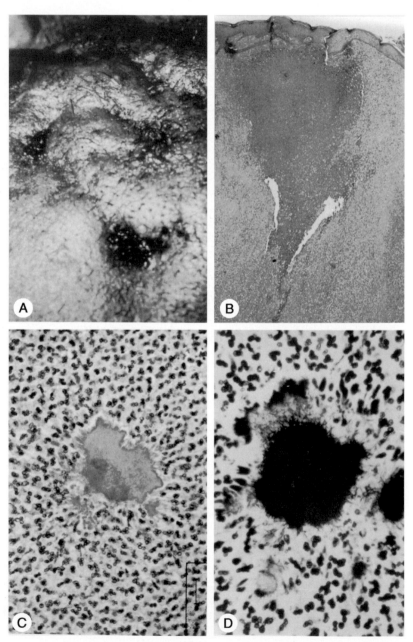

Figure 8–11. Actinomycosis. **(A)** Boggy, indurated facial skin contains several draining sinus tracts. **(B)** Scanning view of a sinus tract that extends from the epidermal layer into deep subcutaneous tissue. The central portion is filled with abscess-like aggregates of neutrophils; the borders of the tract are composed of granulation tissue. **(C)** Closer inspection of the abscess-like zone reveals characteristic sulfur granules of *Actinomyces* (bar = 100 μ). **(D)** Slender filaments extend from the perimeter of the basophilic granule and stain intensely with Gram stain.

Granulocytic Dermatitis ■ 149

Histologically, biopsy of pyoderma is often nonspecific, with neutrophils and mononuclear cells infiltrating diffusely throughout a markedly edematous dermal layer (Fig. 8–10B). Secondary injury to small vessels may result in the mistaken diagnosis of necrotizing vasculitis if the clinical picture and gross appearance of lesions is not fully considered. The overlying epidermis may show ischemic necrosis, basal cell layer vacuolization with incipient or evolving blister formation, or marked pseudocarcinomatous hyperplasia, as is the case in blastomycosis-like pyoderma, in which dermal and intraepidermal microabscesses are also prominent. Dermal abscesses and sinus tracts should always raise suspicion of infection, and the possibility of unusual as well as ordinary infectious causes should be considered in each patient. In cervicofacial actinomycosis, there is an admixture of granulation tissue and chronic inflammatory cells with discrete dermal abscesses and sinus tracts. Within the aggregated neutrophils that form these structures (Fig. 8–11B) there are colonies of basophilic filamentous bacteria averaging about 300 mm in diameter (Fig. 8–11C, D). These structures are highlighted by use of Gram or silver stains.

Rare Disorders

- TRANSIENT NEONATAL PUSTULAR MELANOSIS[19]
- ACROPUSTULOSIS OF INFANCY[20]
- NEUTROPHILIC ECCRINE HIDRADENITIS[21]
- HYPEREOSINOPHILIC SYNDROME[22]
- INTESTINAL BYPASS SYNDROME[23]

There are numerous disorders that qualify as granulocytic dermatitis but are only rarely encountered. Some of

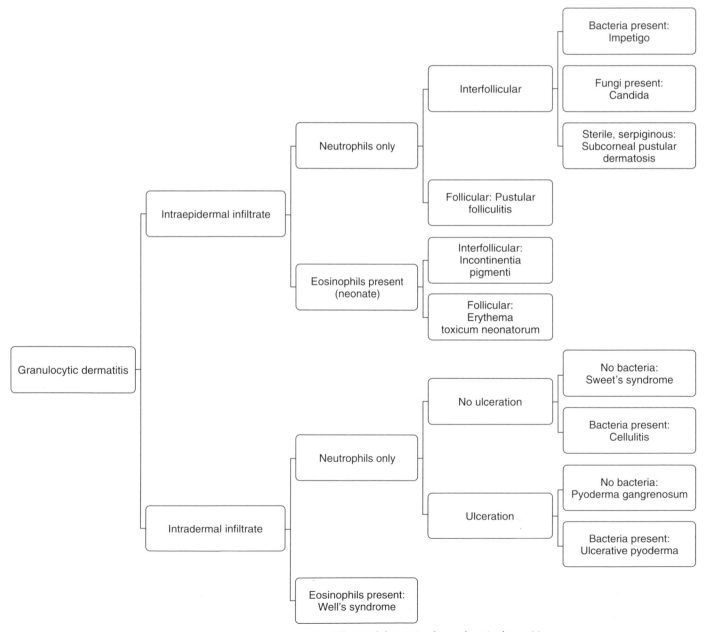

Figure 8–12. Algorithmic approach to differential diagnosis of granulocytic dermatitis.

these have already been mentioned in discussions of more common disorders (e.g., chronic mucocutaneous candidiasis). Others are listed in this section, with references to more comprehensive treatments for purposes of further reading. The complicated associations with other conditions evidenced in this short list provide intriguing clues concerning the pathogenesis of neutrophilic dermatitis in general.

Transient neonatal pustular melanosis, for example, is a curious disorder affecting a small percentage of black newborns in which flaccid vesiculopustules soon develop into hyperpigmented macules. The histology shows intracorneal and subcorneal aggregates of neutrophils and occasional eosinophils. *Acropustulosis of infancy,* on the other hand, consists of recurrent crops of pruritic vesiculopustules involving the distal extremity skin of newborns. The histology may resemble impetigo or subcorneal pustular dermatosis, thus making correlation with clinical information critical to accurate diagnosis.

Neutrophilic eccrine hidradenitis is a disorder that produces erythematous papules and plaques and occurs most often in individuals with myelogenous leukemia after induction chemotherapy. Biopsy, which is usually performed to exclude leukemia cutis, infection, or vasculitis, reveals accumulation of neutrophils about degenerating eccrine coils. *Hypereosinophilic syndrome* is characterized by tissue and organ edema and eosinophil infiltration associated with peripheral blood eosinophilia. The skin and underlying soft tissues may be diffusely edematous and infiltrated by degranulating eosinophils; in some lesions, eosinophils may be sparse, although one of their secretory products, major basic protein, is detectable immunohistochemically. *Intestinal bypass syndrome* is characterized by polyarthritis and vesiculopustules located mainly on the extremities of patients who have undergone jejunal-ileal bypass surgery. Histologically, there is a dermal neutrophilic infiltrate with variable evidence of necrotizing vasculitis. Subepidermal pustules eventually develop in association with marked papillary dermal edema.

DIFFERENTIAL DIAGNOSIS

A simplified schema for the differential diagnosis of granulocytic dermatitis, exclusive of angiocentric granulocytic infiltrates (see Angiocentric Dermatitis), is provided in Figure 8–12. It is critical to appreciate that many of these disorders require close correlation with clinical parameters to reach a definitive diagnosis. However, Figure 8–12 should at least provide a conceptual overview of important branch points in the form of a diagnostic algorithm that is helpful in evaluating the scanning and higher-power histology of the relevant conditions.

SELECTED REFERENCES

1. Dajani AS, Ferrieri P, Wannamaker LW. Natural history of impetigo. Etiologic agents and bacterial interactions. J Clin Invest 1972;51:2863.
2. Elias PM, Levy SW. Bullous impetigo. Occurrence of localized scalded skin syndrome in an adult. Arch Dermatol 1976;112:856.
3. Wuepper KD, Dimond RL, Knutson DD. Studies of mechanisms of epidermal injury by a staphylococcal epidermolytic toxin. J Invest Dermatol 1975;65:191.
4. Sneddon IB, Wilkinson DS. Subcorneal pustular dermatosis. Br J Dermatol 1956;68:385.
5. Sanchez NP, Perry HO, Muller SA. Subcorneal pustular dermatosis and pustular psoriasis. Arch Dermatol 1983;119:715.
6. Maibach HI, Kligman AM. The biology of experimental human cutaneous moniliasis (*Candida albicans*). Arch Dermatol 1962;85:233.
7. Kirkpatrick CH, Rich RR, Bennett JE. Chronic mucocutaneous candidiasis: Model-building in cellular immunity. Ann Intern Med 1971;74:955.
8. Freeman RG, Spiller R, Knox JM. Histopathology of erythema toxicum neonatorum. Arch Dermatol 1960;82:586.
9. Pohlandt F, Harnisch R, Meigel WN, et al. Zum Bild des Erythema toxicum neonatorum. Hautarzt 1977;28:469.
10. Fox AB, Hambrick GW Jr. Recreationally associated *Pseudomonas aeruginosa* folliculitis. Arch Dermatol 1984;120:1304.
11. Pinkus H. Furuncle. J Cutan Pathol 1979;6:517.
12. Cooper PH, Frierson HF, Greer KE. Subcutaneous neutrophilic infiltrates in acute febrile neutrophilic dermatosis. Arch Dermatol 1983;119:610.
13. Cooper PH, Innes DJ Jr, Greer KE. Acute febrile neutrophilic dermatosis (Sweet's syndrome) and myeloproliferative disorders. Cancer 1983;51:1518.
14. Wells GC, Smith NP. Eosinophilic cellulitis. Br J Dermatol 1979;100:101.
15. Newton JA, Greaves MW. Eosinophilic cellulitis (Well's syndrome) with florid histologic changes. Clin Exp Dermatol 1988;13:318.
16. Su WPD, Schroeter AL, Perry HO, et al. Histopathologic and immunopathologic study of pyoderma gangrenosum. J Cutan Pathol 1986;13:323.
17. Lazarus GS, Goldsmith LA, Rockin RE, et al. Pyoderma gangrenosum, altered delayed hypersensitivity, and polyarthritis. Arch Dermatol 1972;105:46.
18. Su WPD, Duncan SC, Perry HO. Blastomycosis-like pyoderma. Arch Dermatol 1979;115:170.
19. Barr RJ, Globerman LM, Werber FA. Transient neonatal pustular melanosis. Int J Dermatol 1979;18:636.
20. Vignon-Pennamen MD, Wallach D. Infantile acropustulosis. Arch Dermatol 1979;122:1155.
21. Harrist TJ, Fine JD, Berman RS, et al. Neutrophilic eccrine hidradenitis: A distinctive type of neutrophilic dermatosis associated with myelogenous leukemia and chemotherapy. Arch Dermatol 1982;118:263.
22. Fitzpatrick JM, Johnson C, Simon P, et al. Cutaneous microthrombi: A histologic clue to the diagnosis of hypereosinophilic syndrome. Am J Dermatopathol 1987;9:419.
23. Morrison JGL, Fourie ED. A distinctive skin eruption following small-bowel by-pass surgery. Br J Dermatol 1980;102:467.

9

Granulomatous Dermatitis

DEFINITIONS AND GENERAL CONSIDERATIONS

The term granulomatous dermatitis is used in this chapter to designate the diverse array of cutaneous inflammatory disorders characterized by dermal and sometimes subcutaneous granulomas. A granuloma is a localized collection of activated histiocytes which may or may not be rimmed by lymphocytes and/or show central necrosis. Activated histiocytes are macrophage-derived cells that ingest either foreign particulates or protein antigens, resulting in attempted lysosomal degradation or antigen processing and presentation. Activated histiocytes often become enlarged, sometimes exhibit multinucleation, and generally show conspicuous eosinophilic cytoplasm resembling epithelial cell cytoplasm. Thus, such cells are often referred to as epithelioid histiocytes.

Particulate material ingested by histiocytes may be birefringent and detectable by polarization microscopy within cytoplasmic granules. Other putative stimuli of epithelioid cell transformation may not be detected, although arrays of lysosomes, presumably activated by these provocative agents, may be visible, as is the case in the star-shaped cytoplasmic asteroid body, often seen in sarcoidosis. Multinucleation within granulomas may be of diagnostic significance, as is the case in cutaneous tuberculosis, in which these cells often have wreath-like configurations of nuclei about the cell perimeter (i.e., Langhans giant cells). Foreign-body giant cells, on the other hand, tend to have more centrally clustered nuclei without a well-defined wreath-like configuration. The presence or absence of central necrosis within granulomas is of limited diagnostic assistance, although the prototypical lesion of sarcoidosis is often described as being composed of predominantly noncaseating, naked (i.e., free of surrounding lymphocytes) granulomas. Granulomas with extensive necrosis, conversely, often suggest the presence of causative organisms, as is the case in mycobacterial and deep mycotic infections. Some granulomas form aggregates about degenerating or "necrobiotic" collagen. Necrobiosis may be associated with mucin deposition, as in granuloma annulare; fibrinoid degeneration of collagen, as seen in a rheumatoid nodule; or sclerosis and homogenization of collagen bundles, as is typical in necrobiosis lipoidica. In all of these disorders, well-formed granulomas are characterized by an array of histiocytes radially arranged about the perimeter of the necrobiotic zone, with the long axes of each cell in parallel (i.e., palisaded granulomas).

The pattern formed by granulomatous inflammation in the skin may be of diagnostic assistance. For example, in sarcoidosis, granulomas may be randomly scattered throughout the superficial and deep dermis, whereas in leprosy they tend to wind around neurovascular bundles in a serpiginous manner. Granulomas in secondary syphilis are poorly formed and tend to be concentrated within the papillary dermis in association with cytotoxic alteration of the basal cell layer. In the case of granulomatous inflammation that accompanies follicular perforation, the histiocytic aggregates are centered about the offending pilar epithelium.

GROSS PATHOLOGY

The gross pathology of granulomatous dermatitis is highly variable. Often, early lesions are covered by a smooth epidermal surface that is unaffected by the underlying dermal inflammation. In advanced disease, ulceration may be present, particularly if there is transepidermal elimination of granulomatous foci or underlying vascular compromise. Although erythema may be present as a result of varying degrees of secondary angiocentric lymphocytic inflammation, the granulomatous foci themselves are not red. Rather, they tend to display a green-yellow hue like apple jelly, especially when background erythema is eliminated by dioscopy (i.e., downward compression over the lesion with a flat glass slide).

In certain lesions, the clinical appearance of granulomatous dermatitis may be very helpful in formulating a differential diagnostic assessment. Chromomycosis, for example, often exhibits numerous black dots on the lesion surface, the result of transepidermal elimination of pigmented spores. Leprosy may present as a plaque with associated anesthesia, indicative of extensive involvement and destruction of underlying cutaneous nerves. Localization of plaques to anatomic sites of environmental and occupational contact may provide important clues to diagnosis, as is the case in zirconium-induced granulomatous dermatitis of axillary skin due to application of antiperspirants. Finally, certain forms of granulomatous dermatitis have a characteristic gross pathologic presentation, as is the case with the circinate dermal papules of granuloma annulare.

GENERAL HISTOLOGY AND TEMPORAL EVOLUTION

Early phases of granulomatous dermatitis may exhibit remarkably nonspecific histologic pictures, often dominated by an angiocentric lymphocytic inflammatory infiltrate, with relatively little in the way of aggregated epithelioid histiocytes. Histiocytic infiltration may be insidious in early stages, as is the case in palisaded granulomatous dermatitis, in which histiocytes are present in small numbers among collagen bundles. As histiocytes begin to aggregate to form discrete granulomas, epithelioid cell transformation accompanied by cytoplasmic eosinophilia and multinucleation may be increasingly apparent. With chronicity, granulomas may be associated with zones of fibrosis and collagen deposition, as is the case in long-standing lesions of silicosis.

HISTOLOGY OF SPECIFIC DISORDERS

Infectious Granulomas[1-6]

- DERMAL AGGREGATES OF EPITHELIOID HISTIOCYTES
- NECROSIS AND MICROABSCESSES MAY BE PRESENT
- ABSENCE OF BIREFRINGENT MATERIAL OR VASCULITIS
- ABSENCE OF PRIMARY PANNICULITIS
- PATIENT OFTEN IMMUNOCOMPROMISED

Granulomas due to infectious agents may result from a variety of organisms. A partial listing of offending agents that must be considered and excluded as causes of granulomatous dermatitis is presented in Table 9–1.

As a general rule, granulomatous dermatitis resulting from infection is rare, although it is frequently considered and excluded by special stains in the differential diagnosis of sarcoidosis, panniculitis in immunocompromised hosts, and even in certain atypical granulomatous responses to foreign material or follicular rupture. The clinical appearance of infectious granulomas may be highly variable, ranging from erythematous plaques and nodules to frank ulcers with purulent drainage and sinus tract formation. Histologically, suspicion of infection is heightened by zones of necrosis, microabscesses, or the general absence of evidence supporting an obvious cause (e.g., the pattern and composition of a specific granulomatous panniculitis, or clear evidence of material that may elicit granuloma formation, such as keratin). Infectious granulomas may be well formed, as is the case in tuberculoid leprosy, or they may be composed of vague ag-

gregates of vacuolated histiocytes, as may be seen in leishmaniasis. Infectious granulomas in immunocompromised hosts may be so poorly formed that only foci of necrosis and admixed acute and chronic inflammatory cells with the vague appearance of loosely aggregated granulomas may suggest the procurement of the appropriate special stains that could result in a life-saving diagnosis.

There are a number of clinical and histologic differential diagnostic features that are helpful in the evaluation of granulomatous dermatitis due to infection. In *cutaneous cryptococcosis*, for example, a biopsy specimen from a cutaneous plaque studded with small papules may reveal diffuse granulomatous inflammation replete with multinucleated giant cells alternating with zones of gelatinous material that is devoid of significant inflammation but contains numerous spores, each surrounded by mucinous capsules (Fig. 9–1). In *histoplasmosis*, similar granulomatous dermal inflammation containing multinucleated giant cells reveals spores even smaller than cryptococci devoid of surrounding mucinous alteration (Fig. 9–2). Pigmented organisms that do not require periodic acid–Schiff (PAS) or silver stains for visualization characterize the granulomatous dermal foci of *chromomycosis* (Fig. 9–3). In *mucormycosis*, vague granulomas within inflamed granulation tissue will harbor large, ribbon-like hyphae that characteristically branch at right angles (Fig. 9–4). *Aspergillosis*, on the other hand, produces variable degrees of granulomatous dermal inflammation containing hyphae that branch at acute angles (Fig. 9–5). *Coccidioides immitis (coccidioidomycosis)* results in giant cells containing large spores which, during multiplication, may contain numerous internal endospores (Fig. 9–6). In ulcerated or draining lesions, diagnostic organisms may be detected near the skin surface as a result of extrusion of dermal inflammatory cells. The organisms of *rhinosporidiosis* are characteristically 6- to 10-μm spores, often within 250- to 350-μm rounded sporangia surrounded by a mixed cellular infiltrate containing granulomatous foci (Fig. 9–7). Unlike the other organisms

Table 9–1. ORGANISMS RESPONSIBLE FOR GRANULOMATOUS DERMATITIS

ORGANISMS	DISORDER
Fungi	
Aspergillus sp	Aspergillosis
Blastomyces dermatitides	Blastomycosis
Candida albicans	Candidiasis
Fonsecaea, Phialophora, and *Cladosporium* sp	Chromomycosis
Coccidioides immitis	Coccidioidomycosis
Cryptococcus neoformans	Cryptococcosis
Histoplasma capsulatum	Histoplasmosis
Rhizopus and *Mucor* sp	Mucormycosis
Rhinosporidium seeberi	Rhinosporidiosis
Sporothrix schenckii	Sporotrichosis
Bacteria	
Calymmatobacterium granulomatis	Granuloma inguinale
Treponema pallidum	Granulomatous syphilis
Mycobacterium tuberculosis	Lupus vulgaris
Mycobacterium marinum	Swimming-pool granuloma
Mycobacterium leprae	Leprosy
Protozoa	
Leishmania sp	Leishmaniasis and kala-azar

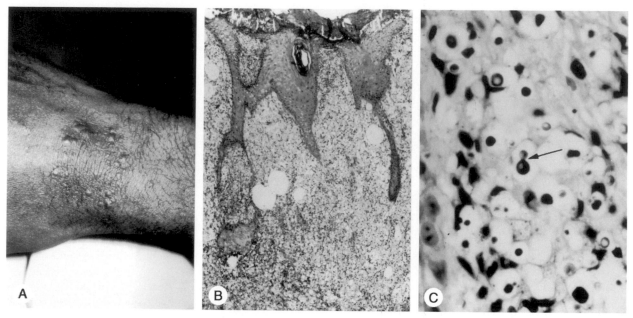

Figure 9–1. Infectious granulomas: Cryptococcosis. **(A)** The skin of a renal transplant patient shows a hyperpigmented plaque studded by small, firm papules. **(B)** A diffusely granulomatous response is present in the dermis, underlying reactive epidermal hyperplasia. **(C)** Periodic acid–Schiff stain reveals a narrow-necked, budding spore *(arrow)* surrounded by a clear halo, representing a mucinous capsule.

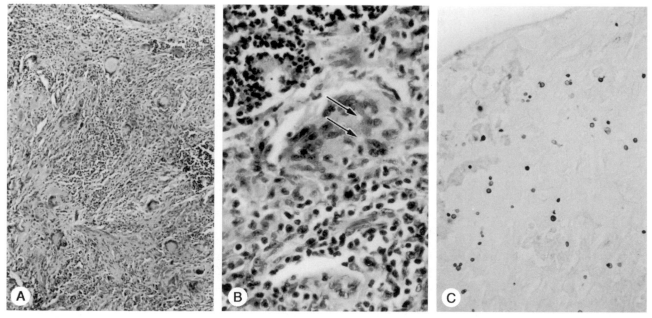

Figure 9–2. Infectious granulomas: Histoplasmosis. **(A)** This lesion on the elbow is characterized by diffuse granulomatous inflammation of the superficial and deep dermis. **(B)** Note the prominent multinucleated giant cells, in which rounded clear zones *(arrows)* are detected. These zones represent cytoplasmic lacunae where spores reside. **(C)** Silver stain reveals numerous spores 2 to 4 μm in diameter.

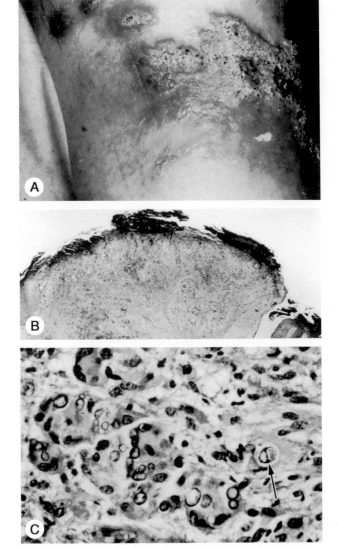

Figure 9–3. Infectious granulomas: Chromomycosis. **(A)** The clinical picture of verrucous nodules and plaques on the lower extremity is typical. **(B)** A biopsy specimen reveals epidermal ulceration bordered by hyperplasia and a dense dermal inflammatory infiltrate composed of noncaseating granulomas as well as aggregates of neutrophils. **(C)** Organisms are endogenously pigmented, copper-colored spores within multinucleated giant cells. They do not reproduce by budding, but rather by formation of septa within individual spores *(arrow).*

listed previously, rhinosporidiosis preferentially affects nasal skin and mucosa, producing pruritus and coryza. *Sporothrix schenckii* infection also results in a characteristic clinical picture, with ascending lymphatic involvement from the inoculation site often resulting in linear dermal nodules (Fig. 9–8A). The organisms of *sporotrichosis* are 4- to 6-μm, round-to-ovoid spores, sometimes accompanied by characteristic cigar-shaped or radially arranged buds (Fig. 9–8B–D).

All *mycobacterial infections* of skin are characterized by small, variably beaded, acid-fast bacilli within histiocytes comprising granulomatous lesions. Organisms may be few in number, and are often best detected in zones that border regions of necrosis or in the setting of immunosuppression. The most common form of cutaneous tuberculosis, *lupus vulgaris,* is characterized by well-formed tuberculoid dermal granulomas on head and neck skin (Fig. 9–9). *Atypical mycobacterial infections,* such as swimming-pool granuloma caused by *Mycobacterium marinum,* may show mixed inflammatory infiltrates containing neutrophils and little in the way of well-formed granulomatous inflammation at sites of

dermal inoculation (Fig. 9–10). The clinical hallmark of *tuberculoid leprosy,* the anesthetic patch or plaque, may contain coalescent, noncaseating granulomas that course along dermal neurovascular bundles in a serpiginous pattern. Organisms are generally not detected by special histologic stains. The more diffuse infiltrative lesions of *lepromatous leprosy* are characterized by poorly organized dermal infiltrates of finely vacuolated histiocytes, or lepra cells, replete with *M. leprae* organisms.

It is beyond the scope of this chapter to provide specific details concerning the many forms of granulomatous dermatitis caused by infectious agents. However, when faced with granulomatous inflammation that is either suspected clinically of being of infectious origin or has histologic features that do not fit well with noninfectious causes of granulomatous inflammation, special stains (e.g., PAS and silver) as well as acid-fast reagents should be obtained. Table 9–2 is a summary of the salient features of the more common causes of infectious granulomatous inflammation in skin and can be used as an adjunct to evaluating the results of these stains within the context of histologic and clinical parameters.

Text continued on page 161

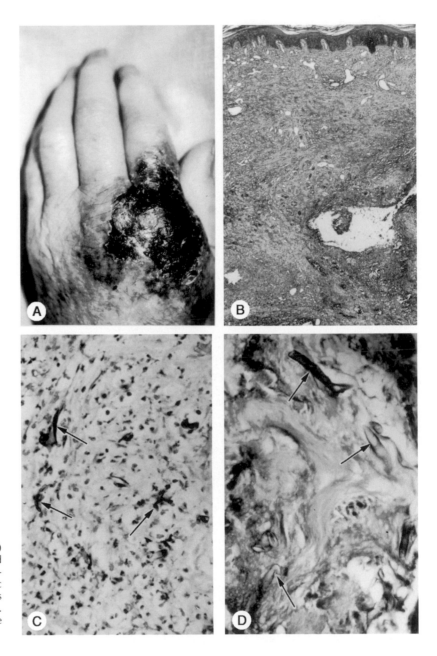

Figure 9–4. Infectious granulomas: Mucormycosis. **(A)** Necrotic and ulcerated plaque on the dorsum of the hand of an immunosuppressed patient. **(B)** Diffuse, vague, granulomatous inflammation; granulation tissue; and cystic necrosis are present in the dermis. **(C)** Silver stain reveals twisted, ribbon-like hyphae *(arrows)* in the deep dermis. **(D)** In a necrotic region, pleomorphic, nonseptate hyphae *(arrows)* are also observed by periodic acid–Schiff stain.

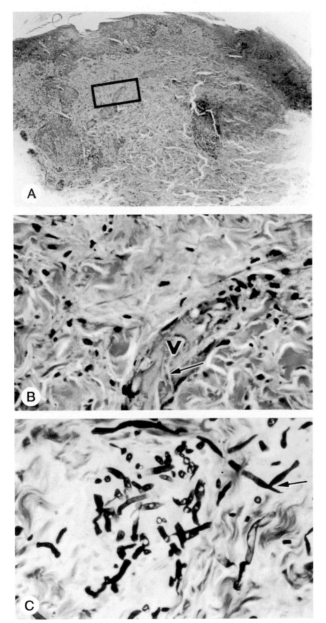

Figure 9–5. Infectious granulomas: Aspergillosis. **(A)** At scanning magnification, there is a patchy, vague granulomatous infiltrate within the superficial and deep dermis. **(B)** Closer inspection of the region enclosed in **A** reveals hyphae *(arrow)* within small vessels (v), indicative in this case of thromboembolic dissemination to the skin. **(C)** Silver stain reveals numerous septate hyphae that branch at acute angles *(arrow).*

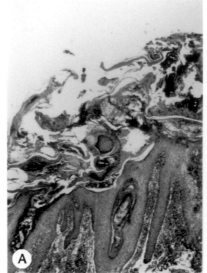

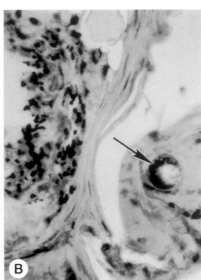

Figure 9–6. Infectious granulomas: Coccidioidomycosis. **(A)** A biopsy specimen of a tender, ulcerated, verrucous nodule in a patient with systemic coccidioidomycosis. The inflammatory infiltrate in the dermis is mixed and focally granulomatous with focal caseous necrosis; the epidermis shows reactive hyperplasia similar to that seen in early blastomycosis. **(B)** Within the stratum corneum, a sporangium containing endospores *(arrow)* is identified.

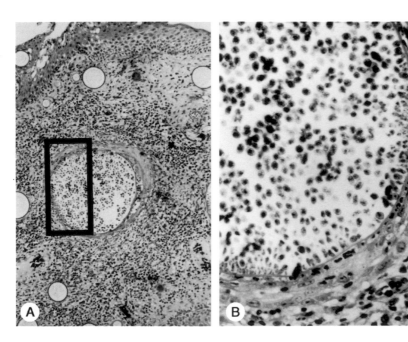

Figure 9–7. Infectious granulomas: Rhinosporidiosis. **(A)** There is a dermal mixed inflammatory infiltrate with focal granulomas and multinucleated histiocytes. **(B)** The sporangia, enclosed in **A** and enlarged in **B,** contain thousands of spores enclosed by a cellulose-like wall.

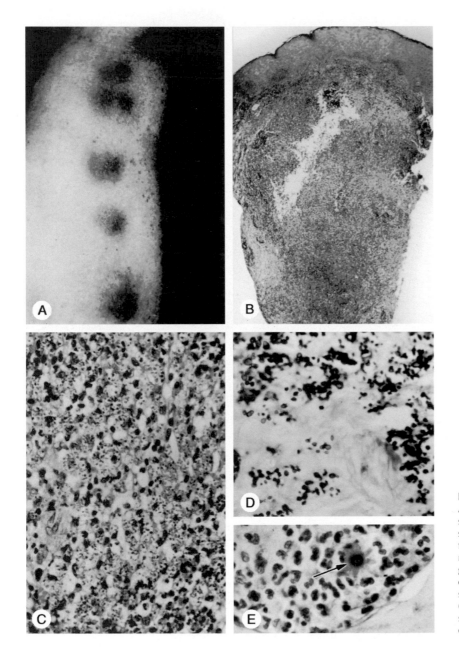

Figure 9–8. Infectious granulomas: Sporotrichosis. **(A)** A linear array of erythematous nodules drain a primary site of infection in a patient with lymphocutaneous sporotrichosis. **(B)** At scanning magnification, the inflammatory infiltrate is composed of lymphocytes, neutrophils, plasma cells, and monocytes, with foci of granuloma formation. **(C)** The histiocytic component of the inflammatory infiltrate contains numerous spores, which stain positively by periodic acid–Schiff **(D)**. **(E)** Asteroid bodies *(arrow),* which are central spores with homogeneous eosinophilic radiations, are occasionally observed.

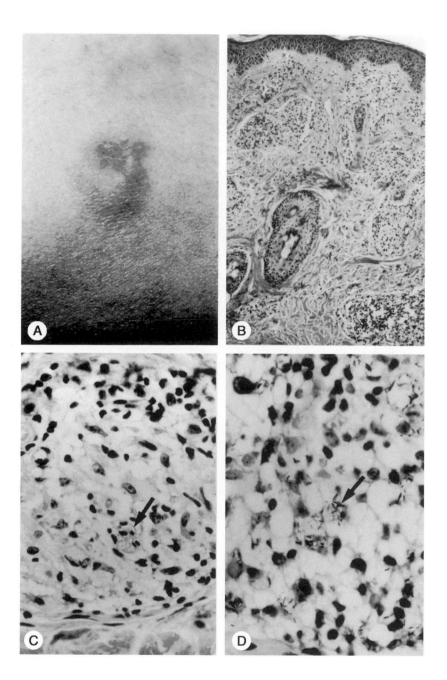

Figure 9–9. Infectious granulomas: Tuberculosis. (A) Erythematous papules and small nodules are present. (B) A biopsy specimen demonstrates a superficial and deep dermal mononuclear cell infiltrate. (C) On higher magnification, these foci are predominantly epithelioid histiocytes and lymphocytes. In contrast to tuberculoid leprosy, dermal nerves (arrow) are not damaged. (D) Acid-fast stain reveals characteristic mycobacteria within dermal histiocytes (arrow).

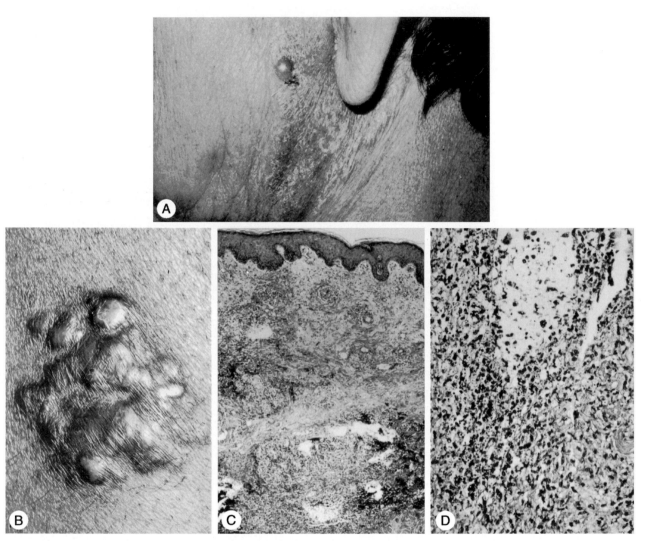

Figure 9–10. Infectious granulomas: Atypical mycobacteria. Primary innoculation sites may manifest as **(A)** solitary nodules or **(B)** multiple nodules, sometimes in linear array mimicking sporotrichosis. **(C)** Histologically, there is a mixed inflammatory infiltrate within the superficial and deep dermis, which may contain vaguely granulomatous foci and necrosis **(D).** Over time, classic epithelioid granulomas may supervene.

Table 9–2. DIFFERENTIAL FEATURES IN GRANULOMATOUS DERMATITIS

DISORDER	ORGANISMS	INFLAMMATION	CLINICAL APPEARANCE
Fungi			
Aspergillosis	Silver-positive septate mycelia, 45-degree angle branching	May be minimal; vessel emboli and intramural growth	Necrotic eschar
Blastomycosis	PAS- and silver-positive 10-μm spores with broad-based buds	Granulomas, microabscesses, epidermal hyperplasia	Verrucous plaques, pustules, ulceration
Candidiasis	PAS- and silver-positive pseudoseptate mycelia, 90-degree angle branching, 4–6-μm spores	Granulomas, epidermal hyperplasia, subcorneal pustules	Beefy red scaling plaque, peripheral pustules
Chromomycosis	Cooper-colored, 6–12-μm spores, division by septation	Mixed inflammation, epidermal hyperplasia; transepidermal elimination of spores	Verrucous plaque covered with black dots (i.e., surface spores)
Coccidioidomycosis	PAS- and silver-positive spherule ≤80 μm containing 2–5-μm endospores	Mixed inflammation, variable epidermal hyperplasia	Verrucous papules and plaques
Cryptococcosis	PAS- and silver-positive 3–20-μm spores with narrow-based buds, mucin-positive capsule	Granulomatous or noninflammatory, gelatinous	Plaques, ulcers, molluscum-like papules
Histoplasmosis	3-μm H&E- and Giemsa-positive encapsulated spores (capsule is silver-positive)	Mixed inflammation with granulomas, or sheets of histiocytes with impaired immunity	Ulcerated papules and plaques
Mucormycosis	PAS- and silver-positive 30-μm-diameter nonseptate mycelia, 90-degree angle branching	Mixed inflammation, vessel invasion	Indurated nodules and ulcers
Rhinosporidiosis	H&E-positive 250–350-μm sporangia containing 6–12-μm spores	Mixed inflammation, epithelial hyperplasia	Papules, nodules, and polyps of nasal epithelium
Sporotrichosis	PAS-positive 4–6-μm spores, cigar-like bodies, asteroid-like bodies	Mixed inflammation, microabscesses, organisms difficult to find	Cutaneous nodules with lymphatic distribution, plaques
Bacteria			
Granuloma inguinale	Giemsa- or silver-positive intracellular 10–20-μm bacilli (i.e., Donovan bodies)	Mixed inflammation with large histiocytes containing organisms	Ulcerated genital, inguinal, or perianal nodule
Granulomatous syphilis	Silver-positive corkscrew-like spirochetes, mostly within epidermis	Superficial dermal granulomas, cytotoxic pattern, plasma cells	Multiple nodules or plaques
Lupus vulgaris (*Mycobacterium tuberculosis*)	Acid-fast beaded bacilli within giant cells or at zones of necrosis	Tuberculoid granulomas, Langhans giant cells	Red-brown nodule or plaque on head or neck
Swimming-pool granuloma (*M. marinum*)	Acid-fast beaded bacilli, slightly larger than *Mycobacterium tuberculosis*	Mixed inflammation, tuberculoid granulomas rare, focal necrosis	Nodule or plaque often on arm or hand, may show lymphatic spread
Leprosy	Acid-fast intracellular bacilli	Tuberculoid cells or sheets of foam cells (i.e., lepromatous); nerve destruction	Anesthetic plaque or diffuse skin thickening
Protozoa			
Chronic leishmaniasis	Giemsa-positive 2–4-μm round intracellular organisms	Microtubercles with epithelioid histiocytes and Langhans cells	Scaling plaques

Infectious causes of granulomatous dermatitis are important to keep in mind, because accurate diagnosis often relies on ordering a special stain, and such a measure may result in lifesaving therapeutic intervention. It is recommended that infectious granulomatous dermatitis be strongly considered when histologic evidence of granuloma formation is encountered in the following settings:

- Clinical suspicion of infection
- Unusual occupational or travel history
- Immunocompromised patient
- Dermal granulomas without obvious cause
- Granulomatous panniculitis without clear-cut clinico-pathologic diagnosis of primary panniculitis
- Microabscesses or necrosis

It must be emphasized that definitive exclusion of an infectious cause for granulomatous dermatitis does not depend solely on obtaining negative special stains. Culture of fresh biopsied tissue is generally a much more sensitive means of excluding organisms. Therefore, cultures should be a component of the diagnostic evaluation of potentially infectious forms of granulomatous infiltration of the skin when infection is suspected based on existing clinical or histologic parameters.

Foreign-Body Granulomas[7]

- EPITHELIOID HISTIOCYTES AND FOREIGN-BODY–TYPE GIANT CELLS
- NEUTROPHILIC ABSCESSES IN ACUTE LESIONS
- FOLLICULAR DESTRUCTION OR SINUS TRACT FORMATION
- BIREFRINGENT MATERIAL IN DERMIS

Foreign-body granulomas are probably the most common form of granulomatous dermatitis. Although they are biologically trivial in comparison to infectious granulomas, their accurate diagnostic recognition may save considerable cost and time in excluding other causes of this form of dermal inflammatory reaction. For the purposes of this brief discussion, foreign bodies are defined as any material extrinsic to the viable layers of the skin that may provoke a granulomatous response. Accordingly, both wood splinters and acellular mature keratin protein, which normally does not come into contact with viable dermal cells, are considered in this section.

The clinical appearance of a foreign-body reaction is generally nonspecific, consisting of a region of induration, erythema, and pain. If the particulate material elicits abscess formation, lesions may become pustular and drain. Foreign-body granulomas may be confused clinically with more serious conditions, including painful primary skin tumors, nodular variants of deep fungal infection, and metastases at the site of the removal of a previous skin tumor. Foreign-body reactions to keratin protein extruded into the dermis as a consequence of follicular cyst rupture are commonly encountered in melanocytic nevi, in which nevus cells have mechanically resulted in follicular stasis and rupture. Such events result in pain and erythema in the nevus which may be confused with host response to a melanocytic dysplasia or malignancy. Sites of previous surgical manipulation are prone to retention of suture material which may result in a foreign-body response when incompletely absorbed (i.e., suture granuloma; Fig. 9–11A). Large epidermal inclusions and pilar cysts may remain indolent for years only to undergo rupture spontaneously or after minor trauma, producing exquisitely tender nodules that require surgical removal for relief.

Histologically, acute evolutionary phases of foreign-body granulomas may be predominated by dermal infiltration by neutrophils forming abscesses and an associated granulation tissue response; granulomas may be inconspicuous at this stage. Over time, epithelioid granulomas predominate, demarcating the site of persistent foreign material, such as a retained suture (Fig. 9–11B, C). Multinucleated or foreign-body histiocytes containing many centrally-located nuclei, in

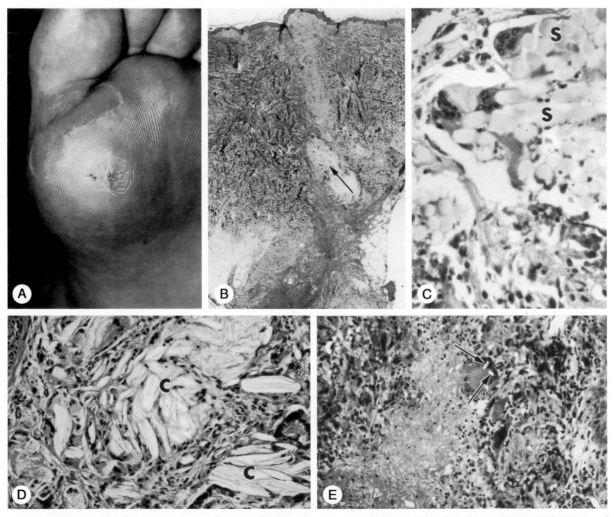

Figure 9–11. Foreign-body granulomas. **(A)** A granuloma at the site of previous surgical removal of a plantar wart reveals **(B)** scar formation associated with granulomatous inflammation to foreign material *(arrow)*. **(C)** Retained suture material (S) is present within foci of fibrosis and granulomatous inflammation. **(D)** Foreign-body giant cell response to site of cyst rupture demonstrates cleft-like spaces **(C)** formed by cholesterol from membranous cyst contents. **(E)** Polarization microscopy of foreign-body reaction at the site of traumatically introduced foreign material reveals birefringent material as clear clefts *(arrows)* within multinucleated histiocytes.

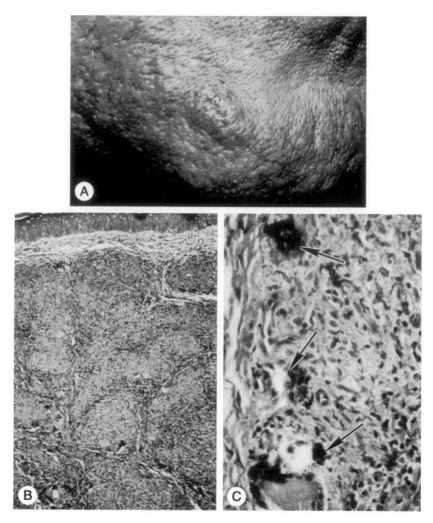

Figure 9–12. Silica granulomas. **(A)** Delayed hypersensitivity response to silica occurred many years after its local introduction into the dermis. **(B)** Well-formed granulomas within the superficial and mid-dermis mimic sarcoidosis. **(C)** Sites of deposition of refractile silica crystals *(arrows)*, associated with brown hemosiderin, are visible even by routine microscopy. Polariscopy, clinical history, and occasionally x-ray dispersive electron microscopy for elemental analysis may facilitate accurate diagnosis.

contrast to Langhans-type histiocytes, which contain peripherally marginated nuclei, are generally observed and may contain clefts or vacuoles that include refractile or stainable foreign material (Fig. 9–11*C, D*). Keratin generally appears as lamellar flakes, which initially stain pink and, over time, develop a pale blue tinctorial quality. Birefringent material that escapes scrutiny by routine microscopy may be detected with the use of polarization lenses (Fig. 9–11*E*). In certain situations, multiple levels through the specimen block may be required to identify foreign material responsible for the granulomatous reaction.

It is important to remember that environmental and industrial exposure to foreign materials that become entrapped in the dermis may result in granulomatous dermatitis. For example, traumatic introduction of oils into the dermis will produce histiocytic infiltrates containing cytoplasmic vacuoles of varying diameter, resulting in a ''Swiss-cheese'' appearance (i.e., paraffinoma). A similar histologic picture may be produced after rupture of iatrogenically introduced silicone implants. Immunologically mediated granulomatous responses are elicited by mineral elements such as silica (Fig. 9–12), zirconium (Fig. 9–13), aluminum, and beryllium. Silica, a component of glass, may elicit a granulomatous immune response many years after lying dormant in a dermal scar. Zirconium, a component of certain antiperspirant prep-

arations, is a cause of granulomatous axillary dermatitis as well as hidradenitis suppurativa, which actually represents a deep, chronic, granulomatous reaction to follicular, not apocrine or eccrine glandular, rupture.

Sarcoidosis[8–10]

- SUPERFICIAL AND DEEP DERMAL EPITHELIOID GRANULOMAS
- MINIMAL OR ABSENT RIM OF LYMPHOCYTES ABOUT GRANULOMAS (I.E., ''NAKED TUBERCULES'')
- CASEATION NECROSIS OFTEN ABSENT
- DERMAL NERVES PRESERVED
- SPECIAL STAINS AND CULTURES NEGATIVE FOR ORGANISMS

Sarcoidosis is a systemic granulomatous disorder that commonly affects skin. The underlying cause of sarcoidosis is not known, although it is often assumed that this disorder results from a host immune reaction to an as yet obscure environmental protein or infectious agent. Patients may present with bilateral involvement of hilar lymph nodes, producing a characteristic ''butterfly'' pattern on radiographic ex-

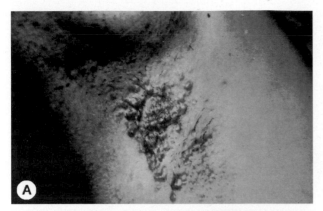

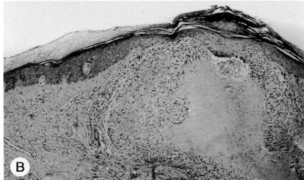

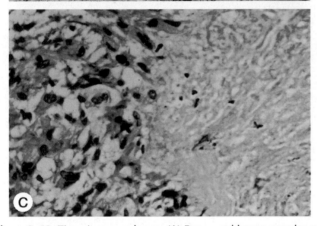

Figure 9–13. Zirconium granulomas. **(A)** Boggy, red-brown papules are present at the site of application of zirconium-containing antiperspirant. **(B, C)** Epithelioid granulomas have foci of central caseous necrosis. Although zirconium and beryllium usually do not cause necrosis, this case of zirconium-induced granulomatous dermatitis demonstrated prominent zones of necrosis.

amination. Sarcoidal granulomas may affect a number of viscera, including heart, liver, and lungs.

Cutaneous involvement in sarcoidosis is evidenced by red-brown plaques which are sometimes annular (Fig. 9–14A). *Lupus pernio* is a clinical term referring to sarcoidosis involving the facial skin, particularly the nose, cheeks, and ears. Occasionally, sarcoidosis presents as superficial papules or deep subcutaneous nodules.

Histologically, scanning magnification reveals coalescent pale pink granulomas within the superficial and deep dermis (Fig. 9–14B). At this power magnification, a differential diagnosis of infection, including tuberculoid leprosy,

is often entertained. On closer inspection, the granulomas are observed to be composed of eosinophilic epithelioid histiocytes, some of which are multinucleated (Fig. 9–14C). Generally, the rim of lymphocytes that surrounds the granulomatous foci is inconspicuous to absent, although exceptions do exist. Many of the granulomas are devoid of central necrosis, although small foci of caseation may be detected in sarcoidosis in about 10% of cases, in my experience. Nerves in neurovascular bundles are not infiltrated by inflammatory cells, nor do they exhibit degenerative alterations, as is the case in tuberculoid leprosy. Multinucleated histiocytes may contain eosinophilic stellate inclusions (i.e., asteroid bodies), representing a peculiar structural presentation of engulfed collagen, and rounded, laminated inclusions (i.e., Schaumann bodies), presumably representing degenerating or residual lysosomes.

Special stains are generally performed when the granulomatous dermatitis of sarcoidosis is encountered, and these stains are uniformly negative, as are cultures of fresh biopsied tissue. Without special stains and sometimes supportive cultures, it is impossible to exclude fungal or mycobacterial infection based on routine histology alone. Sarcoidal granulomas should be polarized to exclude the presence of birefringent foreign material as a causative agent. Accordingly, although cutaneous sarcoidosis has certain typical clinical and histologic features, it is generally a diagnosis of exclusion for the dermatopathologist.

Palisaded Granulomas

Granuloma Annulare[11, 12]

- ANGIOCENTRIC DERMATITIS WITH FOCAL INTERSITIAL HISTIOCYTIC INFILTRATION IN EARLY LESIONS
- DERMAL MUCINOUS DEGENERATION (I.E., NECROBIOSIS)
- HISTIOCYTIC AGGREGATION AT PERIMETER OF DERMAL NECROBIOSIS IN ESTABLISHED LESIONS

Granuloma annulare, along with rheumatoid nodule and necrobiosis lipoidica, are referred to as palisaded granulomas because of the vague suggestion of parallel alignment of histiocytes that form at the perimeter of zones of altered collagen in established lesions. Each of these conditions, however, has a distinctive clinical and histologic appearance, and they represent different cutaneous disorders. Granuloma annulare presents clinically as multiple asymptomatic, flesh-colored dermal papules, usually grouped in a ring-like configuration (Fig. 9–15A). Although papules are occasionally generalized, they most often involve the skin of the hands and feet. A deep variant also exists, resulting in nodules affecting the dermis and subcutaneous fat of children and rarely adults. The clinical differential that accompanies a biopsy specimen of granuloma annulare may be quite diverse, including dyshidrotic eczema, scabies, folliculitis, and insect bites.

The histologic appearance of early lesions of granuloma annulare may be extremely subtle. There is a superficial perivascular lymphocytic infiltrate that may dominate the

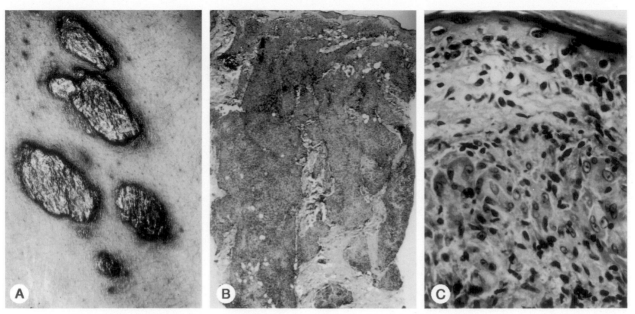

Figure 9–14. Sarcoidosis. **(A)** Erythematous plaques raise the clinical differential of lupus erythematosus, sarcoidosis, or infection. **(B)** Scanning magnification reveals numerous confluent granulomas within the superficial and deep dermis. **(C)** High magnification demonstrates epithelioid granulomas devoid of both significant central necrosis (noncaseating granulomas) and a substantial peripheral rim of lymphocytes (naked granulomas). Special stains and culture of fresh tissue in sarcoidosis are invariably negative for organisms.

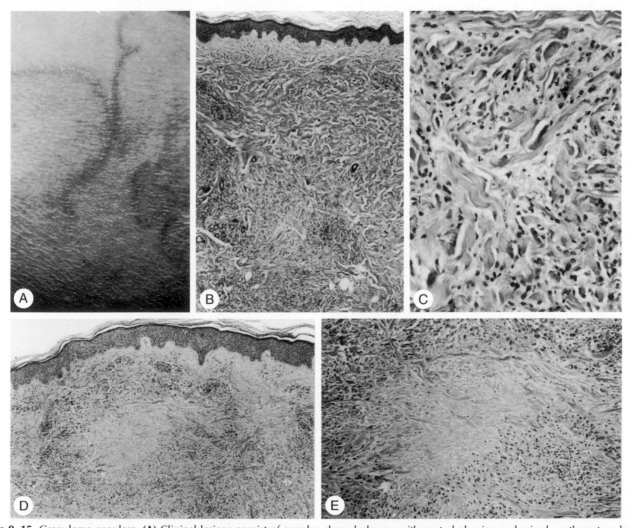

Figure 9–15. Granuloma annulare. **(A)** Clinical lesions consist of annular, dermal plaques with central clearing and raised, erythematous borders. **(B, C)** Early lesions typically show an interstitial pattern of infiltration by inflammatory cells. **(C)** Mononuclear cells are present among collagen bundles in association with variable mucin deposition. **(D, E)** Well-developed lesions show zones of mucinous necrobiosis of collagen, surrounded by mononuclear cells with an infiltrative pattern similar to that described in **B** and **C.** About the perimeters of zones of necrobiotic collagen are palisades of monocytes, forming a vaguely granulomatous pattern of inflammation.

165

pattern, leading to the unfortunate diagnosis of chronic dermatitis. Generally, however, there will also be subtle zones of associated superficial dermal hypercellularity resulting from infiltration or "meandering" of histiocytes within foci of collagen showing associated mucin deposition (Fig. 9–15*B, C*). In some lesions, these areas may initially mimic the subtle proliferation of dermal fibroblasts that accompanies an early dermatofibroma. The mucin is best observed with the $40\times$ lens as delicate, beaded strands of pale blue-grey material separating the affected collagen bundles, which themselves may be pale, fragmented, or enlarged. In lesions undergoing rapid acute evolution, neutrophils with nuclear fragmentation and occasional eosinophils may also be present in the areas of degenerating matrix.

Established lesions of granuloma annulare, on the other hand, are quite characteristic clinically and histologically and for this reason are seldom biopsied. Scanning magnification reveals discrete dermal zones of pallor surrounded by a mantle of mononuclear cells (Fig. 9–15*D*). The central zone is composed of degenerating collagen bundles, mucin, and, occasionally, residual cellular debris. The mantle is formed by a zone of histiocytes and lymphocytes, sometimes admixed with multinucleated giant cells. In rare lesions, the histiocytes actually have long axes aligned in parallel and radiating outward from the central zone of collagen degeneration.

In the setting of subcutaneous granuloma annulare, the central zone of matrix degeneration tends to be hypereosinophilic and relatively devoid of mucin. These palisaded granulomas may resemble rheumatoid nodules, and careful clinicopathologic correlation is required to formulate a definitive diagnosis. Superficial zones of degenerating collagen may be eliminated transepidermally in granuloma annulare, resulting in reactive epidermal hyperplasia and hyperkeratosis overlying what otherwise are typical dermal alterations of this disorder.

Rheumatoid Nodule[13, 14]

- SUBCUTANEOUS NODULES ASSOCIATED WITH RHEUMATOID ARTHRITIS
- OCCURRENCE OVER BONY PROMINENCES
- SHARPLY DEMARCATED DERMAL ZONES OF FIBRINOID NECROBIOSIS
- RIM OF HISTIOCYTES AND MONONUCLEAR CELLS AT PERIPHERY

Rheumatoid nodules generally present as firm, asymptomatic, flesh-colored nodules that overlie bony prominences such as the elbow or foot (Fig. 9–16*A*). They are generally seen in individuals with rheumatoid arthritis, although they have also been reported in patients with rheumatic fever and in those with lupus erythematosus. Occasionally, children and adults will develop subcutaneous nodules with features of rheumatoid nodules in the absence of systemic disease. Such lesions most probably represent subcutaneous variant forms of granuloma annulare, as discussed previously.

Biopsy specimens of rheumatoid nodule reveal geographic zones of fibrinoid necrobiosis within the dermis (Fig. 9–16*B*). In these zones, normal reticular dermal collagen is transformed to a granular-to-amorphous, highly eosinophilic material that resembles fibrin. Mucin deposition, as seen in dermal forms of granuloma annulare, is not present. Some

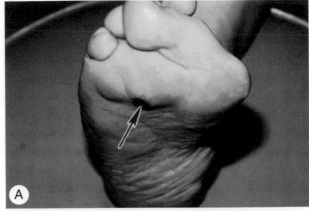

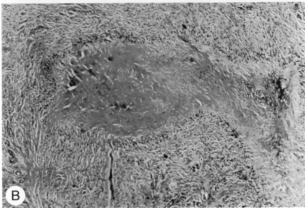

Figure 9–16. Rheumatoid nodule. **(A)** Firm nodules *(arrow)* are associated with the metacarpophalangeal joints on the plantar aspect of the foot of this patient. **(B)** The pathology consists of zones of fibrinoid necrobiosis, surrounded by palisades of histiocytes and a fibrotic stroma.

lesions also demonstrate nuclear debris in the foci of degenerating collagen. The granulomatous component consists of a mantle of histiocytes and lymphocytes identical to that described for fully evolved lesions of granuloma annulare. In lesions that have been chronically traumatized, striking fibrovascular proliferation may accompany some of these inflammatory foci.

Necrobiosis Lipoidica[15, 16]

- SQUARE OR RECTANGULAR BIOPSY SPECIMEN
- HORIZONTAL STRATIFICATION OF INFLAMMATION AND MATRIX DEGENERATION
- INFLAMMATORY COMPONENT: VAGUE GRANULOMAS ADMIXED WITH LYMPHOCYTES AND PLASMA CELLS
- MATRIX COMPONENT: SCLEROSIS AND THICKENING OF DERMAL COLLAGEN
- EPIDERMAL ATROPHY AND SUPERFICIAL DERMAL TELANGIECTASIA

Previously termed necrobiosis lipoidica diabeticorum, it is now recognized that this disorder frequently occurs independent of diabetes mellitus. The gross pathology typically involves indurated plaques affecting skin overlying the anterior tibial compartment (Fig. 9–17*A*). Plaques have a yellow-brown hue and generally exhibit clinical features of epidermal atrophy and telangiectasia. The perimeter of the plaques may be slightly raised and show a violaceous hue.

At scanning magnification (Fig. 9–17B), the biopsy specimen demonstrates a square or rectangular contour similar to that typically seen in scleroderma, the localized form of which necrobiosis lipoidica may clinically resemble. An important diagnostic feature at this magnification is the tendency for the inflammatory and sclerotic mesenchymal components of the lesion to be demarcated into horizontal strata or layers beneath the atrophic overlying epidermis. At higher magnification (Fig. 9–17C), the inflammatory strata are composed of an admixture of histiocytes, lymphocytes, and occasional plasma cells. The strata composed of altered dermal matrix consist of sclerotic collagen bundles exhibiting widening and homogenization.

Elastolytic Granulomas[17]

- PATCHY MONONUCLEAR DERMAL INFILTRATE CONTAINING MULTINUCLEATED HISTIOCYTES
- PHAGOCYTOSIS OF DERMAL ELASTIC FIBERS BY HISTIOCYTES
- COLLAGEN ALTERATIONS OF PALISADED GRANULOMAS ABSENT

The original descriptions of elastolytic granuloma used the term actinic granuloma, implying that this unusual inflammatory process was incited by actinically altered dermal elastic tissue. It is now recognized that this process may affect non–sun-exposed skin, and that severe actinic elastosis is not common to all lesions. Clinically, one or more erythematous plaques develop, often on the skin of the face or neck, although extremity skin may also be involved. Over time, as inflammation subsides, diminished elastic recoil may be observed clinically (Fig. 9–18A). Histologically, there is a patchy mononuclear cell infiltrate within the superficial dermis (Fig. 9–18B). Multinucleated histiocytes within the infiltrate may contain asteroid bodies similar to those observed in sarcoidosis. The diagnostic hallmark is incorporation of dermal elastic fibers into the cytoplasm of the histiocytes via phagocytosis (Fig. 9–18C).

Although localized plaques of elastolytic granulomatous dermatitis, also called giant cell elastolytic granulomas, are relatively uncommon, the reaction pattern of granulomatous elastolysis may be observed as an incidental finding in a number of disorders, including actinic keratoses, persistent insect-bite reactions, and certain variant forms of cutaneous T-cell dyscrasia (i.e., granulomatous slack skin). It is therefore useful to recognize the pattern of granulomatous elastolysis, lest it be confused with other forms of granulomatous dermatitis. Accordingly, an additional component of the diagnostic algorithm in approaching granulomatous dermatitis is to determine whether elastic fiber phagocytosis is a prominent feature of the histiocytic response.

Rare Disorders

- NECROBIOTIC XANTHOGRANULOMA[18] (see Chap. 19)
- TERTIARY SYPHILIS[19]
- GRANULOMATOUS CHEILITIS[20]
- WEGENER GRANULOMATOSIS[21]
- ALLERGIC GRANULOMATOSIS[22]
- LETHAL MIDLINE GRANULOMA[23]

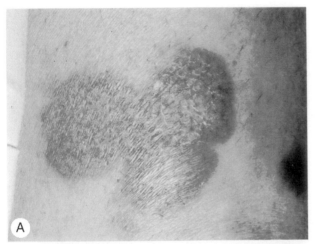
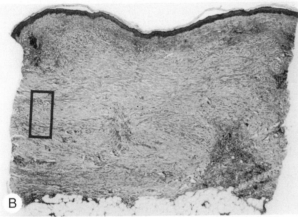
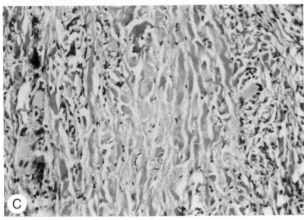

Figure 9–17. Necrobiosis lipoidica. **(A)** The gross pathology consists of pale, erythematous plaques with telangiectasia and an atrophic, overlying epidermal layer. Lesions often affect the anterior aspects of the lower extremities. **(B)** Histologically, layers of inflammation alternate with broad zones of fibrosis in the horizontal plane. **(C)** Higher magnification of the enclosure in **B** demonstrates a central zone of fibrotic dermis sandwiched between two bands of inflammatory infiltrate composed of lymphocytes and histiocytes, some of which are multinucleated. The apparent vertical stratification of these zones is the result of 90-degree rotation of the rectangular enclosure in **B**.

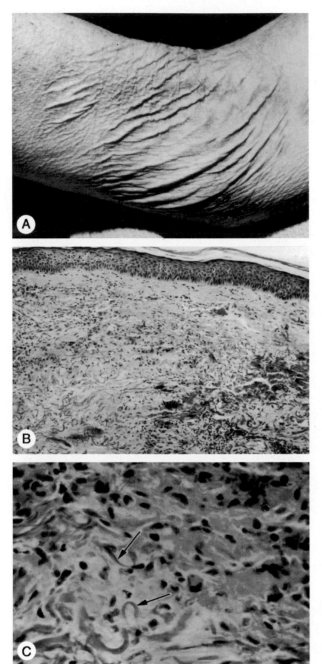

Figure 9–18. Elastolytic granuloma. **(A)** The clinical appearance demonstrates the consequence of loss of dermal elastic recoil; the lesion is more wrinkled and redundant than the surrounding, unaffected skin. **(B)** A biopsy specimen reveals a patchy granulomatous infiltrate within the dermis. **(C)** On higher magnification, this infiltrate demonstrates phagocytosis of altered and fragmented elastic fibers *(arrows)* by histiocytes within the granulomas.

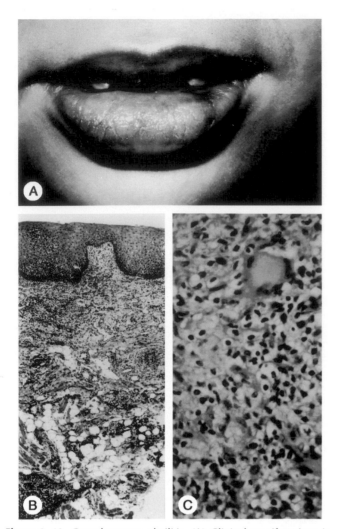

Figure 9–19. Granulomatous cheilitis. **(A)** Clinical manifestations include development of permanent swelling and induration of the lips. **(B, C)** Biopsy specimens reveal multiple sarcoidal granulomas within submucosal connective tissue. Extension into fat or underlying muscle may occur.

These disorders are all exceedingly rare. They all, however, fall within the boundaries of the differential diagnosis of granulomatous dermatitis when it is broadly defined. The following brief summaries highlight several salient points for each condition and serve as a springboard for referral to more comprehensive texts that deal with uncommon forms of granulomatous dermatitis.

NECROBIOTIC XANTHOGRANULOMA. Large indurated plaques with epidermal atrophy and telangiectatic vessels occur primarily on the trunk skin of individuals with paraproteinemia. Granulomatous bands of inflammatory cells replete with foreign-body–type and Touton-type giant cells separate superficial and deep dermal collagen replaced by hyalinized matrix.

TERTIARY SYPHILIS. Annular nodules or punched-out ulcers contain sarcoidal epithelioid granulomas, sometimes with massive geographic zones of central caseous necrosis.

GRANULOMATOUS CHEILITIS. Also called Miescher-Melkersson-Rosenthal syndrome. Chronic lip enlargement correlates with submucosal infiltration by sarcoidal granulomas (Fig. 9–19).

WEGENER GRANULOMATOSIS. Triad of (1) necrotizing granulomatous lesions of the upper and lower respiratory tract; (2) widespread necrotizing vasculitis; and (3) necrotizing glomerulonephritis. Zones of necrosis are juxtaposed with mixed inflammatory infiltrates containing numerous giant cells (Fig. 9–20). Vasculitis also may be prominent.

ALLERGIC GRANULOMATOSIS. Also termed the Churg-Strauss syndrome, it consists of (1) preceding history of asthma; (2) circulating and tissue eosinophilia; (3) pulmonary infiltrates; (4) small vessel vasculitis; and (5) connective tissue palisaded granulomas. Zones of dermal degeneration containing fragmented eosinophils and surrounded by palisaded granulomatous inflammation accompany cutaneous vasculitis.

LETHAL MIDLINE GRANULOMA. Edema and ulceration of nasal skin and mucosa leading to local destruction involving bone and cartilage is associated with obliterative small vessel mononuclear cell inflammation and scattered atypical mononuclear cells within a mixed interstitial inflammatory infiltrate.

DIFFERENTIAL DIAGNOSIS

Like other disorders discussed in this book, there are basic histologic features that are pivotal to an initial differential diagnostic approach to granulomatous infiltrates. The pivot points in diagnosing granulomatous dermatitis include the presence or absence of foreign bodies, the results of

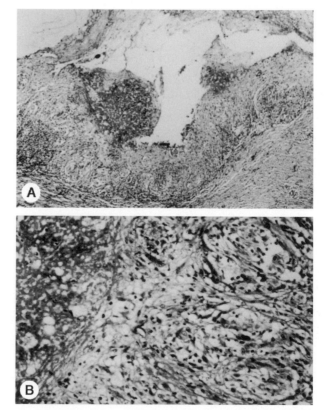

Figure 9–20. Wegener granulomatosis. **(A)** At scanning magnification, there is epidermal and dermal ulceration associated with a brisk, underlying inflammatory infiltrate. **(B)** Characteristic features at higher magnification include geographic zones of fibrinoid necrosis *(upper left)* bordered by a loosely aggregated granulomatous response.

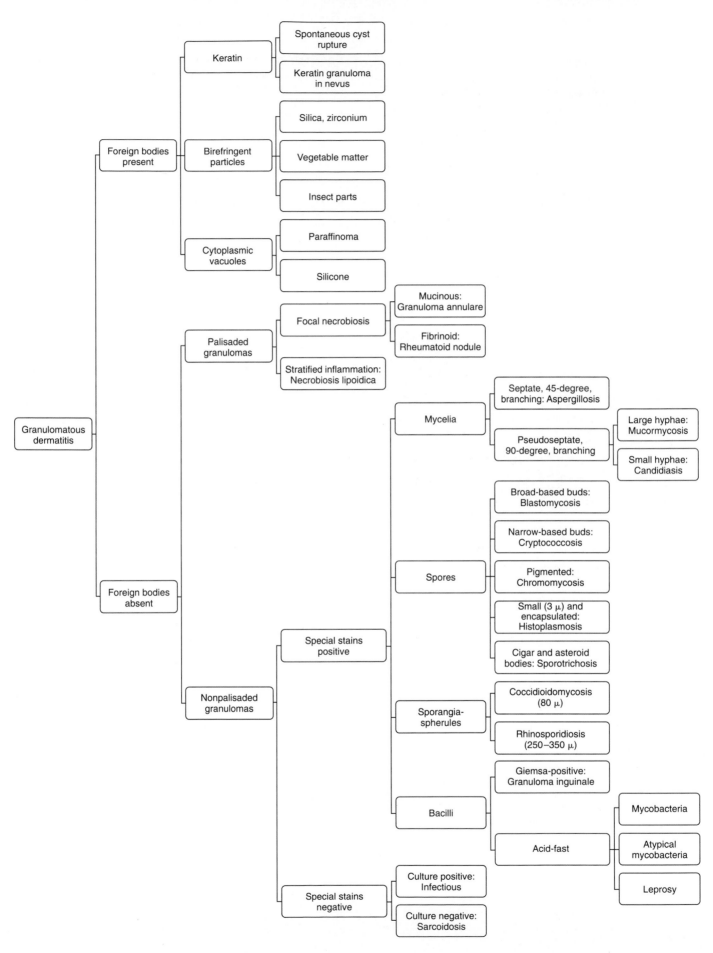

Figure 9–21. Algorithmic approach to differential diagnosis of granulomatous dermatitis.

special stains, and whether the granulomas represented are palisaded or tuberculoid in character. Such features permit an algorithmic approach that will begin to focus the differential on additional discriminating features, resulting in formulation of the most precise diagnosis or limited differential diagnosis possible. Clinicians both expect and appreciate this type of analysis, rather than the generic labeling of a biopsy specimen as granulomatous dermatitis without additional clarification. Atypical presentations and chronologic factors may conspire to confound the use of an algorithm that relies on characteristic features of well-developed, classic lesions. However, such a method provides a conceptual foundation upon which diagnostic nuances and subtleties may be affixed by the individual dermatopathologist. Figure 9–21 represents an algorithmic summary of a few of the histologic features that may facilitate an initial diagnostic approach to more common forms of granulomatous dermatitis.

SELECTED REFERENCES

1. Chu AC, Hay RJ, MacDonald DM. Cutaneous cryptococcosus. Br J Dermatol 1980;103:95.
2. Batres E, Wolfe JE Jr, Rudolph AH, et al. Transepithelial elimination of cutaneous chromomycosis. Arch Dermatol 1978;97:38.
3. Moskowitz LB, Ganjei P, Ziegels-Weissman J, et al. Immunohistochemical identification of fungi in systemic and cutaneous mycoses. Arch Pathol 1986;110:433.
4. Grossman ME, Silvers DN, Walther RR. Cutaneous manifestations of disseminated candidiasis. J Am Acad Dermatol 1980;2:111.
5. Santa Cruz DJ, Strayer DS. The histologic spectrum of cutaneous mycobacterioses. Hum Pathol 1982;13:485.
6. Sehgal VN, Jain MK. Tissue section Donovan bodies, identification through slow-Giemsa (overnight) technique. Dermatologica 1987;174:228.
7. Jaworsky C. Analysis of foreign materials in skin. Clin Dermatol 1991;9:157.
8. Vainsencher D, Winkelmann RK. Subcutaneous sarcoidosis. Arch Dermatol 1984;120:1028.
9. Olive KE, Kataria YP. Cutaneous manifestations of sarcoidosis. Arch Int Med 1985;145:1811.
10. James DG, Williams WJ. Immunology of sarcoidosis. Am J Med 1982;72:5.
11. Patterson JW. Rheumatoid nodule and subcutaneous granuloma annulare. A comparative histologic study. Am J Dermatopathol 1988;10:1.
12. Thyresson HN, Doyle JA, Winkelman RK. Granuloma annulare. Histopathologic and direct immunofluorescence study. Acta Derm Venereol (Stockh) 1980;60:261.
13. Dubois EL, Friou GJ, Chandor S. Rheumatoid nodules and rheumatoid granulomas in systemic lupus erythematosus. JAMA 1972;220:515.
14. Horn RT Jr, Goette DK. Perforating rheumatoid nodule. Arch Dermatol 1982;118:696.
15. Quimby SR, Muller SA, Schroeter AL. The cutaneous immunopathology of necrobiosis lipoidica diabeticorum. Arch Dermatol 1988;124:1364.
16. Oikarinen A, Mortenhumer M, Kallionen M, et al. Necrobiosis lipoidica: Ultrastructural and biochemical demonstration of a collagen defect. J Invest Dermatol 1987;88:227.
17. O'Brien JP. Actinic granuloma. Arch Dermatol 1975;111:460.
18. Finan MC, Winkelmann RK. Histopathology of necrobiotic xanthogranuloma with paraproteinemia. J Cutan Pathol 1987;14:92.
19. Tanabe JL, Huntley AC. Granulomatous tertiary syphilis. J Am Acad Dermatol 1986;15:341.
20. White IR, Souteryrand P, MacDonald DM. Granulomatous cheilitis (Miescher). Clin Exp Dermatol 1981;6:391.
21. Fienberg R. The protracted superficial phenomenon in pathergic (Wegener's) granulomatosis. Hum Pathol 1981;12:458.
22. Churg A. Pulmonary angiitis and granulomatosis revisited. Hum Pathol 1983;14:868.
23. Lober CW, Kaplan RJ, West WH. Midline granuloma. Arch Dermatol 1982;118:52.

10
Cutaneous Panniculitis

DEFINITIONS AND GENERAL CONSIDERATIONS

The term panniculitis implies a primary inflammatory process involving the subcutaneous fat. Panniculitis may arise as an immunologic disorder in which antigenic targets specifically located in characteristic regions of the subcutis (e.g., septa or lobules) are attacked by host inflammatory cells. Alternatively, panniculitis may be the result of ischemia to the subcutis, with secondary invasion by inflammatory cells. In addition, panniculitis may arise when endogenous enzymes (e.g., as in the case of pancreatitis or pancreatic carcinoma) or exogenous toxic substances gain access to subcutaneous tissue. Finally, infectious processes centered predominantly within the fat or infiltrative processes involving the hematopoietic system may result in secondary inflammatory changes in subcutaneous fat that may closely mimic primary immunologic insults.

Like the epidermis and dermis, the subcutaneous fat reacts to inflammation and trauma in a limited number of ways. Fat becomes neither hyperplastic nor hypertrophied in response to trauma, and extracellular fluid within the fat is usually localized to the adventitial connective tissue which courses through the thin septa that separate lobules composed of confluent aggregates of adipocytes. Fat undergoing necrosis frequently provokes a histiocytic inflammatory response whereby lipid is engulfed by macrophages to form foamy cells similar to xanthoma cells. Zones of fat necrosis frequently resolve with fibrosis, although microcysts may form in regions of fat necrosis prior to infiltration by fibroblasts and vessels. Dissolution of the cell membranes of adipocytes produces pooled regions of lipid frequently referred to as liquefactive fat necrosis. These zones may have a pale blue hue. Accumulation of pale pink material between intact adipocytes often signifies atrophy and a peculiar associated form of fibrosis referred to as hyalinization, which is typically encountered in lupus panniculitis. Degenerating and necrotic adipocytes also may undergo saponification whereby calcium salts are deposited in zones of fat necrosis. Occasionally, the lipid within the degenerating adipocytes may form needle-shaped clefts, as seen in the rare disorder subcutaneous fat necrosis of the newborn and also in sclerosing lipogranuloma, an iatrogenic disorder representing a response to injected oils or paraffin.

GROSS PATHOLOGY

The clinical pathology of most forms of panniculitis is not as characteristic or helpful as the epidermal and dermal alterations that characterize the various forms of superficial dermatitis. Panniculitis is frequently experienced symptomatically before it represents a defined clinical lesion. In general, panniculitis is exquisitely painful and may first be appreciated as a tender zone of deep induration. Such zones tend to be nodular in early stages, although confluence may result in plaque-like zones of cutaneous hardening. Vague erythema often accompanies panniculitis and is testimony to the inflammatory component within the deep tissue. Because most forms of primary panniculitis fail to show significant dermal or epidermal alterations, the cutaneous surface is generally smooth and unremarkable. In disorders such as panniculitis resulting from connective tissue disease (e.g., lupus panniculitis), dermal and epidermal alterations may be present, providing diagnostic information which paradoxically may occasionally mask the presence of an underlying component within the subcutis.

Early acute lesions of panniculitis are characterized by exquisitely painful zones of nodular induration with or without accompanying erythema. More chronic lesions tend to be considerably less symptomatic. Because panniculitis frequently resolves with some degree of lobular or septal sclerosis, induration may persist long after the onset of tenderness and erythema. Although panniculitis may occur anywhere on the body, there appears to be a predisposition for involvement of the lower extremities. It is fascinating to observe that although fundamental differences between the subcutaneous fat and adipose tissue at extracutaneous sites (e.g., pericardium, omentum) have not been identified, the primary panniculitides discussed herein have a predisposition for selective involvement of the adipose layer that underlies the dermis. Accordingly, systemic forms of panniculitis in

173

which fat cells at extracutaneous sites are also targeted by inflammatory mechanisms are extremely rare.

GENERAL HISTOLOGY AND TEMPORAL EVOLUTION

Histologically, panniculitis is conveniently divided into septal and lobular forms (Fig. 10–1). The prototype of septal panniculitis is erythema nodosum, and the prototype of lobular panniculitis is erythema induratum. In septal panniculitis, the earliest inflammatory cells are generally neutrophils admixed with lymphocytes and monocytes. These inflammatory cells infiltrate about small venules, which are present in greatest concentration within the connective tissue septa separating lobules and within the paraseptal regions of the lobule. The early inflammatory infiltrate may diffusely involve the septa and be accompanied by significant quantities of edema and fibrin, which expand the septa to many times their normal width. Within these expanded septa, subacute and more chronic lesions show a predominance of mononuclear cells, which may produce vaguely granulomatous aggregates.

Epithelioid histiocytes as well as multinucleated cells may be observed at this juncture. With chronicity, fibrosis generally follows septal panniculitis, and the deposition of abnormal collagen conforms to the architecture of the zones of previous inflammatory infiltration. Accordingly, old septal panniculitis shows expansion of septa by fibroblasts, proliferating vessels, and collagen.

Early forms of lobular panniculitis are also composed of neutrophils admixed with mononuclear cells, but these inflammatory components infiltrate more diffusely throughout the central portions of the fat lobule. Although the septa may be involved, the bulk of the inflammatory cells in lobular panniculitis are not present in the peripheral regions or septal components of the affected subcutis. As time passes, mononuclear cells may predominate, and in certain forms of lobular panniculitis (e.g., erythema induratum), frank epithelioid granulomas with caseation necrosis identical to that occurring in pulmonary tuberculosis are identified. Although vasculitis may be observed in some forms of lobular panniculitis, the affected vessels generally reside within septa. Inflammatory infiltration of the lobule frequently results in secondary degeneration and necrosis of adipocytes, and in

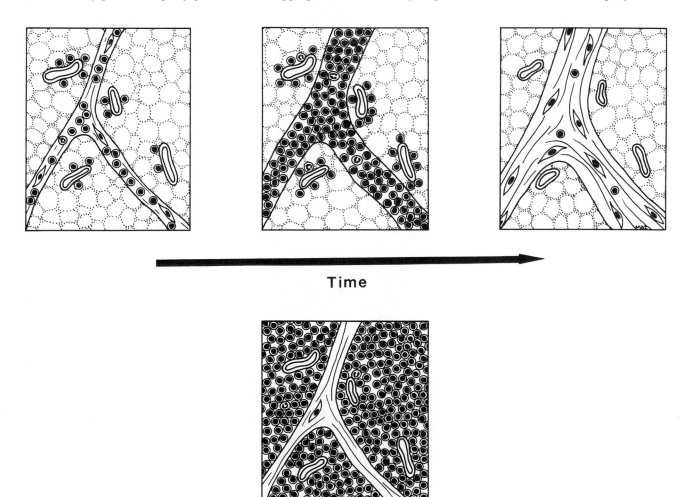

Time

Figure 10–1. Schematic representation of the temporal evolution of septal panniculitis. The earliest inflammatory events involve small venules within septa and in paraseptal adipose tissue *(left)*. This inflammation results in gradual widening of the septum as it becomes filled with mononuclear cells *(upper middle)*. At this point, perivenular inflammation in paraseptal adipose tissue may also be prominent, but this limited involvement of the lobule should not be confused with true lobular panniculitis *(lower middle)*, in which lobules are diffusely involved by inflammation and septa are relatively spared. With chronicity, the septum may become permanently thickened by scar tissue *(right)*.

such regions lipid-laden macrophages, microcysts, and fibrosis are commonly identified. Chronic lesions of lobular panniculitis may show diffuse fibrosis of the lobule, and in extreme cases lobules may be almost entirely replaced by collagen and proliferating fibroblasts. In more subtle forms of lobular panniculitis, in which atrophy predominates over necrosis, hyalinized sclerosis between adipocytes may be observed, as in lupus panniculitis. Figure 10–1 summarizes the temporal evolution of primary septal panniculitis.

HISTOLOGY OF SPECIFIC DISORDERS

Erythema Nodosum[1-3]

- SEPTAL PANNICULITIS
- LITTLE OR NO DERMAL INVOLVEMENT
- LITTLE OR NO VASCULITIS

- NEUTROPHILS IN EARLY LESIONS
- MONONUCLEAR CELLS, EOSINOPHILS, PLASMA CELLS IN LATE LESIONS
- PARASEPTAL PERIVENULAR INFLAMMATION
- SEPTAL FIBROSIS WITH CHRONICITY

The clinical features of erythema nodosum are suggested by its name, which describes a zone of redness (erythema) that takes the form of a hard lump (nodosum). Patients frequently present with bilateral nodules measuring 1 cm to several centimeters in size affecting lower extremities. Individual nodules are indurated, slightly raised, often poorly defined, and exquisitely tender to pressure (Fig. 10–2A). Typically, lesions are warm to the touch and may show variability in color from pink-red to a slightly greenish hue resembling a bruise or hematoma. Lesions typically evolve over a course of 3 to 6 weeks. Women are affected more often than men by a 6:1 ratio. Erythema nodosum is a disorder typically seen in young adults, and interestingly, is most

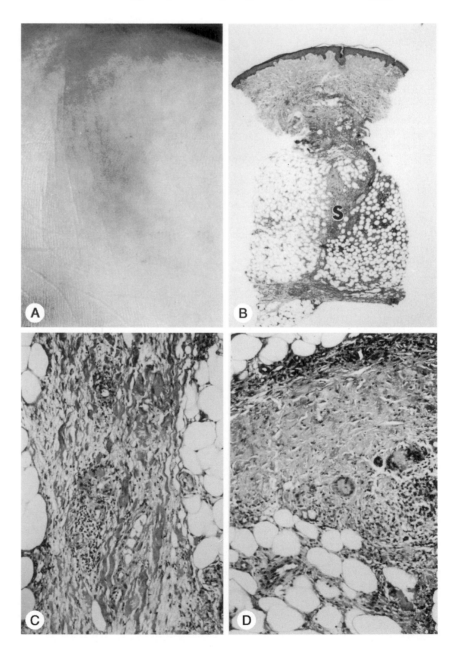

Figure 10–2. Erythema nodosum. **(A)** A poorly defined, erythematous, painful, deep-seated nodule is typical of early disease. **(B)** Scanning magnification reveals inflammation and expansion of a septum (s) within the subcutis. There is also some degree of paraseptal lobular involvement, perhaps accentuated by a tangential plane of section. **(C, D)** Inspection at higher magnification reveals granulomatous aggregates within edematous septa, perivenular lymphocytic infiltrates, variable numbers of eosinophils, and occasional giant cells. Vasculitis is not present.

often encountered during the first 6 months of each calendar year.

Although it is generally believed that erythema nodosum is the result of an immunologic attack centered within the subcutaneous fat, its etiology appears to be multifactorial. The development of erythema nodosum is associated with coexistent tuberculosis, preceding streptococcal infection, sarcoidosis, infection by *Yersinia enterocolitica,* Crohn disease, toxoplasmosis, and rarely, with other infections such as granuloma inguinale and cat-scratch fever.

At scanning magnification, erythema nodosum is the prototypical septal panniculitis (Fig. 10–2B). There is an inflammatory infiltrate which preferentially although not exclusively tracks down the branching septa that separate the lobules of the subcutaneous layer. This inflammatory infiltrate results in prominence and widening of the subcutaneous septa and is best appreciated when septa are perpendicularly sectioned; tangential sections through widened septa may occasionally give the false impression of a more lobular infiltrative process. Because accurate representation of septa within sections is critical to the appreciation of septal panniculitis by scanning magnification, biopsy specimens that include the bulk of the subcutaneous tissue are required for accurate evaluation and differential diagnosis of the various forms of panniculitis. Although inflammatory cells are most typically concentrated within septa, aggregates of inflammatory cells, generally lymphocytes and plasma cells, may also be seen about small venules within the paraseptal fat. These perivenular inflammatory aggregates may give the impression at scanning magnification that the inflammatory infiltrate has spilled over from the septa into the adjacent fat or that the panniculitis is both septal and lobular (Fig. 10–2B).

At higher magnification, the individual septa are involved by neutrophils, lymphocytes, mononuclear cells, and plasma cells, and vasculitis is notably absent (Fig. 10–2C, D). The initial expansion of septa in acute lesions is the result of the inflammatory infiltration, edema fluid, and fibrin splaying apart adjacent collagen fibers within the septa. Over time, mononuclear cells and lymphocytes predominate, and epithelioid cells with multinucleation may be identified (Fig. 10–2D). Although these zones may suggest tuberculoid granulomas, frank caseation necrosis, as is typical in erythema induratum, is not observed. Latter stages also frequently show the beginning of septal fibrosis. The fibrosis typically involves deposition of collagen bundles centrally within widened septa, with the persistence of inflammatory infiltrates and granulomatous foci at the perimeter of the septa and in the paraseptal fatty tissue. The overlying dermis and epidermis, as well as the adnexal structures present within the dermis, are uninvolved by the inflammatory infiltrate in erythema nodosum. This is an important negative finding, because certain infections and secondary inflammatory processes involving the subcutis may closely mimic erythema nodosum with regard to the changes within the subcutaneous layer. These mimics, discussed primarily under infectious panniculitis and factitial panniculitis, generally also show involvement of the dermis and epidermis, providing important and clinically critical diagnostic clues.

Subacute nodular migratory panniculitis is a variant of erythema nodosum. This condition frequently occurs unilaterally on the lower legs and is observed predominantly in middle-aged women. Grossly, small nodular lesions may enlarge to form by confluence sharply circumscribed, asymptomatic, indurated plaques with central clearing. The histology is remarkably similar to that of erythema nodosum, and the differential diagnosis depends on clinical factors (e.g., age, unilateral occurrence) and a more chronic course in subacute nodular migratory panniculitis.

Erythema Induratum[4]

- LOBULAR PANNICULITIS
- LITTLE OR NO DERMAL INVOLVEMENT
- NODULAR VASCULITIS, ESPECIALLY IN EARLY LESIONS
- TUBERCULOID GRANULOMAS
- CASEATION NECROSIS MAY BE PRESENT
- MONONUCLEAR CELLS PREDOMINATE

The clinical manifestations of erythema induratum include the initial occurrence of bilateral, well-defined nodules 1 cm to several centimeters in diameter, usually affecting the lower legs. These nodules frequently enlarge, become bright red, and may soften centrally (Fig. 10–3A). As in the case of erythema nodosum, young women are preferentially affected. Associated conditions include tuberculosis and exposure to cold or damp working conditions. The disease runs a chronic course over several years, and symptoms and signs are generally worse during the winter months. Resolution may occur, with pigmented scarring.

Histologically, erythema induratum is the prototypical disorder of lobular panniculitis. At scanning magnification (Fig. 10–3B), early lesions show a patchy inflammatory infiltrate within the fat lobules without specific or preferential involvement within septa. At higher magnification (Fig. 10–3C), the inflammatory infiltrate is seen between adipocytes, and as lesions progress the infiltrate becomes diffusely present throughout the lobule. The inflammatory cells are initially composed of an admixture of neutrophils and lymphocytes. Later, lymphocytes and mononuclear cells with epithelioid forms predominate. Early lesions are typically associated with necrotizing vasculitis involving small- to medium-sized arteries and veins (Figs. 10–3C and 10–4A). Vessel walls are infiltrated by lymphocytes and neutrophils, and zones of fibrinoid necrosis and fibrosis may be observed. Vascular thrombosis is also focally present.

In older lesions, vasculitic involvement may be more difficult to identify. With chronicity, the lobular panniculitis of erythema induratum is predominated by lymphocytes and epithelioid histiocytes with variable degrees of fibrosis (Fig. 10–4C). On close inspection, zones of caseous necrosis may be observed (Fig. 10–4B); occasionally, these zones are extensive and geographic. These zones may be rimmed by epithelioid histiocytes with solitary or multiple nuclei; these more chronic manifestations are indistinguishable from involvement of fat by tuberculous infection. For many years, erythema induratum was regarded as a direct manifestation of pulmonary tuberculosis involving subcutaneous fat. However, intact organisms are not identified in the caseating granulomas of erythema induratum. On the other hand, it remains unknown whether erythema induratum represents an unusual

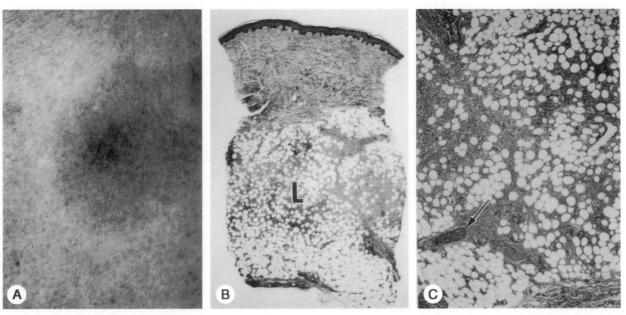

Figure 10–3. Erythema induratum. **(A)** The gross pathology consists of indurated, erythematous, painful lesions; there is a dusky purple center surrounded by a pale pink rim of erythema. **(B)** Biopsy specimens reveal diffuse inflammation within the lobule (L). **(C)** In contrast to erythema nodosum, vascular injury is focally observed *(arrow)*.

allergic manifestation stimulated by a number of environmental antigens, including those related to tuberculous infection.

Although with chronicity, the lobular panniculitis that typifies erythema induratum may result in diffuse fibrosis of the subcutaneous fat, residual inflammatory foci may persist, providing diagnostic clues regarding the inflammatory insult that preceded. However, in end-stage lesions, diffuse fibrosis of the lobule is not considered sufficiently specific to permit

a diagnosis of erythema induratum. In such cases, additional sampling of more recent lesions is recommended for more definitive diagnostic evaluation. As is the case in erythema nodosum, erythema induratum may be mimicked by a number of traumatic or infectious insults to adipose tissue. Accordingly, it is important to note the absence of alterations within the overlying epidermis and dermis in erythema induratum, again signifying primary panniculitis centered exclusively within the subcutaneous layer.

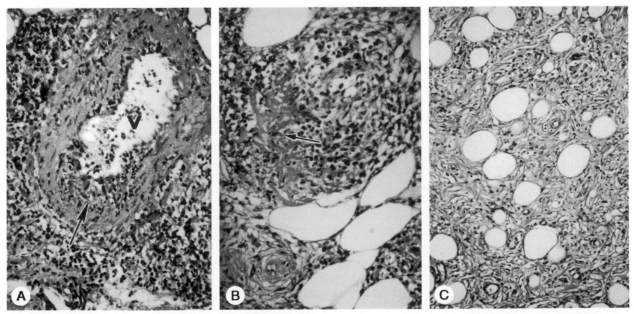

Figure 10–4. Erythema induratum. Higher magnification of the inflammatory infiltrate reveals **(A)** diffuse vasculitis *(arrow)* and **(B)** necrosis within granulomatous foci *(arrow)*. **(C)** Older lesions may show diffuse fibrosis within the lobule.

Polyarteritis Nodosa with Panniculitis[5]

- SEGMENTAL INFILTRATION OF DEEP VESSEL WALLS
- NEUTROPHILS AND MONONUCLEAR CELLS PREDOMINATE
- INTIMAL PROLIFERATION AND ORGANIZATION (LATE)
- FOCAL PANNICULITIS WITH GRANULOMATOUS FAT NECROSIS
- TRUE TUBERCULOID GRANULOMAS ABSENT

It is important to realize that ischemic changes within the fat may produce changes of lobular panniculitis that may be difficult to distinguish from erythema induratum. Ischemia may result from primary vasculitis, and such lesions frequently occur in association with cutaneous polyarteritis nodosa (see Chap. 7). Clinically, polyarteritis nodosa (Fig. 10–5A) manifests as multiple nodules within the subcutaneous tissue, frequently arranged along the course of arteries. Although this is described as the classic clinical appearance of polyarteritis nodosa, several major textbooks of clinical dermatology point out that these diagnostic features are present only in rare patients, and the more common clinical presentation of cutaneous polyarteritis nodosa consists of chronic or chronic-recurrent inflammatory papules and nodules with less specific patterns of distribution. Although any medium- or small-sized muscular artery may be affected, there appears to be a predisposition for skin involvement of the lower extremities; hence, the potential for confusion with forms of primary panniculitis. Because of the protean nature of the clinical manifestations of polyarteritis nodosa, the information that accompanies a biopsy specimen may or may not refer to the possibility of panniculitis.

The ability to diagnose polyarteritis nodosa at scanning magnification largely depends on the adequacy of the biopsy

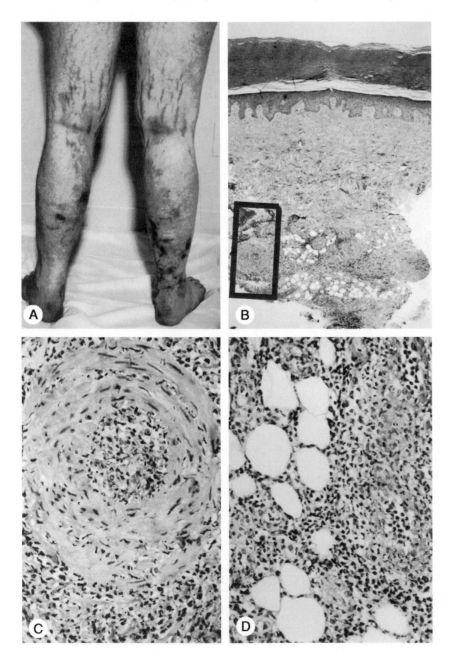

Figure 10–5. Panniculitis associated with polyarteritis nodosa. **(A)** The lower extremities of this transplant patient are enlarged and indurated due to diffuse panniculitis. Focally, overlying skin has broken down, suggesting associated ischemia. The striae on the posterior thighs are a result of chronic treatment with corticosteroids. **(B–D)** Biopsy specimens from the foot reveal both (**B,** *enclosed in rectangle,* **C**) vasculitis and **(D)** secondary lobular panniculitis, characterized by both neutrophils and mononuclear cells. The affected vessels were confirmed to be medium-sized arteries by elastic tissue stains which allowed detection of residual, albeit fragmented, internal elastic laminae. Although erythema induratum also may show vasculitis and panniculitis, both arteries and veins are involved, and the primary lobular panniculitis is granulomatous, often resembling infection with tubercle bacilli.

specimen. The inclusion of one or more medium-sized muscular arteries in the specimen produces a picture of prominence and expansion of the arterial walls by inflammatory cells accompanied by associated secondary lobular panniculitis (Fig. 10–5B). This picture closely mimics that of erythema induratum with vasculitic involvement (early nodular vasculitis stage) at low-power magnification. On closer inspection, there is necrotizing vasculitis involving small- to medium-sized arteries (Fig. 10–5C). This vasculitis is characterized by frequently segmental infiltration of expanded arterial walls by mixed inflammatory cells consisting predominantly of neutrophils and mononuclear cells, fibrinoid necrosis, and in more chronic lesions, zones of fibrosis and intimal proliferation, which also may display a segmental pattern within the vessel wall. This segmental pattern, whereby only a portion of an artery represented in cross section or longitudinal section is pathologically altered, is an important clue to the diagnosis of polyarteritis nodosa; the vasculitic involvement of arteries in the nodular vasculitis phase of erythema induratum tends to be more circumferential and diffuse within the portions of vessel wall represented in tissue sections. The degree of intimal proliferation in chronic lesions of cutaneous polyarteritis nodosa may be striking and may produce obliterative changes, another important clue to this diagnostic entity.

Closer inspection of the panniculitis associated with polyarteritis nodosa will show permeation of the subcutaneous lobule by neutrophils and mononuclear cells (Fig. 10–5D), frequently associated with granulomatous aggregates of lipid-laden histiocytes and zones of fat necrosis. True tuberculoid granulomas, in which epithelioid histiocytes with abundant granular eosinophilic cytoplasm are tightly aggregated and occasionally arranged about caseation necrosis, are absent. This absence of true tuberculoid granulomas within the lobules of the subcutaneous fat is an important differential feature separating polyarteritis nodosa with panniculitis from erythema induratum in the nodular vasculitis phase. Thus, it is convenient to conceptualize polyarteritis nodosa as a primary immunologic event in which the walls of small- to medium-sized muscular arteries are primarily targeted, and in which secondary ischemic and inflammatory necrosis and inflammation of the lobule of subcutaneous fat supplied by these arteries occurs. On the other hand, in erythema induratum, both arterial and venular walls and foci within the subcutaneous fat lobule are targeted for immunologic injury, resulting in the formation of markedly activated histiocytic aggregates (i.e., epithelioid granulomas). As a general rule, arteritis predominates over panniculitis in polyarteritis nodosa, whereas panniculitis is a major component of the pathology in erythema induration.

Lupus Panniculitis[6, 7]

- DERMIS USUALLY INVOLVED
- MIXED SEPTAL AND LOBULAR PANNICULITIS
- LYMPHOCYTES AND PLASMA CELLS PREDOMINATE
- HYALINIZED FAT NECROSIS AND ATROPHY
- NECROTIZING VASCULITIS ABSENT
- MUCIN DEPOSITION PRESENT

Lupus panniculitis, associated with lupus erythematosus and typically involving the deep dermis and subcutis, most frequently affects middle-aged women. The gross pathology demonstrates discrete, erythematous, often tender subcutaneous nodules that most frequently affect the trunk, upper extremities, and face (Fig. 10–6A). Patients may have either pure cutaneous (i.e., discoid) or systemic lupus erythematosus. Because lupus panniculitis, also referred to as lupus profundus, may be the initial presenting sign of systemic lupus erythematosus, awareness of this entity is critical both with respect to patient care and to avoid confusion with other forms of lobular panniculitis, which may mimic this disorder.

At scanning magnification, there is a patchy inflammatory infiltrate within the deep dermis and subcutis (Fig. 10–6B). Septa are not preferentially involved, and lobules are only focally infiltrated at sites of perivascular clusters of mononuclear cells. The epidermis is generally uninvolved. If hair follicles or eccrine coils are included, mononuclear cell aggregates may occasionally be situated about these structures as well. At higher magnification, sites of inflammatory infiltration demonstrate variable atrophy of subcutaneous tissue. This is manifested by variability in size of individual adipocytes and by spaces between adipocytes filled with homogeneous pale pink material (Fig. 10–6C), a finding sometimes referred to as hyalinized sclerosis. The latter alterations within the subcutaneous fat are characteristic findings of diagnostic importance in lupus panniculitis. The inflammatory component generally consists of lymphocytes, occasional histiocytes, and often, plasma cells. An additional finding of diagnostic significance is interstitial mucinosis, particularly within the deep dermis, which interfaces with the affected subcutis (Fig. 10–6D). Mucin is recognized as pale blue-gray, stringy material within interstitial spaces separating collagen bundles. Mucin may also be detected within septa separating subcutaneous lobules in lupus panniculitis.

Enzymatic Panniculitis[8, 9]

- LOBULAR NECROTIZING PANNICULITIS WITH VARIABLE MIXED INFLAMMATORY INFILTRATE
- VASCULITIS ABSENT
- LIQUEFACTIVE FAT NECROSIS
- MICROCYSTS WITHIN FAT
- SAPONIFICATION WITH CALCIFICATION
- FIBROSIS AND ATROPHY WITH CHRONICITY

The histopathology of enzymatic fat necrosis consists of typical liquefactive degeneration and fat necrosis associated with variable foci of reactive mixed neutrophilic and lymphocytic inflammation. Necrotic adipocytes may be replaced entirely by homogeneous, pale blue material, producing ghost-like remnants of previous cellular elements (Fig. 10–7A). Foci of granular, deep blue-purple deposits representing sites of dystrophic calcification within saponified fat are frequently encountered. As the degenerative process continues, small microcysts may also develop within the involved subcutis. Vasculitis is not observed in enzymatic fat necrosis. In older lesions, which unfortunately are seldom available for biopsy due to the grave implications of the underlying pathology, variable degrees of fibrous replacement of the previously necrotic lobule may be observed.

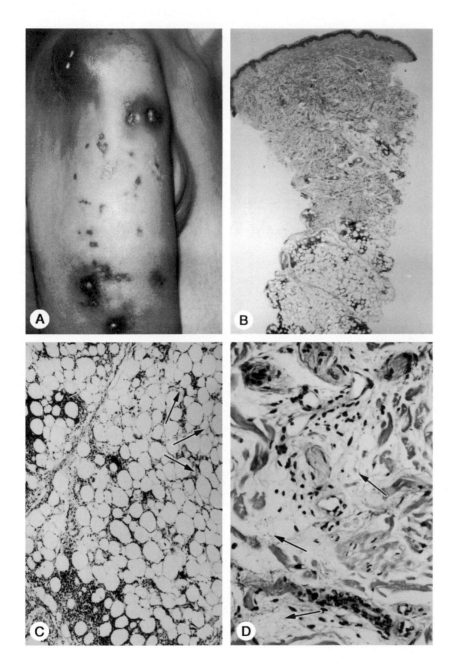

Figure 10–6. Panniculitis of lupus erythematosus. **(A)** Multiple erythematous nodules are present, many with central ulceration. **(B)** Scanning magnification of an early lesion shows deep dermal and subcutaneous aggregates of mononuclear cells. Eccrine coils, when present, are also frequently involved by the inflammatory infiltrate. **(C)** Lymphocytes and plasma cells predominate in this focus; adipocytes within the lobule are variably atrophic and separated by characteristic, pale, hyalinized matrix *(arrows)*. **(D)** Thin, beady strands of mucin are conspicuous about neurovascular bundles and eccrine epithelium *(arrows)*.

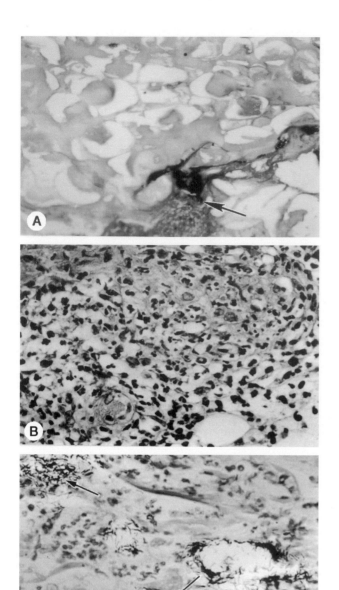

Figure 10–7. Enzymatic and infectious panniculitis. **(A)** Panniculitis of pancreatitis and pancreatic carcinoma is characterized by hyalinized, coagulative necrosis of adipocytes within the lobule and associated saponification with calcification *(arrow)*. **(B)** Mixed inflammation in a fat lobule without a specific pattern of primary panniculitis prompts special stains for fungi and mycobacteria. **(C)** In this case, atypical mycobacteria *(arrows)* were detected in large numbers.

Infectious Panniculitis[10, 11]

- PATIENT OFTEN IMMUNOCOMPROMISED
- MAY MIMIC SEPTAL OR LOBULAR PANNICULITIS
- STELLATE OR ZONAL MICROABSCESSES
- TUBERCULOID GRANULOMAS OR VASCULITIS MAY BE PRESENT
- DERMIS OFTEN INVOLVED
- CULTURE OF FRESH TISSUE CONFIRMATORY

Infectious panniculitis is most commonly encountered in the setting of immunodeficiency. Like other forms of panniculitis, it presents as regions of erythematous, tender induration that may mimic large vessel vasculitis, primary lobular or septal panniculitis, cellulitis, or septic embolic events with subsequent tissue ischemia. The buttocks, thighs, or distal lower extremities are often involved.

The diagnosis of infectious panniculitis, like that of factitial panniculitis, is suspected when the pattern at scanning magnification or the composite cellular elements on inspection at higher magnification do not seem to correlate with a specific diagnosis. The picture is therefore often mixed, with elements of both septal and lobular panniculitis present. Inspection of the inflammatory components may reveal admixtures of acute and chronic inflammatory cells, frank or poorly formed granulomas, or neutrophilic microabscesses (Fig. 10–7B). Because these lesions often develop in immunocompromised patients, the histologic clues indicative of cause (e.g., neutrophils for bacteria, granulomas for deep fungi) may be absent or misleading. One helpful feature in differentiating both infectious and factitial panniculitis from primary panniculitis is the frequent involvement of the dermis by inflammatory cells in the former two conditions. Special stains often will demonstrate organisms in infectious panniculitis (Fig. 10–7C), although culture of fresh biopsy tissue may be required when the number of organisms is low or when organism morphology has been altered by partial treatment.

Factitial Panniculitis[12]

- FEATURES OF MORE THAN ONE TYPE OF PRIMARY PANNICULITIS
- REFRACTILE OR BIREFRINGENT PARTICLES
- HEMORRHAGE OR HEMOSIDERIN WITHOUT VASCULITIS
- ADMIXTURE OF ACUTE AND CHRONIC CHANGES
- SCLEROSING LIPOGRANULOMATA MAY BE PRESENT
- EPIDERMIS AND/OR DERMIS OFTEN INVOLVED

The diagnosis of factitial panniculitis is often problematic, both clinically and histologically. Injected substances that have been reported to induce panniculitis include organic materials including milk and fecal matter, certain drugs, and oily materials. Clinically, the patients develop nodules that may spontaneously drain pus, indurated plaques, ulcers, and zones of scarring. Generally, the areas of involvement are accessible to autoinjection (Fig. 10–8A).

Histologically, there is often a nonspecific or mixed histologic picture that does not correlate with known patterns of primary panniculitis (Fig. 10–8B). For example, there may be both septal and lobular involvement, dermal involvement, or an admixture of acute and chronic inflammation. Granulomas, zones of fat necrosis, and microabscess may be observed, and birefringent particulate material introduced at the injection site also has been reported. If silicone has been injected, the histologic picture of a *paraffinoma* is encountered. This consists of rounded lipid droplets of variable size surrounded by fibrosis and inflammation. At scanning mag-

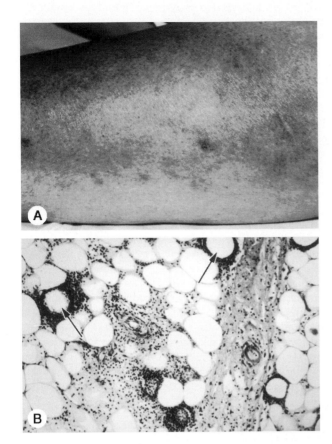

Figure 10–8. Factitial panniculitis. **(A)** Indurated, erythematous skin with residual small papules and pinpoint scabs representing injection sites. **(B)** Panniculitis is both septal and lobular, and inflammatory cells are focally tightly clustered about individual cells *(arrows)*, potentially indicating uneven distribution of the injected toxic material.

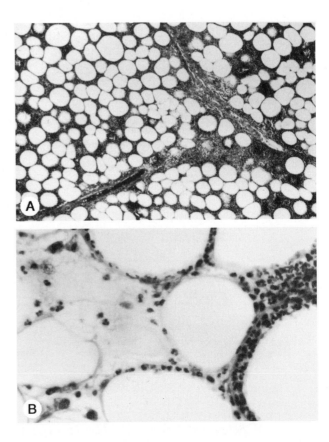

Figure 10–9. Relapsing febrile nodular nonsuppurative panniculitis. In the earliest stages, characteristic histologic changes include diffuse lobular infiltration by inflammatory cells, predominantly **(A)** neutrophils and **(B)** foci of degenerating adipocytes *(left)*. In contrast to infectious panniculitis, discrete microabscesses do not occur.

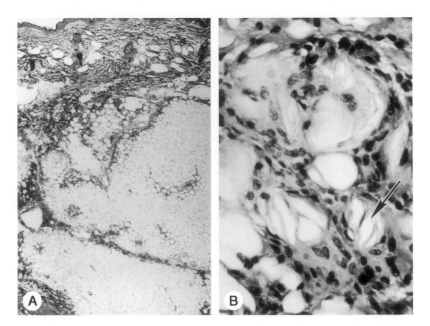

Figure 10–10. Subcutaneous fat necrosis of the newborn. **(A)** Mixed inflammatory cells are centered about lobular aggregates of degenerating subcutaneous fat. **(B)** Individual adipocytes contain characteristic clefts within their cytoplasm *(arrow)*, which on polarization of frozen sections, represent birefringent crystals.

nification, this pattern imparts a ''Swiss-cheese'' appearance. The droplets are differentiated from adipocytes by their irregularity in size and absence of nuclei.

Rare Disorders

- WEBER-CHRISTIAN DISEASE[13]
- SUBCUTANEOUS FAT NECROSIS OF THE NEWBORN[14]
- SCLEREMA NEONATORUM[15]
- COLD PANNICULITIS[16]
- α_1-ANTITRYPSIN DEFICIENCY[17]

Weber-Christian disease, also known as relapsing febrile nodular nonsuppurative panniculitis, is characterized by the clinical appearance of crops of tender subcutaneous nodules preferentially but not exclusively involving the lower extremities. The syndrome also involves recurrent mild fever. Patients of any age or gender may be affected, although middle-aged women appear to be particularly susceptible. Histologically, lesions evolve from a short initial phase characterized by neutrophilic lobular panniculitis with admixed mononuclear cells (Fig. 10–9), to a diagnostic phase characterized by lobular infiltrates of foamy macrophages, to a third phase showing lobular fibrosis with admixed lymphocytes and plasma cells.

Subcutaneous fat necrosis of the newborn is clinically characterized by the appearance of multiple subcutaneous nodules and plaques soon after birth. Histologically (Fig. 10–10), there is a mixed inflammatory infiltrate centered about lobular aggregates of degenerating subcutaneous fat. Individual adipocytes contain characteristic clefts within their cytoplasm which, on polarization of frozen sections, are revealed to represent birefringent crystals.

Sclerema neonatorum, on the other hand, is a diffuse induration of the subcutaneous tissue of newborns, producing a waxy appearance and consistency. Histologically, there is little inflammation; thus sclerema neonatorum does not rep-

resent a true primary panniculitis. Rather, individual adipocytes contain prominent intracytoplasmic, needle-shaped clefts, which correlate with an abnormal ratio of intracellular unsaturated:saturated fatty acids (Fig. 10–11).

Cold panniculitis, also most often observed in infants,

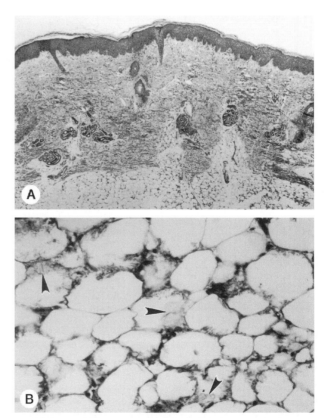

Figure 10–11. Sclerema neonatorum. **(A)** In contrast to subcutaneous fat necrosis of the newborn, inflammation in sclerema neonatorum is inconspicuous to absent; therefore, it does not represent a true panniculitis. **(B)** Individual adipocytes contain fine, needle-shaped clefts at the cell perimeter *(arrowheads)*.

generally occurs as indurated nodules on the cheeks after exposure to cold. Histology reveals cysts resulting from rupture and coalescence of adipocytes, rimmed by mixed inflammatory cells consisting of lymphocytes, histiocytes, neutrophils, and sometimes eosinophils.

α₁-Antitrypsin deficiency produces a nodular panniculitis with a tendency to ulcerate and discharge oily material. This disorder should be suspected in all cases of ulcerative panniculitis. The clinical picture and histology may be indistinguishable from Weber-Christian disease during early evolutionary phases; extensive necrosis of subcutaneous fat may ensue.

DIFFERENTIAL DIAGNOSIS

Although the differential diagnosis of panniculitis may seem to be a complicated issue, the diagnostic clues are quite straightforward. On examining a biopsy specimen, it must first be determined whether the specimen displays an adequate quantity of subcutaneous tissue, including intact lobules and septa. If not, further attempts to stretch the limits of diagnostic certainty based on incomplete data may prove hazardous. If the specimen adequately represents subcutaneous fat, it is advisable to determine at scanning magnification whether the inflammatory process is exclusively (or nearly so) confined to the fat, or whether there is significant dermal involvement. In the latter case, it should be considered that the process may not represent a primary panniculitis, and infection and factitia should be considered. Lupus panniculitis also may show dermal involvement. If the infiltrate is predominantly centered in the fat, it is helpful to determine whether it is primarily septal (erythema nodosum) or primarily lobular (erythema induratum versus other disorders). In the case of lobular involvement with vasculitis, it should be remembered that segmental vasculitis with unimpressive lobular inflammatory changes suggests polyarteritis nodosa, whereas well-established granulomatous lobular panniculitis with diffuse vasculitis suggests the nodular vasculitis phase of erythema induratum. In instances in which the pattern of inflammatory composition does not fit clearly into these categories, or when intracytoplasmic clefts, saponification, or hyalinization affect adipocytes, rare and unusual forms of panniculitis should be entertained, and close correlation of findings with clinical parameters (e.g., age, existence of connective tissue disease, presence of enzyme excess or deficiency) should be established.

SELECTED REFERENCES

1. Winkelmann RK, Forstrom L. New observations in the histopathology of erythema nodosum. J Invest Dermatol 1975;65:441.
2. Niemi KM, Forstrom L, Hannuksela M, et al. Nodules on the legs. Acta Derm Venereol (Stockh) 1977;57:145.
3. Salvatore MA, Lynch PJ. Erythema nodosum, estrogens, and pregnancy. Arch Dermatol 1980;116:557.
4. Thompson R, Urbach F. Erythema induratum. Int J Dermatol 1987;26:402.
5. Goslen JB, Graham W, Lazarus GS. Cutaneous polyarteritis nodosa. Arch Dermatol 1974;110:407.
6. Izumi AK, Takiguchi P. Lupus erythematosus panniculitis. Arch Dermatol 1983;119:61.
7. Sanchez NP, Peters MS, Winkelmann RK. The histopathology of lupus erythematosus panniculitis. J Am Acad Dermatol 1981;5:673.
8. Cannon JR, Pitha JV, Everett MA. Subcutaneous fat necrosis in pancreatitis. J Cutan Pathol 1979;6:501.
9. Hughs PSH, Apisarnthanarax P, Mullins JF. Subcutaneous fat necrosis associated with pancreatic disease. Arch Dermatol 1975;111:506.
10. Prystowski SD, Vogelstein B, Ettinger DS, et al. Invasive aspergillosis. N Engl J Med 1976;295:655.
11. Lloveras J, Peterson PK, Simmons RL, et al. Mycobacterial infections in renal transplant recipients. Arch Intern Med 1982;142:888.
12. Forstrom L, Winkelmann RK. Factitial panniculitis. Arch Dermatol 1974;110:747.
13. Forstrom L, Winkelmann RK. Acute panniculitis. Arch Dermatol 1977;113:909.
14. Tsuji T. Subcutaneous fat necrosis of the newborn. Light and electron microscopic studies. Br J Dermatol 1976;95:407.
15. Kellum RE, Ray TL, Brown GR. Sclerema neonatorum. Arch Dermatol 1968;97:372.
16. Solomon LM, Beerman H. Cold panniculitis. Arch Dermatol 1963;88:897.
17. Su WPD, Smith KC, Pittelkow MR, et al. Alpha-1-antitrypsin deficiency panniculitis. Am J Dermatopathol 1987;9:483.

III

Neoplasms

11
Epidermal Tumors

DEFINITIONS AND GENERAL CONSIDERATIONS

Tumors of the surface epidermis are potentially the most diagnostically problematic conditions in dermatopathology. Major issues, such as the difference between benign and malignant lesions, arise routinely in this group of disorders. Moreover, many of the neoplasms have ambiguous or vague architectural or cytologic features that defy accurate classification. One major problem is the fact that chronically inflamed keratoses acquire a degree of reactive atypia that may superficially mimic carcinoma. In this chapter, specific examples of this potential pitfall are addressed, and criteria are established for differentiation of reactive nuclear alterations from true dysplasia and anaplasia within keratinocytes.

In describing cutaneous epidermal neoplasms, it is important to understand the meaning of the words dysplasia, anaplasia, and atypia. The same issues, of course, also relate to tumors of adnexal epithelium and melanocytes, which are discussed in Chapters 12 and 13. For the purposes of this discussion, the word *dysplasia* (from the roots *dys,* meaning abnormal or faulty, and *plasis,* meaning development or molding) refers to cytologic and architectural characteristics with some but not all of the characteristics of malignancy. *Anaplasia* refers to the prototypical malignant cell, which is devoid of significant differentiation. *Atypia,* perhaps the most problematic of these terms, simply means not typical or not normal. In a sense, dysplastic cellular processes are atypical. However, the term atypia encompasses much more than dysplasia. There are, for example, the reactive atypia of an inflamed epithelial neoplasm or a re-epithelializing ulcer base and the degenerative atypia of virally infected or metabolically poisoned cells. Understanding and correct use of these terms are critical to an algorithmic approach to the differential diagnosis of cutaneous epithelial tumors.

GROSS PATHOLOGY

There is no single common link that unifies the gross pathology of epithelial neoplasms. Many tumors produce ex-

cessive keratin, and therefore abundant scale may predominate the clinical picture, as is the case in squamous cell carcinomas. Other lesions grow in an endophytic manner, provoking stromal and vascular alterations which contribute to the clinical picture, as in the telangiectatic pearly papules and nodules of many basal cell carcinomas. A wide variety of epidermal neoplasms may mimic melanocytic tumors because of endogenous pigmentation incorporated into their epithelial elements. Examples of this phenomenon include pigmented basal cell carcinomas and seborrheic keratoses. Other neoplasms proliferate within or directly beneath the epidermal surface, and associated inflammation and scale may result in a clinical lesion that resembles a form of primary dermatitis, as may be the case in superficial forms of basal cell carcinoma and squamous cell carcinoma in situ. Because of the multitude of clinical appearances that may characterize epithelial neoplasia, an overview of potential variations in gross pathology is essential.

In certain instances, the gross pathology is absolutely essential to establishing a specific diagnosis. An example is the warty dyskeratoma, which may mimic the histology of the well-developed lesions of Darier disease. Because the former generally is a solitary lesion, whereas the latter consists of numerous small hyperkeratotic papules, the clinical information makes possible a final diagnostic refinement that results in the assignment of a precise diagnosis.

GENERAL HISTOLOGY AND TEMPORAL EVOLUTION

The general histology of epidermal neoplasms is basic; tumors generally recapitulate either squamoid or basaloid cells. Squamoid cells are polyhedral and contain abundant cytoplasm and well-defined intercellular junctions, as is the case for cells normally composing the stratum spinosum. Basaloid cells are small, round cells with relatively scant cytoplasm and inconspicuous intercellular attachments, as is found normally in the cells of the stratum basalis. Prototypes for benign epithelial squamoid neoplasms are keratoacan-

187

thoma or verruca. A nonirritated seborrheic keratosis is an example of a benign epithelial basaloid neoplasm. Squamous cell and basal cell carcinomas represent examples of malignant epithelial tumors that differentiate along these two different yet related epidermal layers.

The temporal evolution of epithelial neoplasms differs considerably depending on the lesion. Whereas certain seborrheic keratosis may remain stable, others appear to undergo a form of inflammatory regression, perhaps ultimately to yield nondescript residual zones of verrucous epidermal hyperplasia. Similar alterations may occur in verrucae as a result of either host immune responses or simple loss of viral activity over time, resulting in a verrucous keratosis without specific findings of active human papillomavirus (HPV) effect. Accordingly, it is possible that verrucous epidermal proliferation is a final common pathway for a variety of senescent benign keratoses. Perhaps the most remarkable evolutionary sequence observed in benign epithelial neoplasms involves the keratoacanthoma. Early lesions are characterized by endophytic tongues of proliferative tumor epithelium; midstage lesions are less proliferative and appear to be directed toward the production of a central keratin plug via trichilemmal (i.e., hair follicle-like) keratinization; and old lesions show involution consisting of development of an inflamed and fibrotic underlying stroma which pushes upward to flatten the endophytic epithelial component, avulsing the keratin plug. This latter process is associated with transepidermal elimination of elastic fibers. Many epithelial polyps become progressively infiltrated with fat as they age or, via torsion, infarct and fall off. Epithelial malignancies, such as basal cell carcinoma, may have an indolent course, with extremely slow progression over time. Invasive squamous cell carcinomas will grow inexorably if left untreated, and if tumor size increases significantly, metastases may occur.

HISTOLOGY OF SPECIFIC DISORDERS

Epidermal Nevi and Hamartomas[1, 2]

- VERRUCOUS EPIDERMAL HYPERPLASIA
- VARIABLE ANOMALIES IN ASSOCIATED ADNEXAL EPITHELIUM
- ALTERED SUPERFICIAL DERMAL MESENCHYME

Epidermal nevi and hamartomas are presumed to be *congenital* neoplastic proliferations of benign epidermal cells. Often, the clinical appearance is of a linear, keratotic plaque, and the histology typically shows a verrucous epidermal architecture similar in appearance to some seborrheic keratoses. Nevus sebaceus represents a mixed epidermal and pilosebaceous nevus, and accordingly, it is discussed in the chapter on benign tumors of the pilosebaceous apparatus (see Chap. 12).

Epidermal nevi occur in either a localized or generalized form. Localized epidermal nevi, a term that connotes a birthmark, not a melanocytic tumor, appear as linear streaks anywhere on the body, formed by coalescent, often hyperkeratotic papules (Fig. 11–1A). Most lesions are asymptomatic, although inflamed lesions (i.e., inflammatory linear verrucous epidermal nevi [ILVEN]) may be pruritic. Generalized

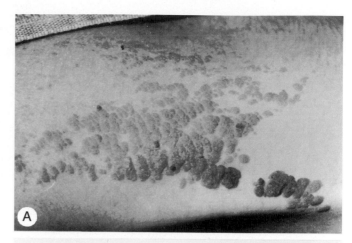
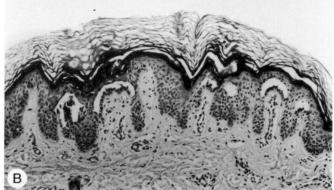
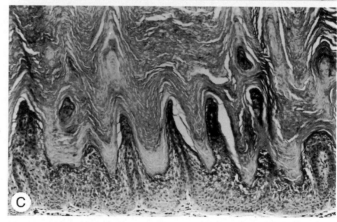

Figure 11–1. Epidermal nevus (i.e., hamartoma). **(A)** Clinical appearance of epidermal nevus. Typical lesions are grouped, keratosis-like plaques arranged in linear array. **(B, C)** Histologically, verrucous acanthosis begins abruptly and is accompanied by variable degrees of hyperkeratosis. Lesions may closely resemble seborrheic keratosis, and correlation with clinical parameters is generally required in formulating a correct diagnosis.

(''systematized'') epidermal nevi consist of multiple streaks, often in parallel arrangement, that extensively involve the body surface. These streaks may be unilateral or bilateral, and in some instances, large segments of the skin surface are involved. Systematized epidermal nevi may be associated with mental retardation, seizures, and neural deafness.

Most epidermal nevi exhibit papillary epidermal hyperplasia that is both exophytic and endophytic (Fig. 11–1B, C). Subtle alterations of the associated superficial dermal connective tissue or anomalous follicular differentiation suggest that the lesions represent cutaneous hamartomas, in which epidermal elements predominate. Cytologically, epidermal nevi are composed of benign keratinocytes arranged in the normal pattern of basaloid, spinous, granular, and cornified layers. Occasional lesions closely resemble seborrheic keratosis. Reaction patterns of *epidermolytic hyperkeratosis,* focal *acantholytic dyskeratosis,* and *cornoid lamella formation* all may be present in epidermal nevi, and may dominate the histologic picture in some lesions.

Epidermal nevi may be misdiagnosed as *seborrheic keratoses.* Avoidance of this error is possible by recognizing that the former lesions are usually present in young individuals. Moreover, there may be associated adnexal or mesenchymal anomalies in epidermal nevi that are not ordinarily present in seborrheic keratoses. Some lesions may demonstrate only papillary epidermal hyperplasia and accordingly be confused with old verrucae, acanthosis nigricans, hyperkeratotic histologic variants of seborrheic keratoses, or a number of other less commonly encountered conditions. Detailed clinical information is therefore important in the accurate histologic recognition of many epidermal nevi.

Acanthosis Nigricans

- VERRUCOUS EPIDERMAL HYPERPLASIA
- BASAL CELL LAYER HYPERPIGMENTATION
- CLINICAL ASSOCIATION WITH MALIGNANCY OR ENDOCRINE ABNORMALITIES

Acanthosis nigricans is discussed in Chapter 19 in relation to its association with visceral malignancy. This condition often presents as hyperpigmented verrucous plaques in intertriginous skin (Fig. 11–2A). The relatively nonspecific histology of acanthosis nigricans is emphasized in this chapter with regard to the differential diagnosis of verrucous epidermal hyperplasia. Most often, acanthosis nigricans is confused histologically with epidermal nevi or hyperkeratotic variants of seborrheic keratoses (Fig. 11–2B). Clinical correlation is important in differentiating acanthosis nigricans from these entities.

Seborrheic Keratosis[3–7]

- ABRUPT PROLIFERATION OF BASALOID CELLS
- VERRUCOUS, VARIABLY ENDOPHYTIC ARCHITECTURE
- HORN CYSTS AND PSEUDO–HORN CYSTS
- SQUAMATIZATION AND REACTIVE ATYPIA WHEN IRRITATED

These lesions characteristically occur in middle-aged and elderly individuals and consist of multiple, benign, localized neoplastic proliferations of basaloid keratinocytes, often with associated hyperkeratosis and hyperpigmentation. They arise spontaneously and are most numerous on the trunk, although the extremities, head, and neck may be involved. In patients of African descent, multiple small lesions that typically appear on the face have been termed *dermatosis papulosa nigra.* Clinically, seborrheic keratoses appear as round, flat, coin-like plaques that vary in size from several millimeters to centimeters (Fig. 11–3A). They exhibit a uniform tan-to-dark-brown color and usually have a velvety-to-granular surface. Small, pore-like ostia impacted with keratin, a feature helpful in differentiating these pigmented lesions from melanomas, are often present. The explosive onset of hundreds of seborrheic keratoses in association with internal malignancy is known as the *sign of Leser-Trélat.*

At scanning magnification, most seborrheic keratoses are exophytic and sharply demarcated from the adjacent epidermis (Fig. 11–3B, C). Tumors are composed of sheets of small basal cells containing variable melanin pigmentation, a factor that contributes to the brown coloration observed clinically. The associated dermal stroma typically forms a hyalinized mantle along the basal cell layer, a helpful diagnostic feature when dealing with minute curettings (Fig. 11–3D). Exuberant keratin production generally occurs at the surface of seborrheic keratoses (Fig. 11–3E), and small keratin-filled

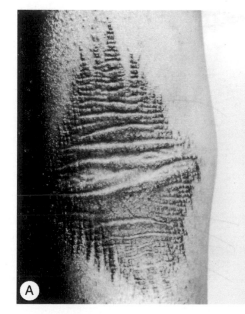
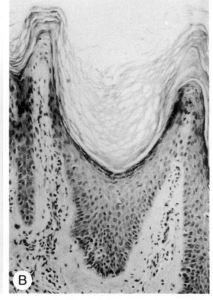

Figure 11–2. Acanthosis nigricans. **(A)** This hyperpigmented plaque is characteristically located in a flexural crease or intertriginous region. **(B)** Histologically, there is verrucous epidermal hyperplasia with hyperkeratosis. Findings may be subtle, appear nonspecific, or be mistaken for an epidermal nevus or seborrheic keratosis.

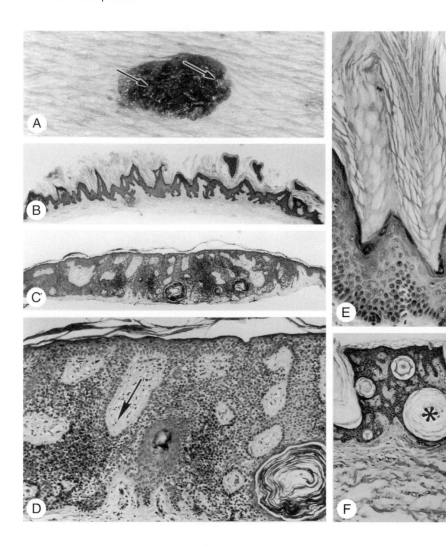

Figure 11–3. Seborrheic keratosis. **(A)** Gross pathology of seborrheic keratosis is a well-defined, hyperkeratotic, pigmented plaque that appears to be stuck on to the epidermal surface. Keratotic plugs *(arrows)* may be helpful in distinguishing these lesions from those of melanocytic origin. At scanning magnification, seborrheic keratoses may have **(B)** an exophytic verrucous surface or **(C)** show endophytic growth. **(D)** Common to all lesions is proliferation of benign basaloid epithelial cells, which resemble normal stratum basalis. The associated dermis *(arrow)* is thickened and hyalinized just below the dermal-epidermal junction of the tumor. This is an important diagnostic clue when dealing with curetted, tangentially-oriented fragments. **(E)** The scale of seborrheic keratosis is generally hyperkeratotic, with a prominent, basketweave appearance. **(F)** Prominent keratin-filled horn cysts are present within the tumor (*) or communicate with the epidermal surface (i.e., pseudohorn cysts; *arrow).*

cysts (i.e., horn cysts) and downgrowths of keratin from the surface of the lesion into the main tumor mass (i.e., pseudo–horn cysts) are characteristic features (Fig. 11–3*F*). Pseudo–horn cysts represent the keratin-filled ostia that are appreciated clinically on the surface of the lesion.

Variant forms of seborrheic keratosis include large cell acanthoma (Fig. 11–4*A*), irritated seborrheic keratosis (Fig. 11–4*B*), seborrheic keratosis with intraepidermal epithelioma or "clonal" pattern (Fig. 11–4*C*), and adenoidal seborrheic keratosis (Fig. 11–4*D*). When seborrheic keratoses become inflamed, they undergo squamous differentiation and become characterized by foci of whirling squamous cells resembling eddy currents (see Fig. 11–4*C*). Such lesions, termed *irritated seborrheic keratoses,* may be confused with squamous cell carcinoma as a result of the reactive atypia they contain. Separation of the nuclear atypia that may be seen in irritated seborrheic keratoses from the dysplasia and anaplasia of squamous cell carcinoma depends on recognition of cytologic details critical to the differentiation of reactive atypia from preneoplastic dysplasia and anaplasia of malignancy (Table 11–1).

Seborrheic keratoses that involve the epithelium of hair follicles often proliferate in an endophytic manner and exhibit squamous differentiation in association with inflamma-

tion. These lesions are termed *inverted follicular keratoses. Melanoacanthoma* is a rarely encountered variant of seborrheic keratosis in which pigmented, dendritic, benign melanocytes proliferate in association with relatively amelanotic, neoplastic, basaloid epithelial cells.

Seborrheic keratoses are indolent neoplasms that are easily treated by curettage or locally destructive measures. Malignant degeneration is exceedingly rare, although a few instances of associated basal and squamous cell carcinoma have been observed.

Table 11–1. CYTOLOGIC CHARACTERISTICS OF REACTIVE ATYPIA VERSUS DYSPLASIA-ANAPLASIA

CHARACTERISTICS	REACTIVE ATYPIA	DYSPLASIA-ANAPLASIA
Nuclear-cytoplasmic ratio	Normal	Increased
Nuclear contour	Smooth	Angulated
Nuclear membrane	Thin, uniform	Thick, irregular
Chromatin	Delicate, evenly dispersed	Coarse, clumped
Nucleolus	Markedly enlarged	Markedly enlarged
Cytoplasm	Often amphophilic	Often eosinophilic

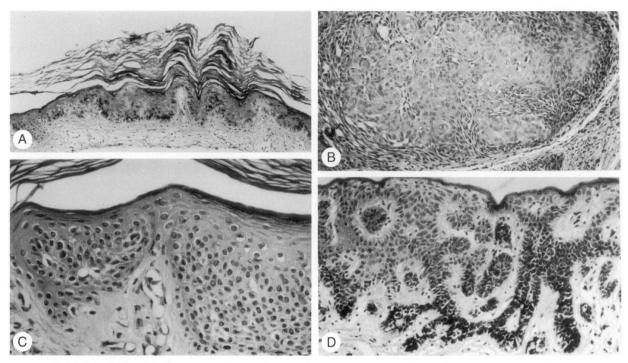

Figure 11–4. Variant forms of seborrheic keratosis. **(A)** Large cell acanthoma is composed of squamoid cells several times the diameter of normal keratinocytes within the adjacent stratum spinosum. **(B)** Irritated seborrheic keratosis is characterized by prominent squamatization and eddy formation. **(C)** In intraepidermal epithelioma pattern, basaloid elements are nested within an otherwise normal epidermal layer. **(D)** In the adenoidal variant, there are heavily melanized endophytic cords of pigmented neoplastic epithelium within the superficial dermis.

Fibroepithelial Polyps

- PEDUNCULATED, CIRCUMSCRIBED NEOPLASMS, OFTEN ON A STALK
- COVERED BY STRATIFIED SQUAMOUS EPITHELIUM
- CORE OF FIBROVASCULAR TISSUE AND SOMETIMES FAT

Variously termed skin tag, acrochordon, and squamous papilloma, these neoplasms commonly occur with advancing age on the trunk, axilla, head, and neck skin. Clinically, they are sessile or pedunculated, soft, flesh-colored, slow-growing tumors (Fig. 11–5A). Eruptive fibroepithelial polyps may be associated with the acute onset of other benign epidermal neoplasms (e.g., seborrheic keratoses) and are a presumed consequence of production of epidermal growth factors by unrelated primary neoplasia.

At scanning magnification, fibroepithelial polyps consist of a mantle of variably reactive epidermis covering a protuberant fibrovascular core (Fig. 11–5B). Within this core, mature adipose tissue and occasionally nerve fibers may be observed. Some fibroepithelial polyps may be confused clinically with polypoidal types of malignant melanoma, neurofibromas, polypoid dermal nevi, and pedunculated hemangiomas. Enlarging lesions present cosmetic problems that necessitate their removal. Spontaneous infarction may lead to clinical concern due to pain and abrupt change in color and sometimes may complicate histologic interpretation; this event frequently precipitates surgical excision of fibroepithelial polyps.

Clear Cell Acanthoma[8-10]

- EPITHELIAL NEOPLASM WITH ABRUPT DEMARCATION
- GLYCOGENATED, CLEAR SQUAMOUS CELLS
- FIBROVASCULAR STROMAL RESPONSE WITHIN SUPERFICIAL DERMIS
- ''PERCOLATING'' NEUTROPHILS WITHIN TUMOR

Clear cell acanthomas are relatively uncommon neoplasms that occur predominantly in middle-aged and older individuals, usually on the lower extremities. The lesions frequently have an eroded, oozing, erythematous surface (Fig. 11–6A). A typical clinical differential diagnosis includes basal cell carcinoma of the lower extremities, pyogenic granuloma, and eccrine poroma. Lesions generally grow slowly, are generally but not invariably solitary, and are usually smaller than 2 cm in diameter.

At low-to-medium magnification, clear cell acanthomas characteristically appear as well-demarcated, downward (i.e., endophytic) proliferations of glycogenated squamoid cells within the epidermal layer (Fig. 11–6B). The endophytic component, consisting of elongated rete ridges, is associated with enlarged, thinned dermal papillae containing dilated vessels which may communicate with the eroded surface. Periodic acid–Schiff (PAS) stain reveals that tumor cells contain abundant quantities of cytoplasmic glycogen. A characteristic feature is the percolation of neutrophils within intercellular spaces of the tumor and within overlying parakeratotic scale (Fig. 11–6C). Melanin pigment is diminished or

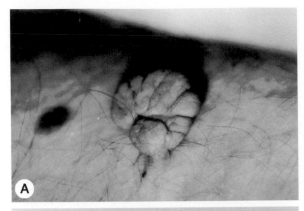

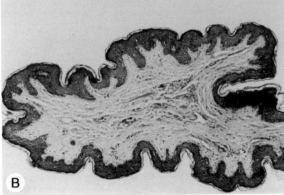

Figure 11–5. Fibroepithelial polyp. **(A)** These common, pedunculated lesions may have a smooth or bosselated surface. Those with a slender stalk may undergo ischemic necrosis due to torsion. **(B)** Histologically, a fibrovascular core is covered by a normal or acanthotic epidermal layer. When the epithelial elements resemble seborrheic keratosis (see Fig. 11–4), such lesions are designated as pedunculated seborrheic keratoses.

absent within tumor cells, indicating an apparent defect in melanocyte-keratinocyte melanin transfer in this neoplasm.

The differential diagnosis of clear cell acanthoma includes eccrine poroma, glycogenated seborrheic keratosis, and even psoriasis. Eccrine poromas may be distinguished from clear cell acanthoma by detection of ductular differentiation in the former. Seborrheic keratoses lack the characteristic prominent and vascularized dermal papillae of clear cell acanthoma, and usually retain focal basaloid differentiation. Moreover, clear cell acanthomas do not form horn and pseudo–horn cysts, as do most seborrheic keratoses. Psoriasis does not exhibit prominent cytoplasmic glycogenation of abrupt demarcation, although it shares many similarities with clear cell acanthoma, including parakeratotic scale containing neutrophils, downward elongation of rete ridges, and prominent dermal papillae containing ectatic and tortuous vessels.

Keratoacanthoma[11–16]

- CUP-SHAPED SQUAMOPROLIFERATIVE NEOPLASM
- CENTRAL CORNIFIED PLUG WITHIN CRATER
- LARGE KERATINOCYTES WITH GLASSY CYTOPLASM

- TRICHILEMMAL KERATINIZATION
- NEUTROPHILIC MICROABSCESSES AND TRANSEPIDERMAL ELIMINATION OF ELASTIC FIBERS

Keratoacanthomas generally involve the skin of the face or dorsal aspects of the upper extremities and infrequently affect non–sun-exposed skin. Lesions begin as small keratotic papules that enlarge rapidly over the course of several months. Mature tumors have a crater-like topography with a centrally located defect filled with a keratotic plug (Fig. 11–7A). Men are preferentially affected by a 3:1 ratio, and typi-

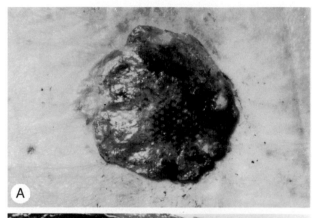

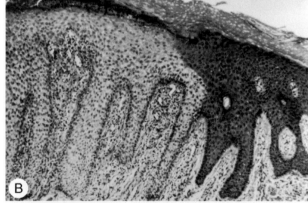

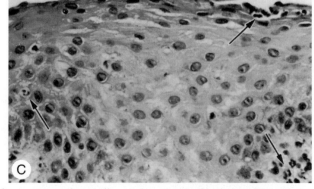

Figure 11–6. Clear cell acanthoma. **(A)** This lesion from the lower extremity demonstrates a typical oozing surface; the clinical impression was basal cell carcinoma. **(B)** The biopsy specimen reveals a well-demarcated endophytic neoplasm sharply juxtaposed with the adjacent epidermis because of the clear, highly glycogenated cytoplasm of the tumor cells. **(C)** An additional diagnostic feature is the presence of neutrophils *(arrows)* that percolate within the epithelial elements of this neoplasm.

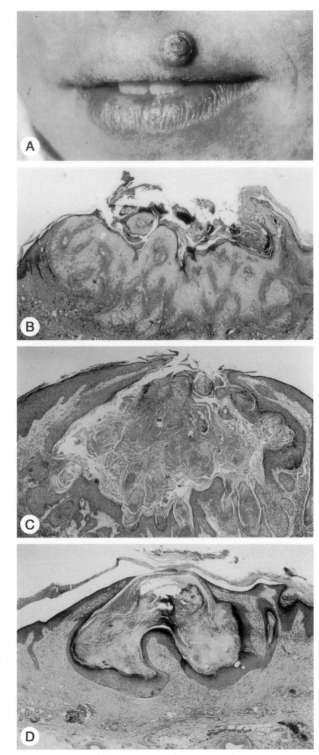

Figure 11–7. Keratoacanthoma: Natural evolution. **(A)** This crater-like nodule has a prominent central keratin plug which, upon histological examination, forms much of the tumor mass. The histologic sequential evolution of this neoplasm can be defined in stages: **(B)** early, proliferative stage, in which epithelial elements predominate; **(C)** middle stage, in which the well-formed keratotic crater is surrounded by endophytic lobules of proliferating epithelium; and **(D)** regressing late phase, with fibrosis at the base of the lesion, attenuated epithelial elements, and incipient extrusion of the central keratotic plug.

cal lesions range in size from 1 to 2.5 cm. Giant keratoacanthomas are rare tumors that may exceed 5 cm in diameter and are locally destructive. Lesions on the nose, the ear, or the vermilion border of the lip also may be locally destructive, as may keratoacanthomas that arise in subungual skin. The natural history of common keratoacanthomas involves spontaneous regression if left untreated. In addition to regression, the characteristically rapid clinical growth (a history of

growth over a few weeks is the rule) is a distinctive biological feature of this neoplasm.

At scanning magnification, there is an exophytic and endophytic neoplasm with a typical cup shape that is sharply demarcated from the surrounding epidermis and dermis (see Fig. 11–7A–C). Centrally within the neoplasm is a crater filled with eosinophilic laminated keratin, although this may be inconspicuous in early lesions (Fig. 11–7B) or suboptimally sectioned specimens. This crater is partially enclosed by well-defined lips that form the superficial border of the tumor. At the base of the tumor, interfacing with dermal connective tissue, are proliferating lobules of epithelium that may extend well into the reticular dermis, although bilateral symmetry is generally maintained. As keratoacanthomas regress, the proliferative epithelial component becomes less prominent and eventually flattens out above a zone of prominent fibrovascular proliferation (Fig. 11–7D).

Cytologically, keratoacanthomas are composed of large squamous epithelial cells that contain abundant cytoplasmic glycogen, imparting a characteristically glassy quality (Fig. 11–8). Cells at the periphery of proliferating lobules are more basaloid (Fig. 11–8C), and if this feature is maintained throughout the neoplasm, it may be helpful in separating keratoacanthoma from well-differentiated cup-shaped squamous cell carcinoma. Some degree of reactive cytologic atypia is invariably present, and although mitoses may be observed, large numbers of atypical mitotic figures are unusual and should raise suspicion of malignancy. Reactive atypia is characterized by cells with uniformly large, ovoid nuclei with smooth, regular contours; a peripherally marginated chromatin pattern which forms a thin, uniform band along the nuclear membrane; delicately dispersed heterochromatin; and prominent, eosinophilic nucleoli. Keratin formation within these tumors is "abrupt," without an intervening granular cell layer (Figure 11–8D). Numerous neutrophils may percolate in the intercellular spaces of tumor lobules,

focally forming discrete microabscesses (Fig. 11–8C). Transepidermal elimination of elastic fibers throughout the tumor may be prominent (Fig. 11–8A, B), and may correlate with the early stages of lesional regression. Accordingly, this feature has also been advocated as a means of discriminating between keratoacanthoma and well-differentiated squamous cell carcinoma.

Table 11–2 summarizes salient features of keratoacanthoma and cup-shaped squamous cell carcinoma. Although these differential features may be used in combination with clinical parameters to assign a likely diagnosis, it is frequently impossible to diagnose keratoacanthoma based on histology alone.

Warty Dyskeratoma[17, 18]

- FLAT OR SHALLOW CUP-SHAPED VERRUCOUS TUMOR
- SUPRABASAL ACANTHOLYSIS WITH CLEFT FORMATION
- DYSKERATOTIC ACANTHOLYTIC CELLS ABOVE INTACT BASAL CELL LAYER
- HYPERKERATOSIS

Warty dyskeratomas typically occur on sun-exposed, hair-bearing surfaces of adults, although their potential relation to actinic keratoses, which may also show focal acantholysis and dyskeratosis, is conjectural, and oral lesions

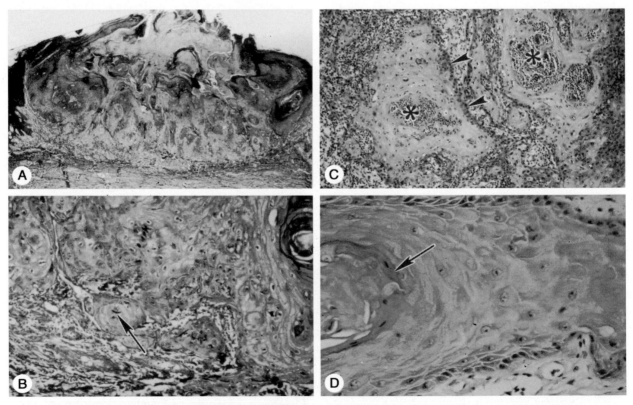

Figure 11–8. Keratoacanthoma: Distinguishing characteristics. **(A)** Lesions are bilaterally symmetrical; often contain **(B)** elastic fibers *(arrow)* and **(C)** neutrophilic microab... esses (*) within their epithelial elements; retain a more basaloid layer at the perimeter of endophytic, pseudoinvasive epithelial lobules *(arrowheads)*; and **(D)** exhibit glassy, homogeneous cytoplasm with abrupt keratinization *(arrow)* devoid of an intervening granular layer (i.e., trichilemmal keratinization).

Table 11–2. CLINICAL AND HISTOLOGIC FEATURES OF KERATOACANTHOMA AND WELL-DIFFERENTIATED SQUAMOUS CELL CARCINOMA*

FEATURES	KERATOACANTHOMA	INVASIVE SQUAMOUS CELL CARCINOMA
Growth rate	Rapid	Gradual
Basaloid layer in proliferating endophytic lobules	Consistent	Inconsistent
Involvement of lower one third of reticular dermis or extension below sweat glands	Unusual	May be observed
Cup-shaped architecture	Usually	Variable
Glassy cytoplasm	Always	Variable
Abrupt (trichilemmal) keratinization	Prominent	Often absent
Nature of keratotic plug	Often hyperkeratotic	Often parakeratotic
Transepidermal elimination of elastic fibers†	Yes	Absent or inconspicuous
Neutrophilic microabscesses	Often	Variable
Eosinophils in stromal infiltrate	Variable‡	Often numerous
Plasma cells in infiltrate	Variable	Often numerous
True single-cell invasion of stroma	Never	May be present

*No single feature has been shown to permit distinction between these two entities in the absence of definitive stromal invasion.
†Usually present only in regressing lesions.
‡Extrusion of naked keratin into dermis may elicit eosinophils, regardless of cause.

have been described. Lesions appear as solitary, elevated, keratotic papules or nodules, occasionally with an umbilicated center (Fig. 11–9A).

Architecturally, lesions are well-demarcated, endophytic proliferations of squamous epithelium that may appear to have replaced preexisting hair follicles (Fig. 11–9B). Condensed orthokeratin forms centrally and above suprabasal clefts, which are readily apparent at scanning magnification. At higher-power magnification, these clefts are clearly formed by acantholysis of suprabasal cells (Fig. 11–9C). Many of the acantholytic cells are also dyskeratotic, appearing as large, eosinophilic, rounded cells with perinuclear halos (i.e., corps ronds) and small, densely eosinophilic, ovoid cells containing pyknotic, flattened nuclei in association with a partially acantholytic stratum granulosum and parakeratotic stratum corneum (i.e., corps grains). The features therefore are similar to those seen in Darier disease, and if specimens are evaluated in the absence of clinical history, many biopsy specimens of warty dyskeratoma cannot be absolutely differentiated from a well-formed lesion occurring in Darier disease (see Chap. 19). The underlying superficial dermis usually shows an exaggerated papillomatous pattern, with each papilla covered by a single layer of intact nonacantholytic basal cells.

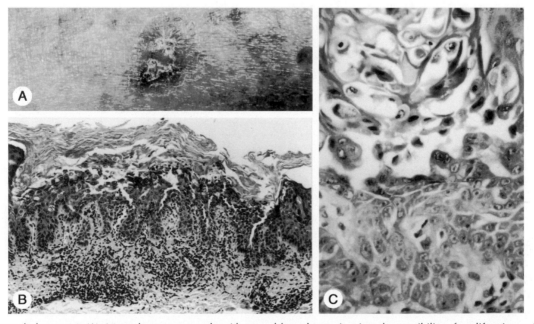

Figure 11–9. Warty dyskeratoma. **(A)** An erythematous papule with central hyperkeratosis raises the possibility of proliferative actinic keratosis or squamous cell carcinoma. **(B)** A biopsy specimen reveals a verrucous lesion with both exophytic and downward growth into an inflamed dermis. Numerous suprabasal clefts resulting from acantholysis are present. **(C)** Closer examination of the acantholytic tumor cells reveals large, rounded cells as well as small, dense cells arising in association with parakeratotic scale (i.e., corps ronds and corps grains, respectively).

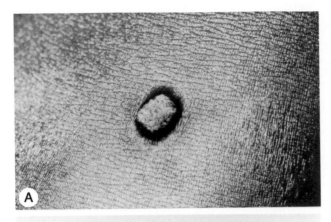

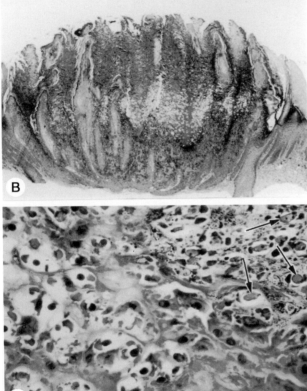

Figure 11–10. Verruca vulgaris. **(A)** The clinical lesion consists of a raised, flat-topped papule with a rough, hyperkeratotic surface. **(B)** Architecturally, lesions are symmetrical verrucous keratoses with prominent exophytic as well as endophytic components. **(C)** Viral cytopathic change is manifested by clearing and pallor of nuclear chromatin *(arrows)*, cytoplasmic swelling and vacuolization, and condensation of cytokeratin to form densely eosinophilic intracellular aggregates.

Verrucae[19–23]

- VARIABLY PAPILLOMATOUS EPITHELIAL PROLIFERATION
- SUPERFICIAL KOILOCYTOSIS
- STEEL GREY INTRANUCLEAR INCLUSIONS
- CYTOPATHIC ALTERATIONS IN CYTOPLASM (CONDENSED KERATIN)
- ENLARGED, ROUNDED KERATOHYALIN GRANULES

Verrucae or warts are divided into four major clinical types. *Verruca vulgaris* and filiform warts are the most common, appearing as circumscribed, papillomatous, hyperkeratotic papules and nodules commonly located on the dorsal aspect of the hands and fingers (Fig. 11–10*A*), although any part of the body surface may be affected. *Plantar warts* characteristically occur as solitary or multiple, poorly defined, hyperkeratotic, painful lesions on the sole of the foot, often involving skin overlying a pressure point (Fig. 11–11*A*). *Flat warts* (i.e., verruca plana) generally occur as mul-

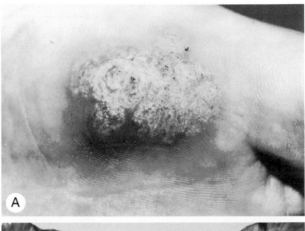

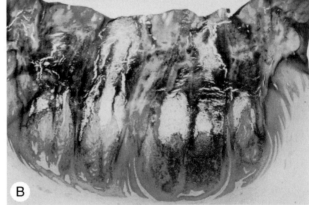

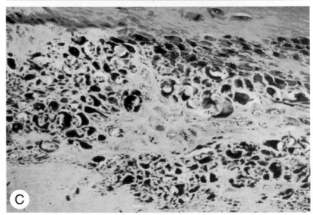

Figure 11–11. Verruca plantaris. **(A)** A slightly raised, hyperkeratotic plaque characteristically affects the ball of the foot; note punctate zones of hemorrhage from superficial wart vessels. **(B)** Histologically, these lesions differ from verruca vulgaris in their mainly endophytic architecture and the prominence of condensed cytokeratin, which sometimes is mistaken for the more rounded molluscum bodies.

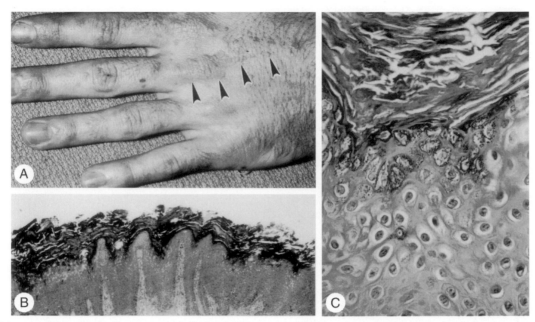

Figure 11–12. Verruca plana. **(A)** Coalescent, raised, flesh-colored papules *(arrows)* are arranged in linear distribution, indicating the path of inoculation. **(B)** The histologic appearance is more subtle than that of verruca vulgaris or palmar or plantar verrucae, with only mild exophytic and endophytic verrucous hyperplasia with associated hyperkeratosis and parakeratosis. **(C)** Cytoplasmic swelling and vacuolization (i.e., koilocytosis) and nuclear pallor within the uppermost epidermal layers are evidence of an active viral cytopathic effect. These cytologic alterations are more subtle than those encountered in most other types of verrucae.

tiple, flesh-colored papules that demonstrate a linear distribution on the dorsa of the hands and feet (Fig. 11–12*A*). Epidermodysplasia verruciformis is a rare condition involving an inherited predisposition to develop flat warts that degenerate into dysplasias and frank carcinomas. *Condyloma acuminatum* appears as a verrucous, cauliflower-like excrescence on anogenital or surrounding skin (Fig. 11–13*A*). Bowenoid papulosis is a form of genital wart with histologic similarities to squamous cell carcinoma in situ. The different clinical types of HPV infection are determined not only by regional differences in their sites of occurrence, but also by the type of virus that elicits each lesion. Table 11–3 summarizes the HPV types associated with various clinical types of warts.

The histology of verruca vulgaris shows crown-like, radiating, fibrovascular spires covered by hyperkeratotic scale and typically surmounted by zones of parakeratosis at the tips of each spire (see Fig. 11–10*B*). The exaggerated dermal papillae that form the inner cores of the epithelial spires characteristically contain dilated, sometimes thrombosed vessels that extend close to the lesional surface. On

inspection at higher magnification, there are enlarged coarse keratohyalin granules, many of which have rounded contours. Cells in the more superficial regions also show cytoplasmic pallor and clearing, a type of koilocytotic change caused by ballooning cytoplasmic degeneration. The most specific finding, however, is the subtle change that may be seen in nuclear chromatin distribution, consisting of pallor and dispersion of chromatin (see Fig. 11–10*C*). This alteration imparts a steel grey appearance to the nuclei of the upper epidermal layers. These inclusions represent aggregates of HPV particles.

Plantar warts are characterized by an endophytic architecture composed of numerous epithelial downgrowths (Fig. 11–11*B*). Lesions are frequently surmounted by a dense hyperkeratotic and parakeratotic scale. In addition to the cytological features mentioned for verruca vulgaris, plantar warts typically have irregular, densely eosinophilic cytoplasmic keratin inclusions affecting the uppermost viable epidermal layers (Fig. 11–11*C*). These inclusions can be differentiated from those seen in *molluscum contagiosum* by their jagged and uniformly eosinophilic appearance.

Table 11–3. CLINICAL FEATURES OF VERRUCAE AND ASSOCIATED HUMAN PAPILLOMAVIRUS (HPV) TYPES

CLINICAL TYPE	HPV TYPE	ANATOMIC SITE	BEHAVIOR
Verruca vulgaris	2, 4, 7	Distal extremities, mucosae	Benign
Plantar wart	1, 2	Soles of feet	Benign
Verruca plana	3, 10	Face, extremities, entire body surface, larynx	Benign
Condyloma acuminata	6, 11	Anogenital region; cervix	Aggressive behavior rare
Bowenoid papulosis	16, 18, 33, 34	Penis, vulva	Aggressive behavior rare
Epidermodysplasia verruciformis	3, 5, 8, 9, 10, 12, 14, 15, 17, 19–29	Entire skin	May progress to malignancy

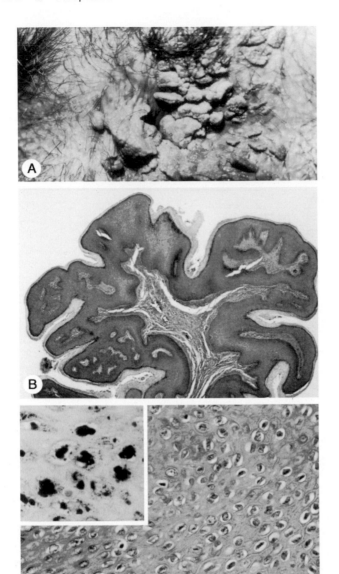

Figure 11–13. Condyloma acuminatum. **(A)** The clinical appearance is characterized by numerous cauliflower-like excrescences affecting anogenital skin. **(B)** Lesional architecture at scanning magnification is that of a fibroepithelial polyp with an elaborate epidermal surface. **(C)** At higher magnification, perinuclear vacuolization, nuclear angulation, and occasional binucleated cells, which collectively indicate koilocytosis, are observed near the surface of the epithelial layer. Immunohistochemical detection of human papillomavirus protein within tumor nuclei *(inset)* confirms the diagnostic impression in difficult cases.

Flat warts are similar to verruca vulgaris in cytologic appearance, although architecturally the papillomatosis and hyperkeratosis are considerably more subtle (Fig. 11–12*B*, *C*). Condyloma acuminata characteristically shows alternating exophytic and endophytic growth of squamous epithelium arranged about complex fibrovascular cores (Fig. 11–13*B*). Early condylomas may resemble seborrheic keratoses or fibroepithelial polyps. Close inspection will generally reveal perinuclear cytoplasmic clearing, irregular nuclear contour, raisin-like nuclei with salt-and-pepper chromatin pat-

terns, and multinucleation of keratinocytes of the upper epidermal layers (i.e., koilocytosis, Fig. 11–13*C*). Mitotic activity may be brisk and frozen in metaphase in lesions that have been previously treated with podophyllin.

Immunohistochemistry for HPV antigens and in situ hybridization for viral message may be used for documentation of HPV in tissue (see Fig. 11–13*C*). These approaches assist both in establishing cause and in defining the type of HPV that is responsible for the wart. In anogenital warts, for example, there is an association between infection by HPV types 16 and 18 and the subsequent development of neoplasia of the uterine cervix.

Many verrucae will spontaneously regress via development of inflammatory changes akin to a delayed hypersensitivity reaction. Others will lose evidence of viral cytopathic change and persist as localized regions of verrucous epidermal hyperplasia. In these instances, it is appropriate to assign a diagnosis of verrucous epidermal hyperplasia consistent with remote HPV effect. This is a reasonable approach when lesions clinically still resemble verrucae and when dilated dermal vessels remain within dermal cores that define residual epithelial spires. Some verrucae age by developing squamous eddies similar to those observed in irritated seborrheic keratoses and inverted follicular keratoses but within the context of the residual architecture of a wart. Others develop glycogenation, mimicking the histology of trichoepithelioma (see Chap. 12), but retaining architectural and stromal landmarks of preexisting HPV effects.

Molluscum Contagiosum

- CUP-SHAPED ENDOPHYTIC TUMOR FORMED BY HYPERPLASTIC, COALESCENT FOLLICULAR INFUNDIBULA
- CENTRAL CORNIFIED PLUG
- INTRACYTOPLASMIC MOLLUSCUM BODIES

Molluscum contagiosum is a common pox virus–induced cutaneous proliferation. Clinically, lesions present as multiple, small, grouped papules anywhere on the body surface but often affecting facial skin. Individual lesions are dome-shaped papules with a central umbilication containing a cornified plug (Fig. 11–14*A, inset*). Histologically, there are endophytic epithelial downgrowths formed by proliferating and coalescent follicular infundibula (Fig. 11–14*A*). Numerous diagnostic molluscum bodies are present both within the cornified material that fills the central crater (Fig. 11–14*B*) as well as within the cytoplasm of the underlying viable keratinocytes. These bodies are round to ovoid and typically are composed of bubbly aggregates of variably eosinophilic material (Fig. 11–14*C*). A characteristic feature of molluscum bodies is their tendency to become less eosinophilic and increasingly basophilic as they ascend from the stratum granulosum into the stratum corneum (i.e., "red in the blue layer, and blue in the red layer").

Multiple or giant lesions of molluscum contagiosum may be seen in the setting of acquired immunodeficiency syndrome. Molluscum bodies should not be confused with the deeply eosinophilic, homogeneous, irregular aggregates of cytoplasmic keratin typical of plantar verrucae.

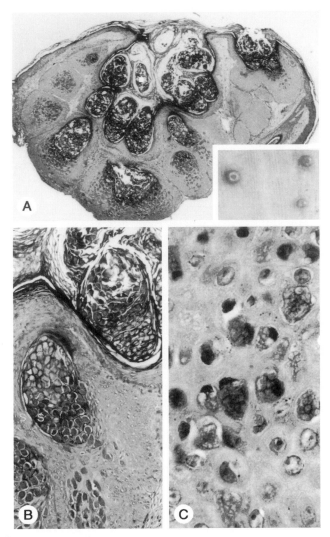

Figure 11–14. Molluscum contagiosum. **(A)** Grouped papules with central umbilication *(inset)* correlates with **(B)** symmetrical downgrowth of epithelium and a central cornified plug containing **(C)** numerous molluscum bodies. These bodies are eosinophilic, rounded cytoplasmic inclusions with a bubbly quality.

Actinic Keratosis[24–31]

- VARIABLE EPIDERMAL ATROPHY OR HYPERPLASIA
- DYSPLASIA OF THE LOWER EPIDERMAL LAYERS
- FOCAL TO DIFFUSE PARAKERATOSIS
- RETENTION OF ENLARGED, HYPERCHROMATIC NUCLEI INTO THE SCALE
- DERMAL ELASTOSIS

Actinic keratoses typically occur as multiple lesions on sun-exposed skin of middle-aged or older individuals, although clinically and histologically similar dysplasias may result from nonactinic factors, such as chronic ingestion of arsenicals or in the setting of immunosuppression (Fig. 11–15). Lesions tend to be erythematous and smaller than 1 cm in diameter. Adherent surface scales impart a roughened, sandpaper-like texture on palpation. Some lesions are pigmented, erythematous, or surmounted by horn-like scale and

are therefore confused with melanocytic neoplasms, dermatoses, or invasive carcinomas, respectively. Actinic cheilitis is a synonym for actinic keratosis involving the vermilion border of the lip.

The architecture of actinic keratoses tends to be either atrophic (Fig. 11–16*A*) or proliferative (Figs. 11–16*B* and 11–17). All actinic keratoses show dysplasia of the lower epidermal layers, first manifested in the basal cell layer, and gradually observed in overlying layers of the stratum spinosum with increasing severity that accompanies clinical evolution of lesions. This dysplasia is characterized by enlarged, irregularly shaped nuclei with diffuse hyperchromasia or coarsely clumped nuclear chromatin patterns. Maturation, the gradual and orderly change from vertical axis of basal cells to horizontal axis of upper stratum spinosum cells, is perturbed (Fig. 11–16*C, D*). Actinic keratoses also characteristically demonstrate abnormalities in stratum corneum formation, as is evidenced by the production of atypical parakeratotic scale. This scale contains tightly aggregated, plump nuclei with diffuse nuclear hyperchromasia. In certain instances in which actinic keratoses are superficially curetted,

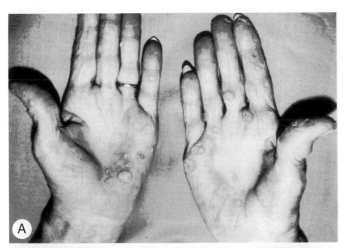

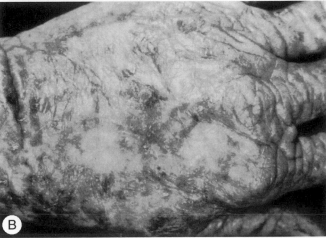

Figure 11–15. Dysplastic keratoses. **(A)** Arsenical keratoses typically involve the palmar surfaces. **(B)** Actinic keratoses are located on the dorsum of the hand and other chronically sun-exposed surfaces. These ill-defined lesions are characterized by coarse adherent scale with a sandpaper-like texture. Some lesions may be raised and erythematous. Also note zones of hyperpigmentation which correlate with actinically induced melanocytic hyperplasia.

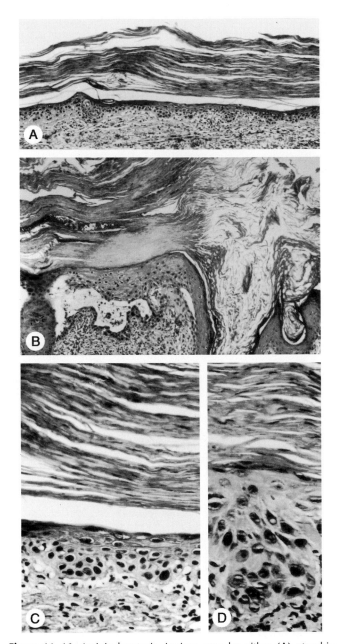

Figure 11–16. Actinic keratosis. Lesions may be either **(A)** atrophic, with loss of epidermal rete ridges and diffuse thinning of the epidermal layer, or **(B)** proliferative, with endophytic budding of atypical basaloid cells. The lesion depicted in **B** also shows suprabasal acantholysis, a frequent finding in actinic keratoses. Note the diffuse parakeratotic scale overlying lesions depicted in both **A** and **B**. **(C, D)** A hallmark of actinic keratoses is dysplasia affecting the lower epidermal layers. This is evidenced by nuclear enlargement, contour angulation, and hyperchromasia. Note that plump, atypical nuclei are also retained in the overlying parakeratotic scale, a diagnostic clue when superficial currettings disclose only stratum corneum and fail to demonstrate full-thickness epidermis.

atypical parakeratotic scale may be the only histologic evidence present, even after multiple levels through the tissue block are examined.

The dermis that underlies actinic keratosis typically shows a variable degree of elastosis (see Chap. 18) and inflammation. In some lesions, the degree of inflammation is intense, and overt cytotoxic alterations are present along the basal cell layer. Such lesions are referred to as lichenoid actinic keratoses. The percent of actinic keratoses that progress to become squamous cell carcinoma and basal cell carcinoma is not known. The finding of zones of near–full-thickness dysplasia in an actinic keratosis warrants the designation of actinic keratosis in transition to squamous cell carcinoma in situ. The majority of actinic keratoses are clinically indolent, however, and many may not become locally aggressive tumors within the lifetime of the host.

Squamous Cell Carcinoma[32–37]

- FULL-THICKNESS EPITHELIAL DYSPLASIA OR ANAPLASIA (IN SITU)
- DYSPLASIA OR ANAPLASIA IN LOWERMOST EPIDERMAL LAYERS WITH SINGLE CELL OR NESTED TRANSGRESSION ACROSS BASEMENT MEMBRANE (INVASIVE)
- HYPERKERATOSIS WITH FORMATION OF ATYPICAL PARAKERATOSIS
- INDIVIDUAL CELL OR ZONAL NECROSIS
- KERATIN PEARL FORMATION

Squamous cell carcinoma occurs in both in situ and invasive forms. Although the in situ form may give rise to invasive lesions, an in situ stage is not requisite for the development of invasive squamous cell carcinoma. Squamous cell carcinoma in situ occurs on sun-exposed skin, although non–sun-exposed sites may also be affected, an event that has been given the appellation of Bowen disease. The gross pathology of squamous cell carcinoma in situ is often in the form of one or several well-demarcated, erythematous and sometimes hyperkeratotic plaques (Fig. 11–18A). Mucosal involvement results in a zone of white, thickened tissue, a nonspecific appearance also caused by a variety of

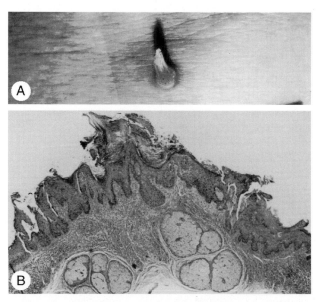

Figure 11–17. Proliferative actinic keratosis with horn formation. **(A)** A cutaneous horn represents a tower of compacted scale and is not entirely dissimilar to a true animal horn. **(B)** Early horn formation is evidenced by a spire of compacted parakeratotic scale eminating from the center of this proliferative actinic keratosis.

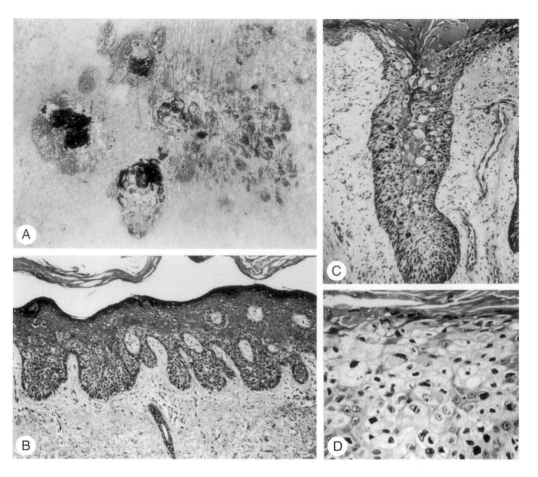

Figure 11–18. Squamous cell carcinoma in situ. **(A)** Clinically, scaling erythematous plaques may be confused with subacute to chronic inflammatory dermatitis. **(B)** Nests of anaplastic keratinocytes are present in an intraepidermal epithelioma pattern within this expanded epidermal layer. **(C)** Growth within the acrosyringium and superficial dermal portion of the eccrine duct may also occur. **(D)** Closer inspection reveals that anaplastic tumor cells are confined to the epidermal layer. These cells are often glycogenated, imparting a relatively clear cytoplasm. Note the absence of a stratum granulosum, with an abrupt transition to atypical, compacted parakeratotic scale.

unrelated disorders and referred to clinically as *leukoplakia.* Invasive squamous cell carcinoma usually appears as an indurated, sometimes ulcerated plaque or nodule surmounted by hyperkeratotic scale (Fig. 11–19A). Well-differentiated, cup-shaped squamous cell carcinomas may have a crater-like architecture and be clinically indistinguishable from keratoacanthoma.

Squamous cell carcinoma in situ is characterized by epidermal thickening by uniformly atypical keratinocytes proliferating at all levels (Fig. 11–18B). This results in complete replacement of the normal epidermal or adnexal architecture (Fig. 11–18C), such that maturation from the basal cell layer to the stratified squamous epithelial layer is no longer appreciated. Malignant cells may be nested within the epidermis and sharply juxtaposed to adjacent, normal appearing epidermal cells in the "intraepidermal epithelioma" pattern. Cytologically, the malignant cells show nuclear enlargement, hyperchromasia, and angulation of contour, and the cytoplasm is often variably glycogenated (Fig. 11–18D). "Buckshot" scattering of profoundly atypical cells may sometimes be observed in the epidermal layer. The stratum corneum is thickened and densely parakeratotic, and the stratum granulosum is generally absent. The superficial dermis contains prominently dilated and proliferating vessels, fibrosis, and a chronic inflammatory infiltrate, possibly representing a localized immune response. All of these features may be observed in *bowenoid papulosis* involving the genitalia, a viral lesion with an indolent course. Fortunately, there are important clinical differences between bowenoid papulosis

and genital squamous cell carcinoma in situ. For example, bowenoid papulosis generally affects younger individuals and appears as multiple lesions.

In the early phases of invasive squamous cell carcinoma, invasion by single cells may be observed to infiltrate a variably fibrotic and vascularized papillary dermis (Fig. 11–19B–D). Irregular sheets, strands, fascicles, and nests of malignant squamous cells may infiltrate the dermis deeply and evoke an exuberant fibroblastic response. This tumor stroma is important in differentiating invasive components of squamous cell carcinoma from reactive processes that may mimic this condition. Cytologically, the invasive cells vary from well to poorly differentiated, although some degree of nuclear atypia is always observed. Nuclei are enlarged and hyperchromatic and demonstrate variably angulated contours; chromatin is often coarsely clumped, and nucleoli may be prominent (Fig. 11–19D), although reactive keratinocytes may also show this latter feature. Keratinization, if present, may be in the form of small, laminated keratin cysts within the tumor lobules (i.e., "pearls") or abortive in the form of single-cell keratinization (i.e., dyskeratosis). Poorly differentiated tumors may show little or no ability to form keratin.

There are a number of rarely encountered forms of squamous cell carcinoma. These include *spindle cell, acantholytic,* and *verrucous* types of squamous cell carcinoma, and *lymphoepithelioma-like carcinoma.* Each of these forms poses its own set of diagnostic challenges. Spindle cell variants often infiltrate a highly reactive stroma insidiously, such that differentiation of malignant epithelial and reactive

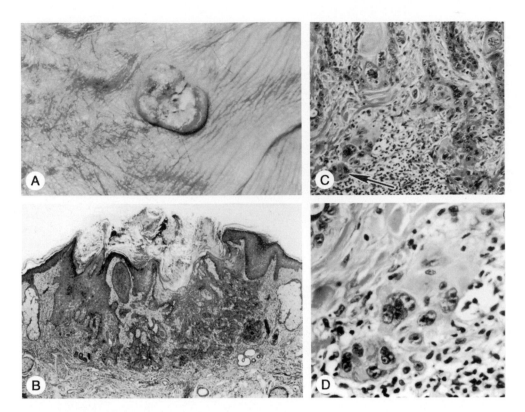

Figure 11–19. Invasive squamous cell carcinoma. **(A)** A raised and asymmetrical facial nodule has a cornified and focally ulcerated center. **(B)** A biopsy specimen reveals endophytic tongues of atypical epithelium within a fibrotic, inflamed dermis. Note the central zone of hyperkeratosis and parakeratosis. **(C, D)** In contrast to keratoacanthoma, true single-cell stromal invasion **(C,** *arrow)* by malignant cells is easily documented.

stromal elements is not always possible. Immunohistochemical detection of cytokeratin may be helpful in this situation. Acantholysis within lobules of squamous cell carcinoma may produce a pseudoglandular pattern and thus mimic adenocarcinoma. Recognition of rounded acantholytic cells within the false lumens is the basis for accurate diagnosis of acantholytic squamous cell carcinoma. Verrucous squamous cell carcinoma is a problematic lesion characterized by deeply invasive, club-like lobules of minimally atypical yet malignant squamous epithelial cells. Recognition of the depth of epithelial penetration, the expansive nature of the deeper components of the endophytic epithelial tongues, and foci of clear-cut dysplasia are essential to accurate diagnostic recognition of verrucous carcinoma. Lymphoepithelioma-like squamous cell carcinoma is recognized as a tumor predominated by reactive small lymphocytes which may mask detection of islands of malignant, invasive epithelium. This tumor is similar to lymphoepithelial carcinoma, which ordinarily arises in nasopharyngeal epithelium.

Basal Cell Carcinoma[38–42]

- NESTS AND CORDS OF ATYPICAL BASALOID CELLS WITH PERIPHERAL PALISADE
- INDIVIDUAL CELL NECROSIS AND MITOTIC ACTIVITY
- VARIABLY MUCINOUS STROMA
- STROMAL-EPITHELIAL SEPARATION ARTIFACT
- ADNEXAL DIFFERENTIATION COMMON

Basal cell carcinoma appears as a well-circumscribed, tan-red plaque (Fig. 11–20A), or a pearly, tan-gray papule that is relatively devoid of scale (Fig. 11–20C). A typical feature is the presence of numerous telangiectatic blood vessels coursing over the tumor papule or nodule. The variant form of basal cell carcinoma termed the *superficial multicentric* variety (see Fig. 11–20A, B) correlates clinically with a relatively large, erythematous, scaling plaque, and therefore may be confused with squamous cell carcinoma in situ, radial growth phase melanoma, or even an inflammatory dermatosis. Basal cell carcinomas exhibit indolent biological behavior, and most lesions are relatively small at the time of clinical attention. However, chronic neglect may result in large, locally destructive tumors (i.e., "rodent ulcers"), with invasion of underlying soft tissue and even bone.

At scanning magnification, basal cell carcinoma characteristically appears as well-defined foci of atypical basaloid cells arising from the epidermis of follicular epithelium (see Fig. 11–20B) or as nests and nodules of basaloid tumor cells within the superficial and deep dermis (Fig. 11–20D). These cells, at low- to medium-power magnification, show a deeply blue hue as a result of sparsity and pallor of cytoplasm and a tendency for the cells at the periphery to be arranged in a palisade (see Fig. 11–20D). At higher magnification, the tumor is composed of a uniform population of basaloid cells with round-to-ovoid nuclei, coarsely clumped nuclear chromatin patterns, and occasional mitotic figures (see Fig. 11–20D). As opposed to the conspicuous nucleoli in squamous cell carcinoma, nucleoli in basal cell carcinoma are not prominent, an important feature in tumors showing a deceptive degree of squamous differentiation. Individual cell necrosis is generally present, a feature, along with mitoses, that is not characteristic of basaloid variants of trichoepithelioma (see Chap. 12). Surrounding the individual nests of tumor cells is a characteristic reactive stroma that contains abundant acid mucopolysaccharides and that frequently splits from the periphery of tumor nodules as an artifact of tissue preparation.

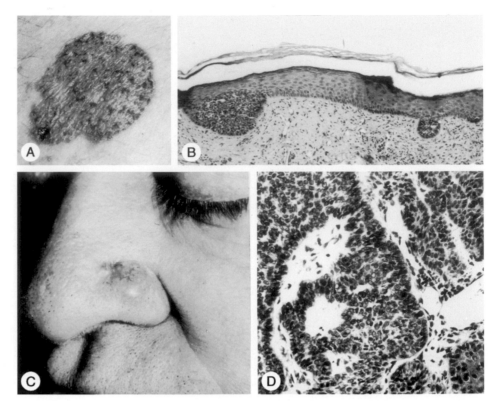

Figure 11–20. Basal cell carcinoma. **(A)** A plaque-like, focally pigmented superficial multicentric basal cell carcinoma. Like some forms of squamous cell carcinoma in situ, such lesions may be confused with dermatitis. **(B)** A biopsy specimen reveals seemingly discontinuous buds of basal cell carcinoma, superficial multicentric type, arising from the epidermal layer. **(C)** A nodular basal cell carcinoma on the nose presents as a pearly lesion with prominent telangiectasia. **(D)** A biopsy specimen reveals strands and nests of basal cells invading a mucinous stroma, which focally separates from the epithelial elements to form clefts (i.e., separation artifact). The tumor islands are characterized by peripheral palisading, focal, single-cell necrosis, and occasional mitotic figures.

This characteristic "separation artifact" is diagnostically important in recognition of basal cell carcinoma histologically. The stroma is also frequently infiltrated by lymphocytes and monocytes, suggesting that host immune mechanisms may in part explain the indolent behavior of basal cell carcinoma.

Adnexal differentiation in basal cell carcinoma is common. The very neoplasm is an imperfect simulation of the relation between germinative hair matrix epithelium and the underlying mucinous follicular mesenchyme. Sebaceous differentiation, abortive eccrine duct formation associated with epithelial mucinosis, and inner and outer root sheath development all may be focally observed within basal cell carcinomas. The presence of mucinous stroma, separation artifact, mitotic activity, and individual cell necrosis, however, all assist in differentiating basal cell carcinoma with prominent adnexal differentiation from benign appendage tumors (see Chap. 12).

Histologic variants of basal cell carcinoma include the *superficial multicentric type* and the *sclerosing type* (Fig. 11–20A, B; Fig. 11–21C). Both lesions are frequently ill-defined clinically, and as a result, they may recur locally because of inadequate excision. The superficial type of basal cell carcinoma is characterized by multiple buds of neoplastic basaloid cells that originate from the basal cell layer of the epidermis (Fig. 11–20B). A characteristic mucinous stroma is associated with each bud, and separation artifact may be seen. The sclerosing or morpheaform type of basal cell carcinoma shows ill-defined cords and streams of cuboidal-to-fusiform basal cells proliferating with a cellular stroma (Fig. 11–21C). The prominence of proliferating fibroblasts within the stroma creates a pseudosarcomatous appearance in which it is difficult to differentiate malignant epithelial cells from stromal

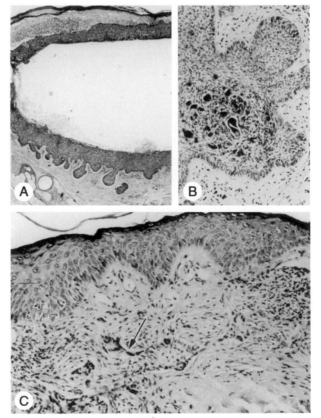

Figure 11–21. Variants of basal cell carcinoma. **(A)** Cystic basal cell carcinoma. **(B)** Pigmented basal cell carcinoma. **(C)** Sclerosing basal cell carcinoma. The latter is composed of thin cords of fusiform tumor cells *(arrow)* that grow insidiously within a cellular, desmoplastic stroma.

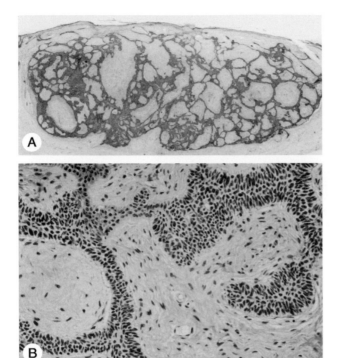

Figure 11–22. Fibroepithelioma of Pinkus. This well-differentiated form of basal cell carcinoma is characterized by a symmetrical proliferation of **(A)** anastomosing, thin epithelial strands within **(B)** a well-developed fibrotic stroma.

components. Margins of such lesions may be exceedingly difficult to evaluate, although immunohistochemistry is useful, as is the case in differentiating epithelial from stromal elements in spindle cell variants of squamous cell carcinoma. Other common variants include cystic basal cell carcinomas, which form as a result of necrosis (Fig. 11–21*A*), and tumors containing abundant melanin pigment (Fig. 11–21*B*). An extremely well-differentiated basal cell carcinoma known as the *fibroepithelioma of Pinkus* (Fig. 11–22), is characterized by numerous anastomosing cords of well-differentiated basaloid

Table 11–4. PROBLEMATIC DIFFERENTIAL DIAGNOSES FOR COMMON EPIDERMAL TUMORS

PROBLEM	SOLUTION
Epidermal nevus versus seborrheic keratosis	Clinical history (congenital in former versus acquired in older individuals in latter)
Clear cell acanthoma versus eccrine poroma	Presence of neutrophils in former and ducts in latter
Keratoacanthoma versus squamous cell carcinoma	History of rapid growth, retention of intact basaloid layer of periphery, absence of significant dysplasia or invasion for keratoacanthoma
Warty dyskeratoma versus Darier disease	Gross pathology: Solitary in former versus multiple lesions in latter
Bowenoid papulosis versus squamous cell carcinoma in situ	Clinical history (bowenoid papulosis: young individuals, multiple lesions)
Basal cell carcinoma versus basaloid trichoepithelioma	Mitotic activity, individual cell necrosis, and mucinous stroma in basal cell carcinoma

cells that arise from the epidermis and proliferate within a delicate network of fibrovascular stroma.

DIFFERENTIAL DIAGNOSIS

From an academic perspective, there are countless differential diagnostic problems that could be generated in a group of neoplasms as diverse and variable as epidermal tumors. The most commonly encountered problematic differential diagnostic issues concerning epithelial neoplasia are summarized in Table 11–4.

SELECTED REFERENCES

1. Basler RSW, Jacobs SI, Taylor WB. Ichthyosis hystrix. Arch Dermatol 1978;114:1059.
2. Ackerman AB. Histopathologic concept of epidermolytic hyperkeratosis. Arch Dermatol 1970;102:253.
3. Holdiness MR. The sign of Leser-Trelat. Int J Dermatol 1986;25:564.
4. Ellis D, Kafka SP, Chow JC, et al. Melanoma, growth factors, acanthosis nigricans, the sign of Leser-Trelat, and multiple acrochordons. A possible role for alpha-transforming growth factor in cutaneous paraneoplastic syndromes. N Engl J Med 1987;317:1582.
5. Mevorah B, Mishima Y. Cellular response of seborrheic keratosis following croton boil irritation and surgical trauma. Dermatologica 1965;131:452.
6. Mehregan AH. Inverted follicular keratosis. Arch Dermatol 1964;89:229.
7. Mishima Y, Pinkus H. Benign mixed tumor of melanocytes and malpighian cells. Arch Dermatol 1960;81:539.
8. Degos R, Civatte J. Clear-cell acanthoma: Experience of eight years. Br J Dermatol 1970;83:248.
9. Fine RM, Chernosky ME. Clinical recognition of clear-cell acanthoma (Degos). Arch Dermatol 1969;100:559.
10. Hu F, Sisson JK. The ultrastructure of pale cell acanthoma. J Invest Dermatol 1969;52:185.
11. Bart RS, Popkin GL, Kopf AW, et al. Giant keratoacanthoma. J Dermatol Surg 1975;1:49.
12. Macaulay WL. Subungual keratoacanthoma. Arch Dermatol 1976;112:1004.
13. Ghadially FN. The role of the hair follicle in the origin and evolution of some cutaneous neoplasms of man and experimental animals. Cancer 1961:14:801.
14. Kern WH, McGray MK. The histopathologic differentiation of keratoacanthoma and squamous cell carcinoma of the skin. J Cutan Pathol 1980;7:318.
15. Chalet MD, Connors RC, Ackerman AB. Squamous cell carcinoma and keratoacanthoma: Criteria for histologic differentiation. J Dermatol Surg 1975;1:16.
16. Giltman LI. Tripolar mitosis in a keratoacanthoma. Acta Derm Venereol (Stockh) 1981;61:362.
17. Harrist TJ, Murphy GF, Mihm MC. Oral warty dyskeratoma. Arch Dermatol 1980;116:929.
18. Syzmanski FG. Warty dyskeratoma. Arch Dermatol 1957;75:567.
19. Orth G, Jablonska S, Breitbard F. The human papillomaviruses. Bull Cancer (Paris) 1978;65:151.
20. Lutzner MA. The human papillomaviruses. Arch Dermatol 1983;119:631.
21. McCance DJ. Human papillomaviruses and cancer. Biochemica et Biophysica Acta 1986;823:195.
22. Pfister P. Human papillomaviruses and genital cancer. Adv Cancer Res 1987;48:113.
23. Jaworsky C, Murphy GF. Special techniques in dermatology. Arch Dermatol 1989;125:963.
24. Brownstein MH, Rabinowitz AD. The precursors of cutaneous squamous cell carcinoma. Int J Dermatol 1979;18:1.
25. James MP, Wells GC, Whimster IW. Spreading pigmented actinic keratosis. Br J Dermatol 1978;98:373.
26. Cataldo E, Doku HC. Solar chelitis. J Dermatol Surg Oncol 1981;7:989.

27. Bart RS, Andrade R, Kopf AW. Cutaneous horn. Acta Derm Venereol (Stockh) 1968;48:507.
28. Hirsch T, Marmelzat WL. Lichenoid actinic keratosis. Dermatol Int 1967;6:101.
29. Shapiro L, Ackerman AB. Solitary lichen planus-like keratosis. Dermatologica 1966;132:386.
30. Scott MA, Johnson WC. Lichenoid benign keratosis. J Cutan Pathol 1976;3:217..
31. Chernosky ME, Freeman RG. Disseminated superficial actinic porokeratosis (DSAP). Arch Dermatol 1967;96:611.
32. Penn I. Neoplastic consequences of transplantation and chemotherapy. Cancer Detect Prev 1987;1:149.
33. Cooper KD, Fox P, Neises G, Katz SI. Effects of ultraviolet radiation on human epidermal cell alloantigen presentation: Initial depression of Langerhans-cell function is followed by the appearance of T6-Dr+ cells that enhance epidermal alloantigen presentation. J Immunol 1985;134:129.
34. Granstein RD. Epidermal I-J-bearing cells are responsible for transferable suppressor cell generation after immunization of mice with ultraviolet radiation-treated epidermal cells. J Invest Dermatol 1985;84:206.
35. Granstein RD, Askari M, Whitaker D, Murphy GF. Epidermal cells in activation of suppressor lymphocytes: Further characterization. J Immunol 1987;138:4055.
36. Kawashima M, Favre M, Jablonska S, et al. Characterization of a new type of human papilloma virus (HPV) related to HPV 5 from a case of actinic keratosis. Virology 1986;154:389.
37. Swanson SA, Cooper PH, Mills SE, Wick MR. Lymphoepithelioma-like carcinoma of the skin. Modern Pathol 1988;1:359.
38. Southwick GJ, Schwartz RA. The basal cell nevus syndrome. Disasters occuring among a series of thirty-six patients. Cancer 1979;44:2294.
39. Murphy GF, Kruzinski PA, Myzak LA, Ershler WB. Local immune response in basal cell carcinoma: Characterization by transmission electron microscopy and T6 monoclonal antibody. J Am Acad Dermatol 1983;8:477.
40. Guillen FJ, Day CL, Murphy GF. Expression of activation antigens on T cells infiltrating basal cell carcinomas. J Invest Dermatol 1985;85:203.
41. Pinkus H. Premalignant fibroepithelial tumors of the skin. Arch Dermatol Syphilol 1953;67:598.
42. Metcalf JS, Maize JC. Histopathologic considerations in the management of basal cell carcinoma. Semin Dermatol 1989;8:259.

12
Adnexal Tumors

DEFINITIONS AND GENERAL CONSIDERATIONS

The subject of adnexal neoplasia is one of the most difficult topics in dermatopathology. This is partially because of the enormous number of individual tumors and variant forms and the complicated nomenclature. In addition, many systems of classification have relied on presumed histodifferentiation and histogenesis, an approach with clear limitations in light of recent evidence indicating ambiguous and multiple differentiation pathways for many lesions. In general, adnexal tumors of the skin do not derive directly from mature appendageal epithelium; rather, they originate from totipotential stem cells and differentiate along adnexal pathways. This explains why many adnexal tumors bear little resemblance to their mature counterparts and how multiple differentiation pathways may occur simultaneously in the same lesion.

In this text, cutaneous adnexal neoplasms are classified according to the following patterns, without regard to histodifferentiation: (1) partially and fully cystic tumors; (2) tumors forming small nests, cords, and ducts; (3) tumors forming sheets and large nodules; and (4) infiltrative, malignant tumors. This approach permits elimination of a large number of adnexal neoplasms at a glance, and limits the diagnostic algorithm to a manageable number of possibilities. Although only the more common tumors are discussed, this chapter addresses the vast majority of the adnexal neoplasms encountered in routine practice.

It should be emphasized that when an adnexal neoplasm that does not conform completely to the diagnostic criteria outlined in these pages is encountered, it need not represent a new or rare entity. It is more likely that such a neoplasm is a variant of a more common tumor form. Adnexal tumors often show hybrid features; for example, co-occurence of spiradenoma and cylindroma in one tumor, or a cyst with mixed infundibular and trichilemmal differentiation. Such lesions should be described as exhibiting mixed features, and their diagnoses therefore appropriately combine more than one entity. A more critical issue, however, is deciding whether an adnexal tumor is benign or malignant. In general, the presence of mitotic activity and individual cell necrosis favors a malignant process, although exceptions do exist (e.g., numerous mitoses in early pilomatricomas, necrosis in proliferating variants of trichilemmal cysts).

Accurate identification of adnexal neoplasms is important, despite the frequent comment that once a skin appendage tumor has been deemed benign or malignant, precise classification does not matter. It is requisite that adnexal tumors be classified and differentiated from other tumors with different biological behaviors (e.g., trichoepithelioma versus basal cell carcinoma; proliferating trichilemmal cyst versus squamous cell carcinoma). Certain adnexal tumors occur in the setting of well-recognized syndromes associated with internal disease (e.g., trichilemmomas and sebaceous epitheliomas in the setting of breast and gastrointestinal carcinoma, respectively). Certain adnexal tumors may be inherited and occur as multiple lesions (e.g., cylindroma) that require clinical monitoring, follow-up, and often, repeated surgical intervention. Some adnexal tumors arise in the setting of lesions potentially programmed for malignant degeneration (e.g., a syringocystadenoma arising in a nevus sebaceus, a hemartoma that also frequently gives rise to basal cell carcinoma).

GROSS PATHOLOGY

The gross pathology of most adnexal tumors is singularly unimpressive. The majority consist of flesh-colored papules and nodules. Lesions may be solitary or multiple, and are generally firm in consistency. Calcified tumors (e.g., calcified cysts, pilomatricomas) may be rock hard. Better differentiated adnexal tumors may be recognized grossly via extrusion of manufactured products, as is the case with trichofolliculoma, which contains a central pore from which emanates a wooly tuft of white hair shafts. Occasionally, adnexal tumors are painful, providing a clue to their diagnosis; this is the case with eccrine spiradenoma. Malignant adnexal neoplasms are generally poorly demarcated, asymmetrical, and often show central ulceration. However, these tumors may be subtle, appearing only as vague zones of induration, as is the case with microcystic adnexal carcinoma (i.e., sclerosing sweat duct carcinoma).

GENERAL HISTOLOGY AND TEMPORAL EVOLUTION

The general histology of adnexal tumors often reflects varying degrees of normal appendageal differentiation. For example, tumors with marked cytoplasmic glycogenation resulting in pale cell or clear cell change (e.g., some nodular hidradenomas, poromas, and trichilemmomas) are generally recapitulating the normally glycogenated follicular outer root sheath or the embryonic acrosyringium. Benign and malignant tumors with granular eosinophilic cytoplasm and foci of bleb formation of the luminal membranes lining gland-like spaces are generally indicative of apocrine differentiation. Sebaceous features consist of cytoplasmic vacuolization, which typically indents the nuclear contour. The stroma of some adnexal tumors consists of a distinctive, fibrotic, eosinophilic mantle that envelops the epithelial elements. Recognition of this typical stroma is of assistance in differentiating many basaloid adnexal neoplams from basal cell carcinoma. Other tumors, such as the mixed tumor, are characterized by a myxoid and chondroid stroma so diagnostically distinctive and prominent that it frequently overshadows the epithelial elements.

The temporal evolution of most adnexal tumors is indistinct and does not contribute to their differential diagnostic recognition. Exceptions include the trichilemmal cyst, which with age and possibly inflammatory stimuli may form a proliferating trichilemmal cyst and eventually the solid pilar tumor of the scalp; and the pilomatricoma, which in early stages is predominated by basaloid cells and in later stages consists primarily of anucleate cells resembling hair cortex.

HISTOLOGY OF SPECIFIC DISORDERS

Partially and Fully Cystic Tumors

Epidermal Inclusion Cyst[1]

- SQUAMOUS EPITHELIAL-LINED CYST, SOMETIMES WITH CONTINUITY WITH FOLLICULAR INFUNDIBULUM
- INTACT GRANULAR CELL LAYER
- FILLED WITH LAMINATED KERATIN
- ABSENCE OF ADNEXAL OUTGROWTHS

The majority of epidermal inclusion or follicular infundibular cysts form as a result of progressive cystic ectasia of the infundibulum of the hair follicle as a result of mechanical occlusion of the follicular orifice or in association with inflammation or scarring of the follicle (e.g., as in cystic acne). Most of these cysts are therefore retention cysts rather that true inclusion cysts. Some, however, result from included epithelium, as in the case of cysts at the sites of trauma. Lesions appear clinically as dermal or subcutaneous, skin-colored, firm nodules of variable size involving the head, neck, and trunk, although any hair-bearing site may be involved. Minute, spontaneously-arising, follicular infundibular cysts involving vellus hairs of the face are referred to as milia cysts. Secondary milia may result from superficial dermal scarring or blistering with dermal involvement. Epidermal inclusion cysts may become exquisitely painful upon rupture, necessitating immediate medical attention. On surgical excision, these cysts often are shelled out from the surrounding dermis, and unless the entire lining is removed, the cysts may recur.

At scanning magnification, epidermal inclusion cysts consist of rounded, keratin-filled cavities within the dermis (Fig. 12–1). Large cysts may extend into the deep dermis

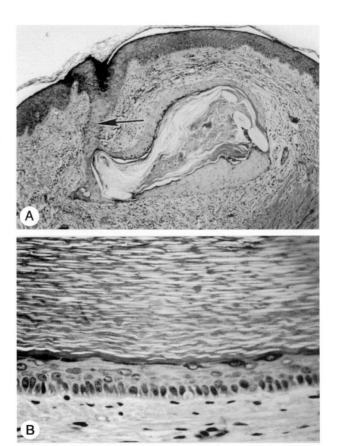

Figure 12–1. Epidermal inclusion cyst (i.e., infundibular cyst). **(A)** This cyst arises from epithelium of the follicular infundibulum *(arrow);* therefore, its wall resembles surface epidermis. **(B)** At higher magnification, the wall has a thin but well-developed stratum granulosum, and the keratin produced is laminated orthokeratin.

and abut the subcutaneous fat. Communication with the overlying epidermis via a small keratin-filled channel may be observed in early lesions (see Fig. 12–1A). Epidermal inclusion cyst contents consist of loosely packed lamellae of keratin that tend to fall out during processing, in contrast to the trichilemmal cyst, which is filled with homogeneous, eosinophilic material. At higher magnification, the cyst wall resembles follicular infundibular epithelium and the surface epidermis, with a well-developed granular cell layer separating the squamous epithelium that forms the cyst wall and the keratin within the cyst cavity (see Fig. 12–1B). At sites of rupture, there is extrusion of keratin into the adjacent dermis, which provokes a foreign-body–type granulomatous response, frank abscess formation, or edematous granulation tissue.

Pilar Sheath Acanthoma[2]

- FOLLICULAR INFUNDIBULAR PORE THAT COMMUNICATES WITH THE EPIDERMAL SURFACE
- BROAD-BASED DERMAL INVAGINATION
- VARIABLE PLATE-LIKE PROLIFERATION OF CYST WALL
- FILLED WITH LAMINATED KERATIN

Pilar sheath acanthoma is a follicular infundibular cystic tumor that forms a pore-like epithelial proliferation, often on the upper lip. The dilated pore of Winer (i.e., conical infundibular acanthoma, discussed later) is a related proliferation characterized by a less elaborate epithelial component and deeper, conical extension of the cystic cavity into the dermis. Pilar sheath acanthomas are usually dome-shaped, contain a central keratin-filled plug, are smaller than 1 cm in diameter, and tend to affect the facial skin of middle-aged to elderly individuals.

At low magnification, a keratin-filled cyst extends from the epidermis into the dermis (Fig. 12–2). In tangential sections, tumors appear as mid-dermal cysts. Whereas the architecture of the pilar sheath acanthoma is characterized by a relatively broad, shallow invagination (see Fig. 12–2A), that of the dilated pore cyst is typified by a deep, conical extension (see Fig. 12–2C). Although the inner portion of the cyst wall of pilar sheath acanthoma is formed by flattened keratinocytes that produce keratin in a manner similar to the epidermal surface or follicular infundibulum (i.e., via formation of a granular cell layer), the outer portions of the wall are composed of pale, glycogenated, squamous cells akin to the epithelium of the follicular outer root sheath (see Fig. 12–2B). These cells form numerous elaborate, finger-like, serpiginous and plate-like extensions into the surrounding dermis

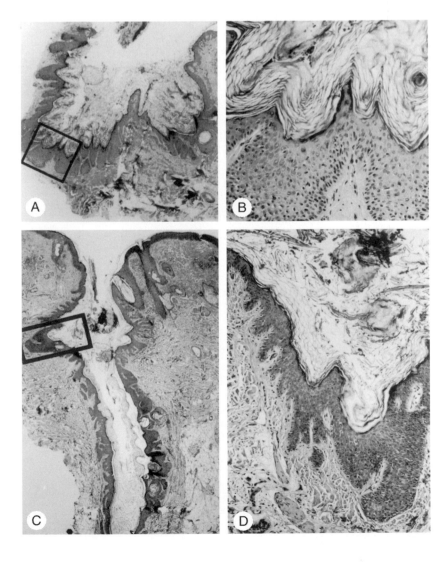

Figure 12–2. Pilar sheath acanthoma and dilated pore. **(A, B)** The pilar sheath acanthoma is a dilated, relatively superficial invagination that produces laminated keratin similar to that within true infundibular cysts. The wall of the tumor, which is enclosed in **A** and magnified in **B,** typically has plate-like outgrowths of glycogenated infundibular epithelium. **(C, D)** The dilated pore of Winer, on the other hand, is a deeper, conical invagination; similar but generally thinner plate-like outgrowths, which are enclosed in **C** and magnified in **D,** are also observed.

and occasionally even into the subcutis. The outermost layer of basal cells that surround these proliferations focally may appear to palisade. Small horn cysts containing laminated keratin may be observed within the proliferating epithelial elements, and abortive secondary follicle formation is sometimes noted.

Dilated Pore[3]

- FOLLICULAR INFUNDIBULAR PORE THAT COMMUNICATES WITH THE EPIDERMAL SURFACE
- DEEP, CONICAL DERMAL INVAGINATION
- VARIABLE, PLATE-LIKE PROLIFERATION OF CYST WALL
- FILLED WITH LAMINATED KERATIN

Dilated pores (i.e., conical infundibular acanthomas) appear as small follicular keratotic plugs (i.e., comedones) centrally located within a skin-colored papule or small nodule on the head or neck. There is no specific age predisposition, and occasionally, multiple lesions have been observed. The architecture of the dilated pore demonstrates a characteristic funnel or cone shape that originates superficially as a dilated follicular infundibulum and extends inferiorly in a tapering fashion into the deep dermis and occasionally into the subcutis (see Fig. 12–2C). Plate- and finger-like projections of squamous follicular epithelium extend from the outer wall of the dilated pore, and in some areas, they may give the impression that they interdigitate with adjacent dermal papilla–like mesenchyme (see Fig. 12–2D).

Trichilemmal Cyst[4]

- THIN-WALLED DERMAL CYST FILLED WITH HOMOGENEOUS, EOSINOPHILIC MATERIAL
- ABSENCE OF GRANULAR LAYER (TRICHILEMMAL KERATINIZATION)
- CYTOPLASMIC GLYCOGENATION
- ROUNDED LUMINAL CELL MEMBRANES

The clinical characteristics of trichilemmal cysts, also called sebaceous cysts, are similar to those of epidermal inclusion cysts, although the vast majority of trichilemmal cysts arise on the scalp. As is the case with epidermal inclusion cysts, trichilemmal cysts often can be shelled out of the dermis at surgery (Fig. 12–3A). If ruptured, these cysts extrude a cheesy, foul-smelling, grumous material.

At low scanning magnification, the trichilemmal cyst differs from the infundibular cyst by virtue of the intact, homogeneous, eosinophilic contents within the cyst cavity (Fig. 12–3B). This material is composed of keratin and lipid and frequently exhibits cholesterol cleft formation. With age, foci of dystrophic calcification may occur. The cyst wall is composed of an outer layer of palisaded basaloid cells and multiple inner layers of large, pale pink, glycogenated squamous cells that form keratin without the genesis of an intervening granular cell layer ("abrupt," or trichilemmal, keratinization) (Fig. 12–3C). The cells lining the cyst frequently display rounded apical membranes, in contrast to the flattened surfaces of the squamous cells that line infundibular cysts. Variable hyperplasia of the cyst wall may be present in some tumors; these are referred to as proliferating trichilemmal cysts (Fig. 12–4). The progression of this process over many years may result in large, bulky tumors that ulcerate and contain zones of pressure necrosis (i.e., pilar tumor of the scalp). Small biopsy specimens that fail to include the smooth, regular, noninvasive perimeter of these tumors may be confused with invasive squamous cell carcinoma.

Steatocystoma[5, 6]

- THIN-WALLED DERMAL CYSTS FILLED WITH PROTEINACEOUS FLUID
- SEBACEOUS LOBULES COMPRESSED ABOUT THE CYST WALL
- CYST LINED BY EPITHELIAL CELLS FORMING THIN, EOSINOPHILIC, LUMINAL CUTICLE

Steatocystomas may occur as solitary or as multiple lesions with an autosomal dominant pattern of inheritance. Lesions appear as rubbery, 1- to 3-cm dermal nodules affecting predominantly skin on the presternal area, upper arms, axillae, and scrotum (Fig. 12–5A). Tumors may become gradually more numerous over time, and total body involvement has been described. On rupture or incision, the cysts are found to contain an odorless fluid, in contrast to the cheesy, rancid material typical of trichilemmal cysts.

At scanning magnification, steatocystoma is characterized by a collapsed cystic space within the mid-dermis, with corrugated infoldings of the cyst wall (Fig. 12–5B). The cyst wall is composed of a single external layer of basaloid cells and several internal layers of squamoid cells that form a thin eosinophilic keratin layer (i.e., cuticle) in a trichilemmal fashion (Fig. 12–5C). By the time of histologic examination, the cyst cavity is either empty or contains scant zones of flocculent to homogeneous eosinophilic secretions. A characteristic feature of the steatocystoma is the presence of mature sebaceous lobules compressed about the outer portion of the cyst wall (see Fig. 12–5C). Small follicular shafts may also originate from the wall and project into the surrounding stroma. This must not be confused with a dermoid cyst, however, which shows sebaceous and follicular outgrowths from what otherwise would be characterized as an epidermal inclusion cyst.

Hair Matrix Cyst

- KERATIN-FILLED CYST WITHIN MID-DERMIS
- CYST WALL COMPOSED OF MULTIPLE LAYERS OF BASALOID CELLS RESEMBLING HAIR MATRIX
- SMALL MICROCYSTS WITHIN WALL

Occasionally, epidermal cysts are characterized by a distinctive wall composed of multiple layers of basaloid cells giving rise to more squamous luminal elements and by production of closely aggregated lamellae of extracellular keratin (Fig. 12–6). The majority of these lesions appear to involve the skin of children and young adults. The basaloid elements of the wall resemble hair matrix epithelium and the basaloid cells that are encountered in pilomatricoma. Small microcysts resembling abortive follicular canals may be observed within the cyst wall (see Fig. 12–6B). Rupture of the wall provokes a florid granulomatous reaction. It is possible that these tumors are forerunners of pilomatricomas in early

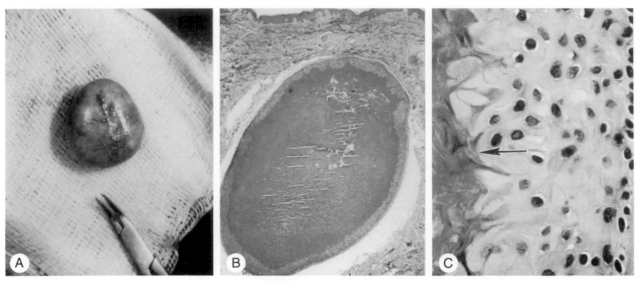

Figure 12–3. Trichilemmal (pilar) cyst. **(A)** These tumors, also called wens and sebaceous cysts, are often shelled out as a cosmetic surgical maneuver or as a result of pain produced after partial rupture. **(B)** At scanning magnification, the cyst is filled with homogeneous keratin admixed with lipid. **(C)** The wall of the cyst recapitulates the portion of the follicle deep to the infundibulum, where trichilemmal, not surface epidermal, keratinization normally occurs. Accordingly, keratin is formed abruptly, without an intervening granular cell layer (*arrow*). Note also the rounded contour of pale cyst epithelial cells as they interface with the cyst contents. The glassy pallor of the cytoplasm is reminiscent of that seen in keratoacanthoma.

Figure 12–4. Proliferating trichilemmal cyst. This cyst shows many of the features depicted in Figure 12–3, although the epithelial elements have begun to proliferate, forming solid ingrowths into the cyst lumen. Over time, continued proliferation will expand the cyst, which will become filled with reactive epithelial elements admixed with zones of pressure necrosis (i.e., pilar tumor). Differentiation from squamous cell carcinoma depends on **(A)** recognition of the smooth outer contour of such tumors and **(B)** detection of zones where trichilemmal keratinization is preserved.

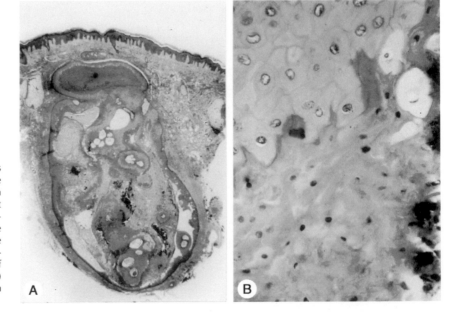

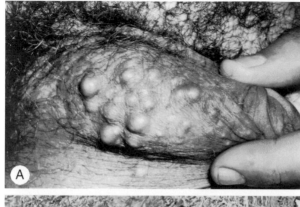

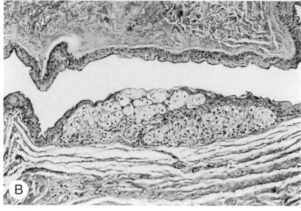

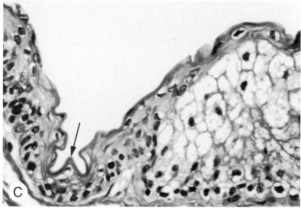

Figure 12–5. Steatocystoma. **(A)** In the clinical form termed steatocystoma multiplex, multiple painless cystic nodules are observed, here on scrotal skin. **(B)** Histologic examination reveals a cystic cavity filled with clear fluid and lined by flattened squamous cells. **(C)** Distinguishing features include compressed sebaceous lobules associated with the cyst wall and a hyalinized inner cuticle (*arrow*) with a corrugated contour.

cystic stages of evolution, and as such, they may be analogous to the spectrum exhibited between trichilemmal cysts and pilar tumors.

Apocrine Cystadenoma[7–9]

- THIN-WALLED CYSTIC TUMOR CONTAINING HOMOGENEOUS, EOSINOPHILIC FLUID, WITH OR WITHOUT CHOLESTEROL CLEFTS
- WALL FORMED BY SEVERAL EPITHELIAL LAYERS

- FOCAL PAPILLATIONS AND EPITHELIAL BRIDGING ALONG CYST LUMEN
- LINING CELLS WITH DECAPITATION SECRETION

Apocrine cystadenomas, also called hidrocystomas, are cystic, simple, nonpapillary or glandular adenomas differentiating toward the apocrine secretory coil. These lesions most often present as blue-black nodules on the face, head, neck, and upper trunk and, because of their color, may be mistaken clinically for malignant melanoma (Fig. 12–7A). Lesions range from several millimeters to several centimeters in diameter, and men and women are equally affected. The average age of occurrence is 55 years.

At scanning magnification, there is a single cystic cavity within the superficial to mid-dermis. The cavity is lined by one to several layers of cuboidal to columnar apocrine-type secretory cells (Fig. 12–7B, C). Cytologically, the lining cells have finely granular, eosinophilic cytoplasm and at least focally exhibit decapitation secretion (see Fig. 12–7C). Small epithelial tufts, but not true papillae with fibrovascular cores, may protrude into the lumen of the cyst. Epithelial elements may also form duct-like spaces as they bridge across the lumenal surface. The outermost portion of the cyst is bordered by a single layer of flattened myoepithelial cells.

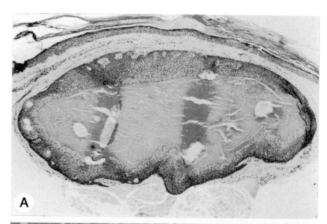

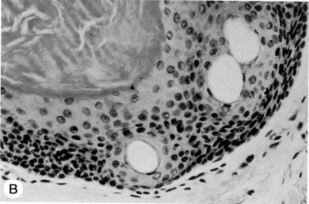

Figure 12–6. Hair matrix cyst. **(A)** These cysts are filled with amorphous, eosinophilic, keratinaceous material and lined by cells that recapitulate normal hair matrix and cortex. **(B)** Occasionally, small cystic lumina may form within the cyst wall. Proliferative counterparts of these cysts may rupture and be responsible for the genesis of tumors called pilomatricoma.

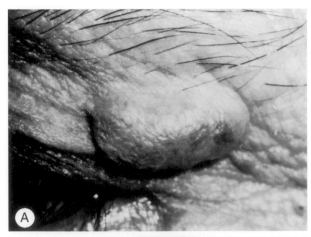

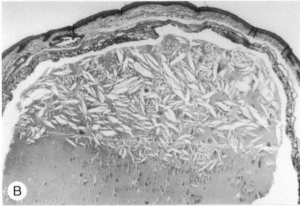

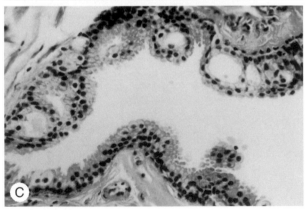

Figure 12–7. Apocrine cystadenoma. **(A)** A semitranslucent cystic nodule with a blue-grey hue arose on the eyelid. **(B)** At low magnification, there is a thin-walled cyst filled with eosinophilic fluid and cholesterol clefts. **(C)** The cyst lining consists of several layers of apocrine-type epithelium, with formation of small papillations and epithelial bridges, and luminal zones of decapitation secretion.

Residua of eosinophilic proteinaceous material, sometimes containing cholesterol clefts, may be present within the cyst cavity. Small apocrine cystadenomas that involve the inner and outer canthus of the palpebral border of the lower eyelid are often referred to as *Moll gland cysts*. Apocrine cytologic features and evidence of proliferation of the lining epithelium (e.g., multiple layers, frond formation) differentiate apocrine cystadenoma from eccrine hidrocystoma, a passive ectasia of the eccrine duct that results from chronic obstruction.

Syringocystadenoma Papilliferum[10, 11]

- CYSTIC NEOPLASM WITH ELABORATE PAPILLARY INFOLDINGS
- OFTEN CONTINUOUS WITH SURFACE EPIDERMIS EXHIBITING PAPILLARY HYPERPLASIA
- LINING COMPOSED OF TWO LAYERS OF CUBOIDAL-TO-COLUMNAR EPITHELIUM
- DECAPITATION SECRETION BY LINING CELLS
- STROMA INFILTRATED BY PLASMA CELLS

Syringocystadenoma papilliferum is a benign, partially cystic, adnexal neoplasm that shows evidence of both apocrine and eccrine differentiation. Most lesions occur on the face and scalp as either skin-colored, often verrucous and scaling nodules or as verrucous and crusted plaques. About one third of all cases of syringocystadenoma papilliferum are associated with a preexisting nevus sebaceus, which is a mixed epidermal and adnexal hamartoma that is often associated with localized scalp alopecia. Lesions associated with nevus sebaceus may manifest in early life as moist keratotic nodules within verrucous plaques, which show a linear or zosteriform distribution. At puberty, these lesions enlarge and become more apparent. Syringocystadenoma papilliferum that is not associated with a preexisting nevus sebaceus usually occurs at or following puberty.

At scanning magnification, syringocystadenoma is first appreciated as a cystic neoplasm within the mid-dermis that is filled with numerous papillary infoldings of the cyst wall (Fig. 12–8A). The epidermis overlying the cyst is often hyperplastic and exhibits a slightly verrucous surface architecture with hyperkeratosis. The superficial portion of the cyst lining may be composed of keratinizing squamous cells contiguous with regions of adjacent epidermal hyperplasia. Communication between the cyst cavity and the epidermal surface may be appreciated. The cyst lining and the lining of the luminal papillary projections are composed of at least two cell layers. The innermost layer is formed by columnar epithelial cells that exhibit focal decapitation secretion. The outermost layer is composed of basaloid to cuboidal epithelial cells. In regions where the lining epithelium appears to be composed of three or more cell layers, small duct-like lumina are frequently seen. The fibrovascular stroma of the tumor is heavily populated by plasma cells (Fig. 12–8B), an important differential diagnostic feature that may be recognized even at low magnification (Fig. 12–9A). Dilated and hyperplastic apocrine glands may be identified in the stroma subjacent to this cystic tumor.

Hidradenoma Papilliferum[12–14]

- CYSTIC NEOPLASM WITH ELABORATE PAPILLARY INFOLDINGS
- OFTEN SEPARATED FROM SURFACE EPIDERMIS, WHICH IS MINIMALLY HYPERPLASTIC
- LINING COMPOSED OF TWO LAYERS OF CUBOIDAL-TO-COLUMNAR EPITHELIUM
- DECAPITATION SECRETION OF LINING CELLS
- STROMA FIBROTIC, NOT INFLAMED

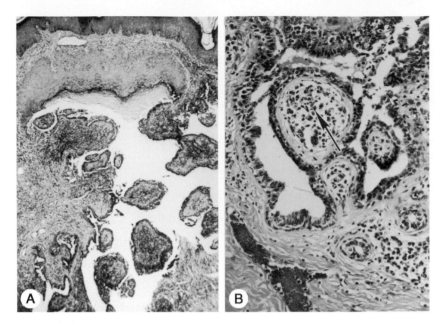

Figure 12–8. Syringocystadenoma papilliferum. **(A)** This cystic and papillary adnexal tumor is characterized by an epithelial lining that may be squamous near the epidermal surface but that becomes cuboidal to columnar over most of the cyst wall. **(B)** Generally, there are two layers of epithelial lining cells with occasional foci of apocrine-type decapitation secretion. The stroma is typically rich in plasma cells (*arrow*) and forms prominent internal papillations into the cyst lumen.

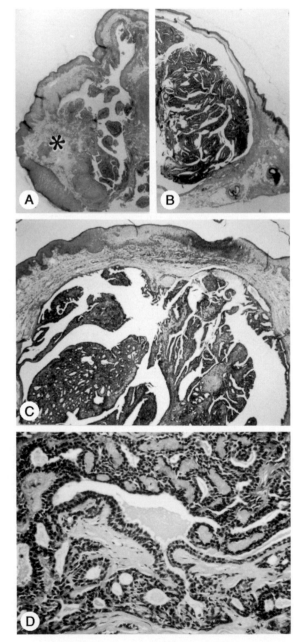

Figure 12–9. Hidradenoma papilliferum. **(A, B)** At scanning magnification, while hidradenoma papilliferum (*right*) has a cystic and papillary architecture that is similar to syringocystadenoma papilliferum (*left*), it is devoid of a stroma filled with plasma cells (* demarcates plasma cell–rich stroma of syringocystadenoma). **(C, D)** The tumor consists of a large cyst with internal papillations that nearly fill its lumen. The covering of the wall and its complex infoldings consist of two layers of cuboidal epithelial cells overlying a condensed, focally hyalinized fibrovascular stroma.

214

Hidradenoma papilliferum usually is detected in Caucasian women over the age of 30 years. Sites of involvement include the labia majora, perineal and perianal skin, and more rarely, the skin of the nipple, eyelid, and external ear canal. Lesions present as solitary, freely movable, skin-colored nodules that range in diameter from several millimeters to several centimeters.

Histologically, hidradenoma papilliferum forms a large, epithelium-lined cyst within the mid-dermis, surrounded by a fibrovascular mantle (Fig. 12–9B). Although the architecture of this partially cystic neoplasm is similar to that of syringocystadenoma papilliferum, these two neoplasms may be differentiated even at scanning magnification by the presence (in syringocystadenoma) or absence (in hidradenoma) of an inflammatory, plasma cell–rich stroma (Fig. 12–9A, B).

At higher magnification, the superficial portion of the cyst may be lined by a single layer of flattened squamous epithelial cells, and occasionally lesions demonstrate continuity with the surface epidermis. Most of the lining, however, is composed of two layers of cuboidal-to-columnar epithelium. As the name implies, the cyst wall protrudes into the lumen at numerous foci as a result of fibrovascular papillae that communicate with the fibrovascular mantle of the cyst (Fig. 12–9C). Elaborate epithelial infoldings and invaginations within individual papilla may impart a glandular appearance (Fig. 12–9D). At high magnification, the lining epithelial cells exhibit apocrine-type decapitation secretion, whereas the underlying cuboidal cells are myoepithelium.

Tumors Forming Nests, Cords, and Ducts

Trichoepithelioma and Trichoadenoma[15–18]

- BASALOID CORDS AND NESTS RADIATING FROM SUPERFICIAL DERMAL FOCUS
- DISTINCT FIBROCOLLAGENOUS STROMA
- HAIR MATRIX DIFFERENTIATION WITHOUT TRICHOGENESIS
- HORN CYSTS SUPERFICIALLY (TRICHOEPITHELIOMA) OR DIFFUSELY (TRICHOADENOMA)

Trichoepithelioma is an often heritable benign follicular neoplasm that incompletely recapitulates elements of the pilosebaceous apparatus. Solitary (nonhereditary) and multiple (autosomal dominant) forms have been described. Solitary tumors appear as pale, skin-colored papules and nodules, sometimes reaching 2 cm in diameter. Facial skin of adults is most commonly involved, and these tumors are not infrequently confused with basal cell carcinoma. In the multiple form, numerous skin-colored papules and nodules smaller than 1 cm develop on the face, scalp, neck, and upper trunk (Fig. 12–10A). Lesions show a predilection for involving the nasolabial folds and preauricular regions. The onset of multiple lesions often occurs during childhood and persists and progresses during adulthood.

At scanning magnification, both solitary and multiple

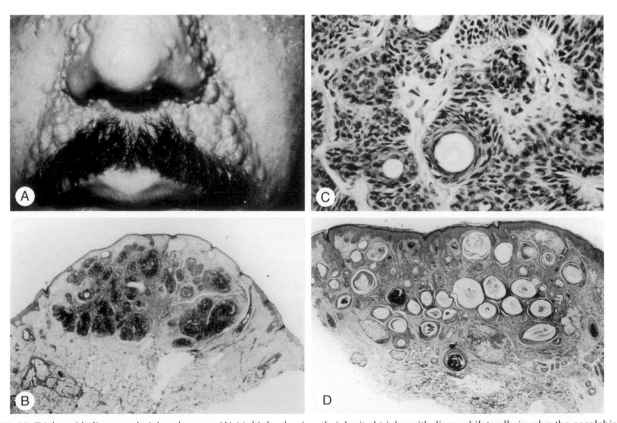

Figure 12–10. Trichoepithelioma and trichoadenoma. **(A)** Multiple, dominantly inherited trichoepitheliomas bilaterally involve the nasolabial folds. **(B)** Scanning magnification reveals symmetrical nests of basaloid epithelial cells within a distinctive eosinophilic stroma. **(C)** At higher magnification, there are nests and cords of basaloid cells forming small horn cysts. Unlike basal cell carcinoma, individual cell necrosis, mitotic activity, and stromal-epithelial separation artifact are not observed. **(D)** Similar tumors that are predominated by horn cysts are termed trichoadenomas.

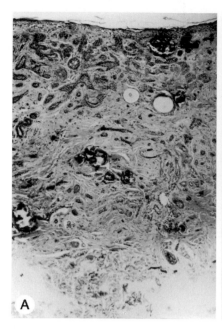
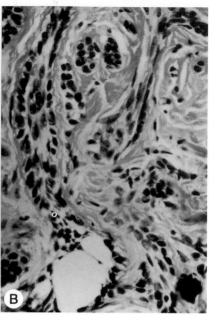

Figure 12–11. Desmoplastic trichoepithelioma. **(A, B)** The features of symmetry, basaloid cords without necrosis of mitoses, and a distinctive fibrotic stroma devoid of separation artifact are maintained, although the stromal component predominates. This results in apparent compression of epithelial elements in a pattern that may resemble sclerosing basal cell carcinoma. The separation that has occurred at the base of **B** is among the epithelial cells, not between stroma and epithelium.

forms of trichoepithelioma show radiating buds, nests, and anastomosing cords of basaloid cells within the mid-dermis. These epithelial elements are invested within a fibrotic stroma (Fig. 12–10B). Many of the basaloid buds resemble hair matrix, although well-formed bulbs and trichogenesis are seldom observed. Multiple, small, keratin-filled cysts are typically present within the epithelial nests (Fig. 12–10C), particularly within the more superficial dermal nests of trichoepithelioma. When these horn cysts predominate, basaloid epithelial elements may be inconspicuous; these lesions are called *trichoadenomas* (Fig. 12–10D). These variant forms occur as small, solitary nodules on the face and occasionally on the trunk.

Another variant of trichoepithelioma is the *desmoplastic trichoepithelioma*, which occurs as a nodular tumor smaller than 1 cm on the faces of young women. The frequent presence of a central zone of depression may result in a resemblance to the morpheiform variant of basal cell carcinoma. Histologically, these lesions also may mimic basal cell carcinoma, forming small cords and nests of basaloid cells embedded within a dense, sclerotic stroma (Fig. 12–11). Trichoepitheliomas and their variants may be differentiated from basal cell carcinoma by their absence of mitoses, individual cell necrosis, and mucinous stroma with foci of separation artifact. However, occasional lesions of solitary trichoepithelioma cannot reliably be distinguished from keratotic basal cell carcinomas. In these situations, complete excision is recommended.

Trichofolliculoma[19, 20]

- BASALOID CORDS AND NESTS RADIATING FROM SUPERFICIAL DERMAL FOCUS
- DISTINCT FIBROCOLLAGENOUS STROMA
- HAIR MATRIX, CORTEX, AND ROOT SHEATH DIFFERENTIATION WITH TRICHOGENESIS
- DILATED PRIMARY FOLLICLE SUPERFICIALLY

The trichofolliculoma is a highly differentiated neoplastic proliferation of actively trichogenic epithelium with differentiation reflecting all portions of the pilosebaceous complex. These tumors present as solitary, skin-colored, 3- to 5-mm nodules that frequently have a central pore or crater from which may emerge a wooly tuft of small white hairs. Architecturally, trichofolliculomas consist of a dilated follicular infundibulum-like pore (i.e., primary follicle) that communicates with the epidermal surface and contains laminated keratin and often multiple small hair shafts (Fig. 12–12A). Numerous secondary follicles bud at the base of this plug within the mid-dermis, producing a radiating pattern. Secondary follicles consist of either rudimentary bulbs of basaloid cells or outer and inner root sheath epithelium (Fig. 12–12B). There also may be focal lipidization within the follicular wall, hair matrix and papilla formation, and trichogenesis. The stroma is fibrotic, and as is the case in trichoepithelioma, it is well demarcated from the adjacent dermis. Conceptually, the trichofolliculoma may be regarded as a well-differentiated counterpart of trichoepithelioma.

Syringoma[21–24]

- MULTIPLE EPITHELIAL CORDS AND NESTS WITHIN DISTINCTIVE COLLAGENOUS STROMA
- TADPOLE- AND COMMA-LIKE CONTOURS OF EPITHELIAL NESTS
- DUCTULAR LUMINA WITHIN SOME NESTS

Syringoma, from the Greek word *syrinx*, meaning tube, refers to a benign adnexal tumor of well-differentiated eccrine ductular elements. Lesions usually occur as multiple papules, often on the face of genetically predisposed individuals. Syringomas appear as small (1 to 3 mm in diameter), asymptomatic, skin-colored papules that may be solitary but often are multiple (Fig. 12–13A). Women are preferentially affected, and lesions begin at puberty and continue to form

*??? BCC: mitoses, individual cell necrosis, separation artifact

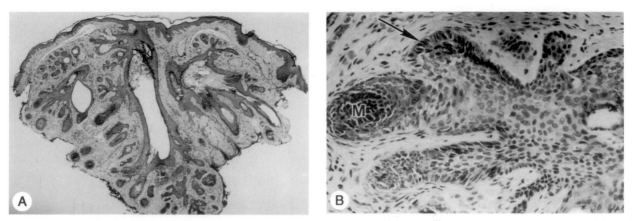

Figure 12–12. Trichofolliculoma. **(A)** Low magnification reveals a central follicular infundibular plug from which radiating cords and branches of pilar epithelium sprout within a distinctive fibrotic stroma. **(B)** Upon closer inspection, hair matrix differentiation (M, *arrow*), hair cortex, and outer root sheath may be observed. In addition, small hair shafts may be detected within central microcysts.

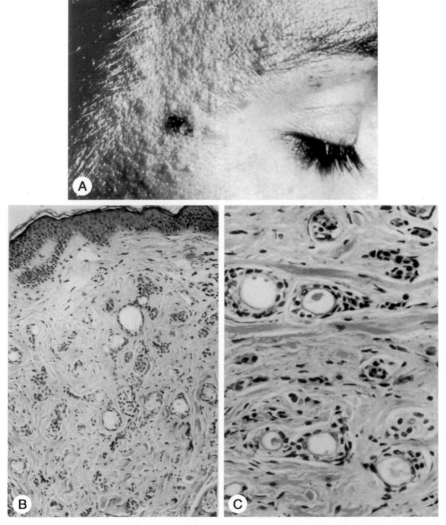

Figure 12–13. Syringoma. **(A)** Multiple, small, flesh-colored papules are present on the temporal skin of this young woman. **(B)** Histologically, small nests and cords of epithelium are embedded within a dense, collagenous stroma. **(C)** Individual cords have central, eccrine-type lumina, and some cords have contours reminiscent of comma- or tadpole-like shapes.

during adult life. Lesions commonly involve skin of the lower eyelids, cheeks, axillae, lower abdomen, vulva, and rarely, acral areas. *Eruptive syringomas* are seen primarily in children and occur as successive crops of lesions on the anterior aspect of the body surface. *Linear syringomas* are aggregated in discrete linear or unilateral zones, reminiscent of the distribution of some epidermal nevi or giant congenital melanocytic nevocellular nevi.

Histologically, scanning magnification reveals numerous small cords and nests forming discrete aggregates within the mid-dermis (Fig. 12–13*B*). Often, these cords appear to originate from overlying keratin-filled cystic epidermal invaginations. Lesions show bilateral symmetry and are embedded within a well-developed, collagenous, eosinophilic stroma (Fig. 12–13*C*). Many of the epithelial nests have contours reminiscent of tadpoles or commas. Ductular lumina are generally observed within many of the nests and may contain homogeneous, eosinophilic, periodic acid–Schiff (PAS)-positive, diastase-resistant secretions. *Clear cell syringomas* are a histologic variant showing the same basic architecture as the common variety. They are composed, however, of highly glycogenated ductular epithelial cells with a swollen, empty appearance of their cytoplasm.

Cylindroma[25–27]

- NUMEROUS, CLOSELY AGGREGATED DERMAL NESTS CONTAINING BASOPHILIC CELLS
- NESTS FIT TOGETHER AS IF PIECES OF A JIGSAW PUZZLE
- DISTINCT COLLAGENOUS STROMA ENVELOPING NESTS
- DUCTULAR LUMINA WITHIN SOME NESTS
- PERIODIC ACID–SCHIFF-POSITIVE GLOBULAR INCLUSIONS WITHIN NESTS

Cylindromas are benign, histologically primitive adenomas thought to be predominantly of apocrine differentiation. They occur in either a solitary form or as multiple, dominantly inherited scalp nodules that lead to progressive disfigurement. Solitary cylindromas tend to involve the face and scalp of older adults and do not show a definite pattern of inheritance. Multiple lesions frequently begin as nondescript, firm, skin-colored scalp nodules (Fig. 12–14*A*). Over time, new cylindromas form, and older lesions grow and coalesce to produce a mutilating turban-like mass (hence the name "turban tumor"). These lesions must be surgically removed, often in multiple stages (Fig. 12–14*B*).

At scanning magnification, cylindromas are characterized by numerous ovoid to polygonal nests of basaloid cells within the superficial and deep dermis (Fig. 12–14*C*). These nests are arranged in close approximation to form a well-circumscribed but not encapsulated tumor mass. Proximity of adjacent nests and their tendency to mold to one another produces the impression that they fit together like pieces of a jigsaw puzzle. Individual nests are surrounded by a thickened zone of hyalinized, eosinophilic collagen and are composed of small basaloid cells and larger pale cells, both of which contain rounded nuclei devoid of atypia (Fig. 12–14*D*). Variable numbers of small, round, hyalinized, eosinophilic bod-

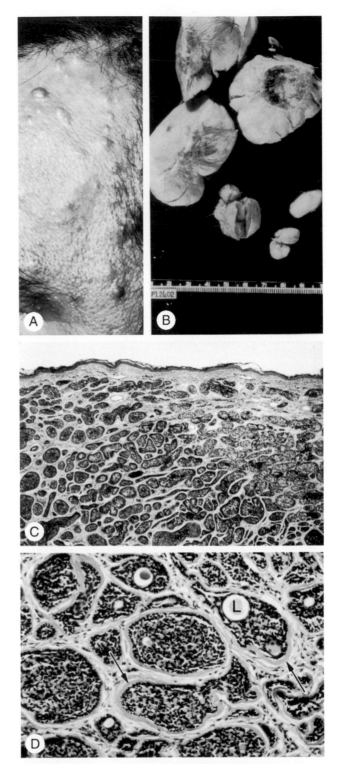

Figure 12–14. Cylindroma. **(A)** Early lesions on the forehead and scalp. Over time, these may enlarge, become confluent, and produce a turban-like deformity. **(B)** For this reason, multiple cylindromas may be cosmetically removed and be submitted for pathological examination. **(C)** At scanning power, individual epithelial islands appear to interlock, as if they are pieces of a jigsaw puzzle. The islands are composed of small basaloid cells admixed with larger pale epithelial cells. **(D)** They contain small duct-like lumina (L) and are surrounded by a cylinder or mantle of hyalinized basement membrane (*arrow*), which, over time, may become incorporated into islands as small, rounded, extracellular bodies.

ies are interspersed among tumor cells. These bodies are believed to originate from incorporation of small fragments of the hyalinized band of PAS-positive, basement membrane–like collagen that surrounds individual nests of tumor cells. Small, duct-like lumina are usually present within tumor nests. Cellular and matrix components that constitute individual nests are nearly identical with those of eccrine spiradenoma at a light microscopic level, although the architectures of these two neoplasms are distinctive.

Papillary Adenoma[28]

- NUMEROUS CORDS, DUCTS, AND GLANDS WITHIN SUPERFICIAL AND DEEP DERMIS
- PAPILLARY FRONDS WITHIN DUCT LUMINA FORMED BY CUBOIDAL EPITHELIUM
- ABSENCE OF NECROSIS, MITOSES, OR CELLULAR PLEOMORPHISM
- DISTINCTIVE FIBROTIC STROMA

The papillary adenoma is a solitary nodular tumor with a predilection for occurrence on the hands and feet. Lesions range from 0.5 to 2 cm in diameter, and individuals with darkly pigmented skin are preferentially affected. Lesions may be present for many months or years prior to excision, and recurrence after treatment is rare.

Histologically, the low-power magnification appearance of papillary adenoma consists of a well-circumscribed, symmetrical proliferation of variably dilated ducts that exhibit focally prominent, intraluminal, papillary, epithelial projections (Fig. 12–15). The tumor is present within the superficial and deep dermis, and contiguity with the overlying epidermis is not seen. Amorphous and granular eosinophilic secretions are present in many of the duct lumens. Small, keratin-filled cysts may also be observed. The adenomatous regions are composed of variably spaced ducts and glands lined by one to several layers of cuboidal epithelium (see Fig. 12–15B). Both ductular and glandular differentiation is observed, and

papillary fronds frequently extend from the luminal cytoplasm of the lining cells. The stroma is composed of eosinophilic fibrovascular tissue with admixed collagen, which distinguishes it from the more cellular stroma of dermal endometriosis (see Chap. 16). Zones showing excessive cellular crowding, poorly formed ducts and glands, and nuclear pleomorphism with numerous mitotic figures should raise the possibility of the more aggressive variant that occurs primarily on the digits of the hand (i.e., aggressive digital papillary adenocarcinoma), primary adnexal carcinoma, or metastatic adenocarcinoma.

Mixed Tumor[29–31]

- MULTIPLE ANASTOMOSING CORDS AND DUCTS WITHIN SUPERFICIAL AND DEEP DERMIS
- WELL-CIRCUMSCRIBED, SYMMETRICAL, NONINFILTRATIVE NEOPLASM
- CHARACTERISTIC STROMA WITH MYXOID AND CHONDROID CHANGE

The mixed tumor of skin (i.e., chondroid syringoma) is a benign eccrine and apocrine appendage tumor with the distinctive diagnostic feature of a variably chondroid stroma. These tumors present clinically as firm, skin-colored, intradermal or subcutaneous nodules on the head and neck. They range between 0.5 and 3 cm in diameter, and the normal-appearing overlying skin surface may be anchored to the underlying nodule.

Histologically, mixed tumors are relatively well circumscribed because their epithelial elements are incorporated within variably mucoid to chondroid stroma (Fig. 12–16A). Mixed tumors form coalescent, symmetrical ovoid to lobulated tumors within the superficial to deep dermis. The symmetry and noninfiltrative pattern of growth are important features in differentiating benign mixed tumors from the rarely encountered malignant variant. The epithelial compo-

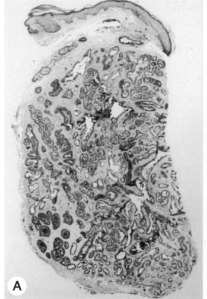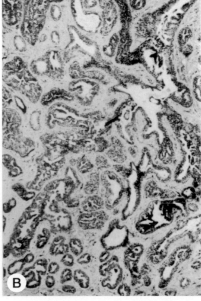

Figure 12–15. Papillary adenoma. **(A)** The tumor is encased in a distinctive fibrotic stroma and consists of anastomosing epithelial nests with prominent glandular differentiation. **(B)** At higher magnification, small internal papillations are seen within glands lined by one to two cuboidal epithelial layers. Foci of apocrine-type secretions may also be detected.

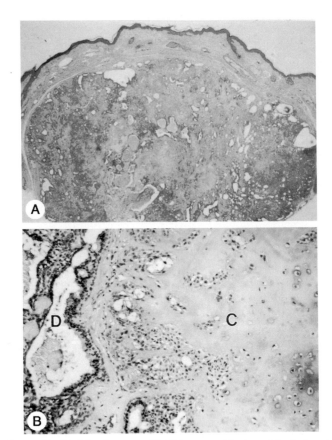

Figure 12–16. Mixed tumor. **(A)** This symmetrical nodule is largely composed of stroma in which small epithelial cords and ducts are dispersed. **(B)** The stromal matrix varies from myxoid to chondroid (C). Epithelial elements show eccrine duct–like differentiation (D) and are lined by one to two cuboidal epithelial layers.

nents of the tumor may assume a branching architecture formed by small to dilated ducts. Alternatively, the epithelial components may be entirely composed of small solid cords and small ducts formed by cells resembling those of a true syringoma. At scanning magnification, the stroma varies from vaguely eosinophilic to basophilic and may appear to represent loose reactive fibrous tissue, pale hyalinized fibrous tissue, myxoid tissue, or true cartilage.

On inspection by higher magnification, the epithelial elements of the mixed tumor are composed of cuboidal cells lining ductular spaces and a variably apparent outer layer of flattened myoepithelial cells (Fig. 12–16*B*). These cells form the walls of small tubular ducts, more elaborate branching tubular lumina, and dilated cystic ducts. The latter are frequently filled with PAS-positive, diastase-resistant material, and although apocrine-like secretion has occasionally been observed, these ducts are generally regarded to show a preponderance of eccrine differentiation by routine light microscopic criteria. The stroma of early lesions is composed of loose connective tissue containing alcian blue–positive, hyaluronidase-resistant acid mucopolysaccharide and delicate stellate fibroblast-like cells that impart a myxoid character. Over time, the cellular components of the stroma become better developed, exhibiting more rounded contours and abundant cytoplasm. In some lesions, these cells are indistinguishable from true chondrocytes (see Fig. 12–16*B*). The associated extracellular matrix acquires a glassy basophilic

to slightly eosinophilic quality resembling that of true cartilage or hyalinized connective tissue. The vast majority of mixed tumors do not recur after surgical excision.

Tumors Forming Sheets and Nodules

Poroma[32–34]

- ABRUPT, PLATE-LIKE DOWNGROWTH FROM EPIDERMAL SURFACE
- CELLS FORMING TUMOR RESEMBLE KERATINOCYTES BUT ARE SMALLER
- PALE, GLYCOGENATED CYTOPLASM
- SPRIALING DUCTS PRESENT FOCALLY AMONG PROLIFERATING CELLS
- VASCULARIZED, FIBROTIC, UNDERLYING DERMIS

Eccrine poroma is a benign, usually solitary appendage tumor characterized by cellular differentiation toward the

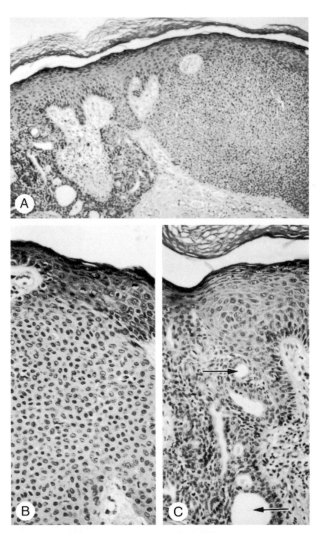

Figure 12–17. Poroma. **(A)** Sheet-like downgrowths of epithelium are observed at scanning magnification. **(B)** The cells forming these downgrowths are polyhedral but smaller than normal keratinocytes. Their cytoplasm is pale as a result of increased glycogen content. **(C)** Foci of spiraling ductular differentiation (*arrows*) are also typically observed.

intraepidermal portion of the eccrine coil (i.e., acrosyringium). The majority of these lesions occur on or near the palms and soles, where eccrine gland density is regionally highest. Other areas may be involved, including the head, neck, and trunk. Affected individuals are generally middle-aged, and the lesions are firm to rubbery, dome-shaped, verrucous or pedunculated nodules that rarely exceed 2 to 3 cm in diameter. Although intrinsically painless, some tumors may become symptomatic as a result of their tendency to erode, with oozing, crusting, and occasionally frank ulceration.

Architecturally, poromas demonstrate primarily endophytic growth by lobular plates of cells that expand initially into the papillary dermis and sometimes into the reticular dermis (Fig. 12–17A). The underlying stroma is richly vascular, and foci of dilated and tortuous vessels are easily observed. Tumor cells are characteristically sharply juxtaposed with their neighbors in the adjacent normal epidermis (Fig. 12–17B), a feature that is readily observed even at low magnification because of the pallor of the cytoplasm of the tumor cells due to their glycogen content. Small eccrine ducts, some with a spiraling architecture, are focally observed in most poromas.

The cells that compose the eccrine poroma are squamoid with inconspicuous intercellular bridges, and generally, they are smaller than midepidermal keratinocytes (see Fig. 12–17B). This cytologic appearance is sometimes referred to as poral epithelium. Eccrine ducts that form within the tumor are lined by a single layer of vaguely cuboidal ductular epithelial cells (Fig. 12–17C). The lumina of these ducts contain a thin, PAS-positive lining (i.e., cuticle) similar to that of normal eccrine ducts. Mitotic figures and individual cell necrosis are rare in benign poromas. The term *hidroacanthoma simplex* has been used to distinguish poromas that display an intraepidermal epithelioma pattern of growth and does not represent an entity that is biologically different from classical poroma.

Trichilemmoma[35]

- PLATE-LIKE ENDOPHYTIC EPITHELIAL DOWNGROWTHS
- EARLY LESIONS SHOW PERIFOLLICULAR PATTERN
- FOCAL-TO-DIFFUSE CYTOPLASMIC PALLOR DUE TO GLYCOGENATION
- VARIABLE PALISADING OF BASAL CELL LAYER AT PERIMETER
- THIN, HYALINIZED STROMAL MANTLE SURROUNDING TUMOR

Solitary trichilemmomas present clinically as verrucous, hyperkeratotic or smooth papules ranging in size from several millimeters to occasionally more than 1 cm. The facial skin is generally affected, and lesions most often occur on the nose, cheek, and upper lip. Multiple trichilemmomas are manifestations of an autosomal dominant condition referred to as *Cowden disease* or syndrome, which is most commonly associated with carcinoma of the breast in females. Other cutaneous manifestations of this syndrome consist of benign verrucous and lichenoid keratotic tumors of the hands and feet (i.e., acral keratoses), punctate keratoses of the palms and soles, papillomatosis of the lips and oral mucosa, and scrotal tongue.

Histologically, there is a well-defined lobular proliferation of glycogenated epithelium that may originate at the shoulder of a follicular orifice and include a portion of a pilosebaceous unit at its base (Fig. 12–18A). Other possibly more advanced tumors are devoid of identifiable preexisting pilar structure (Fig. 12–18B). The surface of the lesion is verrucous and may show increased scale production. The architecture of the trichilemmoma consists of plate-like lobular downgrowth into a fibrovascular stroma. The most peripheral layer is basaloid and may show palisading. A thickened, hyalinized, stromal mantle surrounds this basaloid

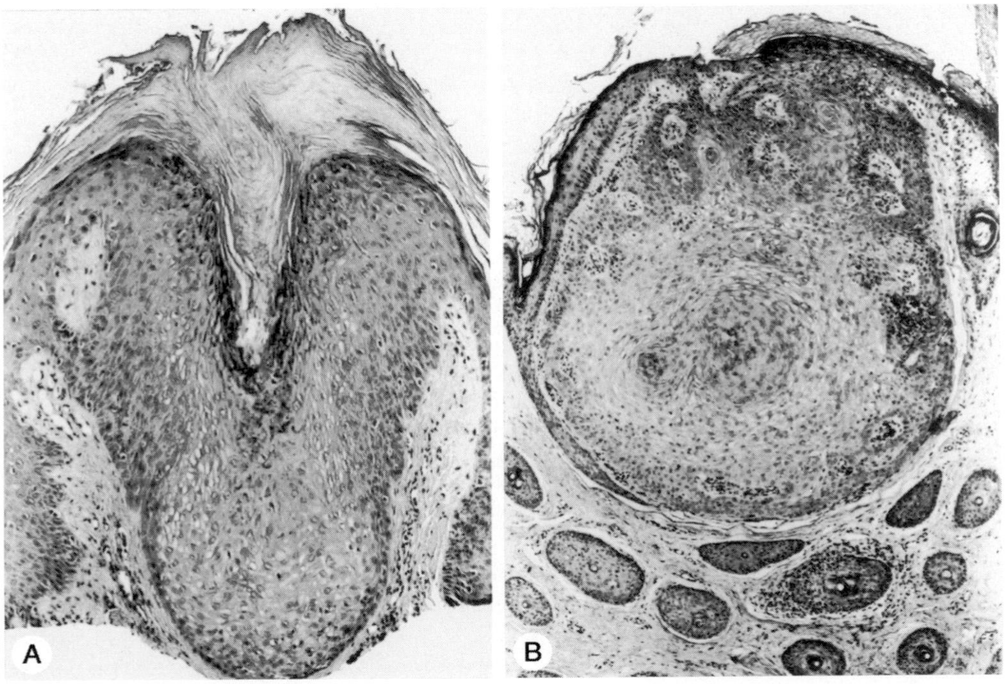

Figure 12–18. Trichilemmoma. **(A)** There is plate-like downgrowth about a follicular infundibulum, which eventually may form **(B)** an expansile nodule within the superficial and deep dermis. With the exception of the basal cells at the periphery, the cells forming this tumor are highly glycogenated, and a thin, hyalinized, stromal mantle usually is present at the dermal-tumor epithelial interface.

layer. Lesional cells are large squamous cells with a pale pink cytoplasm that is PAS-positive, indicating abundant quantities of glycogen. Verrucae may at times acquire cytoplasmic glycogen and mimic the features of trichilemmoma. Trichilemmomas may be differentiated from ordinary verrucae by their formation about follicular infundibula, basaloid palisading at the periphery of tumor lobules, and development of a thickened, hyalinized basement membrane. Although some have posited that all trichilemmomas are the result of human papillomavirus infection, molecular hybridization to detect the viral genome has thus far failed to substantiate this association.

Nodular Hidradenoma[36, 37]

- NODULAR DERMAL NEOPLASM COMPOSED OF SQUAMOID CELLS
- VARIABLE CYTOPLASMIC GLYCOGENATION
- DUCT FORMATION
- FOCALLY HYALINIZED STROMA
- RELATIVE ABSENCE OF MITOSES AND INDIVIDUAL CELL NECROSIS

Nodular hidradenomas, also called clear cell hidradenomas, are benign adnexal neoplasms showing eccrine acrosyringeal differentiation. Nodular hidradenomas are usually solitary, asymptomatic, intradermal nodules measuring between 0.5 and 2 cm in diameter. There is no site predilection, although many of the lesions that have been described appear on the face, scalp, chest, and abdomen. Tumors are usually covered by smooth, normal skin, and variations in coloration from red to blue have been described. Occasional nodular hidradenomas show superficial ulceration by the time the patient presents for evaluation.

At scanning magnification, nodular hidradenomas are usually composed of multiple coalescent nodules surrounded by a collagenous pseudocapsule within the superficial and deep dermis, with occasional involvement of the subcutaneous fat (Fig. 12–19A). Continuity with the overlying epidermis may or may not be seen. Clear cell change as a result of cytoplasmic glycogenation may be inconspicuous or

prominent and easily appreciated as extensive zonal pallor. Small, branching, tubular ducts and large, cyst-like ducts are conspicuous in some tumors and must be sought in others. These ductular elements are lined by cuboidal epithelial cells or columnar secretory cells, respectively. Condensed, eosinophilic, hyalinized stroma forms a mantle at the periphery of the tumor and often extends into the tumor as trabeculae. Solid portions of the tumor are composed of a variable admixture of small basaloid to squamoid polyhedral and fusiform cells. These cell types often exhibit distinct plasma membranes, and there may be striking cytoplasmic clarity as a result of their glycogen content (Fig. 12–19B). Although tumor nuclei may be hyperchromatic and exhibit coarsely clumped chromatin, marked pleomorphism and frequent or atypical mitoses are not observed. If present, the lesion should be considered to have potential for aggressive behavior. An infiltrative pattern on scanning magnification or the presence of necrosis also suggests the possibility of malignancy.

Nodular hidradenomas may occasionally recur subsequent to attempts at local excision. The histology of the recurrences generally resembles that of the primary lesion, although architectural distortion and fibrosis may confound diagnostic interpretation when the histology of the primary lesion is unknown or unavailable. Malignant variants of nodular hidradenoma exist, although the majority of these arise de novo, rather than in association with preexisting benign lesions.

Pilomatricoma[38-39]

- NODULAR DERMAL AGGREGATES OF BASALOID AND SQUAMOID CELLS
- BASALOID CELLS RESEMBLE HAIR MATRIX EPITHELIUM
- SQUAMOID CELLS WITH CENTRAL NUCLEAR "SHADOWS"
- GRANULOMATOUS, FIBROTIC STROMA
- VARIABLE DYSTROPHIC CALCIFICATION AND SOMETIMES OSSIFICATION

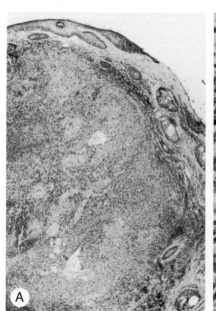
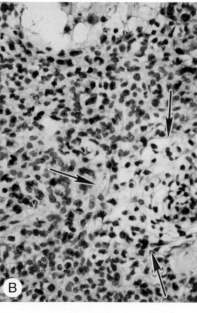

Figure 12–19. Nodular hidradenoma. **(A)** There is a large cellular nodule within the dermis. The nodule may contain variable numbers of eccrine-type ducts, and invaginations of stroma frequently are markedly hyalinized. **(B)** At higher magnification, foci of marked cytoplasmic glycogenation impart striking cytoplasmic clearing (*arrows*). Tumors predominated by this cytologic change have been termed clear cell hidradenomas.

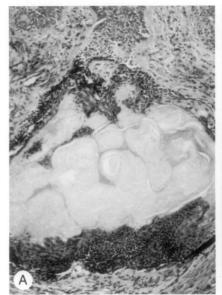
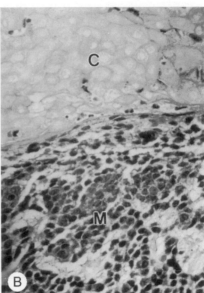

Figure 12–20. Pilomatricoma. **(A)** The tumor consists of a nodular aggregate within a reactive desmoplastic stroma usually containing foreign body giant cells. **(B)** Diagnostic features include anucleate cells exhibiting hair cortex (i.e., shadow cells; C) and hair matrix (M) differentiation. Foci of calcification and even ossification may be present.

Pilomatricomas present clinically as solitary, 0.5- to 3.0-cm, firm, deep-seated, dermal or subcutaneous nodules that are often best appreciated by palpation. Children and adolescents are frequently affected, and tumors have a predilection for occurrence on skin of the face or upper extremities. Multiple lesions and familial patterns of occurrence have been reported, and the hereditary type has been linked to myotonic dystrophy.

Histologically, pilomatricomas appear at scanning magnification as solitary deep dermal or subcutaneous nodules formed by coalescent aggregates of basophilic and eosinophilic material within a fibrotic stroma that frequently contains granulomatous inflammation with foreign-body–type giant cells (Fig. 12–20A). Occasional, presumably early tumors present as simple cystic structures with hair matrix differentiation in the majority of the cells forming the wall (see Hair Matrix Cyst). Eosinophilic foci are composed of squamous cells resembling hair cortex that have lost their nuclei, leaving ovoid, clear zones centrally within the cytoplasm (i.e., ghost or shadow cells). Zones of basaloid cells resembling hair matrix may also be observed, particularly in early tumors (Fig. 12–20B). Basaloid cells are often juxtaposed with shadow cells, as if they were giving rise to the latter. Mitotic activity may be observed in these basaloid regions; however, nuclear atypia or infiltrative growth patterns, as seen in rare malignant variants, are not typical of benign pilomatricomas. As lesions age, shadow cells predominate or are present exclusively, and dystrophic calcification and occasionally metaplastic ossification occur.

Spiradenoma[40, 41]

- NODULAR DERMAL TUMOR WITH VARIABLE VASCULARITY
- EPITHELIAL ELEMENTS COMPOSED OF SMALL BASALOID AND LARGE PALE CELLS
- DUCTS LINED BY CUBOIDAL EPITHELIUM
- HYALINIZED STROMAL INCLUSIONS WITHIN TUMOR

Eccrine spiradenomas are 1- to 2-cm, solitary or rarely multiple intradermal nodules that usually present in children and young adults. Many of these lesions occur on the trunk and extremities, although any site may potentially be affected. Tumor nodules are dome-shaped, skin-colored, and classically painful, a feature potentially related to an often elaborate network of unmyelinated axons and Schwann cells that is present within their investing stroma.

Eccrine spiradenoma presents histologically as a well-circumscribed, round to ovoid, blue nodule with variable vascularity, located within a loose fibrovascular dermal stroma (Fig. 12–21A). Several nodules may be present, and adjacent nodules may coalesce. Rarely, small nests resembling cylindroma are adjacent to an eccrine spiradenoma. Spiradenomas are round to ovoid in shape and may be encapsulated by a thin, hyalinized, eosinophilic mantle. The epithelial cells forming the tumor are characteristically closely packed and consist of three types (Fig. 12–21B,C). The first type of epithelial cell, which tends to predominate, is large and contains a round to ovoid nucleus with evenly dispersed pale chromatin and a scant rim of cytoplasm. The second type, which is admixed with the first to form poorly defined cords, is smaller and contains a round, hyperchromatic, lymphocyte-like nucleus and inconspicuous cytoplasm. The third type, which is the least apparent and only focally present in certain spiradenomas, is a cuboidal to flattened epithelial cell that forms eccrine-type ducts.

Spiradenomas are surrounded by a thin, stromal mantle composed of hyalinized connective tissue that is variably permeated by small, unmyelinated axons. This morphology potentially relates to the frequent clinical symptom of localized pain or discomfort. Small branching stromal septa may extend from this mantle into the tumor parenchyma, where minute rounded fragments of hyalinized stromal matrix appear to be progressively incorporated into the tumor nodule. These hyalinized bodies, each about the size of a tumor cell or small ductular lumen, become evenly distributed throughout the neoplasm, producing a histologic picture that is highly characteristic and is simulated only by one other adnexal tumor at high magnification, the cylindroma.

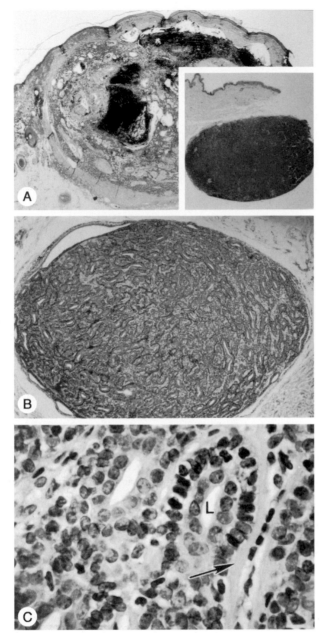

Figure 12-21. Spiradenoma. **(A)** Vascular variant and solid variant (*inset*) of spiradenoma; initial diagnostic impressions at scanning magnification may include glomangioma or lymph node, respectively. **(B)** Spiradenomas are nodular tumors composed of compacted cords of cuboidal epithelium. **(C)** Small eccrine-type lumina (L) and hyalinized matrix (*arrow*) that often forms extracellular rounded bodies similar to those of cylindroma are routinely detected. As in the case of cylindroma, the epithelial cells vary from small basaloid cells to larger, pale, epithelial elements.

Benign Sebaceous Neoplasms[42]

- PERIFOLLICULAR PROLIFERATION OF OTHERWISE NORMAL SEBACEOUS LOBULES (I.E., SEBACEOUS HYPERPLASIA)
- SEBACEOUS HYPERPLASIA IN THE SETTING OF VERRUCOUS EPIDERMAL HYPERPLASIA AND ASSOCIATED ANOMALOUS ADNEXAL DIFFERENTIATION (I.E., NEVUS SEBACEUS)

- LOCALIZED PROLIFERATION OF SEBACEOUS LOBULES WITH BASALOID ELEMENTS LESS THAN 50% OF LIPIDIZED CELLS (I.E., SEBACEOUS ADENOMA)
- LOCALIZED PROLIFERATION OF SEBACEOUS LOBULES WITH BASALOID ELEMENTS GREATER THAN 50% OF LIPIDIZED CELLS (I.E., SEBACEOUS EPITHELIOMA)

Lesions of *sebaceous hyperplasia* are small, pale to yellow papules that generally occur on the faces of older individuals. A central umbilication is characteristic, and chronically sun-exposed skin of Caucasians appears to be most vulnerable to the development of sebaceous hyperplasia. Lesions are often biopsied to exclude basal cell carcinoma, which may demonstrate a similar clinical appearance. Confluence of individual papules of sebaceous hyperplasia on the nose may produce dramatic enlargement known as *rhinophyma*, or "W.C. Fields nose," particularly in individuals prone to acne rosacea (Fig. 12–22A). *Nevus sebaceus* refers to sebaceous hyperplasia occurring in association with a seborrheic keratosis–like zone of epidermal hyperplasia and is often also associated with anomalous adnexal differentia-

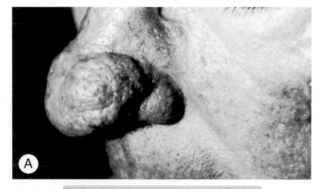

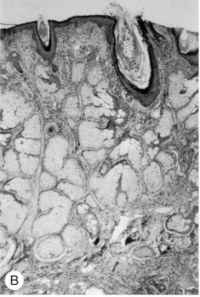

Figure 12-22. Sebaceous hyperplasia. **(A)** Typical rhinophyma, or W.C. Fields nose, is due to extensive sebaceous hyperplasia. **(B)** Histologically, the superficial and deep dermis are crowded with mature sebaceous lobules. Dilated and plugged follicular infundibula are also characteristically seen.

tion (e.g., pilar, apocrine). These lesions are congenital plaques that most often affect scalp or facial skin. Prepubertal lesions, which are devoid of sebaceous activity, present as zones of localized alopecia; peripubertal and postpubertal lesions show in addition to alopecia, plaque-like elevation and a yellow hue as a result of sebaceous growth (Fig. 12–23A). *Sebaceous adenomas* and *epitheliomas* are relatively uncommon, usually solitary, tan-yellow papules that occur on the facial skin of middle-aged and older individuals. As is the case with sebaceous hyperplasia, these lesions are often confused with basal cell carcinoma. Sebaceous epitheliomas have been known to bleed and ulcerate, increasing suspicion

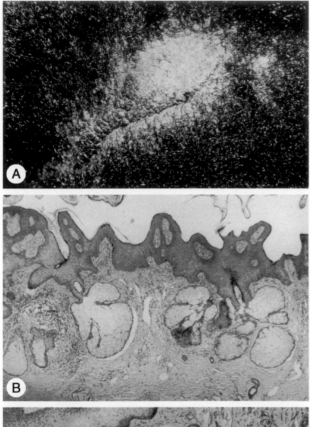

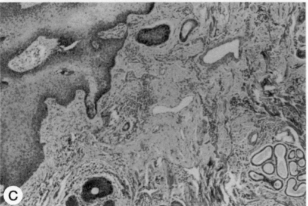

Figure 12–23. Nevus sebaceus. **(A)** Alopecia at the site of a verrucous plaque that has been present since birth. **(B)** A biopsy specimen reveals verrucous epidermal thickening, focal sebaceous hyperplasia, aberrant follicular buds, and anomalous apocrine differentiation for this anatomic site **(C,** *lower right*). **(C)** Often overlooked is the abnormal fibrovascular stroma, a form of dermal hamartoma, that generally accompanies nevus sebaceus.

that they may represent more aggressive tumors, and the occurrence of both tumors has been associated with the co-existence of internal malignancy in a small percentage of patients (i.e., *Muir-Torre syndrome*).

At scanning magnification, hyperplastic sebaceous glands are characterized by a dilated follicular infundibulum plugged with keratin, and enlarged sebaceous lobules that are increased in number (Fig. 12–22B). In a superficial shave biopsy specimen, budding of lobules above a horizontal plane that approximates the origin of the sebaceous duct, as occurs in sebaceous hyperplasia, will result in lipidized cells abnormally associated with epidermal and papillary dermal fragments. Unlike sebaceous adenomas, the basal cell layer of hyperplastic sebaceous glands is not increased. In addition to regions of sebaceous hyperplasia, nevus sebaceus may show sebaceous lobules that empty directly onto a verrucous epidermal surface (Fig. 12–23B). In addition, there may be anomalous pilar epithelial elements resembling embryonic hair germs, apocrine metaplasia, and hamartomatous stromal elements (Fig. 12–23C). Sebaceous adenomas and epitheliomas are well-circumscribed lobular epithelial proliferations that originate from the overlying epidermis and that are characteristically surrounded by a fibrotic, eosinophilic stroma (Fig. 12–24A, C). Sebaceous adenomas consist of multiple, coalescent, sebaceous glands, some of which may show rudimentary or abortive formation of individual lobules and dilated ducts. The cells forming the centers of these lobules are the predominant cell type and are well lipidized. The basaloid cells defining the periphery of the lobules are several layers thick, in contrast to the single basaloid layer of normal or hyperplastic lobules, and may protrude into more lipidized regions (Fig. 12–24B). Sebaceous epitheliomas, on the other hand, show a preponderance (more than 50%) of basaloid cells, and lipidized cells may be only individually scattered throughout the tumor lobules (Fig. 12–24D). In contrast to sebaceous carcinoma, neither tumor demonstrates nuclear atypia, although some examples of sebaceous adenoma and epithelioma show considerable mitotic activity, particularly in the basaloid regions.

Adnexal Carcinoma[43–47]

- INFILTRATIVE DUCTULAR AND GLANDULAR STRUCTURES WITHIN DERMAL COLLAGEN
- FOCAL CONTINUITY WITH EPIDERMIS OR TRANSITIONS WITH BENIGN ADNEXAE
- ASYMMETRY
- MITOSES, SOME ATYPICAL, AND INDIVIDUAL CELL NECROSIS
- PERINEURAL INVASION

Adnexal carcinomas may show sebaceous, eccrine, or apocrine differentiation. Their significance lies in their tendency to metastasize, as opposed to other primary skin epithelial malignancies (e.g., squamous and basal cell carcinoma), and in their tendency to be confused histologically with metastatic carcinoma to the skin.

The majority of *sebaceous carcinomas* occur on the eyelid, where they arise in association with the meibomian glands of the tarsus and the glands of Zeis. The skin of the upper eyelid in women is commonly involved. Lesions are asymptomatic, firm, often ill-defined nodules which may be

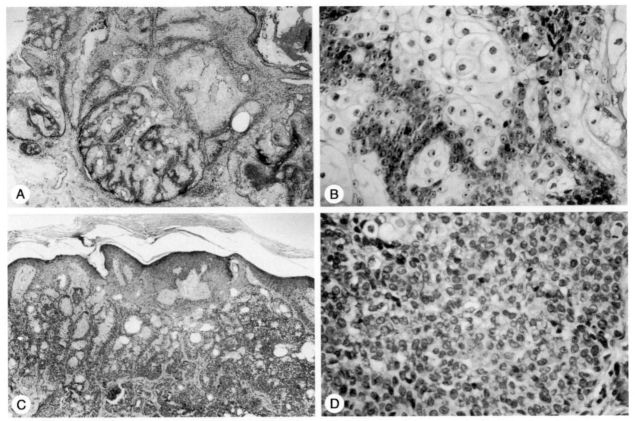

Figure 12–24. Sebaceous adenoma and epithelioma. **(A,B)** Sebaceous adenoma is an endophytic lobulated tumor with prominent central lipidization and only several layers of nonlipidized basaloid cells at the periphery. **(C)** Sebaceous epithelioma has a similar architecture, but **(D)** basaloid cells predominate, and lipidization is only focally observed.

mistaken for chalazion, partially ruptured cysts, or blepharo-conjunctivitis. Individual tumors exceeding 1 cm in diameter are associated with a poorer prognosis than smaller lesions. Sebaceous carcinoma may also be associated with multiple facial sebaceous adenomas, basal and squamous cell carci-nomas, keratoacanthomas, and visceral carcinomas, particu-larly of the gastrointestinal tract (i.e., Muir-Torre syndrome).

Although sebaceous carcinomas retain a vaguely lobular configuration (Fig. 12–25A), many infiltrate as irregular tongues and small clusters of malignant cells into the dermis,

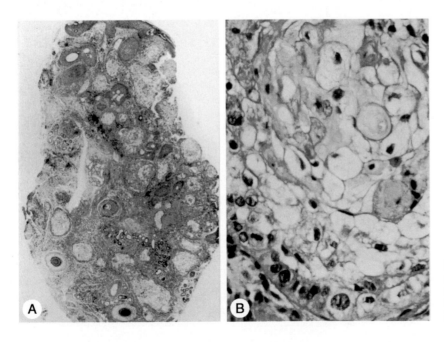

Figure 12–25. Sebaceous carcinoma. **(A)** This poorly defined, deeply infiltrative neoplasm shows **(B)** regions of overt cytoplasmic lipidization. Other examples have a paucity of cytoplasmic lipid, and more resemble poorly differentiated squamous cell carcinoma.

subcutis, and skeletal muscle. Tumor cells are frequently large and squamoid in appearance, and basaloid differentiation and lipidization may be inconspicuous. Zones of necrosis, marked nuclear atypia, and abnormal mitotic figures are all commonly observed (Fig. 12–25*B*). Pagetoid growth of tumor cells in the epidermis or conjunctiva also may occur. Histologic findings that predict a poorer prognosis include pagetoid spread, multicentric origin, lack of differentiation (i.e., sparse evidence of lipidization), extent of local infiltration, and vascular and orbital involvement. Metastases first affect regional lymph nodes of the periauricular, submaxillary, and cervical chains, and visceral spread may ensue in some cases.

Eccrine carcinoma is relatively common with respect to most other variants, and it therefore is regarded as the classic form of adnexal carcinoma. A noteworthy feature is its high rate of metastatic spread. The scanning architecture of eccrine adenocarcinoma may initially resemble that of an infil-

trative poroma (i.e., porocarcinoma; Fig. 12–26*A*), or may mimic a moderately differentiated adenocarcinoma (Fig. 12–26*C*). Eccrine adenocarcinomas are asymmetrical and ill-defined, and they may be formed by diffusely infiltrative neoplastic cells. Contiguity with benign eccrine structures or with the overlying epidermis is generally not seen. Classic adenocarcinoma patterns demonstrate cribriform growth of atypical cells with frequent mitoses. A common feature of all eccrine carcinomas at high magnification is nuclear atypia (Fig. 12–26*B, D*). Many eccrine carcinomas show at least a focal presence of spiraling ductular differentiation, duct formation lined by cuticular material, and zones of cytoplasmic glycogenation. The stroma varies from fibrotic to hyalinized to highly myxoid or even frankly mucinous. Differentiation of eccrine adenocarcinoma from metastatic adenocarcinoma to the skin may be difficult. Careful search for ductular differentiation with PAS-positive cuticle formation may provide strong evidence against metastatic tumor, but the final diag-

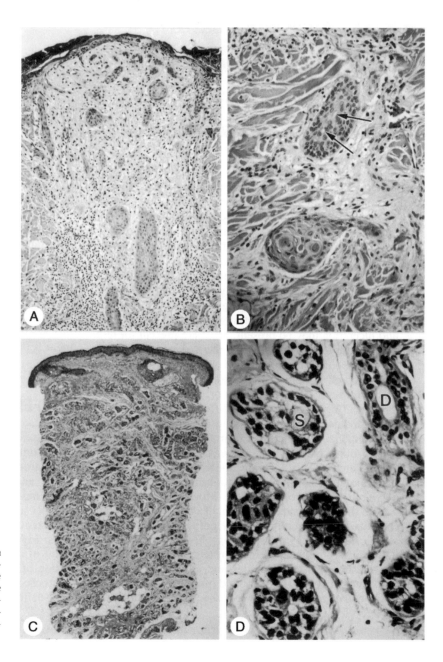

Figure 12–26. Eccrine carcinoma. **(A, B)** Porocarcinoma is characterized by nests and cords of malignant squamous epithelium with focal duct formation (*arrows*). The stroma is mucinous and focally myxoid. **(C, D)** Eccrine carcinoma with foci of dermal ductular (D) and secretory coil (S) differentiation. Note **(C)** the diffusely infiltrative pattern of growth and **(D)** the striking nuclear hyperchromasia.

SELECTED REFERENCES

1. Hashimoto K, Mehregan AH, Kumakiri M. Tumors of Skin Appendages. Boston: Butterworths, 1987:85.
2. Mehregan AH, Brownstein MH. Pilar sheath acanthoma. Arch Dermatol 1978;114:1495.
3. Mehregan AH. Infundibular tumors of the skin. J Cutan Pathol 1984;11:387.
4. Brownstein MH, Shapiro L. The pilosebaceous tumors. Int J Dermatol 1977;16:340.
5. Brownstein MH. Steatocystoma simplex: A solitary steatocystoma. Arch Dermatol 1982;118:409.
6. Hashimoto K, Fisher BK, Lever WF. Steatocystoma multiplex. Hautarzt 1964;15:299.
7. Mehregan AH. Apocrine cystadenoma. Arch Dermtaol 1964;90:274.
8. Kruse TV, Khan MA, Hassan MO. Multiple apocrine cystadenomas. Br J Dematol 1979;100:675.
9. Powell RF, Palmer CH, Smith EB. Apocrine cystadenoma of the penile shaft. Arch Dermatol 1977;113:1250.
10. Rostan SE, Waller JD. Syringocystadenoma papilliferum in an unusual location. Arch Dermatol 1976;112:835.
11. Premalatha S, Raghuveera Rao N, Yesudian P, et al. Segmental syringocystadenoma papilliferum in an unusual location. Int J Dermatol 1985;24:520.
12. Santa Cruz DJ, Prioleau PG, Smith ME. Hidradenoma papilliferum of the eyelid. Arch Dermatol 1981;117:55.
13. Nissim F, Czernoblisky B, Ostfeld E. Hidradenoma papilliferum of the external auditory canal. J Laryngo Otol 1981;95:843.
14. Shenoy YMV. Malignant perianal papillary hidradenoma. Arch Dermatol 1961;83:965.
15. Headington JT. Tumors of the hair follicle. Am J Pathol 1976;85:480.
16. Ziprkowski L, Schewach-Millet M. Multiple trichoepithelioma in a mother and two children. Dermatologica 1956;132:248.
17. Rahbari H, Mehregan A, Pinkus H. Trichoadenoma of Nikolowski. J Cutan Pathol 1977;4:90.
18. Brownstein MH, Shapiro L. Desmoplastic trichoepithelioma. Cancer 1977;40:2979.
19. Pinkus H, Sutton RL Jr. Trichofolliculoma. Arch Dermatol 1965;91:46.
20. Plewig G. Sebaceous trichofolliculoma. J Cutan Pathol 1980;7:394.
21. Hashimoto K, Gross BG, Lever WF. Syringoma: Histochemical and electron microscopic studies. J Invest Dermatol 1966;46:150.
22. Hashimoto K, DiBella RJ, Borsuk GM. Eruptive hidradenoma and syringoma. Arch Dermatol 1967;96:500.
23. Yung CW, Soltani K, Bernstein JE, et al. Unilateral linear nevoidal syringoma. J Am Acad Dermatol 1981;4:412.
24. Kitamura K, Muraki R, Tamura N. Clear cell syringoma. Cutis 1983;32:169.
25. Crain RC, Helwig EB. Dermal cylindroma (dermal eccrine cylindroma). Am J Clin Pathol 1961;35:504.
26. Welch JP, Wells RS, Kerr CB. Ancell-Speigler cylindromas (turban tumors) and Brooke-Fordyce trichoepitheliomas: Evidence for a single genetic entity. J Med Genet 1968;5:29.
27. Urbanski S, From L, Abramowicz A, et al. Metamorphosis of dermal cylindroma: Possible relation to malignant transformation. J Am Acad Dermatol 1985;12:188.
28. Rulon DB, Helwig EB. Papillary eccrine adenoma. Arch Dermatol 1977;113:596.
29. Hirsch P, Helwig EB: Chondroid syringoma. Arch Dermatol 1961;84:835.
30. Headington JT. Mixed tumors of the skin: Eccrine and apocrine types. Arch Dermatol 1961;84:989.
31. Mills SE. Mixed tumor of the skin: A model of divergent differentiation. J Cutan Pathol 1984;11:382.
32. Pinkus H, Rogin J, Goldman P. Eccrine poroma. Arch Dermatol 1956;74:511.
33. Ogino A. Linear eccrine poroma. Arch Dermatol 1976;112:841.
34. Smith JLS, Coburn JG. Hidroacanthoma simplex: Assessment of selected group of intraepidermal basal cell epitheliomata and of their malignant homologues. Br J Dermatol 1956;68:400.
35. Brownstein MH, Mehregan AH, Bikowski J, et al. The dermatopathology of Cowden's syndrome. Br J Dermatol 1979;100:667.
36. Johnson BL, Helwig EB. Eccrine acrospiroma: A clinicopathologic study. Cancer 1969;23:641.
37. Hashimoto K, DiBella RJ, Lever WF. Clear cell hidradenoma: Histologic, histochemical and electron microscopic study. Arch Dermatol 1967;96:18.
38. Chiaramonti A, Gilgor RS. Pilomatricoma associated with myotonic dystrophy. Arch Dermatol 1978;114:1363.
39. Hashimoto K, Nelson RG, Lever WF. Calcifying epithelioma of Malherbe: Histochemical and electron microscopic studies. J Invest Dermatol 1966;46:391.
40. Kersting DW, Helwig EB. Eccrine spiradenoma. Arch Dermatol 1956;73:199.
41. Hashimoto K, Gross BG, Nelson RG, Lever WF. Eccrine spiradenoma. Histochemical and electron microscope studies. J Invest Dermatol 1966;46:347.
42. Rulon DB, Helwig EB. Cutaneous sebaceous neoplasms. Cancer 1974;33:82.
43. El-Domeiri AA, Brasfield RD, Huvos AG, et al. Sweat gland carcinoma. Ann Surg 1971;173:270.
44. Dissanayake RVP, Salm R. Sweat gland carcinoma. Prognosis related to histologic type. Histopathol 1980;4:445.
45. Weigand DA, Burgdorf WHC. Perianal apocrine gland adenoma. Arch Dermatol 1980;116:1051.
46. Warkel RL, Helwig EB. Apocrine gland adenoma and adenocarcinoma of the axilla. Arch Dermatol 1978;114:198.
47. Wick MR, Goellner JR, Wolfe JT III, et al. Adnexal carcinomas of the skin. II. Extraocular sebaceous carcinomas. Cancer 1985;56:1163.

13

Melanocytic Tumors

DEFINITIONS AND GENERAL CONSIDERATIONS

Melanocytic hyperplasias and neoplasms are commonly removed for cosmetic and diagnostic reasons. Although most are benign, many may be confused clinically and histologically with malignant melanoma (heretofore referred to simply as melanoma), the most common potentially fatal neoplasm of the skin. On the other hand, numerous melanoma variants may be mistaken for either benign nevi or other nonmelanocytic tumors. Despite these pitfalls, heightened clinical detection of early lesions has characterized recent advances in this area. Paradoxically, the incidence and mortality of melanoma have risen sharply during recent years. Awareness of melanoma has resulted in more judicious clinical screening and biopsy of early precursor lesions, which may be typified by subtle or ambiguous histologic patterns. Accurate recognition of these patterns is critical to identification of lesions with significant premalignant or malignant potential and to their differentiation from the numerous histologically similar hyperplasias and benign neoplasms of melanocytes.

The term nevus derives from the Sanskrit root "-gna" and the Latin root "-gen," both of which refer to birth. Although most melanocytic nevi and melanomas are acquired during adolescence or adulthood, these lesions are born from a peculiar neoplastic transformation of preexisting melanocytes. As discussed in Chapter 1, melanocytes are dendritic, neural crest–derived cells that normally inhabit the basal cell layer of the epidermis. The purpose of these cells is to synthesize photoprotective melanin pigment, and accordingly, they are evenly dispersed in relatively low numbers (about 1 melanocyte per 10 contiguous basal keratinocytes in truncal skin that is not chronically actinically damaged), with their delicate melanin-laden dendrites extending toward the epidermal surface.

Hyperplasias of melanocytes are manifested clinically as diffuse hyperpigmentation (e.g., tanning) or macular foci of cutaneous darkening (e.g., lentigines). This darkening of skin is associated histologically with an increase in the ratio of melanocytes to basal keratinocytes ($>1:10$) and often with increased melanization of the basal cell layer with thinning and elongation of the rete ridges. Linear hyperplasia of melanocytes within the basal cell layer is referred to as *lentiginous hyperplasia,* from the Latin word "lenticula," referring to a lentil-shaped spot. Lentiginous melanocytic hyperplasia characterizes simple lentigines and may be an integral component of certain acquired nevi, including dysplastic nevi. *Nevus cell transformation* refers to the poorly understood phenomenon whereby dendritic melanocytes become rounded cells that no longer tend to grow in lentiginous patterns but rather nest in aggregations, initially along the dermal-epidermal interface. Over time, most nevi that begin as nests along the dermal-epidermal junction (i.e., *junctional nevi*) invade the underlying dermis, first as nests, and later as cords and single cells, to become *compound nevi.* Eventually, the junctional component is lost, producing pure *dermal nevi.*

The concept of *melanocytic atypia* deserves special attention. For the purposes of this text, atypia connotes abnormal architectural or cytologic development, but not necessarily premalignant alteration. Therefore, nevi recurring in scars; very old nevi with degenerative (i.e., "ancient") changes; and nevi with deep, penetrating patterns are, in a sense, atypical. On the other hand, atypical nevi that share some degree of architectural or cytologic similarity with melanoma are categorized as exhibiting *dysplasia* and are regarded as potentially premalignant.

Melanoma may evolve from benign melanocytes or, more likely, from fields of progressive hyperplasia followed by dysplasia. This concept of tumor progression based on melanocytes has provided a conceptual basis for understanding the origins and natural evolution of a number of neoplastic systems. Early melanoma tends to grow within the epidermis along the lines or radii of a circle (*radial growth*), and does not form expansile nests or nodules, even at a microscopic level (*nontumorigenic growth*). With progression, growth favors vertical spread into the underlying dermis (*vertical growth*), where melanoma cells form expansive and coalescent nests and nodules (*tumorigenic growth*). These

231

simple concepts are of critical biologic importance, because they define stages in the evolution of melanoma without (radial growth) and with (vertical growth) the capacity for metastatic spread.

GROSS PATHOLOGY

The clinical appearance of melanocytic proliferations is usually, but not invariably, distinguished by their ability to synthesize melanin pigment. Freckles and simple lentigines present as tan-brown macules with rounded, relatively uniform borders. Early melanomas may also be macular or very slightly raised, but they show more variegation in pigmentation (from brown to blue-grey to tan) and irregular, often notched borders. Ordinary acquired nevi present as papules or small nodules with uniform color ranging from flesh tones to brown to black. Often, the depth of melanin pigment determines the hue of the lesion, as in the case of blue nevi, in which melanin is concentrated in the deeper dermis, imparting a blue-black color that may be confused with heavily pigmented vertical growth phase melanoma. Less pigmented nevi predominated by spindle and epithelioid cells and associated with highly vascularized stroma (e.g., Spitz nevi) may be pink to red, and the differential diagnosis therefore fre-

quently includes benign vascular tumors. Entirely amelanotic tumors will be flesh-colored, and those with host responses against normal and neoplastic melanocytes may show uniform or asymmetrical vitiligo-like regions (e.g., halo nevi and regressing melanoma, respectively). Congenital nevi often are accompanied by associated hamartomatous anomalies in the surface epidermis, adnexae, or underlying mesenchyme; therefore, these lesions may present as verrucous, hypertrichotic plaques.

A critical issue in biopsy evaluation of a pigmented lesion is knowledge of the site from which the sample was obtained and the clinical impression based on the gross pathologic appearance. For example, it is not uncommon to encounter small biopsy specimens from the periphery of an acral melanoma that contain proliferations resembling lentiginous nevi but which, on complete excision, prove to be misleading and incomplete samples of radial growth phase melanoma. Regressing lesions may clearly present as melanocytic tumors to the clinician only to resemble interface dermatitis to the pathologist unarmed with information relevant to the gross pathology and biopsy site. Nevi from acral and genital skin, as well as the superficial components of many congenital nevi, show architectural features reminiscent of dysplastic nevi; unless clinical information is complete, pathologic evaluation may result in an erroneous

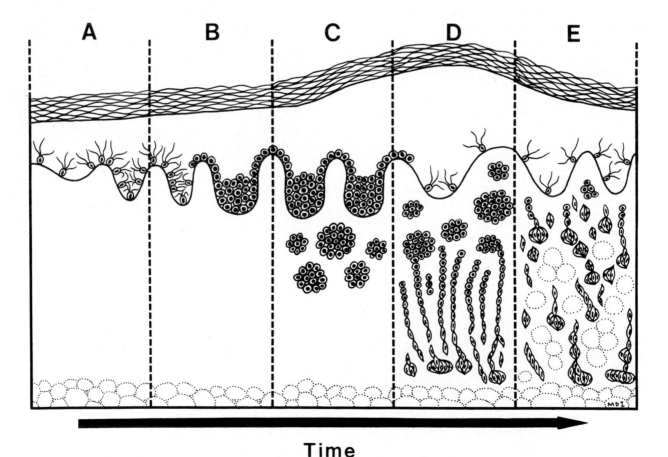

Figure 13–1. Natural evolution of a melanocytic nevus. Proliferation of normal melanocytes along the dermal-epidermal junction (A) leads to lentiginous hyperplasia and eventual nevic cell transformation to form a lentiginous junctional nevus (B). Nested nevic cells at rete tips, over time, grow as nests within the underlying dermis to form a compound nevus (C). The intraepidermal component then involutes (D), and the purely dermal nevus that remains undergoes maturation, evidenced by diminution in size of cells at the base, and eventual diffuse neural transformation of nevic cells within the dermal compartment (E). A minority of nevi will show aberrant growth, developing dysplastic, potentially premalignant features.

diagnostic conclusion. Perhaps in no other area of dermato-pathology is clinicopathologic correlation as essential as in melanocytic tumors.

GENERAL HISTOLOGY AND TEMPORAL EVOLUTION

Figure 13–1 provides a schematic interpretation of the history of a common acquired nevus. Note that the common acquired nevus begins as a zone of noncontiguous lentiginous melanocytic hyperplasia (see Fig. 13–1A), probably on sun-exposed skin, which may be subclinical or correlate with a regular tan macule (i.e., lentigo). With nevus cell transformation, nests of rounded nevus cells form along the dermal-epidermal interface in concert with contiguous lentiginous melanocytic proliferation (see Fig. 13–1B). Over time, similar nests extend from this lentiginous junctional nevus into the superficial dermis, forming a compound nevus (see Fig. 13–1C). As the junctional component is lost, dermal nevus cells extend into the deeper layers, a process often characterized by progressive *maturation* of the more superficial nests of large pigmented nevus cells into deeper cords of relatively nonpigmented nevus cells and finally into deepest fascicles and organoid aggregates of nevus cells with cytologic and histochemical characteristics of neural tissue (see Fig. 13–1D). Maturation is also associated with decreased size of nevus cells as they descend into the dermis. Very old nevi may become entirely neural in appearance (see Fig. 13–1E), and mature fat may be admixed with these transformed nevus cells as lesions involute.

HISTOLOGY OF SPECIFIC DISORDERS

Melanocytic Hyperplasia[1, 2]

- BASAL CELL LAYER HYPERPIGMENTATION
- WITH (LENTIGO) OR WITHOUT (EPHELIS) ASSOCIATED LENTIGINOUS MELANOCYTIC HYPERPLASIA
- VARIABLE MELANIN INCONTINENCE WITHIN PAPILLARY DERMIS
- VARIABLE ASSOCIATED ACTINIC CHANGES

Strictly speaking, an *ephelid* or freckle represents hyper-activity of melanocytes with respect to pigment donation to adjacent keratinocytes, rather than a true hyperplasia, as represented by a *lentigo*. Clinically, simple freckles are light tan, uniform, 2- to 4-mm, pigmented macules with slightly irregular borders. They occur on sun-exposed body surfaces, particularly in lightly pigmented individuals. Lentigines are poorly circumscribed, tan or brown, slightly variegated, 4- to 10-mm macules that occur preferentially on sun-exposed skin (Fig. 13–2A). They may occur indolently with advancing age, or suddenly after actinic damage. Multiple lentigines have been reported consequent to psoralen and UV therapy (i.e., PUVA freckles). Because lentigines are larger and more variegated than true freckles, they are not uncommonly biopsied to exclude melanocytic dysplasia or radial growth phase melanoma, such as lentigo maligna. In certain anatomic sites, lentigines are deeply pigmented, such as the lesion that char-

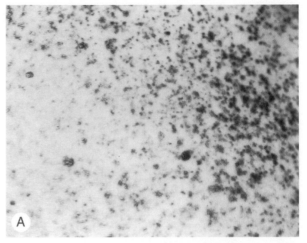
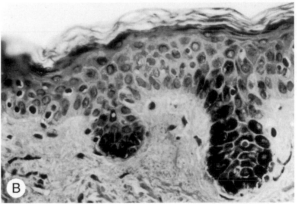
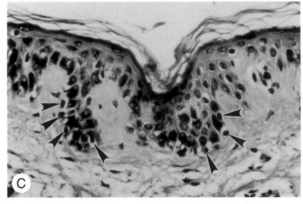

Figure 13–2. Melanocytic hyperplasia. **(A)** Multiple lentigines are present in sun-exposed skin. **(B)** Melanocytic hyperactivity begins as increased pigment donation to basal keratinocytes, resulting in increased basal layer melanization and macular hyperpigmentation, referred to as a freckle or ephelis. **(C)** True melanocytic hyperplasia usually occurs in association with basal cell layer hyperpigmentation, and is manifested by increased numbers of melanocytes at rete tips *(arrowheads)*, producing a lentigo clinically. Unlike a freckle, a lentigo will appear slightly raised with side lighting.

acteristically occurs on the lower lip, termed the *lower labial macule*. This deep pigmentation, as well as irregularities in border, may cause alarm clinically, resulting in biopsy to exclude labial melanoma. Lentigo-like hyperpigmentation associated with increased density of terminal hairs represents a poorly understood acquired hamartoma called *Becker nevus*.

At scanning magnification, a freckle is characterized by basal cell hyperpigmentation, often with accentuation in rete

Table 13–1. DIFFERENTIAL DIAGNOSIS OF EPHELIDES AND LENTIGINES

DISORDER	CLINICAL APPEARANCE	BASAL LAYER	MELANOCYTES
Ephelis	Regular, uniform, tan-brown macule 2–4 mm	Hyperpigmented	Normal
Lentigo	Irregular, variegated macule 4–10 mm	Hyperpigmented; rete thinned and elongated	Hyperplastic
Café-au-lait macule	2 mm or larger	Slightly hyperpigmented	Normal number; macromelanosomes

ridges. At closer inspection, melanocytes are normal in number, and most of the melanin pigment is observed to reside in basal keratinocytes (Fig. 13–2B). In contrast, in addition to basal cell layer hyperpigmentation, a lentigo demonstrates noncontiguous melanocytic hyperplasia (Fig. 13–2C). Rete ridges may be slightly thinned and elongated, and the underlying dermis may show mild fibrosis and melanin pigment incontinence. Melanin granules in both freckles and lentigines tend to be finely particulate. Large, rounded melanin granules may correlate with macromelanosomes. These may be incidental findings in some lentigines, but when they occur in conjunction with the histology of a large freckle, clinical correlation should be sought to exclude the possibility that the lesion sampled was a café-au-lait macule, which potentially may be associated with neurofibromatosis. The clinical and histologic features that separate ephelides from lentigines appear in Table 13–1.

Common Acquired Melanocytic Nevi[3–6]

- SYMMETRICAL PROLIFERATION OF NESTED NEVUS CELLS
- INTRAEPIDERMAL NEVUS NESTS CONCENTRATED AT RETE TIPS
- MATURATION AT BASE
- CYTOLOGY WITH DELICATE CHROMATIN, INCONSPICUOUS NUCLEOLI
- VARIABLE LENTIGINOUS COMPONENT

Common acquired melanocytic nevi are by convention divided into junctional, compound, and dermal types. Other than as an attempt to correlate histology with clinical appearance and to understand the natural progression of these neoplasms, these distinctions are biologically insignificant. A summary of the salient clinical and histologic features of these three forms of acquired melanocytic nevus is provided in Table 13–2.

Junctional nevi present as relatively flat, radially symmetrical zones of hyperpigmentation (Fig. 13–3A). Histologically, their hallmark is the formation of nevus cell nests (arbitrarily defined here as three or more nevus cells in aggregate), preferentially located at the tips of epidermal rete ridges (Fig. 13–3B). Nevus cells are round, uniform cells that contain centrally located nuclei with delicate chromatin patterns, inconspicuous nucleoli, and occasional pseudoinclusions. Pseudoinclusions are invaginations of cytoplasm producing a crisp, rounded, pale, eosinophilic body within a nucleus when viewed in a thin cross section. Because some junctional nevi appear to arise from regions of lentiginous melanocytic hyperplasia which may or may not correlate with clinical lentigines, there may be residual hyperplasia of benign melanocytes along the dermal-epidermal junction (i.e., lentiginous junctional nevus). Unlike junctional nevi, compound nevi are sharply circumscribed, pigmented papules (Fig. 13–4A). Their elevation is attributable to the remarkable tendency of nevus cells to symmetrically invade the underlying dermis (Fig. 13–4B), forming dermal nests and cords of nevus cells that progressively mature as they

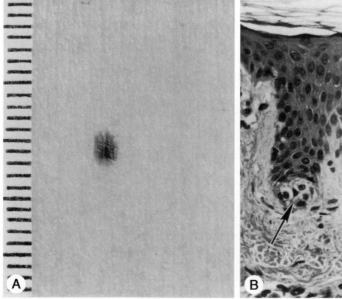
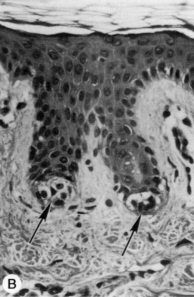

Figure 13–3. Junctional nevus. **(A)** Clinically, junctional nevi are small, slightly elevated, uniformly colored, brown papules. **(B)** Histologically, there are small, rounded nests of nevus cells at the tips of the epidermal rete ridges (*arrows*). The absence of dermal fibrosis or bridging of nests is evidence of aberrant growth.

Table 13–2. DIFFERENTIAL DIAGNOSIS OF ACQUIRED JUNCTIONAL, COMPOUND, AND DERMAL MELANOCYTIC NEVI

TYPE OF NEVUS	CLINICAL APPEARANCE	EPIDERMIS	DERMIS
Junctional nevus	1–4-mm tan-to-dark brown macules or slightly elevated papules	Nests at rete tips; variable lentiginous hyperplasia	Uninvolved
Compound nevus	1–7-mm tan-brown papules	Identical to junctional nevus	Nests (top), cords (middle), neural change (deep)
Dermal nevus	2–7-mm pink-to-flesh-colored papules	Uninvolved	Identical to compound nevus; neural change may predominate

penetrate into the depths of the underlying connective tissue (Fig. 13–4C). This maturation is most pronounced in older lesions that have lost their junctional component (i.e., pure dermal nevi; Fig. 13–5). In these older lesions, superficial junctional nest-like aggregates of nevus cells capable of mel-

anin pigment synthesis (i.e., type A nevus cells) give rise to downgrowth into the dermis by cords of tyrosinase-negative nevus cells which are incapable of pigment synthesis (i.e., type B nevus cells). These type B nevus cells eventually are

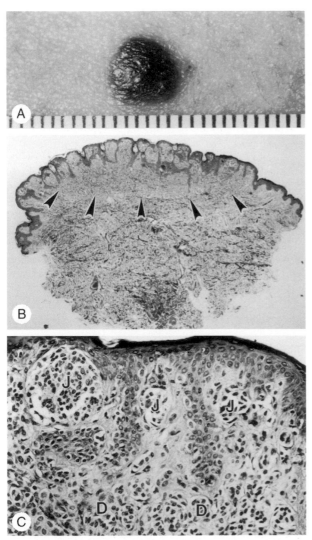

Figure 13–4. Compound nevus. **(A)** In contrast to lentigo and junctional nevus, the compound nevus is more raised and dome-shaped. Note the uniform pigment distribution and symmetry, which are indicators of the benign nature of this process. **(B)** Histologic cross section of a compound nevus shows a symmetrical proliferation of cells at the dermal-epidermal junction and within the superficial dermis, the lower border of which is indicated (*arrowheads*). There often is associated epidermal hyperplasia. **(C)** The nevus is composed of both junctional (J) and dermal (D) nevus cell nests. The dermal nevus nests are routinely smaller than those located at the dermal-epidermal junction.

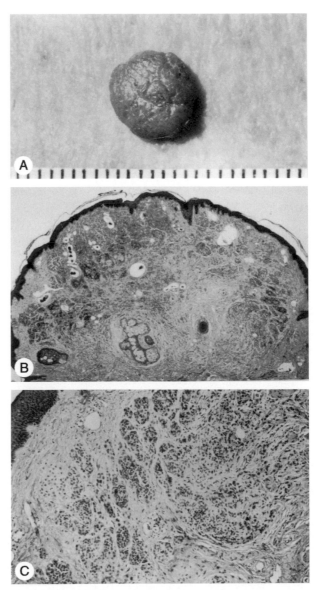

Figure 13–5. Dermal nevus. **(A)** This lesion is larger than the compound nevus depicted in Figure 13–4A. It is lighter in pigmentation and shows an irregular surface texture. However, it retains symmetry and uniformity of residual pigmentation. **(B)** Scanning magnification of a dermal nevus reveals nests within the superficial and deep dermis. **(C)** The nevus cells grow in superficial nests, mid-dermal cords, and as deep dermal, relatively small spindle cells exhibiting neural differentiation (*lower right*).

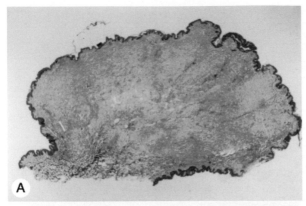

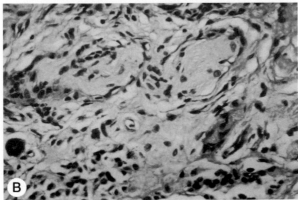

Figure 13–6. Dermal nevus with neurotization. **(A)** At low magnification, this lesion could be mistaken for a pedunculated neurofibroma. **(B)** At higher magnification, nevus cells are fusiform and show prominent neural differentiation, including formation of Meisner corpuscle-like structures. Differentiation from tumors of true neural origin often depends on detection of residua of conventionally nested nevus cells just beneath the dermal-epidermal interface.

destined to become neuroid cells, with spindle-like contours and histochemical profiles akin to neural tissue (i.e., type C nevus cells). Very old dermal nevi, which are devoid of residual epidermal (i.e., junctional) components, are comprised exclusively of type C cells, resulting in confusion between these lesions and neurofibromas (Fig. 13–6A, B). Although both lesions are commonly replete with mast cells, only neurofibromas have small nerve twigs interspersed within the cellular portions of the tumor.

Congenital Melanocytic Nevi[7–9]

- USUALLY COMPOUND NEVI
- ARCHITECTURE OF INTRAEPIDERMAL COMPONENT SIMILAR TO THAT OF DYSPLASTIC NEVI
- DERMAL COMPONENT DEEP AND/OR ASSOCIATED WITH HAMARTOMATOUS GROWTH
- HAMARTOMATOUS COMPONENT CONSISTS OF:
  Adnexal Adventitial Growth
  Adnexal Epithelial Nests

  Perineural Extension
  Vascular Invagination
  Intramuscular Infiltration
- ANOMALOUS EPIDERMAL AND/OR MESENCHYMAL COMPONENT

Clinically, congenital melanocytic nevi typically are present at birth in as many as 1% of all newborns. Like all hamartomas, however, they may become grossly apparent or prominent only months or years after birth. Moreover, they frequently are associated with malformations of other cutaneous structures, including the surface epidermis, adnexae, and dermal mesenchyme. Congenital melanocytic nevi may be large (i.e., giant congenital nevi), may involve the cutaneous surface like an article of clothing (i.e., "garment nevi"; Fig. 13–7A), or may be small, leading to confusion with acquired melanocytic nevi, especially when they are clinically perceptible only an interval after birth. Giant congenital nevi are associated with a clear-cut tendency for malignant degeneration, and removal is generally indicated if staged surgical procedures are feasible. Alternatively, close clinical follow-up and biopsy of regions in which pigmentation or degree of induration changes is indicated.

Microscopically, congenital nevi resemble common acquired nevi in numerous respects. The following features, however, are extremely helpful in the diagnostic recognition of congenital nevi:

1. Lesions are often broad, involving many millimeters of the epidermal surface.
2. The epidermis involved by congenital nevi frequently exhibits a verrucous or seborrheic keratosis–like hyperplasia (Fig. 13–7B).
3. The intraepidermal component of congenital nevi usually demonstrates some degree of anomalous architectural growth, such as bridging and coalescence of adjacent rete ridges.
4. The dermal component of congenital nevi may extend very deeply (Fig. 13–7C) and insidiously as single, mesenchyme-like cells into the dermis (e.g., on the scalp, where nevus cells may even involve the galea aponeurotica).
5. Dermal nevus cells often originate as nests within adnexal epithelium (e.g., eccrine ducts, hair follicles).
6. Dermal nevus cells may invaginate into lymphatic spaces, producing a pseudoinvasive pattern (Fig. 13–7D).
7. Dermal nevus cells frequently infiltrate perineural adventitia (Fig. 13–7E).

It is imperative that congenital nevi are sampled carefully to accurately determine their margins and to ascertain whether malignant degeneration is present. Large lesions should be inked, and representative margins of well-fixed specimens should be liberally sampled. Close examination with a hand lens is indicated to determine regions of nodularity and color variegation within the lesion. Such regions should be selectively examined histologically. Although dogma suggests that the dermal components of congenital nevi, in contrast to acquired nevi, are the first to undergo malignant degeneration, both intraepidermal and dermal nevus cells are susceptible.

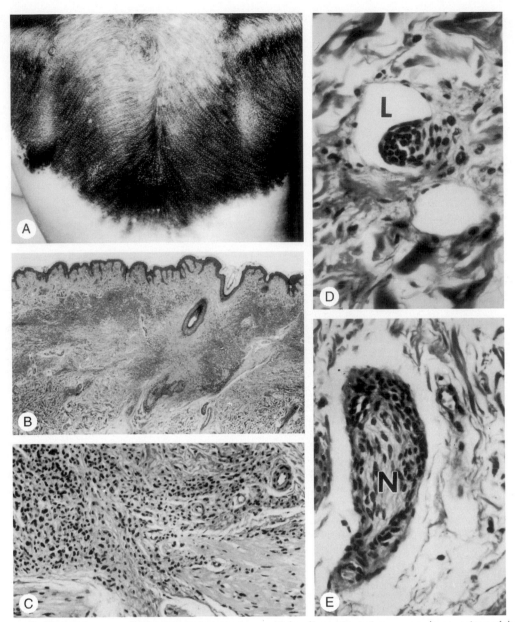

Figure 13–7. Congenital melanocytic nevus. **(A)** Large, garment-type, congenital melanocytic nevi may cover large regions of the body surface and show extensive trichogenesis. **(B, C)** A clue to diagnostic recognition of congenital melanocytic nevi at scanning magnification is the diffusely permeative quality of the dermal component. Congenital melanocytic nevi also commonly show extension about eccrine ducts and neurovascular bundles, nest formation within adnexal epithelium, **(D)** invagination into lymphatic lumina (L), and **(E)** involvement of neural adventitia (N).

Blue Nevus[10, 11]

- HIGHLY DENDRITIC NEVUS CELLS WITHIN DERMAL COLLAGEN
- PROMINENT MELANIZATION OF NEVIC CELL DENDRITES
- ASSOCIATED DERMAL FIBROPLASIA, OFTEN MARKED
- ABSENCE OF INTRAEPIDERMAL COMPONENT
- CELLULAR AND PENETRATING VARIANTS

The gross pathology of the blue nevus is unusual in that it is precisely as the clinical language predicts. Lesions range from 2 to 10 mm, are blue-black papules, and exhibit a symmetrical, dome-shaped architecture with an even, smooth peripheral border. The color of blue nevi is believed to result from reflection and refraction patterns of visible light as it interacts with brown melanin pigment within the deep dermis. However, blue nevi located within the superficial dermis may have a similar clinical appearance. This suggests that the depth of brown pigment within connective tissue is not the sole determinant of the characteristic blue-black color of blue nevi that so often results in confusion with malignant melanoma clinically.

At scanning magnification, blue nevi may be confused with a pigmented scar, dermatofibroma, or spindle cell mel-

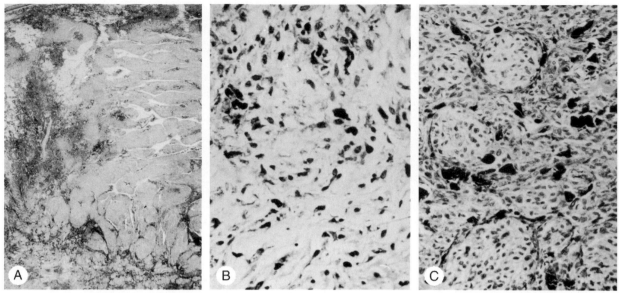

Figure 13–8. Blue nevus and variants. **(A)** This cellular blue nevus contains regions that are typical of ordinary blue nevus (**A**, left side of panel; **B**) and more cellular areas typical of this variant form (**A**, right side of panel; **C**). These lesions may show expansile, asymmetrical growth into the deep dermis and subcutis, mimicking melanoma. **(B)** Ordinary blue nevi are characterized by proliferation of highly dendritic pigmented nevus cells within a fibrotic, superficial to mid-dermal stroma. These cells must be differentiated from pigment-laden histiocytes, which do not display prominent, melanin-containing dendrites. **(C)** Cellular blue nevi are composed of large, nonpigmented epithelioid cells, often admixed with pigmented, dendritic cells.

anoma. Lesions are generally symmetrical and composed of an admixture of pigmented dendritic melanocytes and non-pigmented spindle cells (i.e., fibroblasts). These cells proliferate within the superficial or superficial and deep dermis. At higher magnification, the lesions typically have particulate melanin granules within well-defined, thin dendrites (Fig. 13–8B). This is an important distinction from pigment-laden melanophages that lack these delicate cytoplasmic extensions. Admixture or juxtaposition of these elements with those of conventional acquired melanocytic dermal nevi warrants the designation of *combined nevus* (i.e., dermal nevocellular nevus and blue nevus). Blue nevi are closely related to dermal melanocytomas, in which pigmented dendritic melanocytes are detected beneath the epidermal layer. The three most common forms of dermal melanocytomas are the *mongolian spot*, *nevus of Ito*, and *nevus of Ota*. None of these lesions is common and all involve subtle infiltration of superficial and sometimes deep reticular dermis by pigmented dendritic melanocytes (Table 13–3).

A variant of the blue nevus is the *cellular blue nevus*. Unlike the ordinary blue nevus, this lesion presents as a relatively large (i.e., 1 cm to several centimeters) blue-black, nodular tumor often located in the lumbosacral skin of young adults. Histologically, cellular blue nevi typically involve the full thickness of the reticular dermis, often presenting as dumbell-shaped nodules in cross section. In this manner, an expansile nodule may be formed at the deepest extent of the tumor, producing an alarming appearance at gross sectioning and at low magnification (Fig. 13–8A). Cytologically, tumors are composed of spindle cells at the periphery that is indistinguishable from a blue nevus. The more cellular regions generally predominate toward the center of the lesion (Fig. 13–8C). These areas contain heavily pigmented spindle cells in contiguity with oval to rounded epithelioid cells. These epithelioid cells contain less melanin pigment then the spindle cells, and they have enlarged nuclei with occasionally prominent nucleoli but consistently thin, uniform nuclear membranes and a background of delicate chromatin. Although

Table 13–3. DIFFERENTIAL DIAGNOSIS OF BLUE NEVUS AND DERMAL MELANOCYTOSES

DISORDER	CLINICAL APPEARANCE	HISTOLOGIC APPEARANCE	ASSOCIATIONS
Blue nevus	Blue-black papule or nodule; confused with melanoma	Superficial or superficial and deep proliferation of dendritic, pigmented melanocytes; variable fibrosis	None
Mongolian spot	Congenital blue-black macule on lower back or buttocks	Rare dendritic, pigmented melanocytes in mid-dermis to deep dermis; no melanophages	Infants of Asian descent
Nevi of Ito and Ota	Trigeminal distribution (Ota); supraclavicular and suprascapular (Ito)	Dendritic, pigmented melanocytes diffusely in reticular dermis; melanophages present	Cutaneous and leptomeningeal melanoma (Ota)

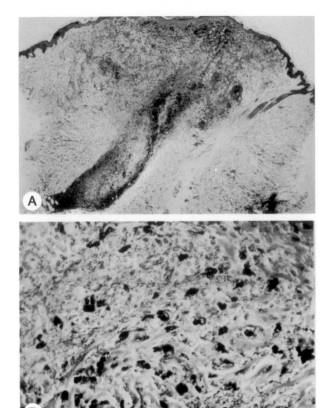

Figure 13–9. Deep penetrating nevus. **(A)** The contour of these nevi, like that of cellular blue nevi, is asymmetrical, with deep extension by tongues pushing into the subcutaneous fat. **(B)** Like cellular blue nevi, lesions are composed of pigmented and relatively nonpigmented cells, although the former tend to be nondendritic in deep penetrating nevi.

cells are found at the dermal-epidermal junction in most cases (Fig. 13–9A). The dermal component varies from variably pigmented spindle and epithelioid cell morphology to smaller, acquired nevic cell differentiation; dendritic pigmented cells, observed in blue and cellular blue nevi, are not present in deep penetrating nevi. Rather, heavily pigmented cells are generally melanophages that lack delicate dendritic extensions. The cytoplasm of these rounded cells is filled with particulate melanin (Fig. 13–9B). Lesional nests may surround skin appendages, and maturation, which consists of gradual diminution in cell size as nevus cells extend more deeply into the dermis, is subtle or incomplete and may lead to confusion with malignant melanoma. In some lesions, more heavily pigmented cells may be preferentially distributed within the deeper confines of the lesion (i.e., the inverted type A pattern). However, mitotic activity is rare to absent; individual cell necrosis is not present; and the nuclear chromatin pattern remains delicate, with thin, uniform nuclear membranes reminiscent of nevus cells. Because cellular blue nevi and deep penetrating nevi are encountered more commonly than is generally appreciated, Table 13–4 presents criteria for their differentiation from nodular malignant melanoma.

Halo Nevus[12, 14]

- COMPOUND NEVI WITH MARKED LYMPHOCYTIC INFILTRATION
- DEGENERATIVE ATYPIA OF NEVUS CELLS
- MELANIN PIGMENT INCONTINENCE WITHIN UPPER DERMIS

The gross pathology of the halo nevus consists of lesions that range from 2 to 10 mm. These nevi are well-circumscribed tan-brown papules, and are characterized by a hypopigmented peripheral zone (Fig. 13–10A). Lesions are generally noted on the trunk and are often first observed during summer months, probably because tanning accentuates the surrounding zone of depigmentation. Most halo nevi disappear over the course of several months, leaving a zone of hypopigmentation (Fig. 13–10B) that eventually repigments. It is generally believed that halo nevi represent a cytotoxic host response to preexisting acquired melanocytic nevi, although most lesions are devoid of associated dysplasia indicative of malignant degeneration which might be expected to stimulate immunosurveillance mechanisms.

Histologically, halo nevi consist of compound melano-

mitoses may be observed, a rate of greater than one mitotic figure per square millimeter (i.e., about 10 high-power fields) should lead to the designation of atypical cellular blue nevus. Because these lesions possess architectural and some cytologic overlap with malignant melanoma, consultation, complete excision, and close follow-up may be indicated for any tumor not fulfilling all of the characteristic clinical and histologic criteria for cellular blue nevus.

An additional, recently recognized variant of the blue nevus is the *deep penetrating nevus.* Clinical lesions most often occur on the head, neck, and shoulder and are commonly confused with blue nevus. Histologically, the architecture is wedge-shaped, and unlike blue nevi, nests of nevus

Table 13–4. DIFFERENTIAL DIAGNOSIS OF CELLULAR BLUE NEVUS, DEEP PENETRATING NEVUS, AND NODULAR MALIGNANT MELANOMA

DISORDER	CLINICAL APPEARANCE	ARCHITECTURE	CYTOLOGY
Cellular blue nevus	Blue-black papule or nodule on lumbosacral skin	Asymmetrical, with endophytic extension into subcutis	Dendritic, pigmented nevus cells and epithelioid, nonpigmented nevus cells
Deep, penetrating nevus	Blue-black papule or nodule on head, neck, or upper extremity	Asymmetrical, with endophytic extension into subcutis	Nondendritic, pigmented melanophages and epithelioid, variably pigmented nevic cells
Nodular melanoma	Blue-black nodule anywhere on body surface	Asymmetrical	Atypia, mitoses, cellular necrosis*

*Features not observed in blue nevi and deep penetrating nevi.

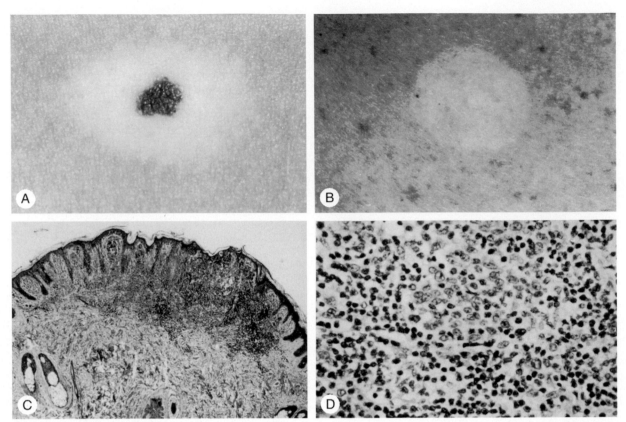

Figure 13–10. Halo nevus. **(A)** A compound nevus is surrounded by a symmetrical, vitiligo-like halo. **(B)** In time, some lesions will regress completely, leaving only a hypopigmented macule. **(C)** At low magnification, a relatively symmetrical compound nevus appears abnormally basophilic because of the associated lymphocytic infiltrate. **(D)** At higher power, individual nevus cells are surrounded by swarms of infiltrating lymphocytes. The normally nested contours of the nevus cell aggregates are jagged and irregular, presumably as a result of partial inflammatory regression induced by the cytotoxic immune response.

cytic nevi that are heavily infiltrated by lymphocytes (Fig. 13–10C). The infiltrating cells permeate the dermal component of the nevus, surrounding individual nevus cells and creating a jagged and irregular contour in an otherwise radially symmetrical lesion (Fig. 13–10D). Because this cytotoxic attack may result in nevus cell injury and death, foci of degenerative atypia and necrosis, which should not be confused with dysplasia and malignancy, may be present. Occasional lesions may be so heavily infiltrated by lymphocytes that nevus cells are only apparent after careful scrutiny, especially for nests along the dermal-epidermal interface. Melanin pigment incontinence is often present in the upper dermis, the sequela of nevus cell destruction.

Spitz Nevus[15–20]

- USUALLY COMPOUND NEVUS WITH SPINDLE AND/OR EPITHELIOID CELL DIFFERENTIATION
- VERTICALLY ORIENTED FASCICLES AND NESTS ALONG THE DERMAL-EPIDERMAL INTERFACE
- DYSKERATOTIC MELANOCYTES (I.E., KAMINO BODIES)
- CLEFTS SEPARATING INTRAEPIDERMAL NESTS FROM KERATINOCYTES

- INFILTRATIVE DERMAL COMPONENT WITH MATURATION
- REACTIVE CYTOLOGIC ATYPIA

The clinical presentation of Spitz nevus (i.e., spindle and epithelioid cell nevus) generally involves the skin of children and young adults. There is a tendency for lesions to be nonpigmented, with underlying vascularity predominating the clinical picture. Accordingly, lesions are often confused clinically with hemangiomas. Occasionally, lesions occur in showers or as primary tumors with peripheral satellites (Fig. 13–11A). Although children are preferentially affected, Spitz nevi may also be observed in adolescents and young and middle-aged adults.

The histopathology of Spitz nevi is characteristic and should not be confused with melanoma, even though these lesions were originally described as "juvenile melanomas." At scanning magnification, lesions are symmetrical compound nevi that may extend either superficially or deeply into the reticular dermis. Some Spitz nevi actually are pure junctional nevi, whereas others are exclusively dermal. Often, there is associated epidermal hyperplasia (Fig. 13–11B). The characteristic diagnostic feature of Spitz nevi is their tendency to be composed of coalescent fascicles of nevus cells, which frequently results in a "raining-down" pattern from the epidermal layer into the dermis (Fig. 13–11C, D). Fascicles may be composed of an admixture of

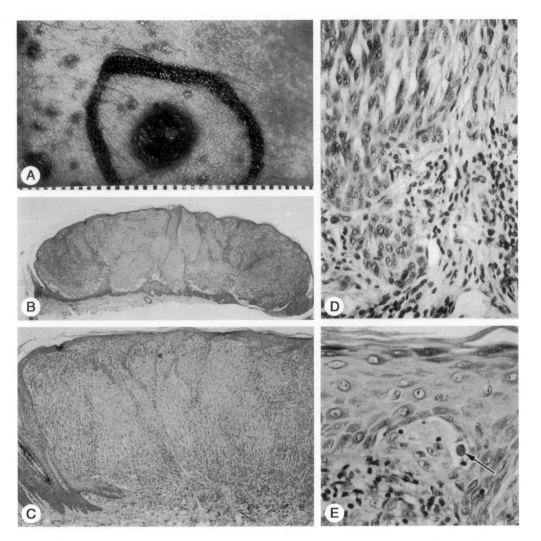

Figure 13–11. Spindle and epithelioid cell nevus. **(A)** This rounded, dome-shaped nevus has a deep red color clinically and is surrounded by a shower of satellite nevi. **(B, C)** Although nevus nests along the dermal-epidermal junction appear large and coalescent, the lesion is bilaterally symmetrical at scanning magnification, and significant pagetoid spread is not observed. **(C, D)** At higher magnification, epithelioid and fusiform cells are arranged in fascicles to produce a "raining-down" pattern. The stroma may be inflamed and often shows hyalinization and proliferation of dilated vessels. **(E)** Along the dermal-epidermal junction, small eosinophilic bodies (i.e., Kamino bodies; *arrow*) representing degenerated nevus cells are frequently observed.

fusiform to epithelioid cells, and intraepidermal nested fascicles are characteristically separated from adjacent keratinocytes by crescent-shaped clefts. Pagetoid spread of single or grouped cells into the overlying hyperplastic epidermal layer may occur, although significant spread to the level of the stratum granulosum is generally absent.

Cytologically, Spitz nevus cells are characterized by enlarged, often pleomorphic nuclei that contain prominent, centrally located nucleoli (see Fig. 13–11*D, E*). Unlike nodular melanoma cells, however, the background chromatin pattern is delicate and evenly dispersed, and the nuclear membrane is uniformly thin and smoothly contoured. The cytoplasm is not granular but rather is filled with a finely fenestrated, net-like array of amphophilic material superimposed on pale pink background. This histologic picture likely reflects abundant ribosomes punctuated by mitochondria and other larger organelles within the cytoplasm of these highly activated cells. Another useful, albeit not entirely specific, feature in Spitz nevi is the finding of eosinophilic bodies along the dermal-epidermal junction (so-called Kamino bodies) (see Fig. 13–11*E*). These bodies are about the size of a solitary nevus cell and are believed to represent the necrotic residua of effete nevus cells of the intraepidermal component. Accordingly, they are analogous to colloid bodies, which may be seen in conditions in which basal keratinocytes

undergo necrosis. The stroma of spindle and epithelioid cell nevi is often vascularized and hyalinized, particularly in the subepidermal region. Older lesions may be exclusively dermal, with nevus cells embedded within a dense fibrotic stroma (i.e., *sclerosing Spitz nevi*).

An important feature of Spitz nevi is their tendency to show maturation at the base of the lesion (see Fig. 13–11*D*). This results in a gradual decrease in cell size as nevus cells grow more deeply into the dermis. Mitotic activity may be observed, particularly within the more superficial nevus cells; however, frequent, deep, or atypical mitoses are not usual and should raise the possibility of melanoma with spindle and epithelioid cell features. Occasional lesions that do not qualify as ordinary Spitz nevi as a result of atypical features (e.g., excessive pagetoid spread, unusually high mitotic rate) are designated as *atypical Spitz nevi,* and conservative reexcision is generally recommended. Diagnostic confusion with nodular malignant melanoma is the most common pitfall; Table 13–5 summarizes the salient differences that separate Spitz nevi from nodular melanoma.

A variant form of Spitz nevus is the *pigmented spindle cell nevus of Reed.* This lesion is relatively small, well-circumscribed, uniformly pigmented, dark brown–black nevus that characteristically is found on the lower extremities of young adult women. Most lesions measure between 3 and

Table 13–5. DIFFERENTIAL DIAGNOSIS OF SPITZ NEVUS AND NODULAR MELANOMA

SPITZ NEVUS	NODULAR MELANOMA
Smaller (often <6 mm in diameter)	Larger (often >6 mm in diameter)
Symmetrical	Often asymmetrical
Epidermal layer hyperplastic	Epidermal layer normal or thinned
Fascicular, raining-down cellular orientation	Random cellular axes
Variable pagetoid spread with upper epidermal layers unaffected	Often marked pagetoid spread with involvement of stratum granulosum
Maturation present	Maturation absent
Tendency to form Kamino bodies	Kamino bodies rare or absent
Mitoses rare, especially in deep layers	Mitoses common, involving deep layers
Atypical mitoses absent	Atypical mitoses may be present
Cytoplasm amphophilic, net-like	Cytoplasm eosinophilic, granular

Recurrent Melanocytic Nevi and Artifacts[21, 22]

- RAPID REPIGMENTATION AFTER EXCISION
- SCAR WITH MELANOPHAGES IN SUPERFICIAL DERMIS
- INTRAEPIDERMAL NESTS PREDOMINATE OVER SINGLE CELLS
- ABSENCE OF CYTOLOGIC ATYPIA OR MITOSES
- PAGETOID GROWTH RARE

There are a number of in vivo phenomena and post-biopsy processing artifacts that must be recognized in the accurate diagnosis of melanocytic nevi. Some of the more common artifacts are those that result from in vivo scarring (i.e., nevus entrapment and recurrent nevus phenomena), occur after freezing of formalin-fixed tissue, and appear as a result of fixation itself.

Nevi may recur after excision for at least two reasons. They may be inadequately excised, which often results in persistence of relatively nonpigmented nevus cells within the forming dermal scar tissue (i.e., nevus entrapment). They also may return as a result of presumed inductive influences exerted by scarring on persistent melanocytes within the overlying epidermis. Such *recurrent nevi* usually result in intraepidermal reappearance of nevus nests even after excision of pure *dermal nevi*. Although both situations may produce nevus aggregates with altered architecture, the recurrent nevus phenomenon is the most problematic in distinguishing the histologic alterations produced from those of melanoma. Clinically, recurrent nevi present with a rapid return of pigmentation at a site of previous nevus excision. This is in contrast to local recurrence of melanoma, which generally occurs more slowly. Recurrent nevi often show irregularities in pigmentation and contour which, along with the rapid clinical reappearance and growth, cause alarm and prompt additional sampling.

The histology of recurrent nevi may have certain features in common with in situ malignant melanoma. These include a diameter greater than 6 mm, confluence and varia-

10 mm and show a smooth, well-defined border. Their deep color and occasional history of rapid growth, however, often raise the clinical concern of melanoma. Histologically, lesions are usually symmetrical and confined to the superficial dermal layers (Fig. 13–12A). The lesional cells are fusiform and may show fascicular, coalescent growth such as that observed in ordinary Spitz nevi (Fig. 13–12B), although prominent clefts separating nevus nests from keratinocytes are uncommon in pigmented spindle cell nevi. Intraepidermal mitoses may be numerous, although dermal mitoses are infrequent. If dermal mitoses are observed, they should raise the possibility of melanoma. Pagetoid spread is not prominent. A characteristic feature of pigmented spindle cell nevi is the presence of variable numbers of markedly pigmented melanophages admixed with the dermal component of the nevus, contributing to the often alarming clinical and histologic impression of a heavily pigmented lesion. The associated nevus cells show evidence of maturation; however, the stroma may be fibrotic and focally may resemble the lamellar fibroplasia observed in dysplastic nevi.

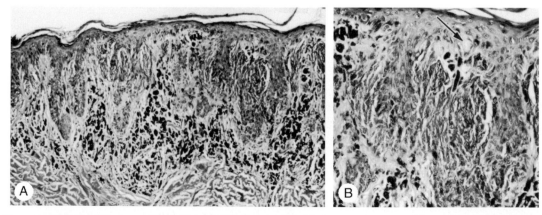

Figure 13–12. Pigmented spindle cell nevus. **(A, B)** These relatively superficial lesions retain some of the architectural and cytologic features of ordinary spindle and epithelioid cell nevi and therefore may be mistaken for dysplastic nevi or malignant melanoma. Lesions are generally symmetrical, composed predominantly by fascicles of spindle cells along the dermal-epidermal junction, and have marked melanin pigmentation, both within nevus cells and within aggregates of melanophages along the base of the dermal component. Note the pale Kamino body (*arrow*) in **B.**

bility in the size and shape of intraepidermal nests, occasional foci of pagetoid growth, and foci of heavy melanin pigmentation. However, in recurrent nevi, nests generally predominate over single cells, mitoses are seldom observed, and there is little or no cytologic atypia (Fig. 13–13A, B). At scanning magnification, the characteristic picture involves nested and occasional single-cell proliferation of nevus cells along a dermal-epidermal interface of a thinned epidermal layer devoid of rete ridges. These epidermal changes, along with the presence of an underlying dermal scar, signify that the anomalous architecture is an artifact of previous trauma to the site. Melanin pigment incontinence is frequently present within the dermis, directly subjacent to the nevus. Occasionally, artifactually distorted, entrapped dermal nevic cells are present within the underlying scar. Although the architectural disarray of the intraepidermal component may cause alarm at low magnification, higher-power magnification will disclose the cells in question to demonstrate their banal nuclear characteristics.

A common artifact hindering interpretation of melanocytic nevi that is observed particularly in winter months in more northern latitudes, is formalin-freeze artifact (Fig. 13–14A, B). This occurs when specimens fixed in formalin partially or completely freeze during transit. The artifact is characterized by striking cytoplasmic vacuolization that preferentially affects cells of the nevomelanocytic series. This results in cell enlargement with partial to complete displacement of cytoplasm and nucleus by single or coalescent, rounded, clear vacuoles. The degree of artifact may be so devastating as to render a nevus or melanoma unrecognizable. This devastating change may be avoided by adding an antifreeze agent to the formalin (e.g., 95% methyl alcohol added to the formalin to a final concentration of 10% methanol).

Some artifacts may be attributable solely to formalin fixation and subsequent tissue processing. This is the case with the ''venetian-blind'' effect observed in dermal nevus cells, in which lymphatic-like horizontal spaces are regularly interposed among cords of nevus cells (Fig. 13–14C). Nevi from women seem to be unusually predisposed to this alteration, which may be analogous to the epithelial-stromal separation artifact typical of basal cell carcinoma (see Chap. 11). Nevi with this change have been mistaken for vascular tumors, a pitfall that can be avoided by recognizing the repeating, horizontally stratified architecture of the artifactual spaces as well as by detecting foci of more superficial nevic nests, which seem to be resilient to cleavage.

Melanocytic Dysplasia and Dysplastic Nevi[23–28]

- NEVUS NESTS ENLARGED
- NEVUS NESTS ORIGINATE IN INTER-RETE SPACES
- NEVUS NESTS BRIDGE ACROSS ADJACENT RETE RIDGES
- RANDOM OR DIFFUSE NUCLEAR ENLARGEMENT, CONTOUR ANGULATION, HYPERCHROMASIA
- LAMELLAR PAPILLARY DERMAL FIBROSIS

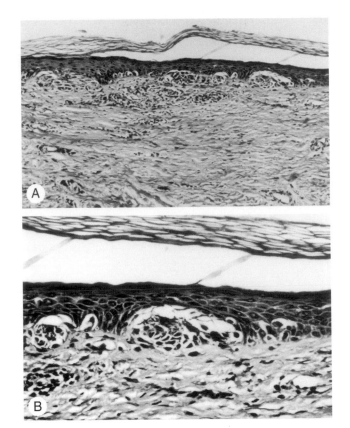

Figure 13–13. Recurrent nevus. **(A)** This lesion is characterized by primarily intraepidermal nevic cell growth overlying a healing scar. **(B)** Nevus cells may be dyshesive and grow in irregular and coalescent nests composed of pigmented cells of variable shapes and sizes; true cytologic atypia or significant pagetoid spread, however, are not observed.

- LYMPHOID INFILTRATE, PIGMENT INCONTINENCE, VASCULAR PROLIFERATION

The concept of melanocytic dysplasia is controversial. However, the notion that at least some benign melanocytic proliferations undergo step-wise alterations that progress from minimally dysplastic lesions to malignancy is now supported by an impressive array of morphologic, antigenic, functional, and genomic data. Because not all nevi with dysplasia are typical dysplastic nevi, the criteria for architectural and cytologic dysplasia, as well as the criteria that must be fulfilled for a designation of dysplastic nevus, are outlined at the beginning of this section and are further elaborated upon in the following text.

It may be helpful in the discussion of melanocytic dysplasia to consider a hypothetical temporal schema of dysplastic alteration (Fig. 13–15). Normal melanocytes along the basal cell layer may proliferate in a noncontiguous lentiginous fashion (stage A), an effect which may be stimulated focally, as in lentigo, or diffusely, as in chronically UV-irradiated skin. Eventually, nevus cell transformation (stage B) may occur at sites of lentiginous hyperplasia, resulting in lentiginous junctional nevi. Aberrant nevus cell growth (stage C) is heralded by the formation of enlarged, coalescent nests; random cytologic dysplasia (i.e., occasional enlarged cells with dark nuclei); and reactive stromal alterations, including lymphocytic infiltrate and lamellar fibroplasia. These

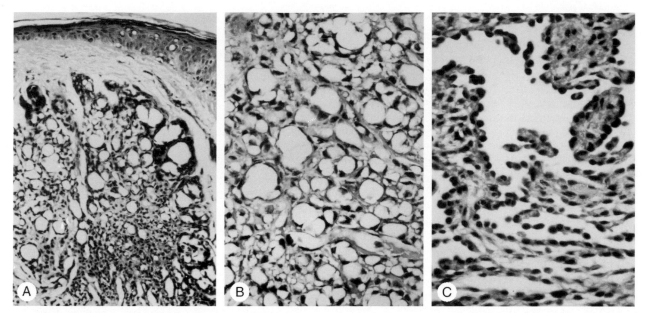

Figure 13–14. Common processing artifacts in nevi. **(A, B)** Coarse vacuolization occurs as a result of freezing followed by thawing of tissue transported in formalin. This artifact is usually seen in winter months, and should not be confused with balloon cell change in melanoma, or with metastatic signet-ring cell carcinoma. Note that in **A** even the more resilient keratinocytes show early vacuolization. **(C)** Lymphatic-like spaces are present in a dermal nevus as a result of dyshesion consequent to tissue preparation. The phenomenon may have a structural basis in impaired cell-cell adhesion between dermal nevus cells arranged in cords, and is responsible for the "venetian-blind" pattern of clefts seen in the dermal components of some ordinary acquired melanocytic nevi.

changes may signify the development of a lesion with the potential for further neoplastic progression, as opposed to involution to a neurotized dermal nevus, as is the case for most melanocytic nevi (see Fig. 13–1). Further tumor progression results in the emergence of a clone of malignant cells (stage D) with the initial ability to proliferate only within or in close proximity to the epidermal layer (i.e., radial growth phase melanoma). Residual remnants of the preexisting nevus may persist in the adjacent epidermis or subjacent dermis. Eventually, additional clones emerge with the selective ability to grow deeply into the dermis as tumorigenic nodules (i.e., nodules larger than intraepidermal nevus nests). These cells also may acquire the ability to invade lymphatic spaces and spread to lymph nodes. Systemic dissemination depends on the ability of invasive tumor cells to enter blood vessels and to metastasize to nonlymphoid viscera. Some melanomas appear to arise independently of a nevus cell intermediate, and thus may progress from stage A directly to stage D.

According to the broad concepts outlined previously, any melanocytic proliferation may have architectural dysplasia, cytologic dysplasia, or both without fully meeting the criteria for a dysplastic nevus. Accordingly, such lesions should be diagnosed descriptively (e.g., lentigo with cytologic dysplasia; compound nevus with architectural atypia). True dysplastic nevi, on the other hand, are diagnosed only by combined clinicopathologic criteria. The clinical criteria (Fig. 13–16A) are as follows:

- ACQUIRED PIGMENTED MACULES AND PAPULES FIRST APPEARING IN ADOLESCENCE
- MOST LESIONS HAVE A DIAMETER BETWEEN 5 AND 12 MM
- MACULAR COMPONENT ALWAYS PRESENT
- PAPULAR COMPONENT OFTEN PRESENT AND CENTRALLY LOCATED WITHIN MACULE
- VARIEGATED TAN-BROWN COLOR ON PINK BACKGOUNND
- IMPALPABLE, IRREGULAR, ILL-DEFINED BORDER

Histologically, scanning magnification reveals a lentiginous junctional or lentiginous compound nevus with architectural atypia consisting of bridging of adjacent nevus nests (Fig. 13–16B, C), origination of nests at rete edges or in inter-rete spaces (recall that normal nests grow from the tips of rete ridges), and expansive nests which may focally erode upward into the epidermal layer. These architectual alterations may be most pronounced at the edge of the lesion, where the macular, intraepidermal component predominates (i.e., the "shoulder" of the lesion). At higher magnification, individual nevus cells may show nuclear enlargement; contour angulation, often to form rhomboidal and rectangular configurations; and dense hyperchromasia, all of which are features of cytologic dysplasia. Cells affected in this manner also frequently show coarsely granulated (i.e., muddy) cytoplasm. Lamellar fibroplasia, consisting of fine lamellae of papillary dermal collagen concentrically encasing the nevus nests, is best appreciated at higher magnification. Less important findings that often accompany lamellar fibroplasia consist of vascular proliferation, a patchy lymphocytic infiltrate, and melanin pigment incontinence.

Fully evolved dysplastic nevi in patients with clinical signs that are compatible with multiple large atypical nevi are diagnosed as lentiginous compound dysplastic nevi. When the clinical history is not fully apparent, it is appropriate to note in the diagnostic report that nevi with this histology may occur as isolated lesions in many individuals, and the biological potential for further dysplastic or malignant

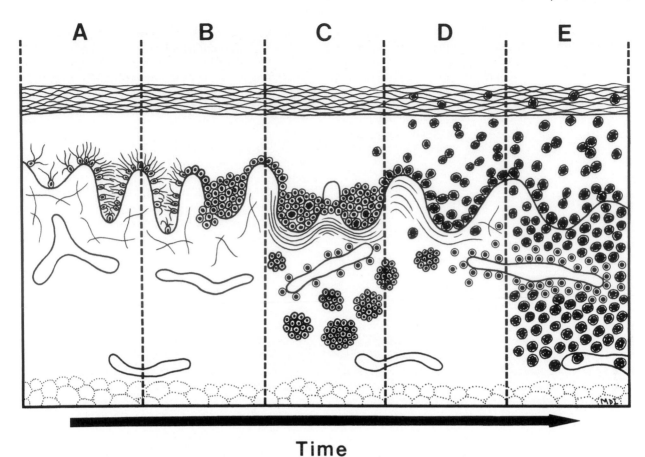

Time

Figure 13–15. Tumor progression to malignant melanoma. Normal melanocytes along the basal cell proliferate in lentiginous fashion (A) and eventually undergo nevus cell transformation (B). Aberrant nevus cell growth (C), consisting of enlarged, coalescent nests, random cytologic dysplasia, and reactive stromal alterations including lymphocytic infiltrate and lamellar fibroplasia, heralds the development of a lesion with the potential for further neoplastic progression, as opposed to involution to a neurotized dermal nevus, as is the case for most melanocytic nevi. Progression results in the emergence of a clone of malignant cells (D) with the ability to proliferate only within or in close proximity to the epidermal layer (i.e., radial growth phase melanoma). (E) Eventually, additional clones emerge with the ability to grow deeply into the dermis as tumorigenic nodules. Such cells also may acquire the ability to invade lymphatic spaces and spread to lymph nodes. Systemic dissemination depends on the ability to enter blood vessels and to metastasize to nonlymphoid viscera. Some melanomas appear to arise independently of a nevus cell intermediate and thus may progress from stage A directly to stage D.

Figure 13–16. Dysplastic nevus. **(A)** The clinical lesion is a large (i.e., >6 mm), asymmetrical, variably pigmented plaque with an irregular, notched border. **(B)** Histologically, there is a lentiginous compound nevus with prominent bridging of nevus nests across adjacent epidermal rete ridges. Some nests also arise aberrantly in interrete spaces (*arrow*). **(C)** Bridging of nests (*arrow*) is associated with lamellar fibrosis of the underlying papillary dermis (*arrowheads*) as well as a variable lymphoid response with pigment incontinence. Cells within the nests show focally enlarged, angulated, hyperchromatic nuclei. This is clearly a very different clinical and histologic picture than that observed for the majority of acquired melanocytic nevi (see Figs. 13–3 through 13–6).

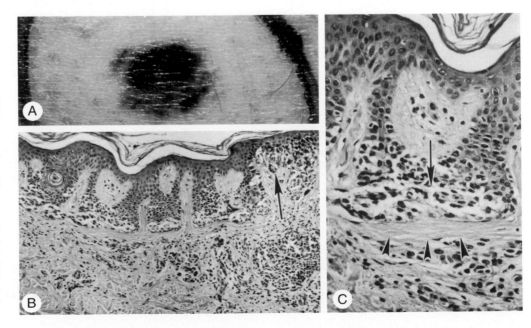

degeneration has not been established in these situations. Dysplastic nevi in individuals with clinical signs consistent with the dysplastic nevus (i.e., heritable melanoma) syndrome but with no family or personal history of melanoma probably have a low prospective lifetime risk (<10%) for the development of melanoma. On the other hand, dysplastic nevi in individuals with clinical signs consistent with the dysplastic nevus syndrome and *with* a family or personal history of melanoma have a high prospective lifetime risk for malignant degeneration (up to 100%).

Radial Growth Phase Melanoma[29–36]

- IRREGULARLY NESTED INTRAEPIDERMAL AND SUPERFICIAL DERMAL GROWTH
- ANOMALOUS INTRAEPIDERMAL PAGETOID AND/OR ADNEXAL SPREAD
- DIFFUSE CYTOLOGIC ANAPLASIA
- VARIABLE HOST RESPONSE

After dysplasia, the next step in tumor progression is radial growth phase melanoma. The radial growth phase is so termed because the tumor spreads centrifugally within the epidermal layer along the radius of an imperfect circle. Rare solitary and clustered cells may also involve the papillary dermis in radial growth (i.e., microinvasive melanoma). Vertical growth phase melanoma, on the other hand, involves tumorigenic dermal invasion in a direction perpendicular to the epidermal surface (discussed later).

Melanomas traditionally have been segregated into morphologic groups based on the presence or absence of a radial growth phase. Lesions that show little or no (<3 rete ridges) evidence of radial growth at the periphery of a vertical growth phase nodule are termed *nodular melanomas.* The vast majority of nodular melanomas were initiated by intraepidermal growth; however, at the time of excision, evidence of this pattern has been obliterated by preferential vertical growth. When radial growth is present, either at the edge of a vertical growth nodule or as pure radial growth disease, it is divided into three categories based upon clinicopathologic features. These categories are superficial spreading melanoma (SSM; Fig. 13–17), lentigo maligna melanoma (LMM; Fig. 13–18), and acral-lentiginous mucosal melanoma (ALMM; Fig. 13–19). Although it is true that not all early melanomas fit neatly into these three categories, many do, and because each lesion has distinctive clinicopathologic fea-

tures, the system remains justified and clinically useful. Moreover, because the morphology of metastases may relate to the type of radial growth within the primary lesion, the system may be critical for establishing the origin of distant tumor deposits, particularly in patients with more than one primary malignancy. Table 13–6 summarizes the salient differences among these three forms of radial growth phase disease.

Superficial spreading radial growth phase is generally characterized by an enlarging plaque that may or may not arise within a preexisting nevus. The gross pathology of lesions is typical, and public awareness of features intrinsic to SSM has resulted in prevention, early detection, and cure. Typical lesions are often larger than 1 cm; have an irregular, notched border; and are a variegated, pink-tan-brown-black color (see Fig. 13–17A). Patients often seek attention because of rapid increase in size of a preexisting lesion, deepening of color in a preexisting lesion, development of pink-white zones within already pigmented lesions, or localized pruritus or pain potentially related to host response. The clinical differential diagnosis that accompanies the pathology requisition may include seborrheic keratosis, pigmented actinic keratosis, or dysplastic nevus.

At scanning magnification, radial growth phase melanoma of the superficial spreading type is characterized by nested and single-cell spread of epithelioid malignant melanocytes within a normal or slightly hyperplastic epidermal layer (see Fig. 13–17B). Pagetoid cells resemble those of mammary and extramammary Paget disease and are present in all layers of the epidermis, including the stratum granulosum. Their presence is an important discriminator between similar spread in Spitz nevi and dysplastic nevi. At slightly higher magnification (e.g., 20×), irregularities in the size and shape of nested malignant melanocytes are encountered (see Fig. 13–17C). For example, whereas ordinary acquired nevi are characterized by uniform, rounded, small nests of nevus cells, SSM is typified by nonuniform, irregular, enlarged nests of atypical cells. Nests in SSM may be observed in all layers of the epidermis in a manner similar to the pagetoid spread of individual malignant melanocytes.

At high-power magnification, SSM cells are characteristically epithelioid in shape, with visible, variably pigmented, granular cytoplasm. Nuclei are large, irregular in size and shape, and contain prominent, often eosinophilic nucleoli. An important feature of melanoma nuclei, with respect to differentiating them from Spitz nevus cells, which

Table 13–6. TYPES OF RADIAL GROWTH PHASE MELANOMA

DIFFERENTIAL FEATURE	SUPERFICIAL SPREADING	LENTIGO MALIGNA	ACRAL-LENTIGINOUS/ MUCOSAL
Site	Trunk, legs, arms	Face, head	Hands, feet, mucosae
Age	Young to middle-aged	Elderly	Variable
Gross appearance	Irregular, variegated plaque	Deeply pigmented macule	Deeply pigmented macule
Time-course	Months to several years	One to several decades	Months to several years
Indicator of vertical growth	Nodule within plaque	Nodule within macule	Often macule remains unchanged
Architecture	Nested and pagetoid intraepidermal spread	Lentiginous intraepidermal spread; epidermal atrophy	Lentiginous intraepithelial spread; epithelial hyperplasia
Cytology	Epithelioid; nuclei vesicular	Variable (often fusiform); nuclei hyperchromatic	Variable (often fusiform); nuclei hyperchromatic

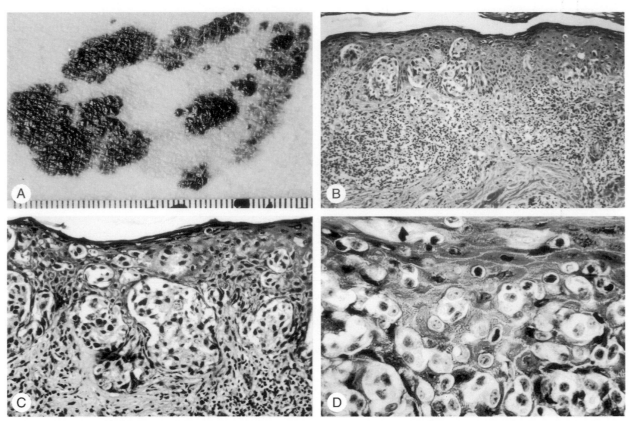

Figure 13–17. Melanoma: Superficial spreading radial growth. **(A)** The gross pathology of this melanoma is characterized by large size, irregularity in border and pigmentation, asymmetry, and striking zones of central regression; compare this clinical picture with the symmetrical and peripheral regression seen in halo nevi (see Fig. 13–10). **(B)** At scanning magnification, there are irregular nests within the epidermis associated with an underlying lymphoid infiltrate. **(C)** At medium-power magnification, irregular and enlarged nests, as well as single cells, are present at all layers of the epidermis, whereas melanocytes in normal skin proliferate along the basal cell layer, and benign nevus cells form nests confined to rete tips. **(D)** Marked pagetoid spread by cells showing fully evolved anaplasia consisting of nuclear enlargement, coarsely clumped and peripherally aggregated heterochromatin, and prominent nucleoli. Pagetoid spread extends upward to involve the stratum granulosum; this event is almost never observed for the rare pagetoid cells that may be seen in some nevi (e.g., spindle and epithelioid cell nevi).

also may have prominent nucleoli, is the presence of coarsely clumped background heterochromatin and irregularly thickened nuclear membranes (see Fig. 13–17D). The cytoplasm of melanoma nuclei is coarsely granulated, as opposed to the finely vacuolated cytoplasm in Spitz nevi. Moreover, dusty

or muddy melanization may be observed in SSM, particularly within the intraepidermal component; this feature is also seen in some dysplastic nevi. Radial growth phase melanoma of the superficial spreading type may arise in association with melanocytic nevus, and in all melanomas, care should be

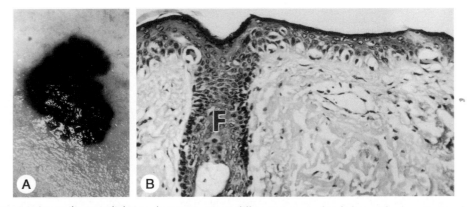

Figure 13–18. Melanoma: Lentigo maligna radial growth pattern. **(A)** A different pattern of radial growth characterizes lentigo maligna, a dark, irregular, ink spot–like, flat plaque that occurs on the sun-damaged facial skin of elderly individuals. **(B)** Histologically, there is contiguous lentiginous proliferation of dyshesive, variably shaped, malignant melanocytes located within an atrophic epidermal layer and involving the infundibular basal cell layer of hair follicles (F). The dermis typically shows solar elastosis. This form of radial growth is distinctive in its clinical appearance, its indolent and prolonged growth characteristics before onset of vertical spread, and the histologic morphology of its radial and vertical growth phase, the latter of which frequently contains spindle cells.

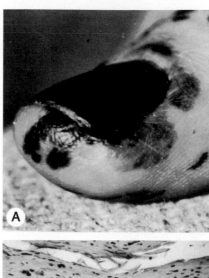
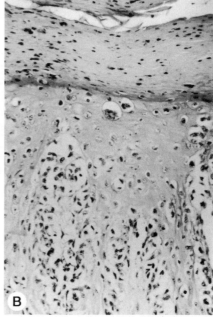

Figure 13–19. Melanoma: Acral-mucosal lentiginous radial growth. **(A)** Melanomas involving the digits, particularly the nail bed, and the mucosal and paramucosal epithelium, often show distinctive clinical and histologic features. Both radial and vertical growth may remain flat and heavily pigmented, obscuring clinical detection of the latter. **(B)** On microscopic examination, the radial growth phase of these lesions resembles that of lentigo maligna, although the malignant cells generally affect a hyperplastic rather than an atrophic epidermal layer. In addition, some acral melanomas also have heavily melanized, relatively thick dendrites that course upward through the thickened epidermis.

Table 13–7. DIFFERENTIAL DIAGNOSIS OF SUPERFICIAL SPREADING MELANOMA IN RADIAL GROWTH PHASE AND DYSPLASTIC NEVUS

DYSPLASTIC NEVUS	SUPERFICIAL SPREADING MELANOMA
Often <1 cm	Often >1 cm
Rete ridges thin and elongated	Rete ridges attenuated
Nests predominate over single cells	Single cells predominate over nests
Pagetoid spread minimal	Pagetoid spread prominent
Intraepidermal mitoses rare	Intraepidermal mitoses in one third of lesions
Most cells not atypical	Most cells atypical
Dermal cells smaller than epidermal cells	Dermal cells similar to epidermal cells

tic nevus) becomes radial growth phase melanoma of the superficial spreading type is subject to some controversy. Table 13–7 addresses common differences between these two entities.

Radial growth phase melanoma of the lentigo maligna type is distinctly different from the superficial spreading variety. The majority of lesions occur on chronically sun-damaged skin, often facial, of elderly individuals. The gross pathology is that of a deeply pigmented, irregular macule resembling an ink stain (see Fig. 13–18A). In lentigo maligna (LM, pure intraepidermal radial growth) lesions may persist with little change for a matter of many years before clinically nodular vertical growth supervenes. This is in sharp contrast to radial growth phase of SSM, which generally lasts for only months to several years before significant risk of vertical growth develops.

Histologically, the proliferating cells of LM involve an atrophic epidermal layer in lentiginous fashion, with characteristic contiguous growth replacing the basal cell layer of the epidermis and infundibulum of hair follicles (see Fig. 13–18B). The underlying dermis generally demonstrates marked solar elastosis. Cytologically, the cells of LM differ from those of SSM by virtue of the features summarized in Table 13–8.

Radial growth phase melanoma of the acral lentiginous/mucosal type (ALMM) is partially distinctive from the other two types already discussed. ALMM tends to occur preferentially on the digits, often involving the nail beds (see Fig. 13–19A), or on mucosal and paramucosal surfaces, including

taken to identify a precursor or associated nevus in the tissue sampled. It is important to recognize that radial growth phase melanoma may be exceedingly focal within a nevus. Melanoma may, for example, be present in only one profile of a serially sampled compound nevus; this makes careful scrutiny of every tissue profile on a slide mandatory for the complete evaluation of any nevomelanocytic neoplasm. Most SSM in the radial phase of growth show some degree of host response, consisting of infiltrative lymphocytic response (i.e., active inflammatory regression) or melanin pigment incontinence, papillary dermal fibrosis, and vascular proliferation and ectasia (i.e., mesenchymal sequela of regression).

The point at which melanocytic dysplasia (e.g., dysplas-

Table 13–8. DIFFERENTIAL DIAGNOSIS OF LENTIGO MALIGNA AND SUPERFICIAL SPREADING MELANOMA IN RADIAL GROWTH PHASE

LENTIGO MALIGNA	SUPERFICIAL SPREADING MELANOMA
Lentiginous growth	Pagetoid growth
Follicular infundibula involved	Follicular infundibula spared
Epidermis atrophic	Epidermis normal or thickened
Individual cells fusiform to stellate	Individual cells epithelioid
Marked retraction around malignant cells	Little retraction around malignant cells
Cytoplasm inconspicuous	Cytoplasm granular, conspicuous
Hyperchromatic nuclei, inconspicuous nucleoli	Vesicular chromatin, prominent nucleoli

the vaginal epithelium. As is the case with LM, the radial growth phase in ALMM is usually a deeply pigmented macule with an irregular border. However, unlike either SSM or LM, types of radial growth, in ALMM, vertical growth often supervenes not with the advent of a nodule, but rather without obvious evidence of a change in the preexisting macule. Therefore, it is difficult to estimate the duration of radial growth of ALMM prior to the onset of growth with metastatic potential. ALMM is more common in people of Asian or African descent. Its existence underscores the critical importance of complete cutaneous and mucosal examination in the screening evaluation for any general medical or dermatologic practice.

The histologic morphology of ALMM in the radial phase of growth is nearly identical to that of LM, with the important exception that the former generally arises in the setting of epithelial hyperplasia rather than atrophy (see Fig. 13–19B). It is critically important to realize that both LM and ALMM may form nest-like aggregates superimposed on a lentiginous growth pattern prior to the advent of dermal microinvasion. This tendency to aggregate within pseudonests may result in an appearance that resembles a dysplastic nevus. However, dysplastic nevi are generally smaller (<1 cm) than melanomas of the radial growth phase type, and the cells composing dysplastic nevi are only focally atypical, as opposed to melanomas, which show diffuse atypia of the cells forming their intraepidermal compartments.

Vertical Growth Phase Melanoma[37–44]

- RADIAL GROWTH MAY (SUPERFICIAL SPREADING, LENTIGO MALIGNA, AND ACRAL-LENTIGINOUS/MUCOSAL MELANOMAS) OR MAY NOT (NODULAR MELANOMA) PERSIST
- TUMORIGENIC DERMAL GROWTH WITH NESTS LARGER THAN THE LARGEST INTRAEPIDERMAL NEST
- CYTOLOGIC ANAPLASIA WITHIN EPIDERMIS AND DERMIS
- LACK OF DERMAL MATURATION
- DEEP DERMAL MITOTIC ACTIVITY

Vertical growth phase melanoma signifies the evolutionary stage in melanoma development in which tumor cells invade the dermis and begin to grow to form expansile (i.e., tumorigenic) nodules. Remember that the occasional melanoma cells that may involve the papillary dermis in radial growth phase disease do not form large nests. Operationally, tumorigenic dermal nodules may be defined as dermal nests that exceed the diameter of the largest intraepidermal nest. Clinically, tumorigenic nodules arising within SSM and LM types of radial growth are observed as papules and nodules within a macular or plaque-like field of preexisting hyperpigmentation (Fig. 13–20A). In heavily pigmented lesions, the extent of dermal involvement within subepithelial strata may occasionally be approximated when surgical excisions are bisected by the pathologist (Fig. 13–20B). Obviously, the entire vertical growth phase nodule must be carefully sectioned and submitted in toto for histologic review to most accurately determine the true extent of invasion.

Histologically, in vertical growth phase melanoma there are one or more nests or nodules of melanoma cells in the dermis, and the papillary dermis is filled and widened by tumor cells (Fig. 13–20C). The dermal nodules often form eccentrically beneath the site of radial growth, and their growth tends to be asymmetrical. The Clark system divides melanoma into levels I and II, which describe radial growth, and levels III through V, which describe vertical growth. Level I indicates in situ spread, and level II indicates in situ plus single-cell involvement of the papillary dermis. Level III indicates filling and expansion of papillary dermis; level IV represents extension into the reticular dermis; and level V describes extension into subcutaneous fat. In addition, it is now considered even more precise to report the depth of invasion as a function of the distance in mm separating the deepest tumor cell from the overlying stratum granulosum.

Cytologically, vertical growth phase melanoma nodules are usually composed of epithelioid malignant melanocytes, although rare variants may show spindle cell and nevus cell morphology (see Rare Disorders and Variants). Typical melanoma cells fail to mature with depth of dermal penetration; the deepest cells are roughly the same size and shape as the more superficial cells. The cytoplasm of typical melanoma cells tends to be granular and variably pigmented. Nuclei are enlarged, irregular, and often angulated in contour, and nuclear membranes are irregularly thickened. Chromatin is coarsely clumped, giving the impression of very dark zones juxtaposed with clear regions, a feature that has been referred to as "vesicular." Nucleoli are large and often eosinophilic, and mitotic activity usually can be detected deep within the vertical growth phase nodule. There may be a lymphoid response at the base of the nodule which occasionally infiltrates into the tumor and surrounds individual tumor cells. Tumor nodules clearly separated from the main tumor mass by normal reticular dermis have been termed microscopic satellites and are believed to confer a poor prognosis.

The histologic reporting of vertical growth phase melanoma remains controversial. Whereas some authorities advocate detailed descriptions enumerating an array of histologic variables that have been shown to provide prognostic insight in their statistical models, others recommend more concise reporting. One approach is to include the most essential information in a brief diagnostic statement, and to provide additional information of proven or potential use in formulating prognosis or treatment protocols in a brief note. Following is an example of this approach for the type of vertical growth phase melanoma that is likely to be encountered in routine practice:

DIAGNOSIS: Malignant melanoma, vertical growth phase type; level IV, measured depth 1.54 mm; all margins clear by at least 1 cm.

NOTE: The vertical growth phase nodule is arising in association with a partially regressed radial growth phase of the superficial spreading type. It is composed of epithelioid cells with numerous (>6/mm²) mitoses and has a lymphoid infiltrate at its base. There is no associated nevus or precursor lesion, and lymphatic invasion or satellite spread distant from the main nodule is not observed.

In general, whereas radial growth phase melanomas do not metastasize after complete surgical removal, vertical growth phase lesions show an increasing tendency to do so as thickness increases. A number of tables are available to

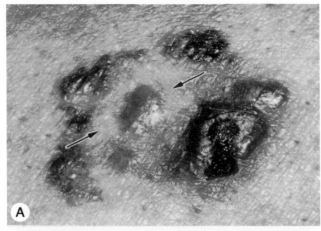

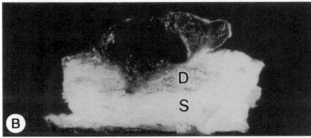

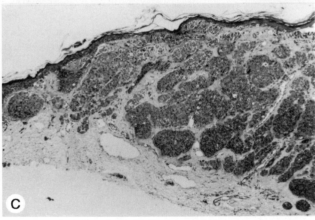

Figure 13–20. Melanoma: Vertical growth phase. **(A)** Development of a nodule within an irregular pigmented plaque heralds the onset of vertical growth. In this case, there is a prominent zone of regression (*arrows*); the lighter nodule central to the regression was composed of a tumoral aggregate of lymphocytes, testimony to the extent of the inflammatory response. **(B)** Cross section of a heavily pigmented, vertical growth phase melanoma shows extensive involvement of the dermis (D) and early involvement of the superficial subcutis (S). **(C)** The microscopic appearance of vertical growth phase melanoma is characterized by downward tumorigenic growth of malignant cells, which expand the papillary dermis and extend into or through the reticular dermis. Note that the dermal nests are considerably larger than ordinary nevus cell or melanoma cell nests that occur at the dermal-epidermal junction, a finding that constitutes tumorigenic growth inherent to vertical growth phase disease.

calculate the prospect of survival based on tumor thickness and other potential variables including mitotic rate, degree of lymphocytic host response, anatomic site, gender, and the presence or absence or regression. Low mitotic rate, presence of brisk lymphocytic infiltration of the vertical growth phase

nodule, relative thinness of the vertical growth phase nodule (<1.70 mm), location on the extremities, female gender, and absence of radial growth phase regression are all indicators of a more favorable prognosis.

Rare Disorders and Variants[45–53]

- REGRESSING MELANOMA
- SMALL CELL MELANOMA
- SPINDLE CELL (DESMOPLASTIC AND NEUROTROPIC) MELANOMA
- "BORDERLINE AND MINIMAL DEVIATION" MELANOMAS
- METASTATIC MELANOMA
- PSEUDOMELANOMA RESULTING FROM MONSEL REACTION

There are enough variants and mimics of melanoma to fill the pages of a separate book. In an attempt to demystify, yet not deemphasize, the more commonly encountered enti-

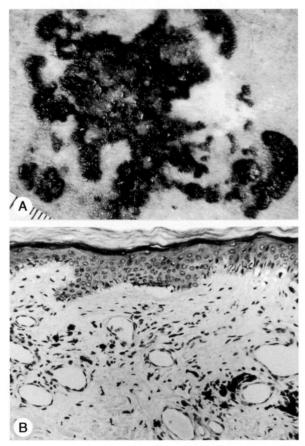

Figure 13–21. Regression in melanoma. **(A)** Extensive regression has produced a "moth-eaten" clinical appearance in this superficial spreading melanoma. **(B)** Examination of the nonpigmented regions internal to the tumor plaque show increased numbers of widely dilated vessels within a fibrotic dermis containing numerous melanophages. Inflammation is minimal at this site, where regression is complete. This may be the only finding at sites where entire lesions have regressed.

ties in this group, this section provides summaries of the salient features inherent in the accurate diagnostic recognition of each lesion.

Regressing melanoma presents a diagnostic problem only when regression is complete or nearly so. Regression clinically takes the form of skin-colored, pink, or gray-blue regions that develop within the radial growth phase of a preexisting melanoma (Fig. 13–21A). Completely regressed primary melanomas may be indistinguishable from normal skin, although subtle alterations in pigment distribution have been detected with the assistance of a Wood light. Histologically, regression is evidenced by papillary dermal deposition of loose, edematous collagen containing increased numbers of ectatic vessels (Fig. 13–21B). Numerous melanophages and residual clusters of lymphocytes are typically entrapped within the abnormal mesenchyme. Lymphocytes may also align along the dermal-epidermal interface, where basal cell layer destruction akin to that seen in lichenoid keratoses may be observed. These features are often observed focally in association with the radial growth phase components of melanomas. When they represent the sole finding in a biopsy or excision specimen, multiple levels should be obtained in an effort to detect small clusters of residual malignant melanocytes.

Small cell melanoma, also referred to as melanoma with nevus cell change, often occurs focally within vertical growth phase melanomas and therefore may be difficult to distinguish from associated nevus cells. Moreover, when small cell change develops near or at the base of a vertical growth

phase nodule, it may mimic cytologic differentiation. Occasionally, an entire vertical growth phase nodule may be composed of small melanoma cells. In general, small melanoma cells are not easily differentiated from nevus cells by the size and shape of their nuclei; rather, they can be differentiated by the diffuse hyperchromasia of small melanoma cell nuclei and the invariable presence of mitotic activity (Fig. 13–22). Also, small melanoma cells usually at least focally show gradual transitions to larger malignant cells.

Spindle cell melanoma, also known as desmoplastic or neurotropic melanoma, is a type of vertical growth phase that often arises in association with LM and ALMM types of radial growth (Fig. 13–23). These lesions may be extremely difficult to recognize histologically, because unlike conventional vertical growth, which tends to enlarge as tumorigenic nodules, spindle cell melanoma tends to be diffusely infiltrative within the collagenous reticular dermal stroma. A helpful diagnostic feature is the frequent presence of lymphoplasmacytic aggregates at the most peripheral extent of the vertical growth phase of spindle cell melanoma (see Fig. 13–23A). Moreover, spindle cell melanoma cells generally do not display vesicular chromatin patterns or prominent nucleoli. Rather, they have enlarged, elongated, somewhat angulated nuclei with diffuse hyperchromasia, although many nuclei are extremely bland and banal in appearance (see Fig. 13–23B–D). A careful search will generally reveal evidence of overlying intraepidermal melanocytic growth consistent with in situ melanoma (see Fig. 13–23B), which is an important feature because amelanotic spindle cell melanoma may

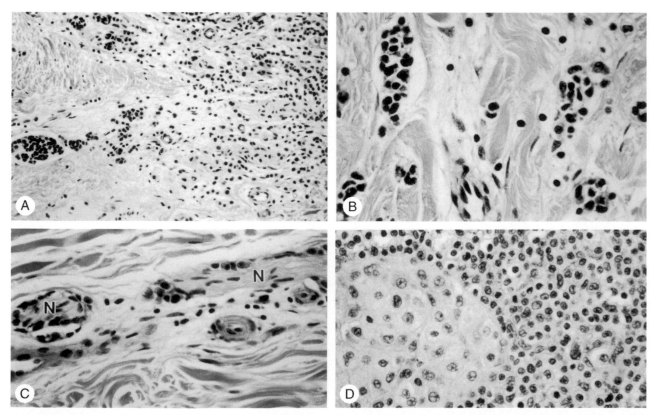

Figure 13–22. Melanoma with small cell differentiation. **(A)** This vertical growth phase nodule has a permeative pattern of dermal infiltration suggestive of a congenital melanocytic nevus. **(B)** Individual cells, however, show nuclear contour angulation and diffuse hyperchromasia. Occasional mitoses are also present (not shown). **(C)** Perineural (N) spread and **(D)** zones where small melanoma cells show apparent transitions with larger, more conventional melanoma cells assist in establishing the diagnosis, although perineural patterns may also occur in congenital nevi.

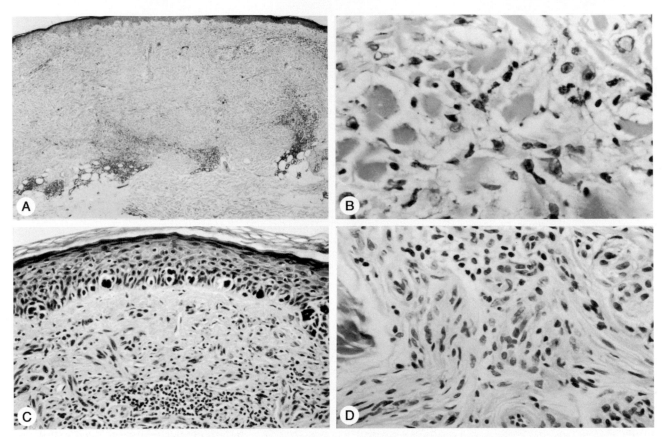

Figure 13–23. Melanoma with spindle cell differentiation. Spindle cell desmoplastic and neurotropic vertical growth phase melanomas often arise in association with lentigo maligna and acral-mucosal lentiginous radial growth. **(A)** A helpful diagnostic feature at scanning magnification is the presence of lymphoid inflammatory infiltrates defining the perimeter of an otherwise vague vertical growth phase nodule. **(B)** In amelanotic lesions, confirmation of melanocytic origin may depend on detection of residual radial growth along the dermal-epidermal interface. **(C)** Individual spindle cells may infiltrate collagen bundles diffusely and show bland nuclei with subtle hyperchromasia. Mitotic figures are generally detected after careful study. **(D)** Zones of true neural invasion characterized by dermal nerve bundles rendered hypercellular by infiltration by malignant spindle cells is also a helpful diagnostic feature.

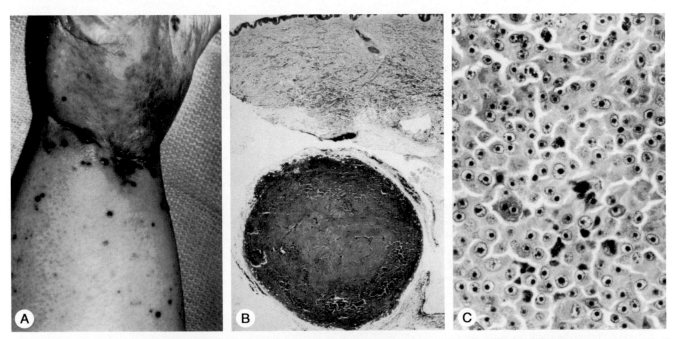

Figure 13–24. Metastatic melanoma. **(A)** Cutaneous metastases of melanoma usually occur in patients with established disease and create few diagnostic problems, as is the case in this patient who has multiple pigmented metastases on a single limb. **(B)** Histologically, there is a large, expansile tumor nodule within the subcutis. **(C)** On higher magnification, this tumor nodule is composed of epithelioid malignant cells containing focal melanin pigmentation. Occasionally, metastases will home to the epidermal layer (i.e., epidermotropic metastases) where they form nests and mimic nevi or primary melanoma. Careful inspection for cellular anaplasia and dermal mitotic activity, as well as close correlation with clinical history, are mandatory for such lesions.

mimic other spindle cell tumors of nonmelanocytic lineage. Desmoplastic spindle cell melanoma is associated with proliferation of plump fibroblasts and collagen deposition, making detection of individual tumor cells even more problematic. Neurotropic spindle cell melanoma may show tumor fascicles mimicking true neural differentiation or extensive neural infiltration (see Fig. 13–23D), a finding that actually is of diagnostic assistance in identifying this problematic melanoma variant.

Borderline and *minimal deviation melanomas* represent a biologically valid concept that has become so misunderstood, it is no longer of practical utility. Early definitions described these melanomas as biologically low-grade neoplasms that seldom metastasized but had a tendency for local recurrence. Histologically, such lesions generally had architectural features of level III (i.e., borderline) or level IV–V (i.e., minimal deviation) tumorigenic melanomas, although they failed to show fully evolved cytologic anaplasia or high mitotic rates. It is therefore likely that this subset of lesions simply represents well-differentiated melanoma variants analogous to the relation between well-differentiated tubular carcinoma of the breast and more commonly encountered infiltrating ductal types.

Metastatic melanoma may present little clinical and histologic diagnostic difficulty in the setting of diffuse cutaneous and extracutaneous dissemination (Fig. 13–24A) or when metastases retain cytologic and biosynthetic (melanogenesis) links to the primary tumors from which they arose (Fig. 13–24B, C). However, metastatic melanoma often represents a diagnostic challenge, particularly when a primary site has not been identified or has regressed completely. In such instances, amelanotic metastatic deposits may be confused with carcinoma or lymphoma, and immunohistochemistry for melanoma-associated antigens (e.g., S100 protein, HMB-45) as well as epithelial (cytokeratin) and hematopoietic antigens (e.g., cytokeratin and leukocyte common antigen, respectively) may be required to define lineage. Certain dermal metastases may be remarkably symmetrical and retain some cytologic features of nevus cells, although mitoses are observed. Other metastases may home to the epidermal layer, forming nevus-like nests or mimicking primary melanoma (i.e., epidermotropic metastases). These lesions may be extremely problematic to diagnose, and clinical history may be required to definitively distinguish these lesions from primary melanoma. One helpful finding in metastatic melanoma is the relative absence of an infiltrative lymphoid response in association with either the epidermotropic or dermal-subcutaneous nodule.

Pseudomelanoma resulting from Monsel reaction most commonly is observed in melanoma reexcisions in which this reagent has been applied to effect hemostasis. Typically, there is a brisk fibrohistiocytic response at the excision site which may have architectural features of a space-occupying lesion (Fig. 13–25A). Many of the histiocytes may be activated, with enlarged nuclei, prominent nucleoli, and occasional mitotic figures. Moreover, they contain particulate residua of iron-containing Monsel solution, resulting in cells that resemble melanized melanoma cells (Fig. 13–25B). Staining with Prussian blue reagent, however, will disclose the pigment to be iron-based rather than melanin (Fig. 13–25C).

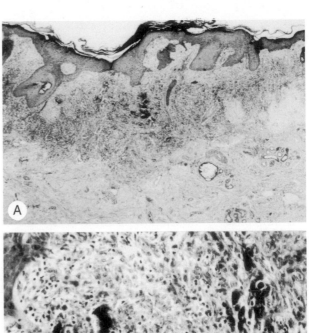

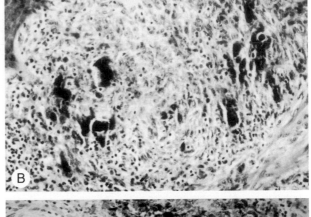

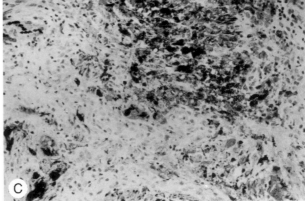

Figure 13–25. Monsel reaction at melanoma excision site. **(A, B)** An excised biopsy site shows epidermal hyperplasia and a brisk dermal reaction consisting of plump fibroblasts and activated epithelioid histiocytes associated with clumped as well as particulate intracytoplasmic brown pigment. Although this histologic picture may resemble that of residual melanoma entrapped within dermal scar tissue, its origin as a cellular reaction to iron-containing Monsel solution is confirmed by **(C)** Prussian blue stain, which reveals that all of the intracellular and extracellular pigment is particulate iron.

DIFFERENTIAL DIAGNOSIS

The differential diagnosis of tumors of the melanocytic series is extraordinarily complex, and it is difficult, if not impossible, to confine it to a simple algorithm. Basic concepts of how melanocytes and nevus cells proliferate and differentiate normally are the best means to facilitate an accurate and measured approach to any lesion. Accordingly, it is recommended that when a problematic pigmented lesion is encountered, the following questions are asked:

- DOES THE LESION GROW IN A BILATERALLY SYMMETRICAL AND ORDERLY MANNER?
- IS THERE CYTOLOGIC AND/OR ARCHITECTURAL EVIDENCE OF MATURATION?
- ARE NEVUS NESTS AND SINGLE CELLS CONFINED TO THE LOWER EPIDERMAL LAYERS?
- IF LENTIGINOUS, DOES THE GROWTH PATTERN ENTIRELY REPLACE THE BASAL CELL LAYER?
- IS THERE A PAPILLARY DERMAL RESPONSE INVOLVING LYMPHOCYTES OR LAMELLAR FIBROSIS?
- ARE THERE DEEP DERMAL MITOSES OR INDIVIDUAL CELL NECROSIS?
- WHAT ARE THE CORRELATIVE CLINICAL CHARACTERISTICS? WAS THE LESION CHANGING?

These are some of the initial branch points that will direct the diagnostician down the correct pathway to determine whether the process is benign, dysplastic, or malignant. Occasional atypical lesions will not fit neatly into these categories, and only clinical outcome will indicate biological potential. Such lesions should prompt a descriptive note, by which complete local excision is recommended.

SELECTED REFERENCES

1. Breathnach AS. Melanocyte distribution in forearm epidermis of freckled human subjects. J Invest Dermatol 1958;29:253.
2. Rhodes AR, Stern RS, Melski JW. The PUVA lentigo: An analysis of predisposing factors. J Invest Dermatol 1983;81:459.
3. Yaar M, Woodley DT, Gilchrest BA. Human nevocellular nevus cells are surrounded by basement membrane components. Immunohistochemical studies of human nevus cells and melanocytes in vivo and in vitro. Lab Invest 1988;58:157.
4. Swerdlow AJ, English J, MacKie RM, et al. Benign melanocytic naevi as a risk factor for malignant melanoma. Br Med J 1986;292:1555.
5. Holman CD, Armstrong BK. Pigmentary traits, ethnic origin, benign nevi, and family history as risk factors for cutaneous malignant melanoma. J Natl Cancer Inst 1984;72:257.
6. Maize JC, Ackerman AB. Pigmented lesions of the skin. Clinicopathologic correlations. Philadelphia: Lea & Febiger, 1987.
7. Clemmensen OJ, Kroon S. The histology of "congenital features" in early acquired melanocytic nevi. J Am Acad Dermatol 1988;19:742.
8. Rhodes AR, Mihm MC Jr. Origin of cutaneous melanoma in a congenital nevus spilus. Arch Dermatol 1990;126:500.
9. Rhodes AR. Congenital nevomelanocytic nevi. Histologic patterns in the first year of life and evolution during childhood. Arch Dermatol 1986;122:1257.
10. Fletcher V, Sagebiel RW. The combined nevus. In: Ackerman AB, ed. Pathology of Malignant Melanoma. New York: Masson, 1981:273.
11. Seab JA, Graham JH, Helwig EB. Deep penetrating nevus. Am J Surg Pathol 1989;13:39.
12. Wayte DM, Helwig EB. Halo nevi. Cancer 1968;22:69.
13. Sutton RL. An unusual variety of vitiligo (leukoderma acquisitum centrifigum). J Cutan Dis 1916;34:797.
14. Schmitt D, Ortonne JP, Haftek M, Thivolet J. Halo nevus and halo melanoma. Immunocytochemical study of the inflammatory cell infiltrate. In: Ackerman AB, ed. Pathology of Malignant Melanoma. New York: Masson, 1981:333.
15. Cullity G. Intra-epithelial changes in childhood nevi simulating malignant melanoma. Pathology 1984;16:307.
16. Kernen JA, Ackerman LV. Spindle cell nevi and epithelioid cell nevi (so-called juvenile melanomas) in children and adults. A clinicopathologic study of 27 cases. Cancer 1960;13:612.
17. Paniago-Periera C, Maize JC, Ackerman AB. Nevus of large spindle and/or epithelioid cells (Spitz's nevus). Arch Dermatol 1978;114:1811.
18. Weedon D, Little JH. Spindle and epithelioid cell nevi in children and adults. A review of 211 cases of the Spitz nevus. Cancer 1977;40:217.
19. Echevarria R, Ackerman LV. Spindle and epithelioid cell nevi in the adult. Clinicopathologic report of 26 cases. Cancer 1967;20:175.
20. Prose NS, Heilman E, Felman YM, et al. Multiple benign juvenile melanoma. J Am Acad Dermatol 1983;9:236.
21. Kornberg R, Ackerman AB. Pseudomelanoma. Recurrent melanocytic nevus following partial surgical removal. Arch Dermatol 1975;111:1588.
22. Park HK, Leonard DD, Arrington JH III, Lund HZ. Recurrent melanocytic nevi: Clinical and histologic review of 175 cases (abstract). J Am Acad Dermatol 1987;17:285.
23. Schmoeckel C. How consistent are dermatopathologists in reading early malignant melanomas and lesions "precursor" to them? An international survey. Am J Dermatopathol 1984;6:13.
24. Rhodes AR, Weinstock MA, Fitzpatrick TB, et al. Risk factors for cutaneous melanoma. A practical method for recognizing predisposed individuals. JAMA J Am Med Assoc 1987;258:3146.
25. Clark WH Jr, Reimer RR, Greene MH, et al. Origin of familial melanomas from heritable melanocytic lesions. Arch Dermatol 1978;114:732.
26. Greene M, Clark WH Jr, Tucker MA, et al. High risk of malignant melanoma in melanoma-prone families with dysplastic nevi. Ann Intern Med 1985;102:458.
27. Elder DE, Goldman LI, Goldman SC, et al. Dysplastic nevus syndrome: A phenotypic association of sporadic cutaneous melanoma. Cancer 1980;46:1787.
28. Bale SJ, Dracopoli NC, Tucker MA, et al. Mapping the gene for hereditary cutaneous malignant melanoma-dysplastic nevus to chromosome 1p. N Engl J Med 1989;320:1367.
29. McGovern VJ. The classification of melanoma and its histologic reporting. Pathology 1970;2:85.
30. Mihm MC Jr, Clark WH Jr, From L. The clinical diagnosis, classification and histogenetic concepts of the early stages of cutaneous malignant melanomas. N Engl J Med 1971;284:1078.
31. Clark WH Jr, From L, Bernardino EA, Mihm MC Jr. The histogenesis and biologic behavior of primary human malignant melanomas in skin. Cancer Res 1969;29:205.
32. Clark WH Jr, Elder DE, Guerry D 4th, et al. A study of tumor progression: The precursor lesions of superficial spreading and nodular melanoma. Hum Pathol 1984;15:1147.
33. McGovern VJ, Cochran AJ, Van der Esch EP, et al. The classification of malignant melanoma, its histological reporting and registration: A revision of the 1972 Sydney classification. Pathology 1986;18:12.
34. Clark WH Jr, Mihm MC Jr. Lentigo maligna and lentigo-maligna melanoma. Am J Pathol 1969;55:39.
35. Clark WH Jr, Elder DE, Van Horn M. The biologic forms of malignant melanoma. Hum Pathol 1986;5:443.
36. Coleman WP III, Loria PR, Reed RJ, Krementz ET. Acral lentiginous melanoma. Arch Dermatol 1980;116:773.
37. Elder DE. Prognostic guides to melanoma. In: MacKie RM, ed. Clinics in Oncology. Philadelphia: WB Saunders, 1984:457.
38. Balch CM, Soong S-J. Characteristics of melanoma that predict the risk of metastasis. In: Costanzi J, ed. Malignant Melanoma, vol 1. The Hague: Martinus Nijhoff, 1983:117.
39. Soong S-J. A computerized mathematical model and scoring system for predicting outcome in melanoma patients. In: Balch CM, Milton GW, eds. Cutaneous Melanoma. Philadelphia: JB Lippincott, 1985:353.
40. Elder DE, Guerry D 4th, Van Horn M, et al. The role of lymph node dissection for clinical stage I malignant melanoma of intermediate thickness (1.51–3.99 mm). Cancer 1985;56:413.
41. Vollmer RT. Malignant melanoma. A multivariate analysis of prognostic factors. Pathol Annu 1989;24:383.
42. Kelly JW, Sagebiel RW, Clyman S, Blois MS. Thin level IV malignant melanoma. A subset in which level is the major prognostic indicator. Ann Surg 1985;202:98.

43. Breslow A. Thickness, cross-sectional areas and depth of invasion in the prognosis of cutaneous melanoma. Ann Surg 1970;172:902.

44. Clark WH Jr, Elder DE, Guerry D, et al. Model predicting survival in stage I melanoma based on tumor progression. J Natl Cancer Inst 1989;81:1893.

45. Reed RJ, Ichinose H, Clark WH Jr, Mihm MC Jr. Common and uncommon melanocytic nevi and borderline melanomas. Semin Oncol 1975;2:119.

46. McGovern VJ. Spontaneous regression of melanoma. Pathology 1975;7:91.

47. Muhlbauer JE, Margolis RJ, Mihm MC Jr, Reed RJ. Minimal deviation melanoma: A histologic variant of cutaneous malignant melanoma in its vertical growth phase. J Invest Dermatol 1983;80(Suppl):63.

48. Conley J, Lattes R, Orr W. Desmoplastic malignant melanoma (a rare variant of spindle cell melanoma). Cancer 1971;28:914.

49. Jain S, Allan PW. Desmoplastic malignant melanoma and its variants. A study of 45 cases. Am J Surg Pathol 1989;13:358.

50. Egbert B, Kempson R, Sagebiel RW. Desmoplastic malignant melanoma. A clinicohistopathologic study of 25 cases. Cancer 1988;62:2033.

51. DiMaiao SM, Mackay B, Smith JL, Dickersin GR. Neurosarcomatous transformation in malignant melanoma. Cancer 1982;50:2345.

52. Reed RJ, Leonard DD. Neurotropic melanoma. A variant of desmoplastic melanoma. Am J Surg Pathol 1979;3:301.

53. Kossard S, Doherty E, Murray E. Neurotropic melanoma: A variant of desmoplastic melanoma. Arch Dermatol 1987;123:907.

14

Lymphoproliferative Tumors

DEFINITIONS AND GENERAL CONSIDERATIONS[1, 2]

Although the notion that skin is a lymphoid organ has emerged only during the past decade, it has gained wide acceptance as a basis for understanding cutaneous immunity and lymphoproliferative neoplasms. Working in concert with draining lymph nodes, the skin is the residence of specialized lymphocytes, histiocytes, and mast cells that compose skin-associated lymphoid tissue (SALT). Benign proliferations, dysplastic proliferations, and frank malignancy of normal lymphohistiocytic constituents of skin commonly occur and present significant diagnostic difficulties, particularly when there is absence of associated lymph node involvement.

Integral to understanding the histopathology and immunoarchitecture of hyperplastic conditions and neoplastic lymphoproliferative neoplasms of the skin is an appreciation of correlative processes in lymph nodes. However, because infiltration of the epidermis and dermis by atypical and malignant lymphohistiocytic cells often results in cytologic and architectural distortion not seen in lymph nodes, distinctive diagnostic challenges are encountered when lymphoproliferative lesions present primarily in the skin. These challenges have been partially addressed by the recent emergence of sophisticated molecular biological techniques for the analysis of clonal lymphoid proliferations. Thus, the accurate diagnosis of lymphohistiocytic tumors of the skin frequently requires a multifaceted approach that combines routine histopathology, refined microscopy (1-μm-section analysis), immunohistochemistry, and molecular analytical techniques.

With the exception of cutaneous T-cell lymphoma (CTCL), the majority of non-Hodgkin lymphomas involving the skin cannot be accurately subclassified based on skin biopsy specimens alone. Although such specimens serve to alert the clinician of the probability of a lymphoproliferative disorder, careful systemic search for clinical evidence of primary lymphoid involvement and, if found, subsequent nodal biopsy, will often permit definitive classification.

GROSS PATHOLOGY

The gross pathology of various lymphoproliferative disorders depends, in large part, on the presence or absence of epidermal involvement. In early stages of CTCL, malignant T cells infiltrate into the epidermal layer, resulting in alterations in surface keratinization. This process correlates with the formation of erythematous, scaling plaques which may be confused with psoriasis, chronic eczematous dermatitis, and other forms of dermatitis. T-cell infiltration of hair follicles may result in mucinous degeneration and localized alopecia. In patients in whom circulating malignant T cells are present (i.e., Sézary syndrome), diffuse erythema and scaling (i.e., erythroderma) may occur. Nonepidermotropic T-cell lymphomas and B-cell lymphomas, on the other hand, tend to form deep dermal nodules beneath an uninvolved epidermal layer. Lesions typically are plum-colored nodules covered by an unremarkable or smooth, glistening epidermal surface. Unfortunately, benign lymphoid hyperplasia within the dermis frequently results in clinical nodules that are indistinguishable from nonepidermotropic lymphomas.

GENERAL HISTOLOGY AND TEMPORAL EVOLUTION

The general histology of reactive and neoplastic lymphoid infiltrates of skin may be predicted based on what is known of lymphoid trafficking patterns in lymph nodes. Normal lymphocyte influx and efflux in nodal tissues occurs at the level of subcapsular microvessels known as high endothelial venules. This angiogenic response is recapitulated in normal and reactive T-cell trafficking in skin, where inflammatory cells tend to cluster about dermal venules. Migration away from venules to produce an interstitial pattern, on the other hand, is regarded as abnormal and is typically observed

257

in both T- and B-cell lymphomas. In normal and reactive lymph nodes, B cells are clustered within follicles and show a spectrum of maturation. Accordingly, reactive B-cell infiltrates in the skin may be nodular and polymorphous, exhibiting small and large, cleaved and noncleaved stages of differentiation. Lymphomas of B cells may also attempt to recapitulate the nodular architecture of normal follicles, although the proliferating cells are monomorphic, representing a clone arrested at a single stage of B-cell ontogeny.

The issue of temporal evolution is most relevant to CTCL, and there are many analogies that exist between the progression of CTCL and the dysplastic nevus–melanoma sequence (see Chap. 13). Early lesions may be clinically and histologically indistinguishable from chronic dermatitis, although certain abnormalities in architecture (i.e., interstitial trafficking pattern) may have begun to emerge. Some of these lesions eventually evolve to become epidermotropic CTCL, a process whereby clonal T-cell populations proliferate horizontally within the epidermal layer in a manner similar to radial growth phase melanoma. In time, T cells begin to grow deeply into the dermis, where destructive nodules may form, an event akin to the emergence of vertical growth within a superficial melanoma. In both neoplastic processes, deep dermal growth correlates with a tendency for systemic dissemination.

HISTOLOGY OF SPECIFIC DISORDERS

Cutaneous Lymphoid Hyperplasia[3, 4]

- SUPERFICIAL AND OFTEN DEEP INFILTRATE
- TENDENCY FOR ANGIOCENTRICITY AND PERIADNEXAL SPREAD
- POLYMORPHOUS CELLULAR COMPOSITION
- VASCULAR PROLIFERATION
- LYMPHOID FOLLICLE FORMATION

Typical clinical lesions of cutaneous lymphoid hyperplasia are single or multiple coalescent erythematous nodules, often located on the face or scalp (Fig. 14–1A). Individual lesions tend to be firm and covered by a smooth, nonscaling epidermal surface. Lesions may be nonpainful, emerge spontaneously, and persist for many weeks or months. Linear or clustered configurations may raise the possibility of florid reactions to arthropod bites, although evidence of precipitating cause is often absent. Unfortunately, many lesions of cutaneous lymphoid hyperplasia may be clinically indistinguishable from B-cell lymphoma, prompting clinical concern and necessitating biopsy examination.

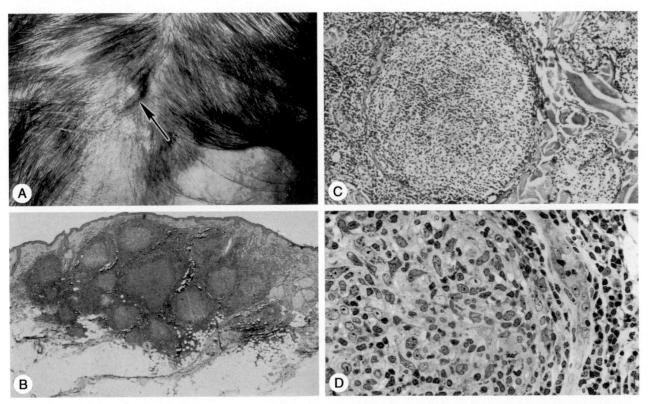

Figure 14–1. Cutaneous lymphoid hyperplasia. (A) Firm, erythematous nodules *(arrow)* on the posterior scalp raised the possibility of lymphoma in this middle-aged woman. (B) A biopsy specimen of a similar lesion shows aggregates of lymphoid follicles within the dermis. (C) At higher magnification, larger cells (i.e., B cells) comprise the central regions of the follicles, whereas smaller lymphoid cells (i.e., T cells) are present about the perimeter. (D) A spectrum of B-cell differentiation is observed within the larger cell component, consisting of smaller and larger lymphoid cells with both cleaved and noncleaved nuclei, occasional immunoblasts, and macrophages containing phagocytized basophilic material (i.e., tingible body macrophages).

At scanning magnification, cutaneous lymphoid hyperplasia reveals symmetrical infiltration of the superficial and deep dermis by cellular aggregates of lymphoid cells (Fig. 14–1B). Although the infiltrate may extend into subcutaneous fat, the epidermis and papillary dermis are generally uninvolved, and adnexal structures are not destroyed. In some lesions, the appearance of variably sized, rounded nodules formed by pale, larger lymphocytes may be appreciated at scanning magnification, raising the possibility of germinal center formation (see Fig. 14–1B). At higher magnification, these follicles are defined by peripheral rims of small lymphoid cells (i.e., T cells) with inconspicuous cytoplasm (Fig. 14–1C, D). The cells composing the follicular nodules demonstrate a spectrum of cytodifferentiation ranging from cells containing small cleaved and noncleaved nuclei to cells containing large cleaved and noncleaved nuclei (see Fig. 14–1D). In addition, occasional plasmacytoid cells, immunoblasts with prominent central nucleoli, and tingible-body macrophages with basophilic debris within their cytoplasm may be seen. Proliferating, arborizing small vessels may also be prominent throughout the regions of lymphoid hyperplasia.

The provocative stimuli of lesions of cutaneous lymphoid hyperplasia are sometimes revealed in the histopathology. For example, the detection of granulomatous foci associated with birefringent material may indicate residua of insect stingers or mouth parts responsible for local antigen injection. Numerous eosinophils and zones of fibrosis may also be present in persistent insect-bite reactions associated with lymphoid hyperplasia. Zones of follicular rupture suggest pilar obstruction with dermal extrusion of noxious follicular contents (i.e., pseudolymphomatous folliculitis).

Lymphocytic Dysplasia "Parapsoriasis" and Cutaneous T-Cell Lymphoma[5–13]

T-Cell Dysplasia

- PERIVASCULAR AS WELL AS INTERSTITIAL PATTERN, ESPECIALLY IN PAPILLARY DERMIS
- COARSE PAPILLARY DERMAL FIBROSIS
- FOCI OF SINGLE-CELL EPIDERMOTROPISM WITH MINIMAL SPONGIOSIS
- RELATIVE ABSENCE OF CYTOLOGIC ATYPIA IN INFILTRATING CELLS
- OFTEN, NORMAL T-CELL IMMUNOPHENOTYPE

Cutaneous T-Cell Lymphoma

- INTERSTITIAL PAPILLARY DERMAL LYMPHOID INFILTRATE WITH FIBROSIS
- EPIDERMOTROPISM WITHOUT SPONGIOSIS
- EPIDERMOTROPIC CELLS AGGREGATED
- EPIDERMOTROPIC CELLS ATYPICAL
- ADMIXED EOSINOPHILS AND PLASMA CELLS
- LATE DISEASE WITHOUT EPIDERMOTROPISM BUT WITH DEEPER DERMAL EXTENSION

Classical CTCL generally, but not invariably, evolves through defined clinical stages: the premalignant dysplasia, and the patch, plaque, and tumor stages (Figs. 14–2A, 14–3A, 14–4A, and 14–5A, respectively). In the dysplastic and patch stages, lesions are barely raised erythematous areas, often with adherent scale. Skin of the trunk and extremities is frequently involved. Lesions wax and wane and often are

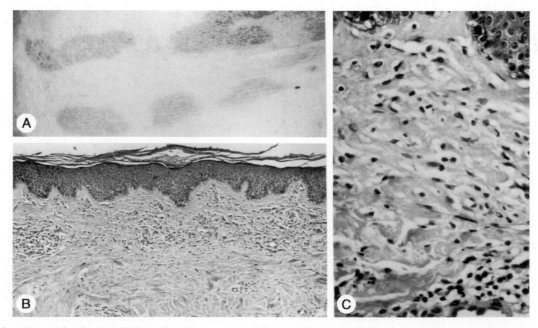

Figure 14–2. T-lymphocyte dysplasia. (A) Often referred to as "parapsoriasis," these large patches and thin plaques are recalcitrant to treatment and may show a poikilodermatous appearance. (B) Histologically, there is a relatively sparse papillary dermal lymphocytic infiltrate beneath an epidermal layer showing diffuse mild hyperplasia and minimal spongiosis. (C) An important histologic clue is the interstitial pattern of lymphocyte infiltration within a diffusely fibrotic papillary dermis. At this juncture, lymphocytes are not predominated by atypical cells with irregular nuclear contours, nor is epidermotropism a prominent feature. Cell marker studies routinely fail to support malignancy in such lesions, although the lymphocyte trafficking pattern is not characteristic of a specific dermatosis (including guttate parapsoriasis, which represents a separate and distinctive entity) and shows signs of chronicity (papillary dermal fibrosis).

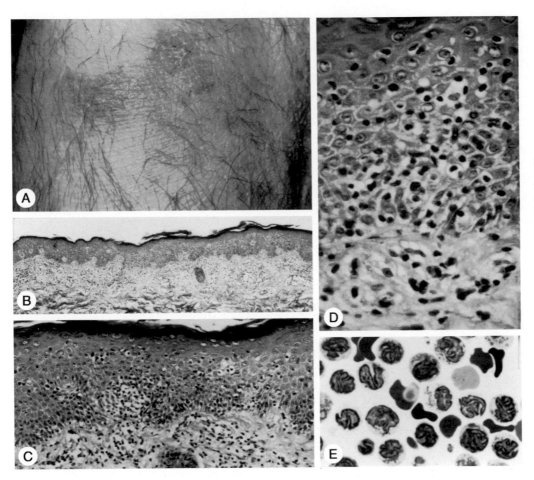

Figure 14–3. Cutaneous T-cell lymphoma, early epidermotropic type. **(A)** The gross pathology is of a chronic, erythematous, scaling patch that is refractory to conventional anti-inflammatory treatment. **(B)** Histologically, there is a sparse band of lymphocytes within a fibrotic papillary dermis, a finding also observed in T-cell dysplasia. **(C)** However, single-cell and clustered epidermotropism is now a prominent feature. **(D)** Epidermotropic cells contain hyperchromatic nuclei with irregular, infolded contours. **(E)** Such cells, upon isolation and thin sectioning, display nuclear convolutions of Sézary cells. Cell marker analysis of such lesions often reveals the epidermotropic compartment to be CD4-positive, with loss of one or more pan-T-cell maturation markers, whereas the dermal component may be of a reactive–T-cell phenotype.

confused with eczematous dermatitis. Early CTCL is frequently refractory to topical anti-inflammatory medications, resulting in clinical concern and often prompting biopsy. Confusing terms such as large-plaque parapsoriasis and parapsoriasis en plaques have been used to refer to early CTCL in the dysplastic and patch stages. Throughout this section, the terms T-cell dysplasia and patch-stage CTCL will be used exclusively for these entities. Because guttate (i.e., small-plaque) parapsoriasis is a benign dermatosis unrelated to CTCL, it is recommended that the term parapsoriasis never be used to refer to T-cell malignancy. Poikiloderma vasculare atrophicans is a variant of early CTCL characterized by cutaneous atrophy (i.e., thinning), telangiectasias, and zones of hyperpigmentation and hypopigmentation.

Plaque-stage CTCL (see Fig. 14–4A) refers to clinical lesions that are raised, indurated, and variable in color, ranging in hue from pink to red to brown-purple. Well-defined plaques, frequently with figurate borders, are the rule; scaling and pruritus are generally more prominent than in the patch stage. Plaques of CTCL may arise de novo or may derive from preexisting patches. Patches and plaques of CTCL are relatively indolent and may progress slowly over many years without systemic spread or the formation of tumoral nodules. Eventually, however, tumor-stage nodules develop in untreated disease. Nodules are firm and dome-shaped, often affecting the face, scalp, and body folds, and they may be indistinguishable from the nodules of B-cell lymphoma (discussed later). The nodular stage correlates with visceral dis-

semination and a poor prognosis. Rarely, tumors may arise de novo, a condition referred to as the "d'emblee" form of CTCL. The advent of multiple de novo nodules occurring in a patient with hypercalcemia should raise the possibility of T-cell lymphoma associated with human T-cell leukemia virus–1 (HTLV-1) retroviral infection. Generalized skin erythema and scaling (i.e., erythroderma) may occur during any of the previously discussed three stages of CTCL or may be the first presenting manifestation of disease. Erythroderma associated with high numbers of circulating tumor cells in the peripheral blood is referred to as Sézary syndrome, a condition that may also raise the differential diagnosis of erythrodermic forms of psoriasis, contact or atopic dermatitis, seborrheic dermatitis, or pityriasis rubra pilaris.

The histologic diagnosis of CTCL in its earliest stages (i.e., dysplastic and plaque stages), when it is most easily and effectively treated, is one of the most challenging tasks in dermatopathology. The architectural and cytologic alterations at these stages are extraordinarily subtle, and special techniques are often required to assist in diagnostic assessment. Moreover, multiple samples, either of various skin sites at one time or of representative lesions sequentially over time, are often required to definitively establish a diagnosis of CTCL. At low magnification, dysplastic-stage (Fig. 14–2B) and patch-stage (Fig. 14–3B) CTCL resemble a low-grade inflammatory dermatitis, with lymphocytes in perivascular array within the papillary dermis, beneath a minimally hyperplastic epidermal layer that exhibits focal hyperkeratosis or parakeratosis. On closer inspection, variable numbers of lymphocytes are also encountered diffusely throughout the papillary dermis (Fig. 14–2C) and within the epidermis, both individually and, rarely, as small aggregates (Fig. 14–3C, D). Three important findings will reliably arouse suspicion of evolving T-cell malignancy at these early stages. First, the lymphocytes that have migrated into the epidermis are not associated with intercellular edema between adjacent keratinocytes (i.e., spongiosis). As discussed in Chapter 3, spongiosis is a characteristic feature of most eczematous dermatoses, particularly at sites of lymphocyte migration into the epidermis; therefore, its absence is helpful in evaluating early CTCL. Second, epidermotropic lymphocytes in patch-stage disease (but often not in dysplastic stages) exhibit nuclear atypia consisting of hyperchromasia and contour irregularities (see Fig. 14–3D, E). These changes may be difficult to appreciate fully in routinely embedded and sectioned specimens, and special adjunctive approaches may be required to evaluate atypia at refined light microscopic and antigenic levels. Third, early CTCL in both the dysplastic and patch stages is almost invariably associated with papillary dermal fibrosis. This fibrosis consists of randomly arranged, coarse, collagen fibers that replace the normally delicate fibrils of the papillary dermis (see Fig. 14–2C).

In the plaque stage of CTCL, which is the prototype for the epidermotropic phase, diagnosis may be established by routine histopathology alone. At scanning magnification, there is an infiltrate of lymphocytes in the lower papillary and upper reticular dermis arranged in a band-like array (Fig. 14–4B). The infiltrate tends to be polymorphous and is composed of enlarged lymphoid cells containing markedly hyperchromatic nuclei with irregular, convoluted nuclear membranes (Fig. 14–4C, D), occasional immunoblast-like cells and even cells resembling Reed-Sternberg variants, plasma cells, and variable numbers of eosinophils. Nonspongiotic foci of the epidermis are infiltrated by cytologically atypical lymphoid cells that form small aggregates and clusters of cells (i.e., Pautrier microabscesses; see Fig. 14–4C) within lacunae resulting from mucinous epidermal degeneration. Similar epithelial infiltration may involve appendages, particularly hair follicles, where extensive mucinous degeneration may produce localized hair loss (i.e., alopecia mucinosa). CTCL occurring on the face or scalp may predominantly or exclusively involve hair follicles, with relative sparing of the interfollicular epidermis.

In the nonepidermotropic or nodular stage (see Fig. 14–5), total sparing of the papillary dermis and epidermis is the rule. Dermal infiltration by sheets and confluent aggregates of tightly compacted lymphoid cells is observed at low-power magnification (Fig. 14–5B). Vessels and appendages may be displaced or destroyed by these infiltrating cells. In contrast to earlier stages, in which reactive cells are often

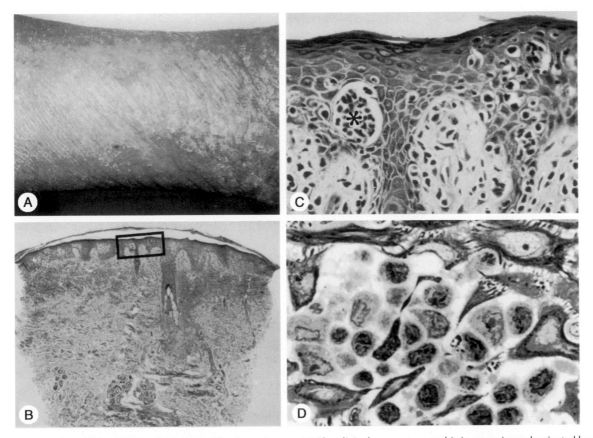

Figure 14–4. Cutaneous T-cell lymphoma, advanced epidermotropic type. **(A)** The clinical appearance at this juncture is predominated by thickened erythematous plaques covered by adherent white scale. **(B)** At scanning magnification, there is a dense band of lymphocytes within the superficial dermis associated with variable epidermal hyperplasia. **(C)** Closer inspection of the portion of the epidermis enclosed in **B** shows well-developed microabscesses of enlarged lymphocytes containing hyperchromatic nuclei. Similar cells are easily detected in the underlying dermis. **(D)** One-micron sections of such lesions confirm the elaborate nuclear convolutions necessary for a diagnosis of lymphoma, although by this evolutionary stage, neither plastic-embedded thin sections nor cell marker analysis is usually required for accurate diagnosis.

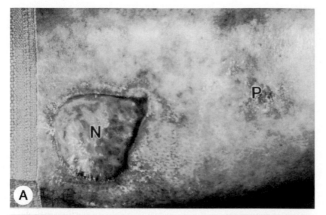

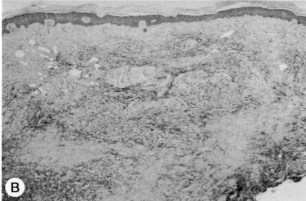

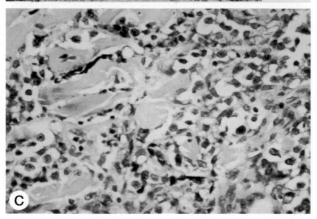

Figure 14–5. Cutaneous T-cell lymphoma (CTCL), nonepidermotropic type. **(A)** An ulcerated nodule (N) has developed within a plaque (P) of epidermotropic CTCL. **(B)** Typical lesions show diffuse infiltration of superficial and deep dermis by malignant lymphoid cells, sometimes accompanied by eosinophils and plasma cells. Note the sparing of the epidermal and papillary dermal layers. **(C)** High magnification reveals malignant cells infiltrating between dermal collagen bundles. Although some lesions are characterized by Sézary cells within the dermis, many contain cells that have undergone transformation to large malignant lymphoid elements which cannot be reliably differentiated from malignant B cells without the assistance of cell marker analysis.

be indistinguishable from B-cell malignancy, which also typically does not demonstrate epidermal involvement.

Diagnostic adjuncts in CTCL include 1-μm-section analysis, cell marker profiling, and molecular biological probes for clonality. Although many laboratories do not have such technologies available, specialized immunodiagnostic facilities are now available in most regions for triage of biopsy tissue. One-μm-section analysis is a means of assessing intricate nuclear convolutions in epidermotropic T cells. Whereas routine sections may be too thick (i.e., approximately 6 μm) to appreciate the complexities of infolded nuclear membranes, sections embedded in plastic resin or JB-4 medium and sectioned at 1-μm intervals (see Fig. 14–4D) increase the sensitivity of detection of cytologic atypia in early epidermotropic T-cell lymphomas. Cell marker analysis using immunoperoxidase detection systems coupled to monoclonal antibody probes is another means of identifying phenotypically abnormal T cells, particularly within the epidermal layer, where they tend to concentrate in early lesions. The dermal component often is a confusing mix of reactive T cells and a minority of malignant T cells. The abnormal clones in early T-cell lymphoma tend to be of the CD4 helper subtype, and often they are lacking in one or more pan-T-cell maturation antigens expressed by mature T cells. In this laboratory, the Leu1–5 series of monoclonal antibodies is used (Leu1, 4, and 5 are markers of pan-T-cell maturation antigens, Leu3 of CD4-positive "helper" T cells, and Leu2 of CD8-positive "suppressor" cells. A typical profile consistent with early T-cell lymphoma consists of predominantly CD4-positive epidermotropic cells (e.g., with a >10:1 CD4:CD8 ratio). In addition, there is often loss of reactivity of many of the cells for one or more of the antigens defined by Leu1, Leu4, or Leu5 antibodies. Finally, molecular detection for T-cell receptor gene rearrangements may be useful, particularly when coupled with polymerase chain reaction (PCR) amplification techniques to enhance sensitivity when only small numbers of cells are present. Although the PCR approach is still in developmental stages with regard to dermatopathology, it holds promise as an important routine diagnostic adjunct in the near future.

Cutaneous B-Cell Lymphoma[14–19]

- NODULAR OR DIFFUSE SUPERFICIAL AND DEEP INFILTRATE
- RELATIVE ABSENCE OF EPIDERMOTROPISM AND PERIADNEXAL SPREAD
- OFTEN, BAND OF SPARING IN PAPILLARY DERMIS (I.E., GRENZ ZONE)
- DESTRUCTIVE RELATIONSHIP TO PRE-EXISTING APPENDAGES AND VESSELS
- MONOMORPHOUS CELLULAR COMPOSITION
- DIFFUSE CELLULAR ATYPIA

B-cell lymphoma of the skin is a relatively rare disorder characterized by progressive, often multifocal infiltration of the dermis and subcutis by malignant lymphocytes of B-cell lineage. Clinically, lesions present as single or grouped, red, violaceous, or plum-colored plaques or nodules (Figs. 14–6A and 14–7A). In contrast to CTCL, in cutaneous B-cell lym-

admixed with malignant T cells, nonepidermotropic variants tend to be predominantly composed of atypical lymphoid cells (Fig. 14–5C). These cells may show considerable variation in size, and their nuclear contour may be jagged, cleaved, or convoluted. Large, immunoblast-like cells are also frequently observed, and some transformed variants may

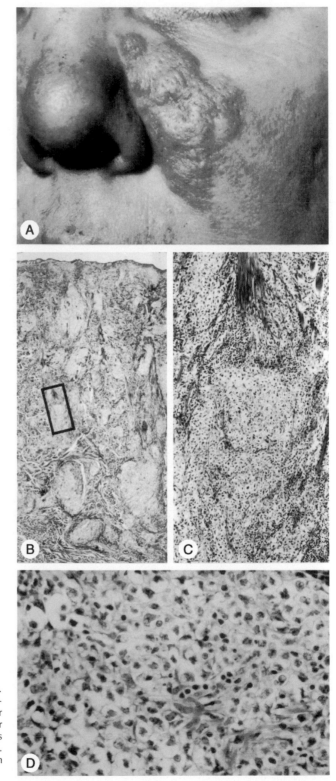

Figure 14–6. Cutaneous B-cell lymphoma, nodular large cell (follicular) type. **(A)** A firm, plum-colored facial lesion is devoid of significant clinical evidence of epidermal involvement. **(B)** The infiltrate has a vaguely nodular quality and is deeply invasive as seen at low magnification. **(C)** Higher-power magnification of the enclosed area in **B** reveals reactive small lymphocytes at the periphery of discrete aggregates of large, malignant lymphoid cells. **(D)** Further magnification of these cells demonstrates nuclear pleomorphism and chromatin aggregation consistent with anaplasia.

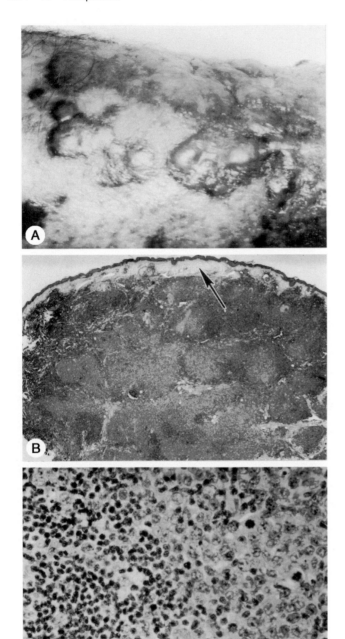

Figure 14–7. Cutaneous B-cell lymphoma, mixed small and large cell type. **(A)** Clinically, lesions are coalescent red-purple nodules covered by an attenuated, shiny epidermal surface. **(B)** An overview of one of the smaller nodules reveals nodular aggregates of cells filling the dermis but sparing the papillary dermis *(arrow)* and epidermis. **(C)** High magnification demonstrates two populations of malignant cells: one composed of monomorphous aggregates of smaller cells with diffuse nuclear hyperchromasia *(left)* and the other composed of larger malignant cells *(right)* similar to those demonstrated in Figure 14–6.

phoma, epidermal alterations manifested by scaling are uncommon. Although any skin surface may be involved, there is a predilection for involvement of the head, neck, and trunk.

The architecture of cutaneous B-cell lymphoma generally shows either diffuse or nodular infiltration of the entire dermis, with sparing of the papillary dermis and epidermal layer (Figs. 14–6*B* and 14–7*B*). Whereas benign lymphoid

hyperplasia within the dermis may show a nodular pattern of growth similar to that observed in B-cell lymphoma; the diffuse, interstitial, nonangiogenic pattern of the latter is distinctly unusual for dermal infiltration by benign lymphocytes.

Cytologically, the infiltrating cells tend to be monomorphous or dimorphous, as compared with reactive B-cell processes that show an admixture of lymphocyte maturational stages (i.e., small and large cells with cleaved and noncleaved nuclei, plasmacytoid or immunoblastic features, and associated cell types such as macrophages and eosinophils). Cytologic composition may be monomorphous (Fig. 14–6*C, D*) or dimorphous (Fig. 14–7*C*) and these relatively homogeneous populations may recapitulate cytologic characteristics of primary nodal counterparts. Although classification based on skin biopsy alone is inappropriate, the following types are represented:

Small B-cell lymphocytic
Plasmacytoid lymphocytic
Immunoblastic sarcoma of B cells
Lymphomas of follicular center cells (FCC)
    Small cleaved cell
    Large cleaved cell
    Small noncleaved cell
    Large noncleaved cell
Lymphoblastic lymphoma (rare B-cell subtypes)

Cutaneous involvement in *small lymphocytic lymphoma* composed of nearly normal-sized lymphocytes may show a nodular or diffuse pattern of dermal infiltration and is particularly problematic, because it is the most likely to be confused with a reactive process. Cytologically, there is a monomorphous infiltrate composed of small, round lymphocytes with dense chromatin, inconspicuous nucleoli, and scant cytoplasm. In *plasmacytoid lymphocytic lymphoma*, the dermis is infiltrated by cells similar to those of small cell lymphoma, although many have features that are intermediate between small lymphocytes and plasma cells. Small, periodic acid–Schiff (PAS)-positive intranuclear inclusions (i.e., Dutcher bodies) are typically present in occasional cells.

FCC lymphomas comprise up to one third of cutaneous non-Hodgkin lymphomas. Small cleaved, large cleaved, and mixed FCC lymphomas grow in diffuse and nodular patterns in the skin and cytologically resemble their nodal counterparts (see Figs. 14–6 and 14–7). Infiltrating cells are composed of monomorphous aggregates of small and/or large cleaved lymphocytes. Reactive T-cell components may be associated with malignant cells in FCC lymphomas involving the skin, leading to diagnostic confusion with benign lymphoid hyperplasias and sometimes necessitating multiple biopsies when clinical suspicion of malignancy is high.

Small noncleaved cell (including *Burkitt lymphoma*) and *large noncleaved cell lymphomas* almost always involve the skin as diffuse, superficial and deep, monomorphic lymphoid infiltrates with sparing of the epidermis. B-cell *immunoblastic lymphoma* is a neoplastic proliferation of immunoblast-like cells that often exhibit plasmacytoid differentiation. These cells are large and contain rounded nuclei with peripherally marginated chromatin, prominent nucleoli, and abundant, amphophilic, pyroninophilic cytoplasm similar to that of immunoblasts. Intermixed neoplastic plasma cells and large immunoblasts are typical and assist in separating this variant from large noncleaved FCC lymphomas.

Table 14–1. FEATURES OF T- AND B-CELL LYMPHOMAS AND BENIGN LYMPHOID HYPERPLASIA

FEATURE	T-CELL LYMPHOMA*	B-CELL LYMPHOMA	BENIGN LYMPHOID HYPERPLASIA
Epidermal involvement	+/−	−	−
Polymorphic infiltrate	+/−	−	+
True germinal centers	−	−	+/−
Pseudogerminal centers†	−	+/−	−
Cerebriform nuclei	+	−	+/−
T-cell infiltrate	+	−	+/−
Abnormal T-cell antigen expression	+	−	−
B-cell infiltrate	−	+	+/−
Monotypic immunoglobulin expression	−	+	−

*Nonepidermotropic variants may be indistinguishable from B-cell lymphoma by routine morphologic criteria.
†May be seen as ''growth centers'' in well-differentiated, small B-cell lymphocytic lymphoma.
+ = present; − = absent; +/− = present or absent.

Because B-cell lymphomas may be indistinguishable from nonepidermotropic CTCL, immunohistochemistry for T- and B-cell typing may be required to define cell lineage. Fortunately, unlike T-cell subtyping, which must be performed on fresh-frozen or Michel-fixed tissue, immunohistochemical differentiation between neoplastic B and T cells may usually be accomplished in formalin-fixed, paraffin-embedded tissue. With regard to differentiation of reactive and malignant B-cell infiltrates, immunohistochemical detection of monotypic kappa or lambda light chain expression by malignant cells is suggestive of a clonal process that is likely to be malignant. Nonetheless, the differential diagnosis between nonepidermotropic CTCL, B-cell lymphoma, and cutaneous lymphoid hyperplasia is often problematic. Table 14–1 highlights some of the salient diagnostic features that distinguish these biologically different entities.

Cutaneous Plasmacytoma[20–23]

- NODULAR DERMAL MONONUCLEAR CELL INFILTRATE
- SEGMENTALLY AGGREGATED HETEROCHROMATIN AT PERIPHERY OF NUCLEUS
- PERINUCLEAR CLEAR SPACE
- MITOTIC FIGURES AND BINUCLEATION WITHIN PLASMA CELLS
- MITOSES AND NUCLEAR ATYPIA
- MONOMORPHIC CYTOLOGY AND LIGHT CHAIN RESTRICTION

Cutaneous plasmacytomas consist of primary and secondary cutaneous infiltrates of benign or malignant bursa-associated lymphocytes (i.e., B cells) with terminal differentiation features of plasma cells. Primary malignant cutaneous plasmacytomas are rare. They may only be so designated if their neoplastic nature has been established and their origin in bone or soft tissue has been excluded. Secondary malignant cutaneous plasmacytomas are, by definition, metastatic lesions that generally are sequelae of multiple myeloma or plasma cell leukemia. As with B-cell lymphoma and acute myeloid leukemia, cutaneous involvement may rarely be the first detectable manifestation of disease. The gross pathology of lesions consists of solitary or multiple plaques and indurated nodules with a red to dull purple hue. Epidermal alterations such as scale or ulceration are usually not present.

At scanning magnification, there is cellular, diffuse or nodular infiltration of the dermis (Fig. 14–8A). The papillary dermis and the epidermis are spared. Plasmacytoid cells forming these infiltrates consist of cells with a benign appearance as well as cells showing angulated nuclear contours, nuclear enlargement, and hyperchromasia (Fig. 14–8B, C). Mitotic figures and binucleated forms are frequently observed. Immunohistochemistry of paraffin-embedded tissue reveals light chain restriction within the cytoplasm of the malignant plasma cells. Malignant cutaneous plasmacytomas may mimic *cutaneous lymphoid hyperplasia* with *plasmacytoid features*. The latter do not exhibit architectural or nuclear atypia and do not demonstrate light chain immunoglobulin restriction. *Benign cutaneous plasmacytomas* resemble lymphoid hyperplasia with plasmacytoid differentiation, although the majority of cells in the former condition appear to be benign plasma cells.

Leukemia Cutis[24, 25]

- ANGIOCENTRIC OR NODULAR DERMAL ARCHITECTURE
- DESTRUCTIVE OR INTERSTITIAL PATTERNS OF INFILTRATION IN ADVANCED LESIONS
- MONOMORPHOUS INFILTRATE IN ACUTE GRANULOCYTIC, LYMPHOCYTIC, AND CHRONIC LYMPHOCYTIC LEUKEMIA
- SPECTRUM OF CELLULAR DIFFERENTIATION IN CHRONIC GRANULOCYTIC LEUKEMIA
- BLAST FORMS IN ACUTE LEUKEMIAS

Leukemia cutis implies secondary infiltration of the dermis by malignant cells of hematopoietic origin in the setting of acute or chronic myelogenous or lymphocytic leukemias. Cutaneous manifestations of leukemia cutis commonly consist of pink-red to purpuric papules and nodules (Fig. 14–9A), although indurated plaques, patches, and ulcers sometimes are observed. In chronic lymphocytic leukemia, erythroderma mimicking Sézary syndrome of cutaneous T-cell lymphoma may be seen. Granulocytic leukemic infiltrates contain abundant myeloperoxidase, imparting a characteristic greenish hue clinically (i.e., chloromas). Any body site may

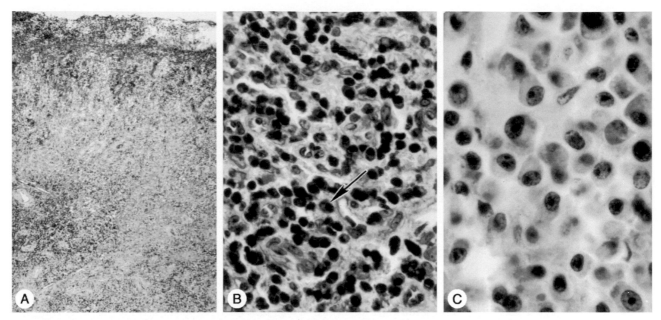

Figure 14–8. Cutaneous plasmacytoma. **(A)** An ulcerated and destructive dermal infiltrate has a diffuse, permeative pattern of infiltration (ulcer surface at top of panel). **(B)** Higher magnification reveals many of the infiltrating cells show eccentric, hyperchromatic nuclei *(arrow)* consistent with plasmacytoid differentiation. Based on a skin biopsy specimen alone, the diagnosis was consistent with malignant lymphoma with plasmacytoid features. **(C)** Cutaneous involvement by multiple myeloma shows more mature plasma cells with prominent, pleomorphic nuclei and focal nuclear hyperchromasia.

be affected, and although cutaneous spread rarely occurs, it generally portends a poor prognosis. Cutaneous lesions may occasionally be the initial clinical sign of leukemia.

Leukemic infiltration of the dermis may mimic benign dermatoses when it has a perivascular pattern or lymphomatous involvement, generally of the B-cell type, when it has a nodular or diffuse pattern (Fig. 14–9B). Cutaneous involvement by chronic lymphocytic leukemia is often indistinguishable from that of small cell (i.e., well-differentiated) lymphocytic lymphoma. The finding of malignant cells within blood vascular lumens, however, is an important clue to the diagnosis of leukemia cutis, as opposed to primary cutaneous lymphoma (Fig. 14–9C). Chronic granulocytic leukemia shows a spectrum of differentiation between mature and immature myeloid forms as well as occasional eosinophilic myeloblasts (Fig. 14–9D); acute granulocytic leukemias contain myeloblasts that are easily confused with large cell lymphoma cells or histiocytic infiltrates.

Langerhans Cell Histiocytosis[26–29]

- VARIABLE ARCHITECTURE (I.E., LICHENOID, NODULAR, OR DIFFUSE)
- EPIDERMOTROPISM OR ADNEXAL INFILTRATION
- LARGE CELLS WITH PALE, INFOLDED NUCLEI AND ABUNDANT PALE PINK CYTOPLASM
- VARIABLE ATYPIA
- ADMIXED EOSINOPHILS IN SOME BUT NOT ALL LESIONS

The biologic behavior of Langerhans cell proliferations in skin varies considerably depending on the clinical situa-

tion in which they arise. Although originally described to involve solitary lytic bone lesions, it is now recognized that "eosinophilic granuloma" involves a number of extraosseous sites, including skin and mucosae. Cutaneous lesions may appear as multiple, crusted papules (Fig. 14–10A, B) or as solitary or multiple nodules. The face and scalp are frequently affected. *Hand-Schüller-Christian disease* is a rare variant of Langerhans cell histiocytosis that affects young children and occasionally adults. Affected individuals classically demonstrate the triad of exophthalmus, diabetes insipidus, and cranial deposits. Multiple skeletal and extraosseous lesions are present, with palpable defects involving the calvarium. Skin of the chest, axillae, and groin are most frequently involved, although other sites may also be affected. Lesions are maculopapular and red to brown in color; nodules and ulcers show a predisposition for the axillae and perineum. *Letterer-Siwe disease* is another rare variant that has a more acute and morbid course than Hand-Schüller-Christian disease. Young children, often younger than 3 years of age, are most often affected. Skin lesions are maculopapular and erythematous, and they frequently show a seborrheic distribution (see Fig. 14–10A, B). Involvement of multiple organ systems is common, with defects similar to those seen in Hand-Schüller-Christian disease. The prognosis is exceedingly poor, and the vast majority of afflicted children succumb within two years of onset.

Variants of cutaneous Langerhans cell histiocytosis, also called histocytosis X, show considerable histologic overlap. The architecture of the infiltrates may be band-like within the superficial dermis, nodular and deep, or diffuse throughout the upper and mid-dermis (Fig. 14–10C). Epidermotropism is frequently encountered with Langerhans cell histiocytosis cells migrating into the epidermal layer (Fig. 14–10C). Hair

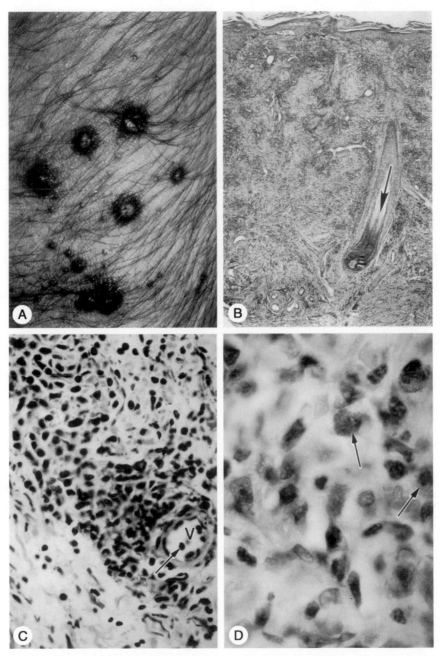

Figure 14–9. Leukemia cutis. **(A)** Hemorrhagic nodules are present in a patient with acute myelogenous leukemia. **(B)** There is diffuse interstitial dermal involvement by leukemic cells; the total absence of an angiocentric pattern of infiltration raises the possibility of hematopoietic malignancy. Arrow denotes distorted, entrapped hair follicle. **(C)** Hyperchromatic mononuclear cells within the dermal interstitium resemble lymphoma cutis; the finding of a malignant cell *(arrow)* within a vessel lumen (V), however, warrants consideration of leukemia cutis, which occasionally may present as cutaneous lesions even before overt dissemination in the peripheral blood. **(D)** Confirmation of acute myelogenous leukemia is made by detection of myeloblasts with eosinophilic cytoplasmic granules (i.e., eosinophilic myeloblasts; *arrows*).

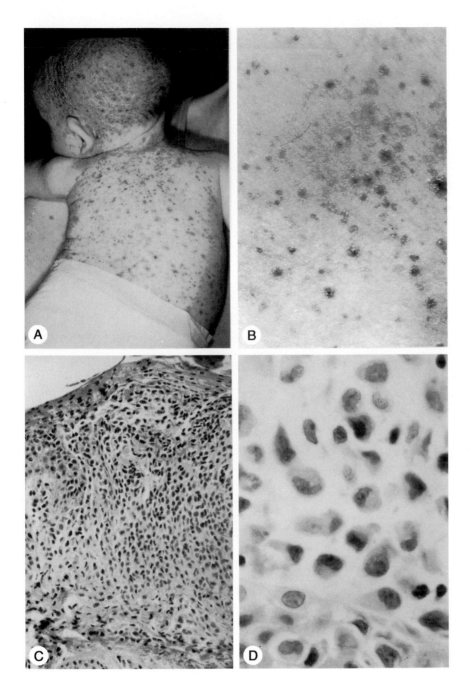

Figure 14–10. Langerhans cell histiocytosis (histiocytosis X). **(A, B)** Eczematous papules mimic infantile seborrheic dermatitis. **(C)** A superficial and mid-dermal mononuclear cell infiltrate with foci of epidermotropism is present. **(D)** The infiltrating cells have pale, focally infolded nuclei and abundant cytoplasm relative to lymphocytes.

follicles may be similarly involved, particularly in axillary and groin skin. Cytologically, the infiltrating cells have pale and ample cytoplasm, and the cell membranes are indistinct (Fig. 14–10D). The nuclei are large and pale, with a typical reniform or infolded nuclear contour. Cytologic atypia and mitotic activity may be seen, but do not appear to reliably correlate with biologic behavior or with the clinical syndromes described previously. An admixture of eosinophils is generally but not invariably observed. Some lesions are entirely devoid of eosinophils, emphasizing the misnomer of eosinophilic granuloma. Multinucleated cells may be encountered in some lesions, and the cytoplasm may occasionally be finely vacuolated, imparting a xanthomatous appearance to the infiltrate.

Immunohistochemistry of lesions of cutaneous Langerhans cell histiocytosis demonstrates positivity for S100 pro-

tein in routinely prepared tissue. Melanocytes and activated histiocytes as well as some carcinoma cells are also S100-positive. A more specific indicator of Langerhans cell histiocytosis cells is detection of the CD1a antigen on the cell surface (Fig. 14–11A, B). This requires fresh-frozen or Michel-fixed and frozen tissue sections and monoclonal antibody reagents to this antigenic determinant (e.g., Leu6 antibody). If Langerhans cell histiocytosis is suspected clinically, it is advised that tissue be triaged for rapid freezing or placed in immunofluorescence transport medium for subsequent freezing and immunohistochemical evaluation of CD1a antigen in the immunopathology laboratory. Ultrastructural evaluation of cutaneous infiltrates in Langerhans cell histiocytosis generally will reveal characteristic tennis racquet–shaped Birbeck granules within the cytoplasm of tumor cells (Fig. 14–11C). The outcome in Langerhans cell histiocytosis

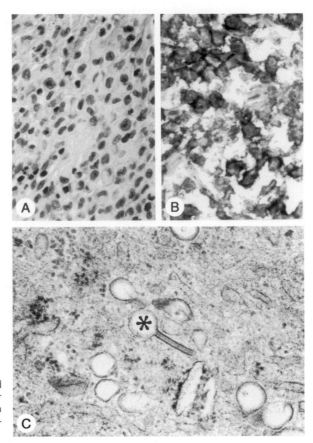

Figure 14–11. Langerhans cell histiocytosis: special studies. **(A)** The histiocytoid dermal infiltrate stains positively for S100 protein in paraffin sections and **(B)** for the cell surface glycoprotein CD1a in frozen sections. **(C)** Diagnostic electron microscopy reveals characteristic tennis racquet–shaped Birbeck granules *(asterisk)* within tumor cells.

appears to depend on at least four clinical variables. These include patient age (older patients tend to do better than younger ones), the number of sites involved (multiple sites suggest a worse prognosis), the speed of progression or treatment response (rapid worsening of clinical course is an unfavorable sign, whereas rapid response to therapy is a good sign), and degree of organ dysfunction (documentation of extent of dysfunction of liver, lung, and hematopoietic system has led to several systems of staging). Thrombocytopenia combined with anemia, jaundice, hepatosplenomegaly, and respiratory disease, in the absence of bone lesions, is generally associated with a fatal outcome.

Regressing Atypical Histiocytosis[30–36]

- DIFFUSE SUPERFICIAL AND DEEP DERMAL INFILTRATE
- EPIDERMAL HYPERPLASIA WITH OCCASIONAL FOCI OF ACANTHOLYSIS AND NEUTROPHILIC MICROABSCESSES
- LARGE, PROFOUNDLY ATYPICAL CELLS, SOME RESEMBLING REED-STERNBERG CELLS
- ADMIXED SMALL LYMPHOCYTES

Regressing atypical histiocytosis (RAH) was first described as a proliferation of histiocytes that formed recurrent noduloulcerative lesions in the skin. Most cases involve young to middle-aged adults, and there appears to be no gender predilection. Individual lesions range between 2 and 10 cm, and primary lesions frequently ulcerate. Single or multiple nodules may be observed at the time of diagnosis, and the extremities are frequently involved. Tumors form rapidly, often over several weeks, and the typical course involves spontaneous regression and recurrence over a period of many months to years. Long-term follow-up has revealed the eventual development of aggressive disease in most cases, which suggests that RAH is really a regressing evolutionary phase of what will progress inexorably to become a fixed T-cell lymphoproliferative disorder.

The prototypic architecture of RAH involves exuberant epidermal hyperplasia associated with dense aggregates of tumor cells (Fig. 14–12A). Tumor cells form expansile aggregates within the dermis, such that even low-power evaluation raises the possibility of hematopoietic malignancy. Cytologically, there is a preponderance of large, atypical mononuclear cells (Fig. 14–12B), many of which demonstrate amphophilic cytoplasm and highly pleomorphic nuclei with irregular contours, vesicular nuclear chromatin patterns, and prominent, centrally located nucleoli (Fig. 14–12C). Lesional cells may be infiltrated by a reactive inflammatory component and exuberant granulation tissue. Perilesional fibrosis, focal tumor cell necrosis, and focal infiltration by eosinophils have all been reported. Molecular biological approaches have shown that the majority of proliferating cells in RAH lesions have aberrant T-cell antigenic profiles and rearrangements of T-cell receptor beta and gamma chain genes, indicating that this neoplasm is most likely of T-cell lineage. High numbers of atypical cells also may express the Ki-1 antigen, a marker also expressed by true Reed-Sternberg cells.

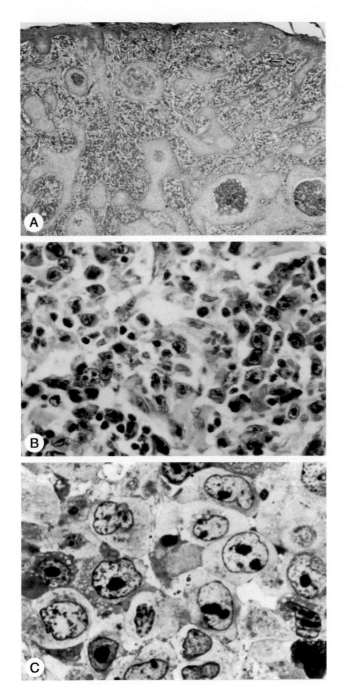

Figure 14–12. Regressing atypical histiocytosis. **(A)** Active lesions show a brisk dermal infiltrate of atypical cells associated with marked overlying epidermal hyperplasia, a finding often associated with growth factors elaborated by an active immune or reparative response. **(B, C)** At progressively higher magnifications, the infiltrative component is composed of enlarged, anaplastic lymphoid cells with an associated infiltrate of reactive benign lymphocytes. Many of the atypical cells share characteristics with Reed-Sternberg variants and are Ki-1 positive by immunohistochemistry.

Lymphomatoid Papulosis[37-40]

- ANGIOCENTRIC, WEDGE-SHAPED, SUPERFICIAL AND DEEP DERMAL INFILTRATE
- VARIABLE EPIDERMOTROPISM
- POLYMORPHOUS INFILTRATE OF VARIABLY SIZED MONONUCLEAR CELLS

- ADMIXED REED-STERNBERG–LIKE CELLS AND EOSINOPHILS
- LYMPHOCYTIC VASCULITIS ASSOCIATED WITH ANGIOCENTRIC DYSPLASTIC CELLS

Lymphomatoid papulosis is a disorder characterized by a chronic clinical course of recurrent, erythematous to hemorrhagic papules and nodules that may ulcerate and generally regress with scarring (Fig. 14–13A). The trunk and extremities are most frequently involved; men outnumber women by 2:1; and systemic examination is characteristically negative for evidence of extracutaneous disease.

At scanning magnification, lesions of lymphomatoid papulosis show characteristic wedge-shaped architecture formed by coalescent angiocentric mononuclear cell infiltrates (Fig. 14–13B). The epidermis may be variably hyperplastic or ulcerated, and epidermotropism may be focally observed. At higher magnification, the infiltrate is polymorphous, composed of an admixture of variably activated lymphocytes, histiocytes, eosinophils, and Reed-Sternberg–like cells. The latter contain large, bilobed nuclei with prominent nucleoli within each lobe (Fig. 14–13C). Although similar cells may also be observed in RAH (discussed previously), lymphomatoid papulosis contains only occasional clusters of these cells and fails to exhibit tumoral dermal infiltration or florid epidermal hyperplasia. Another helpful diagnostic indicator in lymphomatoid papulosis is the presence of endothelial swelling, vacuolization, and focal necrosis in association with intense angiocentric infiltration, which has been termed "dysplastic lymphocytic vasculitis." Finally, it should be noted that the epidermotropic cells in some lesions of lymphomatoid papulosis may involve relatively nonspongiotic foci. Moreover, they may exhibit enlarged, infolded nuclei which may be confused with epidermotropic cells of early CTCL. Such findings must therefore be evaluated within the context of other architectural and cytologic features of the infiltrate in the dermis to enable a diagnosis of lymphomatoid papulosis.

Atypical lymphocytes in lymphomatoid papulosis frequently display elevated helper:suppressor T-cell ratios and defects in mature pan-T-cell antigen expression that suggest cutaneous T-cell lymphoma. The Reed-Sternberg–like cells that characterize some lesions react positively for Ki-1, a Reed-Sternberg cell–associated antigen, and show strong expression of interleukin-2 receptors or T-cell activation complex (TAC). T-cell receptor gene rearrangements have recently been documented in lymphomatoid papulosis as well as in the benign, potentially related dermatosis *pityriasis lichenoides et varioliformis acuta* (see Chap. 6).

Mastocytosis[41, 42]

- CELLULAR TUMORAL (CHILDHOOD) OR LESS CELLULAR (ADULT) DERMAL INFILTRATE
- MAST CELLS WITHIN INTERVENULAR, AS WELL AS PERIVASCULAR, CONNECTIVE TISSUE
- METACHROMATIC GRANULES WITHIN DENDRITIC MAST CELLS
- VARIABLE VASCULAR ECTASIA, ADMIXED EOSINOPHILS, PAPILLARY DERMAL EDEMA
- EPIDERMOTROPISM NEVER SEEN

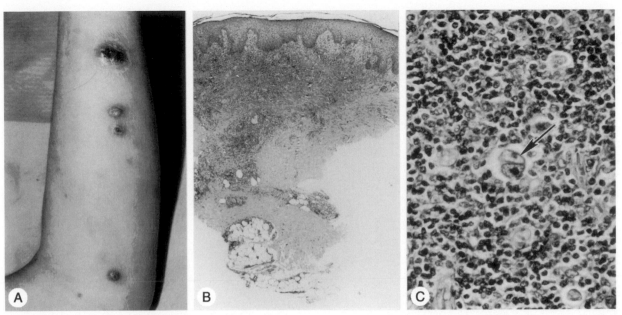

Figure 14–13. Lymphomatoid papulosis. **(A)** Multiple, juicy, erythematous nodules are present on the upper extremity of a young male patient. **(B)** Histologically, there is a wedge-shaped inflammatory infiltrate in the superficial and deep dermis. **(C)** Reed-Sternberg–like cells *(arrow)* are admixed with a pleomorphic infiltrate of lymphoid elements. Lymphomatoid vasculitis is focally present. These lesions exhibit T-cell receptor gene rearrangements, and although most will regress, a minority of patients progress to overt lymphoma.

The term mastocytosis refers to a spectrum of disorders characterized by cutaneous and sometimes extracutaneous mast cell proliferation. A localized form of the disease, termed *urticaria pigmentosa,* predominantly affects the skin of children and accounts for more than 50% of all cases of mastocytosis. Lesions are usually multiple, although solitary mastocytomas may be noted shortly after birth (Figs. 14–14*A* and 14–15*A*). About 10% of patients with mast cell disease have *systemic mastocytosis,* characterized by mast cell infiltration of many extracutaneous organs, including the gastrointestinal tract. Affected individuals often are adults, and unlike localized cutaneous disease, the prognosis is often poor. It is important to point out that although mastocytosis has been divided conceptually into localized cutaneous and systemic forms, most patients with localized disease have subclinical evidence of mast cell aggregates in their bone marrow (i.e., mast cell microgranulomas).

Solitary mastocytomas present as one or several tan-brown nodules that may be pruritic or exhibit blister formation (see Fig. 14–14*A*). In urticaria pigmentosa, lesions are multiple and widely distributed, consisting of round to oval, red-brown, nonscaling urticarial papules and small plaques (see Fig. 14–15*A*). In systemic mastocytosis, skin lesions are similar to urticaria pigmentosa but are accompanied by symptomatic and florid mast cell infiltration of bone marrow, liver, spleen, and lymph nodes. It is presently conjectural as to whether mastocytosis is a true neoplasm or a heterogeneous group of lesions characterized by alterations in mast cell maturation or proliferation within the skin and extracutaneous viscera as a result of abnormalities in the local microenvironment. Evidence supporting the latter possibility exists, however, because normal skin from mastocytosis patients displays abnormalities in epidermally derived mast cell

growth factor as well as in the ultrastructural phenotype of underlying dermal mast cells.

In children, lesions of urticaria pigmentosa frequently present as tumoral accumulations of mast cells within the superficial and mid-dermis (Figs. 14–14*B* and 14–15*B*). These tightly packed cells characteristically have pale-staining, pink cytoplasm and centrally located, round nuclei (Fig. 14–14*C*), and they therefore may resemble nevus cells because of the consistent central localization of the uniform nuclei within the cell cytoplasm. At high-power magnification, faint granularity may be observed within the cytoplasm. These granules become more obvious upon staining with metachromatic reagents such as toluidine blue or Giemsa stains (Figs. 14–14*D* and 14–15*C*). Although the tendency for mast cells to contain numerous metachromatic granules is characteristic and separates them from other lymphoproliferative processes involving the skin, in some cases, the granules may be subtle and difficult to demonstrate. This is partially the result of degranulation of mastocytosis cells as a result of the biopsy technique.

In adult forms of mastocytosis, cutaneous lesions may be extraordinarily subtle, with only slight increases in the numbers of mast cells about superficial vessels. A helpful diagnostic clue is the presence of mast cells within intervenular connective tissue in an interstitial pattern; normal mast cells tend to congregate in the perivascular space. In addition, mast cell profiles after Giemsa staining tend to be dendritic rather than rounded in adult forms of mastocytosis. In all types of mast cell disease, eosinophils may be detected, perhaps as a result of chemotactic factors by degranulating mast cells. The acute and chronic sequelae of mast cell degranulation in the dermis may be present in biopsy specimens and provide additional diagnostic clues. Acutely, there may be

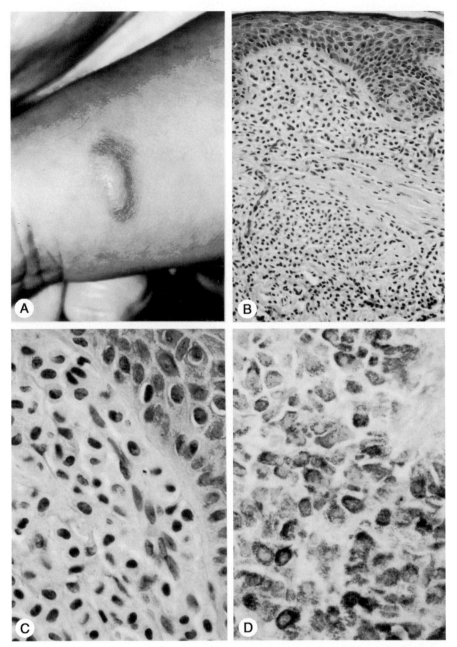

Figure 14–14. Solitary cutaneous mastocytoma. **(A)** A dull-pink nodule from the upper extremity of a 1-year-old child demonstrates a monomorphous dermal infiltrate **(B, C)** that is without epidermotropism and characterized by cells containing evenly spaced nuclei due to a peripheral rim of apparently rigid cytoplasm (i.e., "fried-egg" cells). **(D)** Staining with toluidine blue or with the Giemsa reagent reveals metachromatic cytoplasmic granules typical of mast cells.

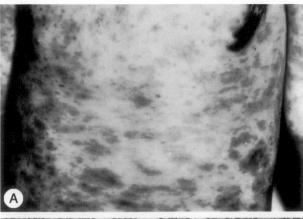

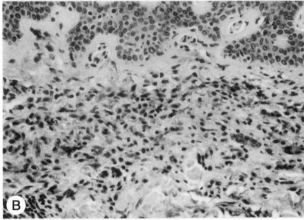

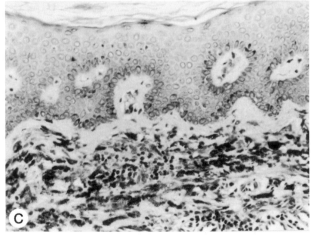

Figure 14–15. Urticaria pigmentosa. **(A)** The clinical appearance in this child consists of hyperpigmented macules and plaques; stroking of the cutaneous surface induces urticarial wheals (i.e., Darier sign). **(B)** Histologically, there are variable numbers of cells within the superficial dermis in an interstitial pattern. These cells exhibit poorly defined, granulated, dendritic cytoplasm. In adults, the increased number of cells may barely exceed normal numbers within the superficial dermis. **(C)** Metachromatic stains reveal positive mast cell granules within the majority of infiltrating cells. There is also increased melanin within basal keratinocytes, possibly the result of increased expression of growth factors that affect both mast cells and melanocytes.

dermal edema and lymphatic ectasia similar to that observed in ordinary urticaria. More chronically, some lesions develop varying degrees of dermal fibrosis. Solitary lesions in which this later response predominates have been termed sclerosing mastocytomas.

True Histiocytomas[43, 44]

- TUMORAL SUPERFICIAL AND DEEP DERMAL INFILTRATION
- POLYMORPHOUS INFILTRATES WITH ADMIXED EOSINOPHILS AND NEUTROPHILS
- MULTINUCLEATED CELLS WITH PERIPHERAL WREATH OF VACUOLIZATION (I.E., XANTHOGRANULOMA)
- MULTINUCLEATED CELLS WITH RED-PURPLE, GRANULAR CYTOPLASM (I.E., RETICULOHISTIOCYTOMA)

The most common purely histiocytic infiltrates of skin are the xanthogranuloma and the reticulohistiocytoma. Xanthomas, which may have implications for hyperlipoproteinemia, are discussed in detail in Chapter 19. Clinically, xanthogranuloma most frequently involves infants and young children (i.e., juvenile xanthogranulomas), although adults are also affected. Lesions often arise during the first 6 months of life; there is no gender predilection; and systemic lipid abnormalities are absent. Tumors are usually small (i.e., several millimeters in diameter), yellow-red papules (Fig. 14–16A) that tend to occur on the head and upper trunk.

At scanning magnification, xanthogranulomas are characterized by symmetrical aggregates of infiltrating cells that form a dome-shaped papule within the superficial and middermis (Fig. 14–16B). Extension into the subcutaneous fat may occur in some lesions. Early evolutionary stages are characterized by an admixture of foamy histiocytes with acute and chronic inflammatory cells, including eosinophils. Lipid-laden cells and multinucleated cells may be only focally present in early lesions. With time, characteristic Touton giant cells appear. These cells have a wreath-like configuration of nuclei about the cell perimeter, surrounded by coarse, cytoplasmic vacuoles (Fig. 14–16C). The presence of Touton giant cells is an important differentiating feature between xanthogranulomas and tumoral xanthomas (Fig. 14–17), which are less polymorphous and composed predominantly of mononuclear foam cells.

Reticulohistiocytoma refers to a benign dermal proliferation of histiocytes with characteristic pink, ground-glass cytoplasm. These lesions generally are observed in middle-aged individuals, and women are preferentially affected. Individual tumors may be solitary (Fig. 14–18A) or multiple (Fig. 14–19A), and the latter are associated with destructive arthritis (Fig. 14–19B) and intermittent fevers. Lesions tend to occur on the hands, arms, and face, and present as firm, yellow-tan papules and nodules (see Fig. 14–18A).

At scanning magnification, reticulohistiocytoma is characterized by well-defined, symmetrical dermal nodules, often with an attenuated overlying epidermis (Fig. 14–18B). It is noteworthy that neither xanthogranuloma nor reticulohistiocytoma is associated with inductive epidermal hyperplasia, as is the case with benign fibrous histiocytoma (see Chap. 15). Cytologically, the tumor cells contain one or more nuclei and ample amounts of bright pink, PAS-positive, finely granulated cytoplasm that produces a ground-glass appearance (see Fig. 14–18C). Touton giant cells are not observed, although early lesions may have a background of acute and chronic inflammatory cells similar to that seen in xanthogranulomas.

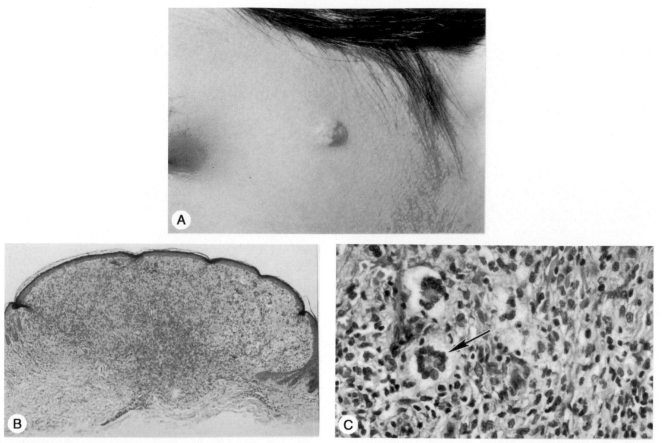

Figure 14–16. Xanthogranuloma. **(A)** There is a yellow-white, firm nodule on the temporal skin of this 4-year-old girl. **(B)** A biopsy specimen reveals a superficial and deep dermal infiltrate of mononuclear cells. **(C)** On higher magnification, the infiltrate demonstrates characteristic Touton giant cells *(arrow)*. These cells are characterized by a wreath of nuclei surrounded by a rim of cytoplasmic vacuolization. Early lesions consisting primarily of focally lipidized histiocytes may be devoid of multinucleated cells and replete with eosinophils.

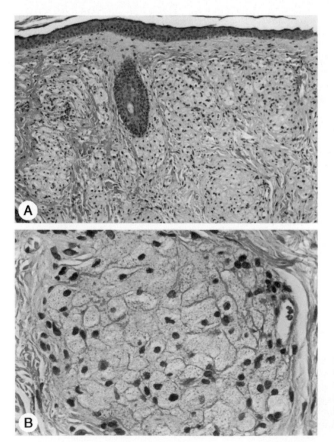

Figure 14–17. Xanthoma. **(A, B)** Collections of lipid-laden histiocytes may occur incidentally or as specific lesion in the setting of hyperlipidemia. They must be differentiated histologically from granular cell tumors, which are composed of cells with cytoplasmic granules, not vacuoles, and from other histiocytic infiltrates that may become lipidized (e.g., xanthomatous variant of Langerhans cell histiocytosis). Correlation with clinical history should prove helpful in resolving these differential diagnostic considerations.

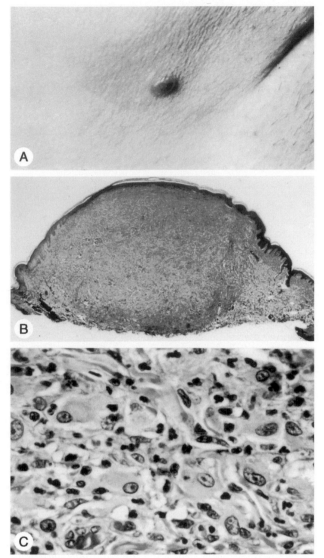

Figure 14–18. Reticulohistiocytoma. **(A)** A small, firm, yellow-tan papule represents a solitary reticulohistiocytoma. **(B)** At low magnification, there is a proliferation of mononuclear and multinucleated, intensely eosinophilic pink-purple cells within the superficial to mid-dermis. **(C)** Cytologically, these cells contain one or more round, benign-appearing nuclei and ample quantities of bright pink, PAS-positive, granulated cytoplasm that produces a ground-glass appearance.

Rare Disorders

Adult T-Cell Leukemia and Lymphoma[45]

Adult T-cell leukemia and lymphoma (ATLL) is a clinical variant of CTCL. ATLL results from HTLV-1 retrovirus infection and has occurred in scattered outbreaks worldwide. Affected patients characteristically present with the explosive onset of variably sized, firm, confluent nodules on the trunk and extremities. Plaques, papules, and nonexfoliative erythroderma may also be seen. Lesions may progress from a few scattered nodules to hundreds of deforming tumors within several weeks. In contrast to classic CTCL, individuals with ATLL demonstrate visceral involvement from the outset. The most common sites of dissemination include the peripheral blood, lymph nodes, bone marrow, gastrointestinal tract,

lungs, leptomeninges, and liver. Lytic bone lesions, hypercalcemia, and elevated serum alkaline phosphatase are often observed at time of presentation.

Most lesions of ATLL histologically resemble those of nonepidermotropic CTCL, although some are indistinguishable from plaque-stage disease. In the peripheral blood, however, ATLL cells are characterized by hyperlobated rather than cerebriform nuclear contours.

Malignant Angioendotheliomatosis (Angiotropic Lymphoma)[46]

Originally believed to represent diffuse neoplastic endothelial proliferation, malignant angioendotheliomatosis is now recognized to be an angiotropic lymphoma. Adults are primarily affected, and there is no gender predilection. Initial skin involvement may consist of erythematous nodules and plaques, which may resemble erythema nodosum or other forms of panniculitis. Histologically, there are numerous hyperchromatic mononuclear cells adherent to the endothelium lining of dermal vascular channels (Fig. 14–20). Occasional vessels will also contain fibrin thrombi. The intimate associations between the adherent atypical mononuclear cells and the endothelial cells may result in the impression that the

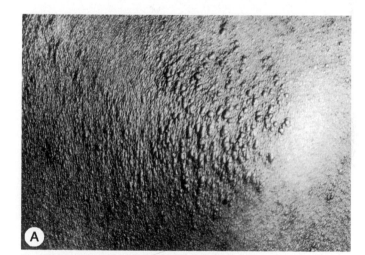

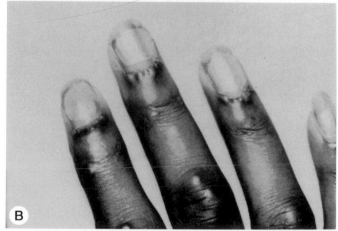

Figure 14–19. Multicentric reticulohistiocytosis. **(A)** Multiple cutaneous papules representing reticulohistiocytomas are associated with **(B)** destructive arthritis.

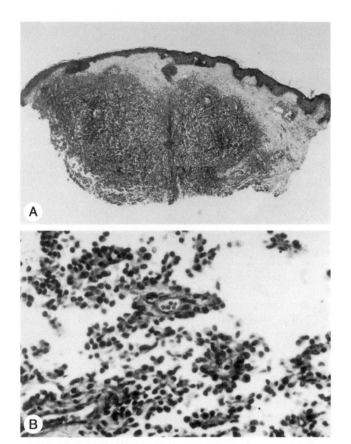

Figure 14–20. Malignant angioendothelioma. **(A)** The dermis is heavily infiltrated by hyperchromatic malignant cells producing a pattern similar to cellular angiosarcoma. **(B)** Atypical cells are aligned along widened vascular spaces. Immunocytochemistry demonstrated these cells to be of lymphoid origin (primarily B cells). The cells are adherent to endothelial cells, mimicking a malignant vascular proliferation.

entire process is endothelial in origin. Immunohistochemical detection of T- and B-cell markers, however, discloses the lymphoid nature of the adherent cell population. Certain lesions have proven to be T-cell lymphomas, whereas others have been marked as B-cell lymphomas. It appears that this rare subset of lymphoma is characterized by unusual expression of adhesive ligands that bond circulating tumor cells to the endothelial surface.

Angioimmunoblastic Lymphadenopathy with Skin Involvement[47]

Angioimmunoblastic lympadenopathy with dysproteinemia is a systemic disorder typified by generalized lymphadenopathy, hepatomegaly, splenomegaly, fever, anemia, and polyclonal gammopathy. Elderly individuals are more commonly affected, and there is no gender predilection. Skin involvement is observed in over one third of cases, and it may precede the development of clinically overt systemic disease. Lesions are polymorphous, ranging from pruritic maculopapular exanthems to papular and nodular eruptions. Histologically, there is a superficial and deep perivascular infiltrate which may be tightly angiocentric and associated with variable degrees of necrotizing vascular injury. Cytolog-

ically, mononuclear cells of variable size and differentiation status predominate. Numerous plasmacytoid cells and immunoblasts are the rule, and their detection, along with associated vascular injury, are of assistance in diagnosing this form of dysplastic lymphocytic vasculitis. Cell marker analysis generally reveals numerous B cells in the dermal infiltrate.

Lymphomatoid Granulomatosis[48, 49]

Lymphomatoid granulomatosis, now recognized as an evolutionary stage of lymphoma from the outset, is characterized by a chronic clinical course with recurrent erythematous to hemorrhagic papules and nodules that may ulcerate and regress with scarring. The trunk and extremities are most often involved, and men are preferentially affected over women by about a 2:1 ratio. Lesions characteristically produce angiocentric, destructive pulmonary lesions, although skin involvement may be the initial presenting sign. Architecturally, the dermal infiltrate is typically composed of coalescent angiocentric aggregates of mononuclear cells that produce a bottom-heavy pattern. Affected vessels often show striking degrees of necrotizing injury; as a result, this disorder has also been classified as a form of dysplastic lymphocytic vasculitis. Individual cells are large and contain hyperchromatic nuclei with a prominent cleft which may be completely folded or unfolded. Cell marker analysis discloses a predominance of T cells in these infiltrates.

"Non-X" Infantile Histiocytoses[28]

There are a number of rare histiocytoses that may also be confused with histiocytosis X. The most confusing diagnostic problem is *Hashimoto-Pritzker disease,* or *congenital self-healing reticulohistiocytosis.* Affected infants have inflammatory nodules at birth or shortly thereafter that spontaneously regress. They are generally free of systemic manifestations, although some may have transient pancytopenia and elevated liver function tests. Dermal and subcutaneous lesions show a mononuclear cell infiltrate, occasionally with epidermotropism and ulceration. The invading cells tend to be more phagocytic than those of histiocytosis X and to have rounded rather than infolded nuclear contours. Unfortunately, Birbeck granules may be detected ultrastructurally in Hashimoto-Pritzker disease as well as in histiocytosis X, and occasional cases with CD1a antigen on infiltrating cells have been described in the former. It remains to be determined whether Hashimoto-Pritzker disease is an unusual congenital variant of histiocytosis X with a variable clinical outcome. Several other histiocytic infiltrates in childhood may be confused with classic Langerhans cell histiocytosis, or histiocytosis X. *Cephalic histiocytosis* is a disorder that produces numerous flat macules and small papules on the head and neck in young children. Although biopsy examination demonstrates a dermal histiocytic infiltrate, these cells lack Birbeck granules. Disorders termed *malignant histiocytosis* or *pure histiocytic lymphoma* could mimic both large cell lymphoma and more anaplastic variants of histiocytosis X. Cell marker and molecular hybridization studies, however, have shown that most of these presumed histiocytic infiltrates are in reality transformed T-lymphocytic processes.

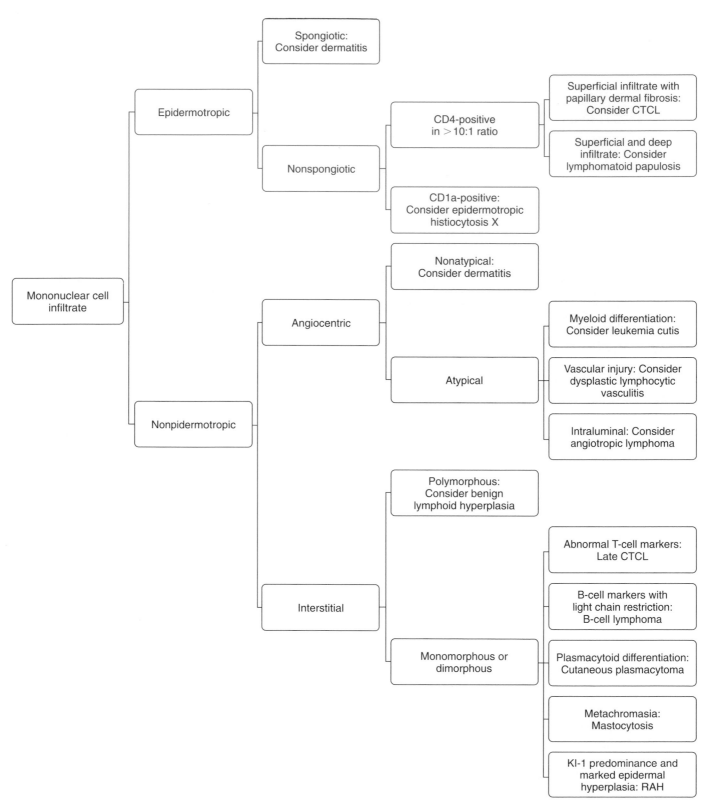

Figure 14–21. Algorithmic approach to cutaneous lymphoproliferative infiltrates.

DIFFERENTIAL DIAGNOSIS

The differential diagnosis of cutaneous lymphoproliferative disorders is a complex issue, and entire books have been devoted to this subject. Figure 14–21, however, attempts to portray a basic approach which may prove useful in initial study of these problematic lesions.

SELECTED REFERENCES

1. Lukes RJ, Collins RD. Immunologic characterization of human malignant lymphomas. Cancer 1974;34:1488.
2. Cossman J, Uppenkamp M, Sundeen J, et al. Molecular genetics and the diagnosis of lymphoma. Arch Pathol Lab Med 1988;112:117.
3. Bernstein H, Shupack J, Ackerman AB. Cutaneous pseudolymphoma resulting from antigen injections. Arch Dermatol 1974;110:756.
4. MacDonald DM. Histopathological differentiation of benign and malignant cutaneous lymphocytic infiltrates. Br J Dermatol 1982;107:715.
5. Knobler RM, Edelson RL. Lymphoma cutis: T-cell type. In: Murphy GF, Mihm MC Jr, eds. Lymphoproliferative Disorders of the Skin. Boston: Butterworths, 1986:184.
6. Sanchez JL, Ackerman AB. The patch stage of mycosis fungoides: criteria for histologic diagnosis. Am J Dermatopathol 1979;1:5.
7. Yamamura T, Aozasa K, Sano S. The cutaneous lymphomas with convoluted nucleus. J Am Acad Dermatol 1984;10:796.
8. Fleischmajer R, Eisenberg S. Sézary's reticulosis. Arch Dermatol 1964;89:9.
9. Murphy GF, Mihm MC Jr. The skin. In: Cotran RS, Kumar V, Robbins SL, eds. Robbins Pathologic Basis of Disease. Philadelphia: WB Saunders, 1989:1293.
10. Shimoyama M, Minato K, Saito H, et al. Comparison of clinical, morphologic, and immunologic characteristics of adult T-cell leukemia-lymphoma and cutaneous T-cell leukemia: a clinicopathological study of five cases. Blood 1983;62:754.
11. McNutt NS, Crain WR. Quantitative electron microscopic comparison of lymphocyte nuclear contours in mycosis fungoides and in benign infiltrates in skin. Cancer 1981;47:698.
12. Murphy GF. Cutaneous T cell lymphoma. Adv Pathol 1988;1:131.
13. McNutt NS. Cutaneous lymphohistiocytic infiltrates simulating malignant lymphoma. In: Murphy GF, Mihm MC Jr, eds. Lymphoproliferative Disorders of the Skin. Boston: Butterworths, 1986:256.
14. Kim H, Dorfman RF. Morphologic studies of 84 untreated patients subjected to laparotomy for the staging of non-Hodgkins lymphoma. Cancer 1974;33:657.
15. Wood GS, Burke JS, Horning S, et al. The immunologic and clinicopathologic heterogeneity of cutaneous lymphomas other than mycosis fungoides. Blood 1983;62:464.
16. Kurtin P, Murphy GF, Mihm MC Jr. Lymphoma cutis: B-cell type. In: Murphy GF, Mihm MC Jr, eds. Lymphoproliferative Disorders of the Skin. Boston: Butterworths, 1986:142.
17. Papadimitriou CS, Muller-Hermelink U, Lennert K. Histologic and immunohistochemical findings in the differential diagnosis of chronic lymphocytic leukemia of the B-cell type and lymphoplasmacytic/lymphoplasmacytoid lymphoma. Virchows Arch (A) 1979;384:149.
18. Burg G, Braun-Falco O. Cutaneous lymphomas, pseudolymphomas, and related disorders. New York: Springer-Verlag, 1983.
19. Michel B, Milner Y, David K. Preservation of tissue fixed immunoglobulins in skin biopsies of patients with lupus erythematosus and bullous diseases. J Invest Dermatol 1973;59:449.
20. Headington JT. Plasma cell tumors of the skin. In: Murphy GF, Mihm MC Jr, eds. Lymphoproliferative Disorders of the Skin. Boston: Butterworths, 1986:160.
21. Swanson NA, Karen DF, Headington JT. Extramedullary IgM plasmacytoma presenting in the skin. Am J Dermatopathol 1981;3:79.
22. Alberts DS, Lynch P. Cutaneous plasmacytomas in myeloma. Arch Dermatol 1978;114:1784.
23. Durie BGM, Salmon SE. A clinical staging system for multiple myeloma. Correlation of measured myeloma cell mass with presenting clinical features, response to treatment, and survival. Cancer 1975;36:842.
24. Su WPD, Buechner SA, Li CY. Clinicopathologic correlations of leukemia cutis. J Am Acad Dermatol 1984;11:121.
25. Buechner SA, Li CY, Su WPD. Leukemia cutis: a histopathologic study of 42 cases. Am J Dermatopathol 1985;7:109.
26. Lichtenstein L. Histiocytosis X: integration of eosinophilic granuloma of bone, "Letterer-Siwe disease," and "Schüller-Christian disease" as related manifestations of a single nosologic entity. Arch Pathol 1953;56:84.
27. Burgdorf WHF. Malignant histiocytic infiltrates. In: Murphy GF, Mihm MC Jr, eds. Lymphoproliferative Disorders of the Skin. Boston: Butterworths, 1986:217.
28. Harrist TJ, Bhan AK, Murphy GF, et al. Histiocytosis X: in situ characterization of cutaneous infiltrates using monoclonal antibodies and heteroantibodies. Am J Clin Pathol 1983;79:294.
29. Murphy GF, Harrist TJ, Bhan AK, Mihm MC. Distribution of T cell antigens in histiocytosis X cells. Quantitative immunoelectron microscopy using monoclonal antibodies. Lab Invest 1983;48:90.
30. Flynn KJ, Dehner LP, Gajl-Peczalska KJ, et al. Regressing atypical histiocytosis: A cutaneous proliferation of atypical neoplastic histiocytes with unexpectedly indolent biologic behavior. Cancer 1982;49:959.
31. McCormick S, Stenn KS, Nelligan D. Regressing atypical histiocytosis. Report of a case. Am J Dermatopathol 1984;6:259.
32. Rilke F, Giardini R, Lombardi L. Recurrent atypical cutaneous histiocytosis. In: Sommers SC, Rosen PP, Fechner RE, eds. Pathology Annual, part 2. Norwalk, Connecticut: Appleton-Century-Crofts, 1985:29.
33. Selch MT, Fu YS. Regressing atypical histiocytosis: a case report following low dose radiation therapy. Int J Rad Oncol Biol Phys 1987;13:1739.
34. Moayed MJ, Kannitakis J, Nabai H, Mauduit G. Regressing atypical histiocytosis (of Flynn): report of a new case. Dermatologica 1987;174:253.
35. Heddington JT, Roth MS, Ginsburg D, et al. Cell receptor gene rearrangement in regressing atypical histiocytosis. Arch Dermatol 1987;123:1183.
36. Heddington JT, Roth MS, Schnitzer B. Regressing atypical histiocytosis: a review and critical appraisal. Semin Diagn Pathol 1987;1:28.
37. Harrist TJ, Murphy GF, Mihm MC Jr. Lymphomatoid vasculitis: a subset of lymphocytic vasculitis. In: Moschella SL, ed. Dermatology Update: Reviews for Physicians. New York: Elsevier, 1982:115.
38. Sanchez NP, Pittelkow MR, Muller SA, et al. The clinicopathologic spectrum of lymphomatoid papulosis: study of 31 cases. J Am Acad Dermatol 1983;8:81.
39. Weiss LM, Wood GS, Trela M, et al. Clonal T-cell population in lymphomatoid papulosis: evidence of a lymphoproliferative origin for a clinically benign disease. N Engl J Med 1986;315:475.
40. Weiss LM, Wood GS, Ellisen LW, et al. Clonal T-cell populations in pityriasis lichenoides et varioliformis acuta (Mucha-Habermann disease). Am J Pathol 1987;126:417.
41. Klaus SN, Winkelmann RK. The clinical spectrum of urticaria pigmentosa. Mayo Clinic Proc 1965;40:923.
42. Mihm MC, Clark WH, Reed RJ, et al. Mast cell infiltrates in the skin and the mastocytic syndrome. Hum Pathol 1973;4:231.
43. Rodriguez J, Ackerman AB. Xanthogranuloma in adults. Arch Dermatol 1976;112:43.
44. Dammert K, Niemi KM. Reticulohistiocytosis (lipoid dermato-arthritis) of the skin and joints. Acta Derm Venereol (Stockh) 1966;46:210.
45. Lichtman AH, Mihm MC Jr, Murphy GF. The role of retroviruses in cutaneous T-cell lymphomas. In: Murphy GF, Mihm MC Jr, eds. Lymphoproliferative Disorders of the Skin. Boston: Butterworths, 1986:205.
46. Bhawan J, Wolff SM, Ucci AA, et al. Malignant lymphoma and malignant angioendotheliomatosis: one disease. Cancer 1985;55:570.
47. Lukes RJ, Tindle BH. Immunoblastic lymphadenopathy: a hyperimmune entity resembling Hodgkin's disease. N Engl J Med 1975;292:1.
48. Katzenstein ALA, Carrington CB, Liebow AA. Lymphomatoid granulomatosis: a clinicopathological study of 152 cases. Cancer 1979;43:360.
49. Murphy GF, Mihm MC Jr. Benign, dysplastic, and malignant lymphoid infiltrates of the skin: an approach based on pattern analysis. In: Murphy GF, Mihm MC Jr, (eds). Lymphoproliferative Disorders of the Skin. Boston: Butterworths, 1986:123.

15
Primary Mesenchymal Tumors

DEFINITIONS AND GENERAL CONSIDERATIONS

Mesenchymal tumors of the skin involve benign and malignant proliferations of endothelial cells, pericytes, and glomus cells; smooth muscle cells; cells of fibrohistiocytic origin; and neural and related supporting cells. The dermis is a fertile source for the development of such neoplasms, because it contains a plentitude of endothelial-lined vessels, vascular and erectile smooth muscle bundles, fibroblasts and fixed histiocytes, and neural elements. Many mesenchymal proliferations in the skin have counterparts in extracutaneous tissues (e.g., leiomyomas, neuromas). However, in almost every case, mesenchymal neoplasms that arise in the dermis have distinctive clinical and histologic features that separate them from their extracutaneous relatives.

In this section, the word hamartoma is used to refer to a malformation of mesenchymal elements normally expected to be present within the dermis. A hamartoma may therefore result from disordered or anomalous differentiation, structural organization, or quantity (i.e., too much or too little) of cellular elements. As is the case in all of dermatopathology, there are many misnomers in the nomenclature of mesenchymal neoplasms of the skin. Perhaps the best example is Kaposi sarcoma, which is not a malignant mesenchymal tumor at all but is rather a variably aggressive, multifocal angioproliferative process, probably resulting from exposure of preexisting vessels to anomalous growth factors. Such terms have not been abandoned, however, because they have gained broad acceptance, and dermatopathologists are aware of the deficits of the terminology. Attempts are made, however, to clarify the biological behavior of all lesions presented, particulary when the names are misleading with regard to histogenesis, pathogenesis, or clinical consequences.

GROSS PATHOLOGY

The gross pathology of mesenchymal neoplasms of the skin is often critical to assembling the clinicopathological criteria necessary for most accurate diagnosis. However, as is too often the case in skin disease, the clinical appearance of certain lesions may be misleading, or result in a differential involving biologically different processes. For example, early Kaposi sarcoma commonly resembles a bruise, and the dermatofibroma variant of benign fibrous histiocytoma may be mistaken for a melanoma. These clinical impressions may be reflected on requisition forms that accompany specimens submitted to the pathologist, and awareness of this clinical mimicry is therefore important from the standpoint of pathologic examination.

Soft tissue tumors involving the skin must be subjected to the same scrutiny that involves gross examination of extracutaneous mesenchymal neoplasms. Specimens should be bread-loafed and care taken to note regions of color change, necrosis, hemorrhage, or cystification. It is often advisable to submit multiple sections, particularly when lesions are large or grossly unusual. Care should be taken to ink margins of primary excisions, and to obtain sections that reflect the adequacy or inadequacy of surgical removal.

GENERAL HISTOLOGY AND TEMPORAL EVOLUTION

The histology of cutaneous mesenchymal neoplasms is so varied that it is impossible to make useful generalizations in a few paragraphs. There are certain features that pathologists have found useful in determining potential histogenesis, however. For example, smooth muscle cells tend to contain

279

nuclei with rounded ends, whereas the ends of nuclei of neural and fibroblastic tumors are often pointed. Nuclei from neural tumors tend to contain pseudoinclusions and to have a wavy, undulant profile, in contrast to fibroblastic cells, which generally show neither of these features. Endothelial cells may be difficult to recognize in poorly differentiated tumors, although their tendency to form blood-filled spaces and occasionally to contain hyalin-like cytoplasmic droplets or intracellular lumenal vacuoles may provide subtle clues to differentiation. Fibrohistiocytic cells may show evidence of cytoplasmic lipidization, a feature that has proven helpful in the diagnostic recognition of certain benign and malignant tumors deriving from this potentially divergent cell lineage.

Whereas certain mesenchymal tumors grow symmetrically larger over time, stabilize, and even eventually involute, others show well-defined stages of tumor progression. Kaposi sarcoma, for example, begins as a relatively flat proliferation of bland spindle cells that evolves from a clinical patch to a plaque. Over time, more atypical cells develop that are capable of forming nodules in the setting of clinically advanced disease. This type of progression is reminiscent of the evolutionary stages of radial and vertical growth phase melanoma or the sequential alterations observed as epidermotropic cutaneous T-cell lymphoma (CTCL) progresses to nonepidermotropic, nodular disease. Because evolutionary stages of cutaneous mesenchymal tumors may be histologically dissimilar, appreciation of the dynamic aspects of tumor progression is particularly germane to soft tissue neoplasia.

HISTOLOGY OF SPECIFIC DISORDERS

Vascular Tumors

Vascular Hyperplasias[1-5]

- PROLIFERATION OF VENULES AND CAPILLARIES WITHIN CONFINES OF PREEXISTING MICROVASCULAR PLEXUS (E.G., ACROANGIODERMATITIS)
- PROLIFERATION OF ENDOTHELIAL-LINED PAPILLARY PROJECTIONS WITHIN PREEXISTING LARGE VESSEL (E.G., INTRAVASCULAR PAPILLARY ENDOTHELIAL HYPERPLASIA)
- TUMORAL PROLIFERATION OF SMALL VESSELS WITHIN EDEMATOUS AND INFLAMED STROMA (E.G., PYOGENIC GRANULOMA)
- PROLIFERATION OF SMALL VESSELS LINED BY PROTUBERANT ENDOTHELIAL CELLS WITH ABUNDANT PINK CYTOPLASM AND ASSOCIATED WITH STROMAL EOSINOPHILS (E.G., EPITHELIOID HEMANGIOMA)

The concept of vascular hyperplasia encompasses proliferation of endothelial cells lining dermal vessels, neovascularization involving growth of entire vascular channels, or a combination of these two entities. These changes frequently accompany inflammatory and reparative processes within the dermis, and in the extreme, they may be confused with true neoplasia. Examples of lesions that fulfill criteria for vascular hyperplasia include *acroangiodermatitis, intravascular papillary endothelial hyperplasia* (IPEH; i.e., Masson tumor), *pyogenic granuloma,* and *epithelioid hemangioma.* Acroangiodermatitis is an exaggerated form of stasis dermatitis (see Chap. 18) that most often affects the lower extremities of elderly individuals. Lesions may be hyperpigmented, purpuric, and indurated, and there may be clinical confusion with conditions such as Kaposi sarcoma, chronic dermatitis, or epidermal and dermal neoplasia. IPEH arises most often in middle-aged and older women, involving skin of the head, neck, and distal extremity (i.e., hand). Lesions usually present as slow-growing, nondescript nodules measuring less than 2 cm in diameter. Pyogenic granuloma frequently affects mucosal membranes and distal extremities, particularly the periungual skin. Lesions exhibit rapid growth, seldom exceed 2 cm in diameter, and typically form pedunculated red to blue nodules that may demonstrate superficial erosion or frank ulceration (Fig. 15–1A).

Epithelioid hemangioma, also known as vegetant intravascular hemangioendothelioma, histiocytoid hemangioma, and angiolymphoid hyperplasia with eosinophilia, most often arises as an asymptomatic, pale red, sessile nodule or as a plaque on the head, neck, or limbs of middle-aged women. *Kimura disease* is a variant of epithelioid hemangioma that affects primarily young men of Asian descent. Lesions are often multiple and involve the head, neck, trunk, and limbs. Pruritus and pain are typical of this variant, and lymphadenopathy and peripheral blood eosinophilia are frequently seen.

Accurate histologic recognition of these disorders is important because they may be confused with angiosarcoma (intravascular papillary endothelial hyperplasia, epithelioid hemangioma) and certain histologic variants of Kaposi sarcoma (acroangiodermatitis, pyogenic granuloma, and epithelioid hemangioma). The pertinent distinguishing histologic features of each condition are presented in the following sections.

Acroangiodermatitis

At scanning magnification, there is an ill-defined plaque within the superficial dermis formed by numerous proliferating vessels. These vessels are small, rounded in contour, and lined by plump endothelial cells. The proliferation typically occupies the stratum normally formed by the superficial vascular plexus, and the proliferating vessels are arranged in small clusters and aggregates that extend as glomeruloid structures within dermal papillae exhibiting edema and fibrosis (see Chap. 17).

Pyogenic Granuloma

In early evolutionary stages, pyogenic granuloma appears as an often ulcerated proliferation of rounded, anastomosing vessels embedded within a markedly edematous stroma that contains both neutrophils and mononuclear cells (Fig. 15–1B,C). Mitotic figures may be prominent, but atypical (e.g., tripolar) mitoses are not observed. Older lesions show less inflammatory change and edema and may be difficult to distinguish from capillary hemangiomas.

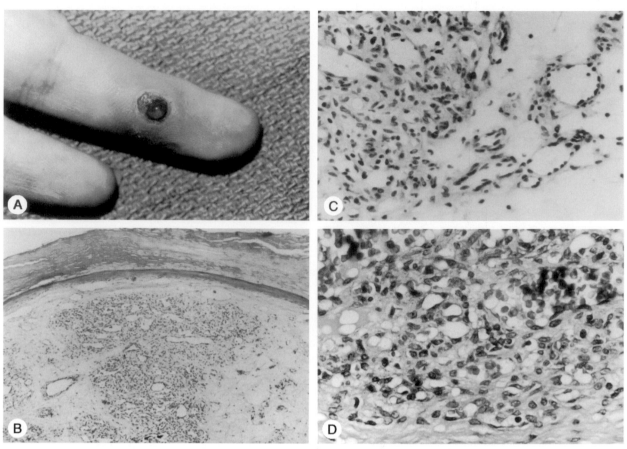

Figure 15–1. Pyogenic granuloma. **(A)** The clinical lesion consists of an ulcerated, gelatinous mass of raised, proliferating tissue. **(B, C)** Earlier lesions are characterized by lobulated aggregates of capillaries within an edematous and frequently inflamed stroma. **(D)** Older lesions may display dense aggregates of benign vessels that are indistinguishable from capillary hemangioma.

Intravascular Papillary Endothelial Hyperplasia

Scanning magnification often demonstrates this endothelial proliferative process to be enclosed within an apparently traumatically distored vascular lumen within the mid- to deep dermis (Fig. 15–2A). The luminal surface of this presumed vessel is characterized by numerous minute papillary projections formed by hyalinized stroma covered by a single layer of flattened endothelium (Fig. 15–2B). Mitotic figures are rare, and nuclear atypia evidenced by hyperchromasia, prominent nucleoli, and irregularity in contour is not observed. Luminal thrombosis is frequently encountered.

Epithelioid Hemangioma

Epithelioid hemangioma generally consists of a poorly circumscribed proliferation of epithelioid or histiocytoid cells associated with variable inflammation within the superficial and deep dermis (Fig. 15–2C). The majority of these cells either line vessel lumens or are present in the perivascular interstitium. They contain enlarged nuclei with vesicular chromatin patterns and conspicuous nucleoli (Fig. 15–2D); mitoses are infrequently observed. The cytoplasm of these cells varies from eosinophilic to amphophilic, imparting an epithelioid or histiocytoid appearance. Although poorly formed vascular spaces may be appreciated, many of the cells

are arranged in ill-defined cords and aggregates. An important clue to the diagnosis is the presence of an associated lymphohistiocytic infiltrate containing a variable number of admixed eosinophils (i.e., angiolymphoid hyperplasia with eosinophilia).

Angiomas and Glomangiomas[6, 7]

- WELL-CIRCUMSCRIBED, SYMMETRICAL ARCHITECTURE
- VARIABLY-SIZED VESSELS LINED WITH FLATTENED ENDOTHELIAL CELLS
- ABSENCE OF MITOTIC ACTIVITY
- VARIABLE PERICYTE COMPONENT SURROUNDING VASCULAR CHANNELS
- MANTLE OF GLOMUS CELLS SURROUNDING ENDOTHELIAL CHANNELS (GLOMANGIOMA)

Hemangiomas are either acquired (Fig. 15–3) or congenital (Fig. 15–4). Congenital hemangiomas show a predilection for the head and neck of female infants, although any site may be affected. Individual tumors are often small, bosselated, and intensely red, hence their name, strawberry hemangiomas. Most of these lesions are *capillary hemangiomas* that completely regress spontaneously by fibrosis within the first decade of life. Larger congenital lesions may produce significant deformity and do not involute (see Fig.

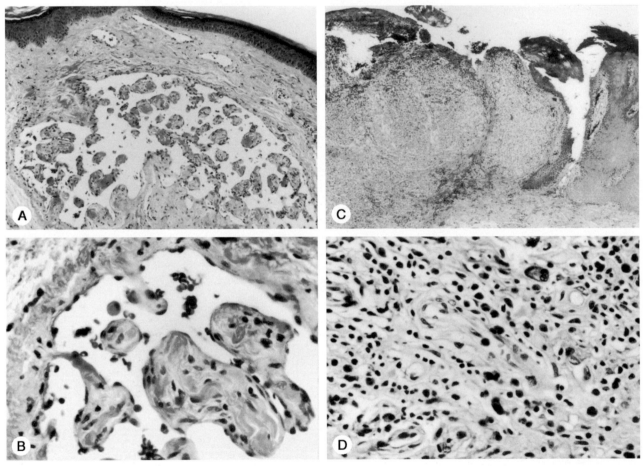

Figure 15–2. Intravascular papillary endothelial hyperplasia and epithelioid hemangioma. Like pyogenic granuloma, these reactive endothelial hyperplasias are characterized by proliferation of benign endothelial cells at sites of inflammation or trauma. **(A, B)** Intravascular papillary endothelial hyperplasia is characterized by papillary projections lined by flattened endothelium within the lumen of a dilated vessel showing perivascular fibrosis and hemosiderin deposition. **(C, D)** Epithelioid hemangioma is characterized in this lesion by a zone of ulceration with underlying granulation tissue containing numerous lymphocytes, eosinophils, and large epithelioid cells both within the stroma and lining the lumens of involved blood vessels.

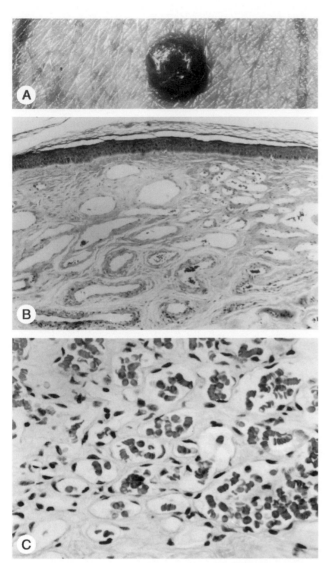

Figure 15–3. Hemangioma. **(A)** A symmetrical, cherry red papule which, on examination of a biopsy specimen, disclosed numerous benign vessels within the superficial dermis. **(B)** Hemangiomas with mixed capillary, arterial, and venous components are characterized by dilated, thick-walled superficial dermal vessels. These lesions result from either long-standing pressure gradients due to chronicity or arteriovenous shunts. **(C)** Capillary hemangioma, consisting of closely aggregated, thin-walled vessels lined with benign, flattened, endothelial cells.

cells devoid of mitotic activity (see Fig. 15–3C). Congenital lesions tend to be lobulated, contain numerous small vessels, and show an associated proliferation of plump pericytes within the perivascular interstitium. Acquired lesions may demonstrate progressive luminal ectasia of the vascular component with age, although vessel walls remain relatively thin throughout the natural evolution of these benign tumors. Hemangiomas with capillary, arterial, and venous components show variable vascular ectasia and vessel wall thickness (Fig. 15–3B). Cavernous hemangiomas are more extensive, deeply infiltrative, and less well-circumscribed within the dermis. These lesions are characterized by proliferation of ectatic vessels with wall diameters that are markedly thicker than those of capillary hemangiomas (see Fig. 15–4B). Intraluminal thrombosis also is frequently observed in cavernous hemangiomas.

There are a number of variant forms of angioma in the skin which deserve brief mention. The *angiokeratoma* is a form of capillary hemangioma–like proliferation in which ectatic, thin-walled, dermal vessels invaginate upward into a hyperplastic, verrucous epidermal layer (Fig. 15–5). There are four clinical settings in which angiokeratomas are observed: (1) diffuse cutaneous involvement of angiokeratoma corporis diffusum associated with Fabry disease; (2) involvement of the dorsa of the fingers and toes (i.e., Mibelli type);

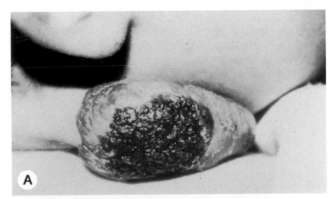

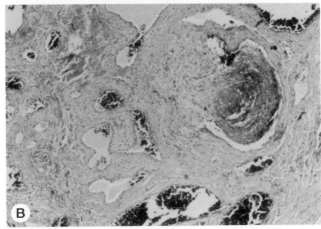

Figure 15–4. Cavernous hemangioma. **(A)** This congenital vascular tumor involving neck skin formed a redundant, pedunculated mass with central foci of deep erythema correlating to superficial vascular proliferation. **(B)** Histologically, there are thick-walled, dilated vessels within a fibrotic dermis. Wall thickening appears to be partially the result of fibroblastic proliferation and collagen deposition. Organizing thrombi are present in some of the vessels.

15–4A); these tumors tend to infiltrate deeply and to be composed of larger vessels (i.e., *cavernous hemangiomas*). These lesions may be associated with multiple enchondromas (i.e., Maffucci syndrome), involvement of the gastrointestinal tract as well as the skin (i.e., blue rubber bleb nevus syndrome), or consumption coagulopathy as a result of intralesional thrombosis (i.e., Kasabach-Merritt syndrome). Capillary hemangiomas also commonly are observed as acquired lesions in middle-aged and older individuals, and face, neck, and trunk skin is particularly affected. These lesions are small, bright red, symmetrical, dome-shaped papules (see Fig. 15–3A), and they are often referred to as senile hemangiomas.

Capillary hemangiomas are well-circumscribed dermal proliferations of small vessels characterized by rounded contours and lined by benign-appearing, flattened endothelial

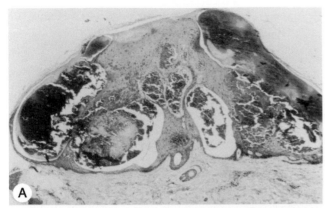

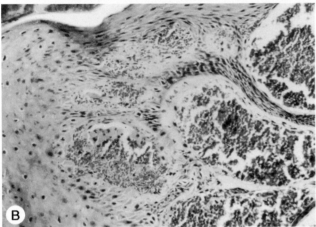

Figure 15–5. Angiokeratoma. **(A, B)** Variably dilated, thin-walled vascular channels, many containing organizing thrombi, are present within the superficial dermis. Characteristic features include overlying verrucous epidermal hyperplasia, which embraces the underlying vascular tumor, and invagination of vessels into the epidermal layer such that some vessels seem to be floating within the epidermis, which is devoid of associated dermal stroma.

(3) scrotal lesions (i.e., Fordyce type); and (4) solitary papular angiokeratoma. *Acquired tufted hemangiomas* demonstrate multiple foci of endothelial and pericyte proliferation within the dermis characterized by formation of semilunar spaces into which more cellular regions protrude (Fig. 15–6). *Arteriovenous hemangiomas* and related malformations consist of aggregates of benign veins and arteries of variable size. Typically, the walls of many of the veins may show degenerative changes as a result of nonphysiologic pressures. *Lymphangiomas* are characterized by thin-walled dermal vessels, often within the most superficial layers of the dermis (Fig. 15–7). These delicate channels may be filled with proteinaceous fluid and occasional lymphocytes, but tend not to be filled with erythrocytes, as is the case in most hemangiomas. In lymphangioma circumscriptum, increased numbers of lymphatic channels within the superficial dermis indent into a hyperplastic epidermal layer in a manner analogous to that seen in angiokeratoma. These lesions may resemble multiple small blisters clinically, and their prominence may wax and wane depending on the degree of lymphatic drainage. *Angiofibromas* are subtle angioma-like proliferations that commonly occur as solitary skin-colored papules on the face, especially the nose (i.e., fibrous papules). In the setting of tuberous sclerosis, multiple angiofibromas,

erroneously termed adenoma sebaceum, may develop (Fig. 15–8A). Histologically, lesions are superficial and mid-dermal proliferations of fibroblasts and small vessels, sometimes associated with concentric fibrosis about hair follicles (Fig. 15–8B, C). A typical feature is the presence of plump stellate cells within the superficial dermis (Fig. 15–8D). *Glomangiomas* may occur as solitary or multiple, often painful nodules with a predilection for skin of the extremities (Fig. 15–9A). Histologically, they are distinguished by large, dilated, irregular vascular spaces surrounded by a mantle of uniform, rounded cells with moderate quantities of eosinophilic cytoplasm, and small, rounded, centrally disposed nuclei (i.e., glomus cells) (Fig. 15–9B, C).

Kaposi Sarcoma[8–12]

- BLAND SPINDLE CELL PROLIFERATION ABOUT SUPERFICIAL VASCULAR AND PERIADNEXAL PLEXUSES
- INTERSTITIAL INFILTRATION, WITH SPINDLE CELLS SURROUNDING COLLAGEN BUNDLES
- FORMATION OF SLIT-LIKE SPACES FILLED WITH ERYTHROCYTES
- INTRACYTOPLASMIC HYALIN INCLUSIONS
- FOCAL HEMOSIDERIN DEPOSITION
- VARIABLE INFLAMMATION; OFTEN, LYMPHOCYTES AND PLASMA CELLS

Kaposi sarcoma, a multifocal angioproliferative process, occurs in two very different biologic forms: one indolent and one aggressive. In contrast to the indolent form that com-

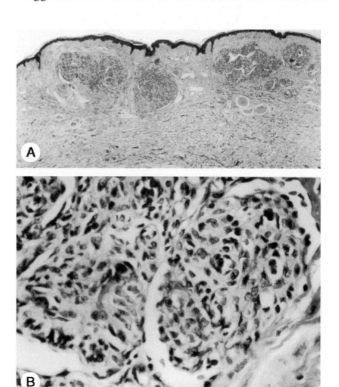

Figure 15–6. Acquired tufted hemangioma. **(A)** At scanning magnification, discrete aggregates of cells are visible in the superficial dermis. **(B)** At increased magnification, the aggregates are observed to contain plump pericyte-like cells that focally bulge into vascular spaces, creating characteristic semilunar contours.

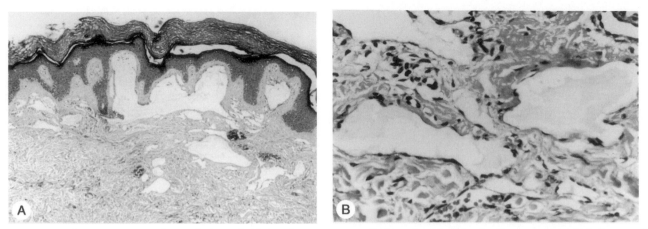

Figure 15–7. Lymphangioma. **(A, B)** Thin-walled vessels filled with proteinaceous fluid but devoid of blood cells are present within the superficial dermis. In lymphangioma circumscriptum, these channels may invaginate into the overlying epidermal layer in a manner similar to that seen in angiokeratoma.

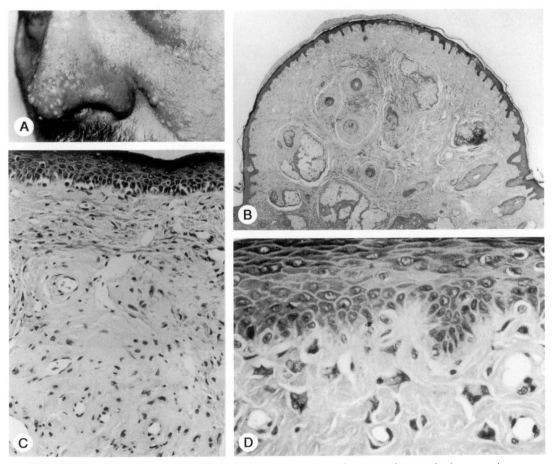

Figure 15–8. Angiofibroma. **(A)** Multiple angiofibromas, also called fibrous papules and erroneously termed adenoma sebaceum, on the nasal and facial skin of a patient with tuberous sclerosis. **(B)** These dome-shaped papules are formed as a result of dermal fibrovascular proliferations, which contain **(C)** small vessels and plump stellate cells within the **(D)** superficial dermis. These stellate cells stain for S100 protein and are believed to be of possible melanocytic derivation (see Chap. 13).

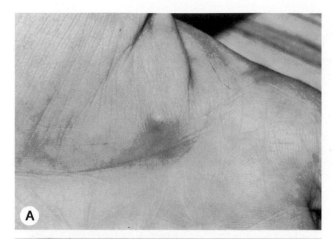

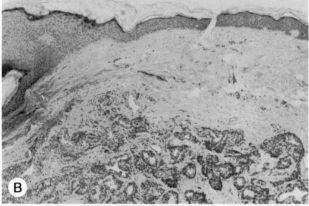

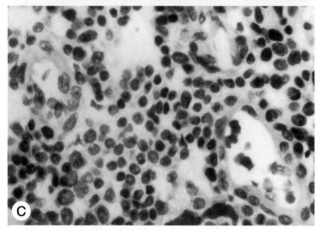

Figure 15–9. Glomangioma. **(A)** A painful dermal nodule with a purple hue is present on the palm skin. **(B)** Biopsy of another similar lesion reveals a collection of mid-dermal vessels surrounded by a cuff of pericytes, imparting the impression of glandular differentiation at low magnification. **(C)** At higher magnification, monomorphic aggregates of rounded-to-cuboidal pericytes containing nevus-like nuclei are intimately associated with an angiomatous dermal proliferation of small vessels.

monly affects elderly individuals, particularly those of Southern European dissent and Ashkenazi Jews, the aggressive form is generally associated with immunosuppression, as in acquired immunodeficiency syndrome (AIDS). Table 15–1 summarizes the clinical and epidemiologic differences between these two distinct angioproliferative processes.

Early lesions of Kaposi sarcoma may appear as a zone

of subcutaneous bleeding or petechial papules. Patches later progress into purpuric plaques (Fig. 15–10A), which sometimes occur at sites of trauma. In the setting of AIDS, facial involvement is common, with a particular predilection for nose skin. Late stages result in hemorrhagic nodules, which may ulcerate. Kaposi sarcoma may be difficult to recognize at any stage of its clinical evolution, and because of its association with AIDS, the differential diagnosis includes a number of uncommonly encountered infectious and neoplastic disorders. Dermatopathologists must be cautious in considering each of these diagnostic possibilities, particularly when early, less-developed stages have been biopsied. A partial list of clinical disorders that commonly may be confused with Kaposi sarcoma in various stages of its evolution includes the following:

Patch Stage
    Bruise or ecchymosis
    Progressive pigmentary purpura (Schamberg disease)
    Postinflammatory hyperpigmentation
    Localized vasculitis
Plaque and Nodular Stage
    Angiosarcoma
    Sarcoidosis
    Cutaneous amyloidosis
    Lymphoma and benign lymphoid hyperplasia
    Atypical dermatofibroma
    Vascularized scar

Early patch-stage Kaposi sarcoma is recognized at scanning magnification by appreciation of a subtle increase in cellularity in the vicinity of the superficial vascular plexus and periadnexal adventitia (Fig. 15–10B). At higher-power magnification, normal vessels characterized by rounded contours and flattened to bulging endothelial cells are surrounded by ill-defined proliferations of bland-appearing spindle cells, some of which appear to form vascular slits or angulated spaces (Fig. 15–10C, D). The superficial vascular plexus also extends around dermal appendages, and thus this angiocentric spindle cell proliferative process may form a mantle about hair follicles and sweat glands within the dermis. Hemosiderin may be detected about the proliferating spindle cells of early Kaposi sarcoma. Moreover, dilated lymphatics and associated inflammatory cells consisting of

Table 15–1. COMPARISON OF CLINICAL FEATURES OF INDOLENT AND AGGRESSIVE FORMS OF KAPOSI SARCOMA

FEATURE	INDOLENT VARIANT	AGGRESSIVE VARIANT
Mean age	41 years	28 years
Gender ratio (M:F)	10:1	3:1
	Insidious	Within 1 year
Presenting sign or symptom	Leg swelling	Lymph node enlargement
Opportunistic infections	Rare	Common
Encephalopathy	Not seen	Often observed
HIV-positive	Minority	Vast majority
Prognosis	Prolonged survival	Poor

lymphocytes and plasma cells are often present in small aggregates at the periphery of lesions.

Plaque and nodular lesions of Kaposi sarcoma tend to reveal more cellular aggregates of spindle cells within the dermis (Fig. 15–11A). These aggregates often retain regions occupied by cytologically bland spindle cells, as evidenced by nuclear pallor and delicate chromatin distribution. However, other zones are composed of spindle cells with more coarsely clumped heterochromatin than is typical of patch or plaque disease, and mitotic figures are usually identified with ease in these regions (Fig. 15–11B). Proliferating cells may form expansive sheets and nodules that contain characteristic slit-like spaces containing erythrocytes configured linearly within these spaces (i.e., ''box-car'' arrangement). These findings in advanced nodular lesions may lead to confusion with a primary spindle cell neoplasm in which recent hemorrhage has occurred, especially leiomyosarcoma. A helpful finding in making an accurate diagnosis of nodular Kaposi sarcoma is the identification of hyaline-like globules within proliferating spindle cells. These cytoplasmic inclusions are believed to represent degenerating membranes of phagocytized erythrocytes and stain positively by PAS. Because of

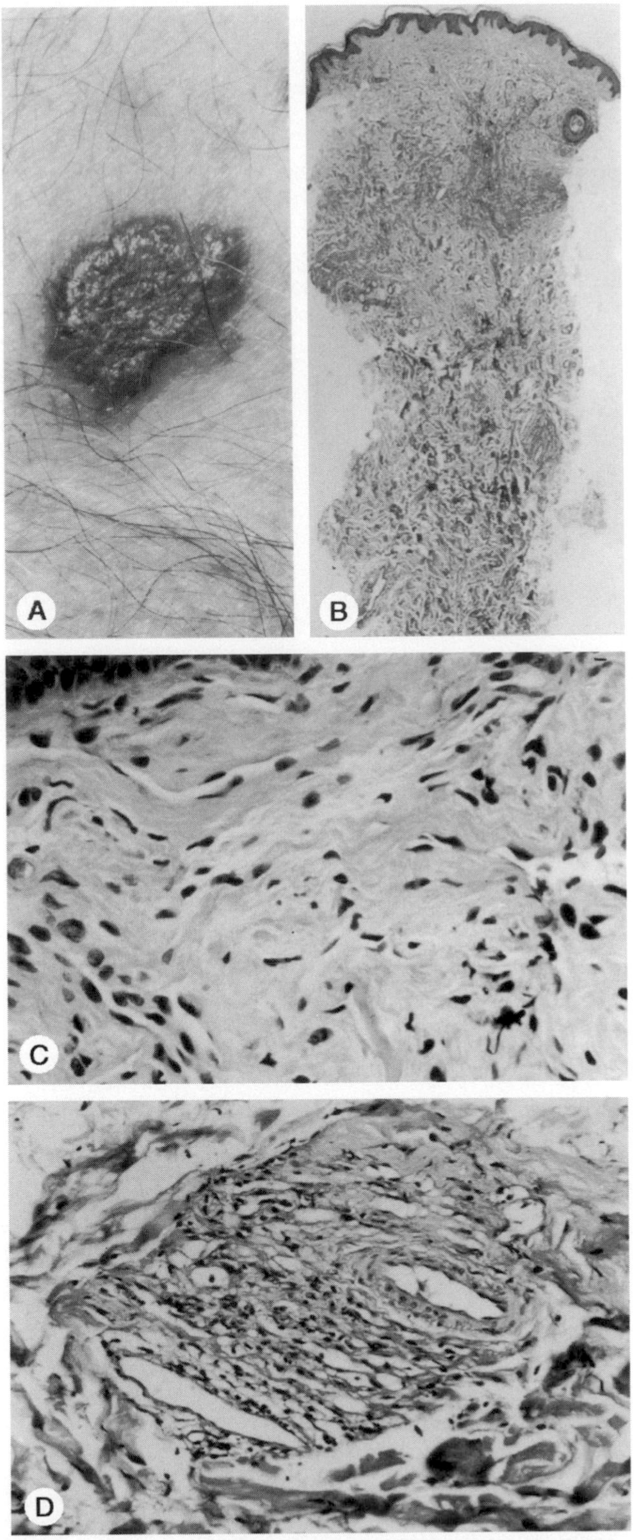

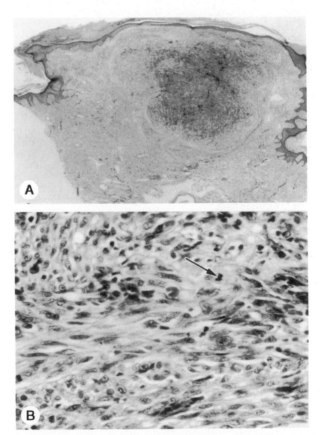

Figure 15–10. Kaposi sarcoma: patch-plaque stage. **(A)** An intensely erythematous, nonblanching plaque is present on the truncal skin of human immunodeficiency virus–positive patient. **(B)** At scanning magnification, there is the impression of increased cellularity in the superficial and mid-dermis. **(C)** This alteration is the result of the proliferation of bland dendritic and spindle-shaped cells about superficial dermal vessels and vessels within periadnexal adventitia. **(D)** Occasional vessels demonstrate striking spindle cell proliferation within the perivascular space.

Figure 15–11. Kaposi sarcoma: plaque-nodular stage. **(A)** A forming mid-dermal nodule is composed of spindle cells. **(B)** Higher magnification exhibits formation of slit-like spaces by cells with more nuclear pleomorphism and atypia than those of the earlier patch-plaque stage. A mitotic figure *(arrow)* can be seen. Other features suggestive of this diagnosis (not illustrated) include the box-car alignment of erythrocytes within vascular spaces, intracytoplasmic hyaline droplets within tumor cells, and perivascular infiltrates of lymphocytes and plasma cells peripheral to the borders defined by neoplastic cells.

the relative specificity of these cytoplasmic inclusions, they are particularly helpful in the recognition of Kaposi sarcoma.

It is important to recognize that unlike the vascular hyperplasia of stasis dermatitis and acroangiodermatitis, the contours of vessels in Kaposi sarcoma are irregular and angulated. Their course is apparently dictated by their tendency to grow along and envelop preexisting reticular dermal collagen bundles. Moreover, the proliferating vessels of early Kaposi sarcoma regularly extend to involve the periadnexal adventitia of dermal appendages. When the inflammatory changes predominate in Kaposi sarcoma, the vascular components are easily overlooked, and a differential diagnosis including superficial inflammatory dermatoses and secondary syphilis may be considered. Recognition that plasma cells are only rarely encountered in the former and that atypical vascular spaces lined by relatively flat, nonobliterative, endothelial cells are unusual in the latter should assist in formulating an accurate diagnosis. Spindle cells in early Kaposi sarcoma tend to insidiously infiltrate about collagen bundles in a manner reminiscent of the collagen infiltration by histiocytes seen in early granuloma annulare or necrobiosis lipoidica. However, in Kaposi sarcoma, these infiltrating cells surround preexisting vessels and are unassociated with mucinous or sclerotic changes in involved connective tissue.

Angiosarcoma[13-19]

- ASYMMETRICAL PROLIFERATION OF IRREGULAR VASCULAR SPACES, CORDS, AND SOLID AREAS WITHIN SUPERFICIAL AND DEEP DERMIS
- TUMOR CELLS DESTROY PREEXISTING STRUCTURES
- BETTER-DIFFERENTIATED REGIONS LINED BY PROTUBERANT ENDOTHELIUM
- TUMOR CELLS MAY LINE INTRALUMINAL STROMAL TUFTS
- MARKED NUCLEAR ANAPLASIA, MITOSES

Most cutaneous angiosarcomas arise de novo on skin of the head and neck of elderly individuals. With the exception of tumors arising in chronically lymphedematous upper extremities in postmastectomy patients, men are preferentially affected by a 2:1 ratio. Lesions begin as single or multiple dusky, erythematous plaques that eventually develop nodules that may ulcerate (Fig. 15–12A). Angiosarcoma arising in the skin and soft tissues of edematous upper extremities following radical mastectomy is referred to as *Stewart-Treves syndrome*. In lymphedematous variants, lesions often present as showers of red-purple nodules involving skin overlying the edematous region.

At scanning magnification, cutaneous angiosarcomas characteristically infiltrate among and dissect between collagen fibers to produce poorly circumscribed and asymmetric zones of dermal hypercellularity (Fig. 15–12B). At the periphery of tumors, dilated lymphatic spaces and associated infiltrates of lymphocytes are often identified. Neoplastic cells focally form angulated and irregular vascular spaces that are inconsistently filled with blood (Fig. 15–12C). The cells lining these spaces form one or more layers, contain

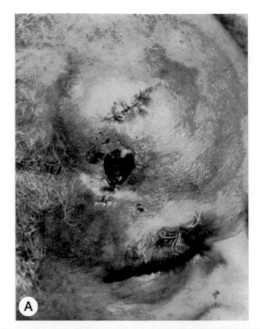

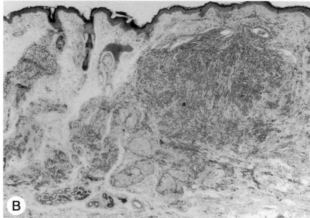

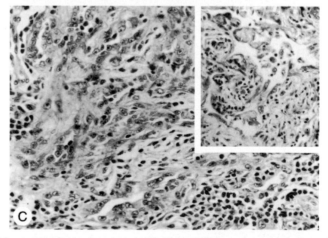

Figure 15–12. Angiosarcoma. **(A)** This extensive, purpuric, indurated plaque on the scalp is typical of a clinical lesion of angiosarcoma. **(B)** Scanning magnification of a biopsy specimen reveals coalescent aggregates of malignant spindle cells within the superficial and deep dermis. **(C)** At higher magnification, atypical spindle cells admixed with lymphocytes form poorly demarcated vascular spaces; papillary fronds formed by bulging tumor cells that extend into vessel lumina also are present *(inset)*.

Table 15–2. DIFFERENTIAL DIAGNOSIS OF ANGIOSARCOMA AND ITS SIMULANTS

	ANGIOSARCOMA	INTRAVASCULAR PAPILLARY ENDOTHELIAL HYPERPLASIA	EPITHELIOID HEMANGIOMA	KAPOSI SARCOMA
Clinical features	Rapid growth, destructive	Nondescript nodule, ? history of trauma	Nodule or plaque, often ulcerated	Purpuric patch or plaque
Architecture	Asymmetrical, irregular vascular spaces	Papillary fronds, preexisting vascular lumen	Symmetrical, ill-defined borders	Asymmetrical, insidious infiltration of dermis
Cytology	Anaplastic, mitoses	Banal, no mitoses	Bulging, plump cells; single, layer; mitoses rare	Banal cells forming slit-like spaces
Associated stroma	Nonspecific	Hyalinized	Mononuclear cells, eosinophils	Plasma cells, dendritic cells

markedly atypical nuclei, and frequently bulge into the lumen or form small tufts (see Fig. 15–12C, inset). The atypical nuclei of the neoplastic endothelial elements are hyperchromatic and irregular in contour, and prominent nucleoli and frequent, occasionally atypical mitotic figures may be observed. Poorly differentiated neoplasms are composed of solid sheets of anaplastic, epithelioid to fusiform cells, leading to confusion with other forms of high-grade carcinomas and sarcomas. Reticulin stain may be helpful in defining vascular boundaries bordered by basement membrane within the solid aggregates of tumor cells. Ultrastructurally, angiosarcomas may demonstrate characteristics of endothelial cells, including the presence of cytoplasmic Weibel-Palade bodies, which are rod-shaped, lysosome-like organelles. Factor VIII-associated antigen is present in some but not all cells of angiosarcoma and may be of limited value in poorly differentiated lesions.

Several angioproliferative disorders that produce histologic findings that mimic angiosarcoma include *epithelioid hemangioma, intravascular papillary endothelial hyperplasia,* and *Kaposi sarcoma.* Salient features that facilitate differentiation from angiosarcoma are listed in Table 15–2.

Smooth Muscle Tumors

Leiomyoma and Angioleiomyoma[20, 21]

- SMOOTH MUSCLE PROLIFERATION WITHOUT ATYPIA OR MITOSES
- POORLY ORGANIZED AND COMPOSED OF BENIGN SMOOTH MUSCLE BUNDLES (PILOLEIOMYOMA AND GENITAL LEIOMYOMA)
- WELL-CIRCUMSCRIBED, SYMMETRICAL DERMAL NODULE FORMED BY BENIGN SMOOTH MUSCLE ENCLOSING INCREASED NUMBERS OF SMALL VESSELS (ANGIOLEIOMYOMA)

Leiomyomas and angioleiomyomas are common dermal and subcutaneous tumors that are composed of benign smooth muscle bundles. Important clinical variants include the following:

1. *Solitary and multiple piloleiomyomas.* Also called arrector pili muscle hamartomas, these neoplasms appear as ten-der intradermal nodules affecting hair-bearing skin surfaces, often the extensor surfaces of the forearms (Fig. 15–13A).

2. *Angioleiomyomas.* These are relatively small (i.e., <4 cm), well-circumscribed, often painful dermal and subcutaneous tumors. They are believed to arise from the walls of preexisting dermal and subcutaneous vessels and show a predilection for occurrence on the lower extremities.

3. *Genital leiomyomas.* These tumors generally present as solitary dermal nodules on skin of the scrotum, labia, and areola. They arise from smooth muscle bundles that typically course through the dermis at these sites, and unlike other variants, they are seldom painful.

At scanning magnification, piloleiomyomas and genital leiomyomas are poorly defined yet symmetrical proliferations of smooth muscle within the superficial and deep dermis (Fig. 15–13B). Angioleiomyomas, on the other hand, tend to be extremely well circumscribed nodules (Fig. 15–14A). All types of leiomyomas are composed of interlacing fascicles and bundles of smooth muscle characterized by elongated nuclei with rounded ends and having ample eosinophilic cytoplasm (Figs. 15–13C and 15–14B). Mitotic activity is generally not observed in benign cutaneous leiomyomas. Smooth muscle bundles, when cut in cross section, may demonstrate a characteristic hollow appearance within each cell profile, and immunohistochemical stains for desmin and smooth muscle actin are positive. As the name implies, angioleiomyomas also have small branching vessels admixed with the interlacing bundles of smooth muscle that form these well-circumscribed tumor nodules (see Fig. 15–14B).

Superficial Leiomyosarcoma[22]

- HYPERCELLULAR, ASYMMETRICAL, INFILTRATIVE DERMAL SPINDLE CELL TUMOR
- PUSHING NODULES AND FASCICLES EXTENDING INTO SUBCUTIS
- MITOSES PRESENT
- NUCLEAR ENLARGEMENT AND HYPERCHROMASIA; RETENTION OF CIGAR SHAPE
- DESMIN POSITIVITY BY IMMUNOHISTOCHEMISTRY

Superficial leiomyosarcoma is divided biologically into those lesions that arise primarily in the dermis (i.e., cutaneous leiomyosarcoma) and those that develop within deeper

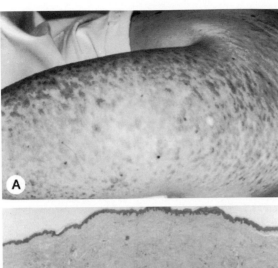

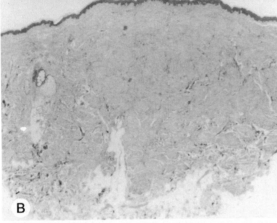

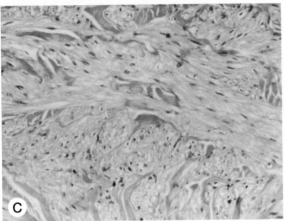

Figure 15–13. Leiomyoma: multiple piloleiomyomas. **(A)** This extremity is affected by multiple red-brown dermal nodules arranged in a linear plaque. **(B)** Histologically, multiple smooth muscle bundles insidiously infiltrate dermal connective tissue. **(C)** At high magnification, smooth muscle cells have elongated, cigar-shaped nuclei with rounded ends in longitudinal section, and in cross section, their cytoplasm appears vacuolated.

tissue (i.e., subcutaneous leiomyosarcoma). Whereas the latter has a poor prognosis with the frequent development of hematogenous metastases, the former has a favorable overall outcome. Cutaneous leiomyosarcomas clinically present as firm dermal nodules that usually span less than 2 cm in diameter. Overlying skin may be depressed or discolored in cutaneous leiomyosarcoma, as opposed to the subcutaneous

variant, in which the skin is uninvolved and freely movable over the nodule.

Histologically, superficial cutaneous leiomyosarcomas are asymmetrical, consisting of infiltrative tumor fascicles with zones of hypercellularity (Fig. 15–15A). Complete replacement of the dermis and infiltration of the subcutis by destructive, pushing fascicles may occur. Although less-differentiated regions may exhibit multinucleation and bizarre nuclear forms, better differentiated zones retain elongated nuclei with rounded ends typical of smooth muscle (Fig. 15–15B). These nuclei differ from those of benign leiomyomas, however, in that they contain coarsely clumped heterochromatin and exhibit numerous mitoses. Tumors confined to the dermis have a low incidence of metastasis, and surgical eradication confirmed by careful pathologic evaluation of all margins is potentially curative.

Fibrohistiocytic Tumors

Hyperplasias and Hamartomas

- FIBROBLASTS AND COLLAGEN BUNDLES IN RANDOM ARRAY PRODUCING A TUMORAL NODULE
- BROAD BANDS OF HYALINIZED COLLAGEN IN A ZEBRA-STRIPE PATTERN (E.G., KELOID)
- ADMIXED, ANOMALOUS NEUROVASCULAR ELEMENTS (E.G., HAMARTOMA)

There are several distinctive types of fibrohistiocytic hyperplasias and hamartomas that are encountered in routine dermatopathology practice. *Keloids* are abnormal hyperplasias of collagen-forming fibroblasts that presumably occur in response to traumatic scarring, although lesions have been reported to occur spontaneously. In North America, the majority of lesions are encountered in adults of African-American ancestry. Clinically, keloids are raised nodules which in early stages may have an erythematous hue, and which may acquire progressive pigmentation over time (Fig. 15–16A). Histologically, there is irregular proliferation of fibroblasts and collagen bundles within the superficial and deep dermis, often covered by an atrophic epidermal layer (Fig. 15–16B). A characteristic feature is the presence of intermixed broad collagen bundles with an eosinophilic, hyalinized quality, imparting a zebra-stripe appearance to the lesion (Fig. 15–16C). A *hypertrophic scar* (Fig. 15–17) resembles a keloid in that the proliferating fascicles of fibroblasts are randomly oriented. Normal scarring results in fibroblasts and collagen strands aligned parallel to the epidermal surface. The thickened, hyalinized collagen bundles typical of keloid formation, however, are entirely lacking in a hypertrophic scar. A connective tissue hamartoma, or nevus, may consist predominantly of abnormal aggregates of fibroblasts and collagen bundles in the dermis (Fig. 15–18). However, as with most hamartomas, there are minor components consisting of abnormal vessels and even nerve bundles which provide the clue that the proliferation is in reality a developmental abnormality, rather than a response to injury or a neoplasm.

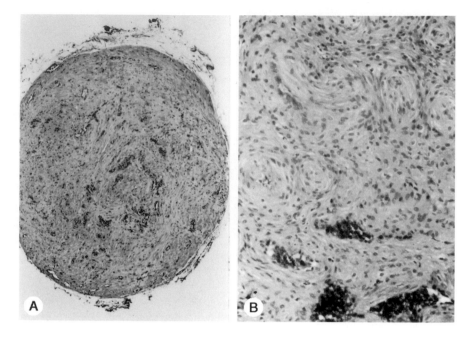

Figure 15–14. Subcutaneous solitary angioleio-myoma. **(A)** This often painful angiomatous variant of leiomyoma was shelled out from the subcutaneous fat at surgery. **(B)** The lesion is a circumscribed, encapsulated tumor formed by proliferation of benign smooth muscle bundles and admixed small blood vessels.

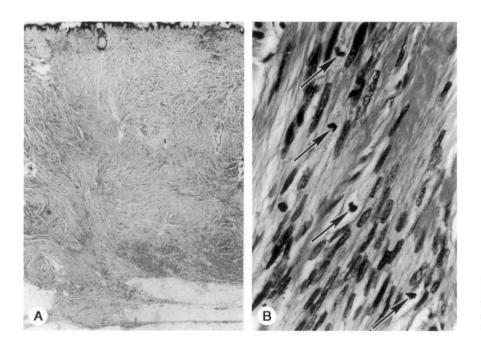

Figure 15–15. Leiomyosarcoma. **(A)** The dermis is diffusely infiltrated by a spindle cell neoplasm that focally extends into subcutaneous fat. **(B)** At high magnification, the fusiform cells composing the tumor are characterized by elongated, cigar-shaped, hyperchromatic nuclei demonstrating numerous mitotoic figures *(arrows)*.

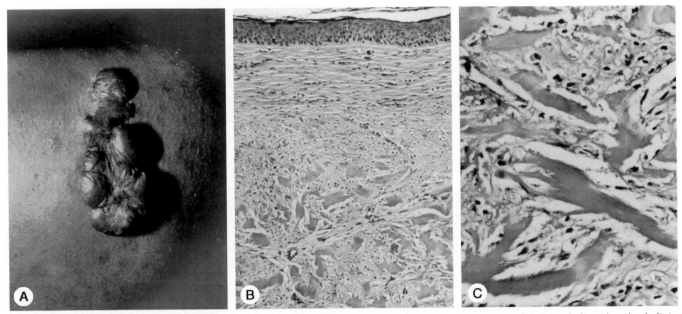

Figure 15–16. Keloid. **(A)** This unique form of proliferative scar results in exophytic plaques and nodules at the sites of clinical and subclinical trauma in genetically predisposed individuals. **(B)** At scanning magnification, there is mid-dermal and deep dermal sclerosis. **(C)** At high-power magnification, proliferating fibroblasts are intermixed with hyalinized and thickened bundles of collagen, producing a zebra-stripe pattern.

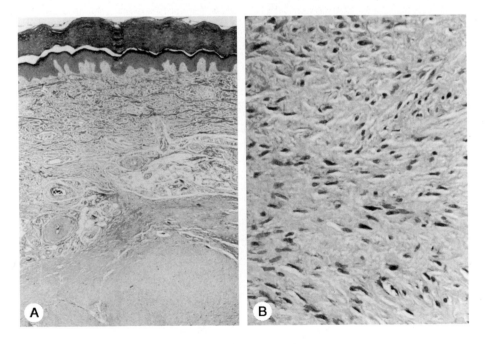

Figure 15–17. Hypertrophic scar. **(A, B)** As opposed to a keloid, hypertrophic scars consist only of interlacing fascicles of fibroblasts and delicate collagen bundles within the mid-dermis and deep dermis. Thickened, hyalinized bands are not present.

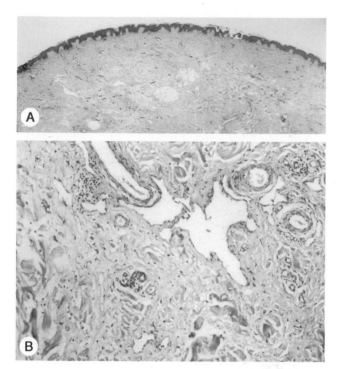

Figure 15–18. Connective tissue nevus (hamartoma). **(A)** Low and **(B)** high magnification reveal a subtle yet anomalous proliferation of vessels, collagen, and associated extracellular matrix elements, as well as lymphatics beneath a diffusely hyperplastic epidermis.

Benign Fibrous Histiocytomas[23–26]

- SYMMETRICAL DERMAL NODULE COMPOSED OF BLAND SPINDLE CELLS
- OVERLYING EPIDERMAL HYPERPLASIA AND BASAL CELL LAYER HYPERPIGMENTATION
- INFILTRATIVE PERIMETER WITH ENTRAPMENT OF COLLAGEN BUNDLES
- VARIABLE NUMBERS OF ADMIXED HISTIOCYTES AND FOAM CELLS
- VARIABLE VASCULARITY AND HEMOSIDERIN DEPOSITION

Benign fibrous histiocytomas, also commonly referred to as dermatofibromas, are common cutaneous neoplasms that most often affect young and middle-aged adults. There is a slight female predominance, and lesions often occur on the lower extremity of people of both genders, although any skin surface may be involved. Tumors are small and slow-growing, arising initially as hard flesh-colored papules that gradually and symmetrically enlarge to become tan to brown nodules (Fig. 15–19A). Although lesions are usually painless, intermittent hyperesthesia and minor pain may be occasionally observed. Benign fibrous histiocytomas are often confused clinically with nodular malignant melanoma. A helpful clinical sign (i.e., Fitzpatrick sign) in differentiating these two entities is the application of centripetal compression radially about the lesion. Whereas nodular melanomas tend to bulge outward with this maneuver, benign fibrous histiocytomas commonly dimple inward as a consequence of their tethering within the deep dermis and subcutaneous fat.

Early benign fibrous histiocytomas are symmetrical, well-circumscribed but not encapsulated proliferations of small fibroblasts admixed with histiocytes within the mid-dermis (Fig. 15–19B). The histiocytic component may be inconspicuous or prominent, and in the latter instance, their histiocytes are frequently vacuolated. Over time, lesions may infiltrate into underlying subcutaneous fat and become less cellular and more collagenous centrally. Cytologically, lesions are formed by small, benign-appearing fibroblasts that typically infiltrate among and surround individual reticular dermal collagen bundles (Fig. 15–19C). Early cellular phases of growth are characterized by zones containing plump fibroblasts, and occasional mitotic figures are observed, although atypical forms are not seen. Vascular proliferation is variable, although some lesions contain significant numbers of small vessels and admixed hemosiderin throughout the tumor nodule; the misnomer sclerosing hemangioma has been used to refer to such histologic patterns. A characteristic diagnostic feature of benign fibrous histiocytomas is the tendency for the overlying epidermis to demonstrate hyperplasia. Hyperplasia may take the form of squamoid, pseudoepitheliomatous hyperplasia, as seen in granular cell tumors, although basaloid hyperplasia resembling primary follicular germ or basal cell carcinoma is also frequently observed. Downward proliferation of hyperpigmented cords of basaloid cells may produces a pattern likened to "dirty fingers."

Dermatofibrosarcoma Protuberans[27–30]

- ASYMMETRICAL PLAQUE OR NODULE COMPOSED OF SPINDLE CELLS
- EXTENSION INTO SUBCUTIS IN HONEYCOMB PATTERN
- PROMINENT STORIFORMING OF TUMOR CELLS
- FOCAL HYPERCELLULARITY AND MITOTIC ACTIVITY

The majority of dermatofibrosarcoma protuberans (DFSP) arise in the third and fourth decades of life, and there

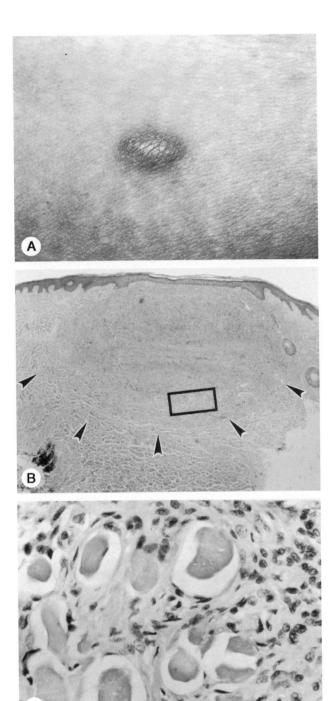

Figure 15–19. Benign fibrous histiocytoma (dermatofibroma). **(A)** Clinically, these lesions appear as firm, brown papules predominantly found on the lower extremities. Inward compression produces dimpling, in contrast to vertical growth phase melanoma, which generally protrudes outward with this maneuver (i.e., Fitzpatrick sign). **(B)** At scanning magnification, there is a subtle spindle cell proliferation within the mid-dermis and deep dermis *(inferior border defined by arrowheads).* The overlying epidermis is generally hyperplastic, although the portion of the epidermis most central to the tumor is attenuated due to pressure atrophy. **(C)** A peripheral region similar to that designated by the rectangle in **B** shows fusiform benign fibroblasts entrapping collagen bundles. Other dermal lesions that result in collagen bundle entrapment include early Kaposi sarcoma, early granuloma annulare, and metastatic carcinoma.

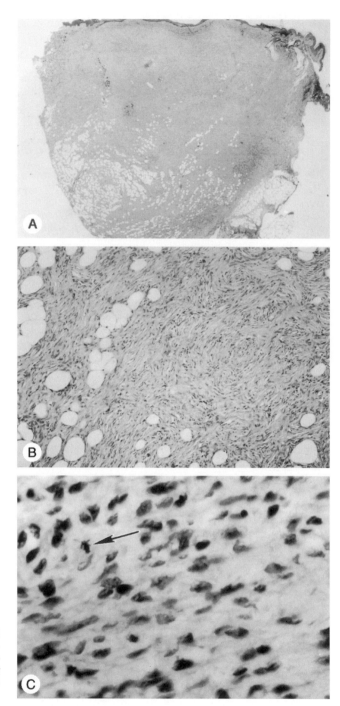

Figure 15–20. Dermatofibrosarcoma protuberans. **(A)** There is diffuse dermal infiltration beneath an attenuated epidermis by a cellular spindle cell neoplasm that characteristically replaces subcutaneous fat to produce a honeycomb pattern. There is a storiform pattern **(B)**, which also may be potentially present in benign fibrous histiocytoma, hypercellularity, and focal dermal mitoses **(C, arrow).**

is a slight male predilection. Tumors initially present as firm, flesh-colored plaques that eventually become lobulated, exophytic nodules. As nodularity supervenes, reddish blue discoloration of the overlying epidermis may be noted, and ulceration is occasionally present. The skin of the chest, back, and thighs is especially prone to the development of DFSP.

The architecture of DFSP at scanning magnification is that of an asymmetrical, expansile, infiltrating cellular nodule within the dermis, usually with extension into the underlying subcutaneous fat and soft tissue (Fig. 15–20A). The majority of proliferating cells are spindle cells with slight nuclear hyperchromasia but with little pleomorphism of nuclear size

and contour (Fig. 15–20B). Cells are characteristically arranged in a pinwheel-like configuration (i.e., storiforming), a pattern that is even better appreciated with reticulin staining. Mitotic figures are present, and atypical mitoses may be seen (Fig. 15–20C). Only rarely are multinucleated tumor cells or necrosis present. In one variant form, the Bednar tumor, small deposits of melanin pigment may be detected in occasional tumor cells, causing confusion with primary spindle cell melanocytic tumors. Unlike melanomas, however, the majority of cells forming DFSP are negative for S100 protein. About 30% of cases of DFSP will recur locally after simple excision. Metastases have been described, but are extremely uncommon.

Atypical Fibroxanthoma[31, 32]

- CELLULAR DERMAL TUMOR WITH ASSOCIATED ELASTOSIS AT PERIPHERY
- ADMIXTURE OF VARIABLY SIZED MONONUCLEAR CELLS, MULTINUCLEATED CELLS, AND FOAM CELLS
- ABSENCE OF CONTINUITY WITH EPIDERMIS OR EVIDENCE OF INTRAEPIDERMAL GROWTH
- PROFOUND NUCLEAR ATYPIA
- BIZARRE, "FIRECRACKER" MITOTIC FIGURES

Atypical fibroxanthoma (AFX) is a nodular tumor that characteristically involves the actinically damaged skin of the head and neck of elderly individuals. Ulceration and bleeding is not uncommon, although individual tumors rarely exceed 2 cm in diameter. The clinical differential diagnosis often involves squamous cell carcinoma, amelanotic melanoma, or solitary metastasis to scalp skin. Accurate diagnosis is important, because AFX usually does not metastasize, although local recurrences may develop after incomplete excision.

At scanning magnification, there is a cellular, symmetrical proliferation of cells within the superficial and deep dermis (Fig. 15–21A) and in some lesions, into the subcutaneous fat. The adjacent epidermis may exhibit reactive changes or an abortive collarette about the perimeter of the tumor nodule, and the adjacent superficial dermis generally demonstrates severe solar elastosis. Cytologic examination reveals cells that vary considerably in size and shape, ranging from elongated spindle cells to plump, often multinucleated histiocytes with profound nuclear atypia (Fig. 15–21B). The spindle cells frequently contain elongated, hyperchromatic nuclei, whereas the multinucleated cells contain irregularly shaped, hyperchromatic to vesicular nuclei, often with prominent nucleoli. Mitotic activity is brisk, and strikingly atypical mitotic figures are characteristic, with some showing distinctive starburst or exploding firecracker patterns. The histiocyte-like cells frequently show cytoplasmic vacuolization. Importantly, the atypical cells of AFX are not continuous with any cell population within the epidermis, militating against the differential diagnostic considerations of squamous cell carcinoma and melanoma. Deeply invasive lesions behave more aggressively and may show biologic characteristics that resemble those of superficial malignant fibrous histiocytoma. Because of the alarming degree of nuclear atypia in AFX and its tendency for spindle cell differentiation, this tumor is frequently confused with anaplastic spindle cell squamous cell carcinoma and spindle cell melanoma. Whereas AFX is variably positive for α_1-antichymotrypsin and negative for S100 protein and cytokeratin, melanomas are generally S100 protein–positive. Spindle cell squamous cell carcinomas show variable keratin immunoreactivity, whereas AFX does not. AFX does not show a prominent vascular component, a finding helpful in its differentiation from metastatic spindle cell renal cell carcinoma, a tumor that not uncommonly metastasizes to the skin of the scalp.

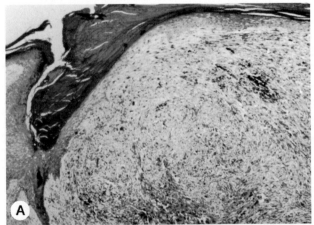

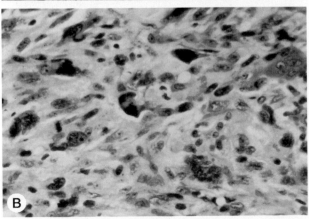

Figure 15–21. Atypical fibroxanthoma. **(A)** A cellular neoplasm of highly pleomorphic cells is present within actinically damaged dermis beneath an attenuated epidermal layer. **(B)** The cells comprising the neoplasm consist of variably pleomorphic fibroblasts and histiocytic cells, some of which exhibit multinucleation, prominent hyperchromasia, and frequent mitotic figures.

Neural Tumors

Neural Hyperplasias

Non-neoplastic proliferations of nerve fibers may result in neuroma-like nodules. *Traumatic neuromas* are nondescript, firm nodules that appear at sites of previous trauma to peripheral nerves. These lesions may be associated with localized pain and anesthesia. *Morton neuroma* refers to a degenerative phenomenon that occurs in skin and soft tissue between the metatarsal heads of the foot. Both traumatic neuromas and Morton neuromas appear to be the result of localized trauma, and both involve proliferation of fibrocollagenous mesenchyme. Traumatic neuroma, however, also involves proliferation of axonal tissue (Fig. 15–22), whereas Morton neuroma involves entrapped, nonproliferative nerve branches with degenerative changes.

Neurofibroma and Neurilemmoma[33–37]

- POORLY DEFINED (NEUROFIBROMA) OR WELL-CIRCUMSCRIBED (NEURILEMMOMA) DERMAL NODULE
- SPINDLE CELLS WITH WAVY NUCLEAR PROFILES PREDOMINATE
- VARIABLE MYXOID STROMA CONTAINING MAST CELLS
- PALISADED NULCEI MAY BE PROMINENT (NEURILEMMOMA)
- MITOSES ABSENT
- SMALL NERVE FIBERS, EITHER WITHIN TUMOR (NEUROFIBROMA) OR AT PERIPHERY OF TUMOR (NEURILEMMOMA)

Neurofibromas and neurilemmomas are benign tumors that predominantly involve proliferation of perineural supporting cells (i.e., Schwann cells). *Neurofibromas* may appear as multiple lesions, particularly in the setting of von Recklinghausen neurofibromatosis (Fig. 15–23A), or as solitary lesions not associated with systemic disease. Any part of the cutaneous surface may be affected, and the age range of patients varies widely. Individual lesions appear as skin-colored, soft papules, nodules, or pedunculated tumors that may be confused with melanocytic nevi or acrochordons. *Neurilemmomas*, also known as *schwannomas*, most commonly affect middle-aged adults and tend to involve skin of the head, neck, and extremities. These lesions are generally solitary and appear as painless, flesh-colored, nondescript papules and nodules (Fig. 15–24A).

At scanning magnification, neurofibromas are well-defined, nonencapsulated often exophytic dermal neoplasms composed of small, variably cellular aggregates of benign-appearing spindle cells embedded within a loose fibrillar, eosinophilic matrix (Fig. 15–23B). Occasional zones may undergo mucinous degeneration, imparting a myxoid quality to these areas. At higher magnification, individual tumor cells have bland nuclear chromatin patterns, often exhibit a wavy nuclear contour, and are devoid of mitotic activity (Fig. 15–23C). Unlike neurotized nevi, which may show a strikingly similar histologic appearance, neurofibromas consistently contain axons forming nerve twigs within the spindle cell

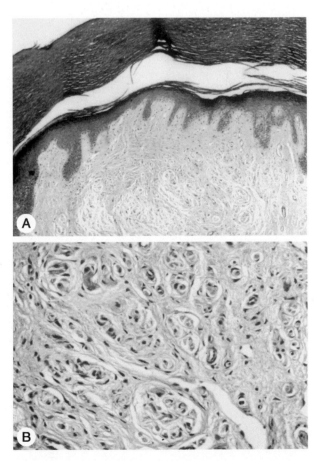

Figure 15–22. Traumatic neuroma. **(A, B)** Numerous nerve fibers are embedded within a sclerotic dermis at a site of repeated trauma or inflammation.

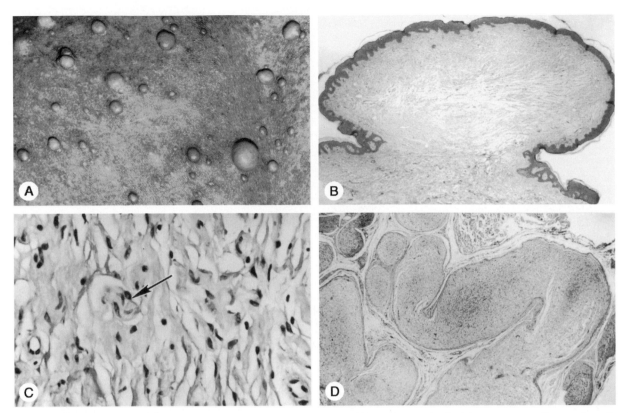

Figure 15–23. Neurofibroma. **(A)** Multiple neurofibromas in the setting of neurofibromatosis. Individual lesions are sessile-to-pedunculated, soft, fleshy tumors. **(B)** At low magnification, a pedunculated neurofibroma shows a loosely arranged stroma partially surrounded by a diffusely hyperplastic epidermal layer. **(C)** At higher magnification, small, bland spindle cells proliferate among wavy collagen bundles, mast cells, and occasional nerve fibers *(arrow)*. **(D)** In a plexiform neurofibroma, a more specific marker for neurofibromatosis based upon a solitary lesion, there are discrete, enlarged nerve bundles in serpiginous array within a loose connective tissue stroma.

component, which is primarily comprised of Schwann cells (Fig. 15–23C). Both nevi and neurofibromas contain numerous mast cells. *Plexiform neurofibromas* are characteristically seen only in von Recklinghausen neurofibromatosis and are composed of cellular and hypertrophied nerve trunks, which ramify in a vermiform manner within the reticular dermis (Fig. 15–23D).

Neurilemmomas are encapsulated dermal tumors that often extend into or primarily arise in the subcutis (Fig. 15–24B). Cytologically, these lesions are biphasic, consisting of cellular zones of spindle cells with nuclear characteristics similar to those of neurofibromas (i.e., Antoni A areas; Fig. 15–24C) and zones of similar spindle cells within an abundant mucinous background (i.e., Antoni B areas). Cellular regions may show parallel alignment of spindle cell nuclei, producing a palisaded pattern, and sometimes two parallel rows of these palisaded nuclei produce small organoid bodies referred to as Verocay bodies (Fig. 15–24D). With aging, isolated nuclei may enlarge and become hyperchromatic, although mitotic figures are virtually never seen (i.e., "ancient change"). This is regarded as a form of degenerative atypia.

Palisaded Encapsulated Neuroma[38]

- WELL-CIRCUMSCRIBED, SYMMETRICAL DERMAL NODULE

- DIFFUSE HYPERCELLULARITY ATTRIBUTABLE TO UNIFORM SPINDLE CELLS IN FASCICLES
- AXON:SUPPORTING CELL RATIO >50%
- MITOSES ABSENT

Palisaded encapsulated neuromas are typically located at mucocutaneous junctions of the facial skin of middle-aged patients. There is no evidence of gender predilection. Lesions characteristically are solitary, painless, flesh-colored papulonodules that are often mistaken for cysts. Histologically, low magnification reveals an encapsulated, nodular tumor composed of spindle cells within the dermis (Fig. 15–25A). At higher-power magnification, these cells are composed of unmyelinated axons that, unlike neurofibromas and neurilemmomas, are present in at least equal proportion to the number of Schwann cells and fibroblastic elements (Fig. 15–25B and C). Proliferating spindle cells may be arranged in coalescent fascicles, and typically show evidence of poorly formed palisaded aggregates (Fig. 15–25C). Mitoses and necrosis are not observed, as is the case in neurofibromas and neurilemmomas.

The occurrence of a well-defined spindle cell neoplasm at mucocutaneous junctions of facial skin should raise the possibility of a palisaded, encapsulated neuroma. S100 stain is helpful in separating this entity from other well-demarcated benign spindle cell tumors that may involve dermal

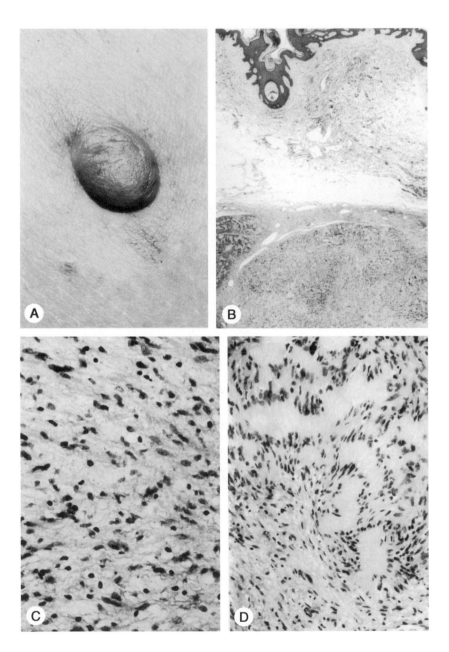

Figure 15–24. Neurolemmoma. **(A)** This soft, fleshy nodule demonstrated a well-demarcated tumor nodule **(B)** within the deep dermis and subcutis. **(C)** At higher magnification, the stroma is composed of neuroid spindle cells within a finely fibrillar matrix and **(D)** zones where spindle cells prominently palisade (i.e., Verocay bodies).

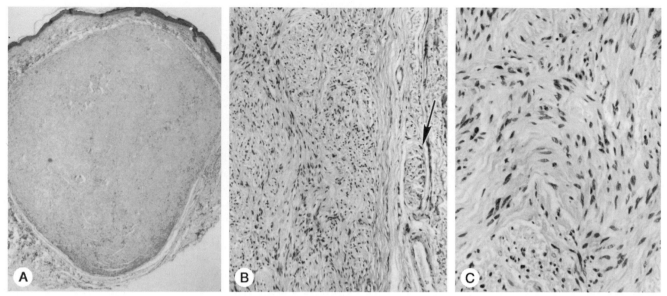

Figure 15–25. Palisaded encapsulated neuroma. **(A)** This uniformly cellular dermal nodule is well demarcated and **(B, C)** is composed of spindle cells and axons in approximately a 50 : 50 ratio. Note the nerve fiber at the perimeter of the tumor *(arrow)*.

tissue (e.g., angioleiomyoma). The identification of a high concentration of axons, facilitated by the use of Bodian stain, aids in excluding other well-circumscribed benign neural lesions that may affect the dermis (e.g., neurilemmoma).

Granular Cell Tumor[39–43]

- SYMMETRICAL PROLIFERATION OF UNIFORM EPITHELIOID CELLS IN SUPERFICIAL AND DEEP DERMIS
- VARIABLE EPIDERMAL HYPERPLASIA
- ABUNDANT, FINELY GRANULAR, PERIODIC ACID–SCHIFF–POSITIVE CYTOPLASM
- EARLY LESIONS SHOW TUMOR CELL INFILTRATES CUFFING DERMAL NERVES

Granular cell tumors most often are encountered in middle-aged women and have a predilection for occurrence on the extremities and tongue. Up to 10% of affected individuals may have multiple neoplasms. Clinically, lesions present as painless, flesh-colored, nondescript nodules that grow slowly and are often present for some time before histologic diagnosis is made. Mucosal involvement is often accompanied by verrucous mucosal thickening, which may be confused with causes of leukoplakia, such as oral squamous cell carcinoma.

Early granular cell tumors appear as perineural collections of plump cells containing small, eccentically-located round nuclei and characteristically granulated pink cytoplasm. This perineural distribution is distinctive in early lesions, and in keeping with the belief that granular cell tumors are of Schwannian derivation. Over time, these tumors enlarge, and cellular aggregates coalesce to form sheets of granular cells throughout the dermis (Fig. 15–26A), often in association with verrucous hyperplasia of the overlying epi-

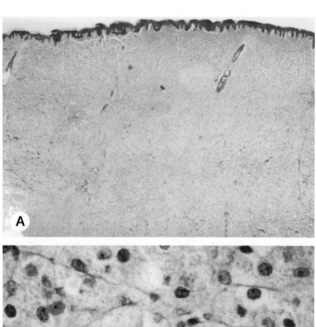

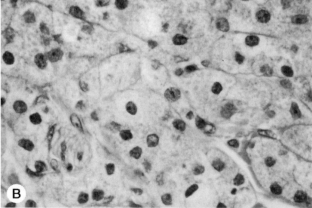

Figure 15–26. Granular cell tumor. **(A)** At scanning magnification, the dermis is diffusely permeated by pale cells beneath an epidermal layer showing marked hyperplasia. **(B)** At high magnification, the tumor cells have distinct cell membranes; finely granular, not vacuolated, cytoplasm; and centrally located, uniform, round nuclei.

dermis. This hyperplasia may be so pronounced, particularly in the oral cavity, that it mimics a well-differentiated, invasive squamous cell carcinoma in superficial biopsy specimens. Cytologically, tumor nuclei are small, round, and centrally located within a finely granulated cytoplasm that stains positively with the PAS reagent (Fig. 15–26B). These cells differ from xanthoma cells, which they may superficially resemble, by having granulated, as opposed to finely vacuolated cytoplasm. Mitoses should not be observed. By electron microscopy, the small cytoplasmic granules within individual tumor cells appear as lysosomes and as laminated membranous aggregates similar to myelin bodies. Immunohistochemically, tumors stain variably for S100 protein.

Neuroendocrine Carcinoma[44–48]

- ASYMMETRICAL DERMAL INFILTRATE WITH DIFFUSE OR TRABECULAR PATTERN
- OCCASIONAL FOCI OF EPIDERMOTROPIC GROWTH
- SMALL TUMOR CELLS WITH HIGH NUCLEAR:CYTOPLASMIC RATIO AND ''WASHED OUT'' CHROMATIN
- MANY MITOSES, AND PROMINENT INDIVIDUAL CELL AND ZONAL NECROSIS

Neuroendocrine carcinomas are primarily neoplasms of the elderly, and men and women are equally affected. These neoplasms are believed to originate from Merkel cells, which normally inhabit the epidermal basal cell layer in low numbers (see Chap. 1). More than one half of these tumors involve the skin of the head and neck, and the remainder affect the lower extremity (about one-fifth), the upper extremity, the buttocks, and miscellaneous other sites. Individ-

ual tumor nodules are generally present for several months to two years before initial presentation and diagnosis. The average neuroendocrine carcinoma is between 0.5 and 9.0 cm and presents as a raised, tender, nodular tumor that clinically may be confused with a boil or blood blister. Color varies from pink to red, and ulceration and superficial hemorrhage are observed frequently. The clinical differential diagnosis may therefore include hemangioma, lymphoma, or angiosarcoma.

Neuroendocrine carcinomas in the skin infiltrate the dermis and subcutis diffusely by sheets of small cells which, at scanning magnification, may appear to be lymphocytes because of their nuclear prominence and scarce cytoplasm (Fig. 15–27A). Zones of necrosis may be apparent even at low-power magnification, and lesions frequently have an asymmetrical profile and an infiltrative border at the periphery. At higher magnification, a minority of tumors show a vague trabecular architecture, the pattern originally described (i.e., trabecular carcinoma of the skin). Tumor cells contain round to slightly ovoid nuclei, scant cytoplasm, frequent mitotic activity, and frequent individual cell and zonal necrosis (Fig. 15–27B). A characteristic feature of neuroendocrine carcinoma is the nuclear chromatin pattern, characterized by pallor due to finely stippled chromatin particles that do not appear to take up hematoxylin avidly. Nucleoli are absent or inconspicuous. Slightly less than 10% of tumors will show pagetoid invasion of the overlying epidermis. By ultrastructural analysis, neuroendocrine carcinomas of skin contain neurosecretory, dense-core granules that, like those of normal Merkel cells, range between 80 and 200 nm in diameter. These tumors also characteristically show aggregated bundles of intermediate microfilaments in a juxtanuclear location. Neuroendocrine carcinomas of skin also show a distinctive pattern of keratin staining consisting of discrete, round, par-

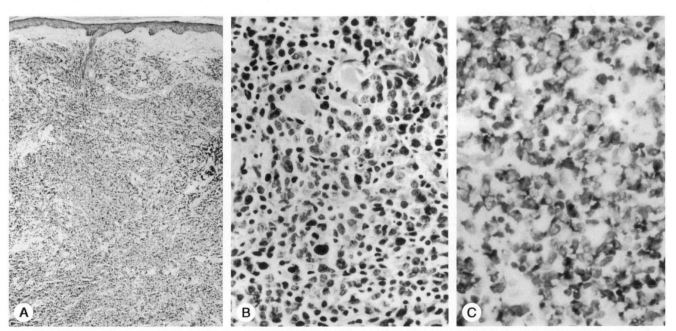

Figure 15–27. Neuroendocrine carcinoma. **(A)** There are confluent nests and inconspicuous trabeculae of small, lymphocyte-like cells within the superficial and deep dermis. **(B)** At higher magnification, there is scant cytoplasm, and nuclei are pleomorphic and exhibit numerous mitotic figures as well as prominent individual cell necrosis. **(C)** Immunohistochemical stain for cytokeratin reveals a characteristic perinuclear zone of positive staining in most cells.

anuclear, inclusion-like globules (Fig. 15–27C). This finding is extremely helpful in separating neuroendocrine carcinomas from other tumors and mimics, such as lymphoma, small cell melanoma variants, and metastatic small cell carcinoma from extracutaneous sites.

Neuroendocrine carcinomas show a marked tendency for recurrence at varying intervals after primary excision. More than one half of patients are noted to have lymph node metastases either at the time of initial diagnosis or within several years after diagnosis.

Neurothekeoma[49]

- WELL-DEMARCATED LOBULES, NESTS, AND CORDS WITHIN MID-DERMIS
- FUSIFORM-TO-EPITHELIOID TUMOR CELLS WITH NUCLEAR PLEOMORPHISM
- OCCASIONAL MITOSES; CELLULAR NECROSIS RARE
- SPINDLE CELL VARIANTS OFTEN SHOW MYXOID STROMA (E.G., NERVE SHEATH MYXOMA)

Neurothekeomas occur at any age, although most are noted in children and young adults. Females are affected over males, and the majority of neoplasms are solitary and localized to skin of the face, shoulders, and upper extremities. Individual tumors are flesh-colored to erythematous soft nodules approximately 0.5 to 2 cm in diameter. Lesions tend to grow slowly, and local recurrence tends to develop only after incomplete excision.

Architecturally, neurothekeomas are composed of symmetrical and well-demarcated lobules, nests, and cords of cells separated by fibrous septa within the mid-dermis (Fig. 15–28A). Tumor cells are fusiform, show pleomorphism in size and shape, contain nuclei with occasional hyperchromasia and mitotic activity, and exhibit focally prominent eosinophilic cytoplasm imparting an epithelioid appearance (Fig. 15–28B). Necrosis or infiltrative destruction of dermal architecture or appendages is not observed. Some tumors have a prominent myxoid background in and around tumor lobules, and a patchy lymphocytic infiltrate may be present. It has been suggested that with aging, the more cellular neurothekeomas acquire an increasingly myxoid matrix and accordingly show histologic features of nerve sheath myxoma.

Tumors of Adipose Tissue: Lipoma[50, 51]

- WELL-DEMARCATED, OFTEN ENCAPSULATED DERMAL OR SUBCUTANEOUS TUMOR
- PREDOMINANT CELL IS MATURE ADIPOCYTE
- DIFFUSE VASCULAR PERMEATION MAY BE PRESENT (E.G., ANGIOLIPOMA)
- SPINDLE CELL DIFFERENTIATION WITH FIBROSIS AND MUCINOUS CHANGE OCCASIONALLY OBSERVED (E.G., SPINDLE CELL LIPOMA)
- OCCASIONAL TUMORS WITH FINELY GRANULATED ADIPOCYTES (E.G., HIBERNOMA)

Lipomas are common neoplasms of subcutaneous fat, and as such, they are frequently encountered by dermatopa-thologists. Although there are numerous rare and exotic subtypes of lipoma, this discussion focuses only on the more commonly encountered variants. *Nevus lipomatosus superficialis* refers to a condition characterized by multiple, brown-yellow, coalescent nodules that form a cerebriform skin surface along the skin folds of the flank, buttocks, and upper portion of the posterior thigh. These are congenital hamartomas, although they may not become apparent until early adulthood. Histologically, the lower- and mid-dermis are replaced by mature fat, and the epidermis may be thrown into a verrucous or bosselated pattern (Fig. 15–29A, B). Ordinary *lipomas* (Fig. 15–29C) and *angiolipomas* (Fig. 15–29D) are common, soft, nodular tumors that occur in adults. They may be confused with cysts or other subcutaneous tumors. Unlike lipomas, angiolipomas tend to be painful. Histologically, both lesions are encapsulated neoplasms composed of mature adipose tissue, although angiolipoma is permeated by small arborizing vessels, many of which may contain fibrin thrombi.

Hibernomas are lipomas of brown or fetal fat. These lesions occur in young adults and are composed of adipocytes containing lipid vacuoles superimposed on a cytoplasm that is granular and eosinophilic because of numerous intracellular mitochondria (Fig. 15–29E). *Spindle cell lipoma* is a distinctive histologic subtype of lipoma that occurs on the

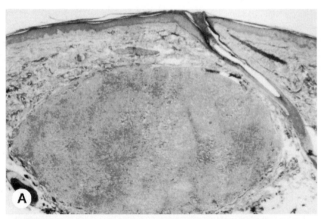

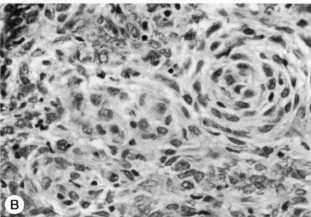

Figure 15–28. Neurothekeoma. **(A)** The tumor is well circumscribed within the mid-dermis. **(B)** This epithelioid variant is composed of clustered nests of round-to-ovoid cells with variable nuclear pleomorphism and occasional mitotic figures. Other foci show cells embedded in a fibrillar matrix. Myxoid variants are composed predominantly of stellate and fusiform cells within a mucinous, myxoid stroma, as well as isolated foci of epithelioid cells.

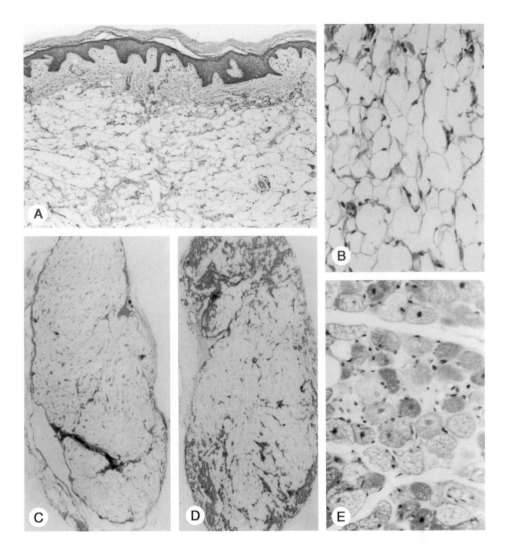

Figure 15–29. Lipoma and variants. **(A, B)** Nevus lipomatosus superficialis, with the lower two thirds of the dermis **(A)** replaced by mature adipose tissue **(B)**. Although both **(C)** lipoma and **(D)** angiolipoma are well-defined encapsulated tumors of mature adipose tissue, only the latter has a significant component of small vessels, often containing thrombi (opaque anastomosing structures concentrated at upper and lower poles of this ovoid tumor). **(E)** Fetal fat is finely vacuolated to granulated fat with a brown clinical appearance and an eosinophilic hue by routine histology. It is found in adults primarily as the main cellular constituent of the lipoma termed hibernoma.

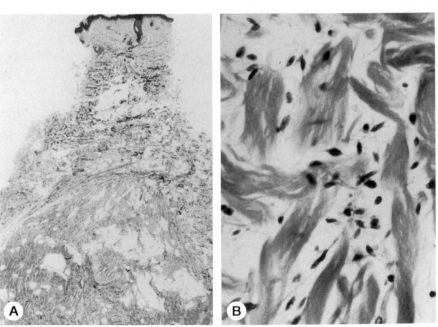

Figure 15–30. Spindle cell lipoma. **(A)** This circumscribed, deep, dermal tumor occurring on the back of an elderly man is composed of mature adipose tissue (clear zones), collagen bundles, and **(B)** numerous spindled fibroblasts within a mucinous stroma. The tumor nodule is also replete with mast cells.

posterior neck and shoulders of middle-aged men. Histologically, these tumors are well circumscribed (Fig. 15–30A) and contain an admixture of mature adipocytes and uniform, collagen-forming spindle cells embedded within a slightly mucinous matrix replete with mast cells (Fig. 15–30B). Despite these zones of cellularity, spindle cell lipomas should not be confused with liposarcomas and are easily cured by local excision.

DIFFERENTIAL DIAGNOSIS

The differential diagnosis of cutaneous mesenchymal tumors is complicated by the fact that nonmesenchymal neoplasms (i.e., epithelial and melanocytic tumors) may mimic spindle cell differentiation. This is particularly problematic when tumors are poorly differentiated. Fortunately, advances in immunohistochemistry have facilitated determination of histogenesis in many problematic mesenchymal tumors of skin. Subclassification relies on detailed knowledge of how tumors of differing lineages are likely to evolve over time (e.g., Kaposi sarcoma) and specific architectural and cytologic features such as the presence or absence of encapsulation, the cellular composition, and the cytologic features. If these characteristics are carefully analyzed, the more common cutaneous mesenchymal neoplasms presented in this chapter should not pose overwhelming difficulties in differential diagnosis or in accurate prediction of biologic behavior.

SELECTED REFERENCES

1. Gottlieb GJ, Ackerman AB. Atlas of the gross and microscopic features of simulators. In: Gottlieb GJ, Ackerman AB, eds. Kaposi's Sarcoma: A Text and Atlas. Philadelphia: Lea & Febiger, 1988:74.
2. Clearkin KP, Enzinger FM. Intravascular papillary endothelial hyperplasia. Arch Pathol Lab Med 1976;100:441.
3. Warner J, Wilson Jones E. Pyogenic granuloma recurring with multiple satellites. A report of 11 cases. Br J Dermatol 1968;80:218.
4. Rosai J. Angiolymphoid hyperplasia with eosinophilia of the skin. Its nosological position in the spectrum of histiocytoid hemangioma. Am J Dermatopathol 1982;4:175.
5. Kuo T, Sayers P, Rosai J. Masson's "vegetant intravascular hemangioendothelioma": a lesion often mistaken for angiosarcoma. Cancer 1976;38:1227.
6. Alessi E, Bertani E, Sala F. Acquired tufted angioma. Am J Dermatopathol 1986;8:426.
7. Johnson WC. The pathology of cutaneous vascular tumors. Int J Dermatol 1976;15:239.
8. Beckstead JH, Wood GS, Fletcher V. Evidence for the origin of Kaposi's sarcoma from lymphatic endothelium. Am J Pathol 1985;119:294.
9. Dictor M. Kaposi's sarcoma. Origin and significance of lymphaticovenous connections. Virchows Arch (A) 1986;409:23.
10. Nickoloff BJ, Griffiths CEM. Factor XIIIa-expressing dermal dendrocytes in AIDS-associated cutaneous Kaposi's sarcoma. Science 1989;243:1736.
11. DeDobbler G, et al. Clinically uninvolved skin in AIDS. Evidence of atypical dermal vessels similar to early lesions observed in Kaposi's sarcoma. J Cutan Pathol 1987;14:154.
12. Safai B, et al. Association of Kaposi's sarcoma with second primary malignancies: possible etiopathogenic implications. Cancer 1980; 45:1472.
13. Wilson Jones E: Dowling Oration 1976: malignant vascular tumors. Clin Exp Dermatol 1976;1:287.
14. Girard C, Johnson WC, Graham JH. Cutaneous angiosarcoma. Cancer 1970;26:863.
15. Hodgkinson DJ, Soule EH, Woods JE. Cutaneous angiosarcoma of the head and neck. Cancer 1979;44:1106.
16. Stewart FW, Treves N. Lymphangiosarcoma in post-mastectomy lymphedema. Cancer 1948;1:64.

17. Enzinger FM, Weiss SW. Malignant vascular tumors. In: Soft Tissue Tumors. St Louis: CV Mosby, 1983:422.
18. Rosai J, Sumner HW, Kostianovsky TJ, et al. Angiosarcoma of the skin. A clinicopathologic and fine structural study. Hum Pathol 1976;7:83.
19. Murphy GF, Dickerson GR, Harrist, Mihm MC. The role of diagnostic electron microscopy in dermatology. In: Moschella S, ed. Dermatology Update. Reviews for Physicians. New York: Elsevier, 1982:370.
20. Fisher WC, Helwig EB. Leiomyomas of the skin. Arch Dermatol 1963;88:510.
21. Hachisuga T, Hashimoto H, Enjoji M. Angioleiomyoma. A clinicopathological reappraisal of 562 cases. Cancer 1984;54:126.
22. Stout AP, Hill WT. Leiomyosarcoma of the superficial soft tissues. Cancer 1958;11:144.
23. Niemi KM. The benign fibrohistiocytic tumours of the skin (review). Acta Derm Venereol (Stockh) 1970;50(Suppl 63):1.
24. Vilanova JR, Flint A. The morphological variations of fibrous histiocytoma. J Cutan Pathol 1974;1:155.
25. Schonfeld RJ. Epidermal proliferations overlying histiocytomas. Arch Dermatol 1964;90:266.
26. Goette DK, Helwig EB. Basal cell carcinoma and basal cell carcinoma-like changes overlying dermatofibroma. Arch Dermatol 1975;111:589.
27. Taylor HB, Helwig EB. Dermatofibrosarcoma protuberans. Cancer 1961;15:717.
28. McPeak CJ, Cruz T, Nicastri AD. Dermatofibrosarcoma protuberans. Z Hautkr 1976;51:583.
29. Brenner V, Schaefler K, Chabra H, et al. Dermatofibrosarcoma protuberans metastatic to regional lymph nodes. Cancer 1975;36:1897.
30. Kahn LB, Saxe N, Gordon W. Dermatofibrosarcoma protuberans with lymph node and pulmonary metastases. Arch Dermatol 1978;114:599.
31. Fretzin DFJ, Helwig EB. Atypical fibroxanthoma of the skin. Cancer 1973;31:1541.
32. Enzinger FM. Atypical fibroxanthoma and malignant fibrous histiocytoma. Am J Dermatopathol 1979;1:185.
33. Jurecka W, Lassmann H, Gebhart W, et al. Classification of peripheral nerve sheath tumors (abstract). Arch Dermatol Res 1977;258:100.
34. Das Guptas TK, Brasfield RD, Strong EW, et al. Benign solitary schwannoma (neurilemmoma). Cancer 1969;24:355.
35. Izumi AK, Rosato FE, Wood MG. Von Recklinghausen's disease associated with multiple neurilemmomas. Arch Dermatol 1971;104:172.
36. D'Agostino AN, Soule EH, Miller RH. Sarcomas of the peripheral nerves and somatic soft tissues associated with multiple neurofibromatosis (von Recklinghausen's disease). Cancer 1963;16:1015.
37. Carstens PHB, Schrodt GR. Malignant transformation of a benign encapsulated neurilemmoma. Am J Clin Pathol 1969;51:144.
38. Reed ML, Jacoby RA. Cutaneous neuroanatomy and neuropathology. Am J Dermatopathol 1983;5:335.
39. Alkek DS, Johnson WC, Graham JH. Granular cell myoblastoma. Arch Dermatol 1968;98:543.
40. Apisarnthanarax P. Granular cell tumor (review). J Am Acad Dermatol 1981;5:171.
41. Moscovic EA, Azar HA. Multiple granular cell tumors ("myoblastomas"). Cancer 1967;20:2032.
42. Al-Sarraf M, Loud AV, Vaitkevicius VK. Malignant granular cell tumor. Histochemical and electron microscopic study. Arch Pathol 1971;91:550.
43. Barr RJ, Graham JH. Granular cell basal cell carcinoma. Arch Dermatol 1979;115:1064.
44. Toker C. Trabecular carcinoma of the skin. Arch Dermatol 1972;105:107.
45. Wick MR, Scheithauer BW. Primary neuroendocrine carcinoma of the skin. In: Wick MR; ed. Pathology of Unusual Malignant Cutaneous Tumors. New York: Marcel Dekker, 1985:107.
46. Gould VE, Moll I, Lee I, Franke WW. Neuroendocrine (Merkel) cells of the skin: hyperplasias, dysplasias, and neoplasms. Lab Invest 1985;52:334.
47. Sibley RK, Dehner LP, Rosai J. Primary neuroendocrine (Merkel cell?) carcinoma of the skin. I. A clinicopathologic and ultrastructural study of 43 cases. Am J Surg Pathol 1985;9:95.
48. Visscher D, Cooper PH, Zarbo RJ, Crissman JD. Cutaneous neuroendocrine (Merkel cell) carcinoma: an immunophenotypic, clinicopathologic, and flow cytometric study. Mod Pathol 1989;2:331.
49. Gallager RL, Helwig EB. Neurothekeoma—a benign cutaneous tumor of neural origin. Am J Clin Pathol 1980;74:759.
50. Enzinger FM, Harvey DJ. Spindle cell lipoma. Cancer 1975;36:1852.
51. Osment LS. Cutaneous lipomas and lipomatosis. Surg Gynecol Obstet 1968;127:129.

16

Metastatic Tumors to Skin

DEFINITIONS AND GENERAL CONSIDERATIONS

Metastatic tumors to the skin represent a diagnostically problematic and diverse group of neoplasms that may mimic primary carcinoma, melanoma, adnexal carcinoma, and sarcoma. Metastatic carcinoma to the skin is relatively uncommon, although the issue arises frequently enough in routine differential diagnosis that its brief consideration is warranted in this text. A small but significant number of patients who succumbed to internal malignancy have evidence of cutaneous metastases. In women, breast carcinoma is the most frequent lesion to spread to the skin, accounting for approximately two thirds of all metastases. Other primary tumor sites that commonly involve metastases to the skin in women include colon cancer, and carcinoma of the lung, ovaries, and melanoma. In men, lung cancer is the most common primary tumor to spread to the skin, accounting for about one fourth of all cases of cutaneous metastasis, followed by colon cancer, malignant melanoma, and oropharyngeal, renal, and gastric carcinoma.

GROSS PATHOLOGY

Metastatic carcinoma may take a number of different clinical forms, including diffuse dermal lymphatic spread, nodular aggregates of tumor within the dermis, or a pattern clinically predominated by a desmoplastic response. When diffuse lymphatic dissemination occurs, edema and inflammation frequently dominate the clinical picture, producing brawny induration and a peau d'orange appearance to the epidermal surface. This latter feature results when superficial dermal edema occurs about follicular ostia, rendering them prominent and patulous. Emboli of tumor cells within blood vessels may lead to associated telangiectasias or overt zones of infarctive tissue necrosis. Carcinomas that produce desmoplasia result in firm induration and, in some instances, depression of the involved site (e.g., carcinoma en cuirasse). Metastases may vary in size and shape, may be flesh-colored to hemorrhagic, and may show ulceration. Metastases may clinically mimic inflamation and edema, fibrosis, vasculitis, or a wide variety of primary cutaneous tumors.

GENERAL HISTOLOGY AND TEMPORAL EVOLUTION

The general histology of metastatic carcinoma to the skin is problematic, because there is no single factor common to all or even most lesions. Carcinomas that infiltrate the dermis unassociated with any suggestion of epithelial or adnexal origin are perhaps prototypical of a metastasis. However, most lesions are considerably more protean. For example, both metastatic carcinomas and melanomas may home to and infiltrate the epidermal layer, closely mimicking their primary cutaneous counterparts. Certain tumors elicit such an exuberant desmoplastic reaction that the tumor cells become inconspicuous. One of the greatest diagnostic challenges inherent in understanding the histologic patterns of metastatic tumors to the skin is the fact that they share no general histologic features that are of diagnostic assistance. The temporal evolution of metastatic tumors is even more problematic, because most tumors simply enlarge in size or undergo partial necrosis over time rather than evolve through defined and progressive stages, as do many of their primary malignant counterparts.

HISTOLOGY OF SPECIFIC DISORDERS

"Benign Metastases": Endometriosis[1, 2]

- IRREGULAR GLANDS WITHIN MID-DERMIS
- EPITHELIAL CELLS RESEMBLE A PHASE OF NORMAL MENSTRUAL CYCLE
- CUFF OF BASOPHILIC SPINDLE (STROMAL) CELLS AT PERIMETER OF GLANDS

Endometriosis involving the skin clinically presents as a single, brown-blue, painful nodule ranging up to 6 cm in diameter. Adult women are exclusively affected, and lesions are often present as implants in a surgical scar or in the

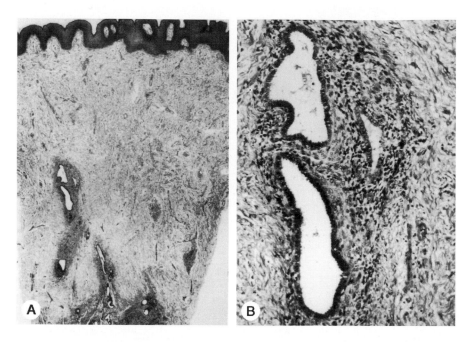

Figure 16–1. Cutaneous endometriosis. (**A**) Within the mid-dermis to deep dermis, there are glands surrounded by a cellular cuff. (**B**) These glands, some of which show early cystic dilation, are composed of nonciliated columnar epithelium. The cuff does not represent inflammation or a desmoplastic response to metastasis but rather is normal endometrial stroma with foci of hemorrhage and hemosiderin deposition.

umbilical region. Lesions typically enlarge and become even more painful during menstruation. Biopsy of involved skin demonstrates glandular lumens of irregular size and shape within the mid-dermis (Fig. 16–1A). The epithelium lining the glands is identical to that of the endometrial cavity, and depending on its stage of cyclic responsiveness, there may be numerous mitoses in the proliferative phase, cytoplasmic vacuoles and lumenal secretion in the secretory phase, or necrosis and sloughing in the menstrual phase. The most characteristic diagnostic feature of cutaneous endometriosis, however, is the presence of a cuff of basophilic spindle cells about each gland (Fig. 16–1B). This cuff represents endo-

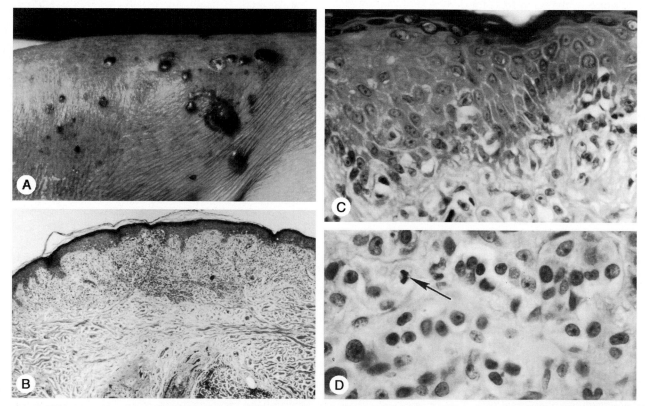

Figure 16–2. Epidermotropic metastases: melanoma. (**A**) Multiple pigmented papules and nodules are covered by a shiny, focally ulcerated epidermal surface. At (**B**) scanning and (**C**) midrange magnification, nested and solitary malignant melanocytes are observed along the dermal-epidermal interface with focal extension into the epidermal layer. Although the silhouette portrayed in **B** is deceptively symmetrical, (**D**) the cytology of the nodule shows variable cellular atypia of the nested melanoma cells and occasional mitotic figures (**D,** *arrow*).

metrial stroma, which accompanies the glandular epithelium in implants of endometriosis.

Epidermotropic Melanoma[3]

- ABSENCE OF INFILTRATIVE LYMPHOCYTIC RESPONSE
- THINNING OF INVOLVED EPIDERMIS
- INWARD ORIENTATION OF RETE RIDGES AT PERIMETER OF TUMOR NODULE
- ABSENCE OF INTRAEPIDERMAL SPREAD LATERAL TO TUMOR NODULE

Although metastases are often suspected in patients with high-risk primary melanomas who develop dermal nodules, it must be remembered that about 4% of patients with metastases have no identifiable primary tumor. Lesions may present as single or multiple, skin-colored or pigmented, firm papules and nodules (Fig. 16–2A). Ordinary metastases demonstrate dermal nodules of melanoma cells without evidence of intraepidermal or adnexal origin. In addition, metastases frequently fail to show an infiltrative lymphocytic response, as do many primary vertical growth phase melanomas. Epidermotropic metastases are especially difficult to identify, because tumor cells infiltrate the epidermal layer in a manner similar to primary lesions (Fig. 16–2B, C). Moreover, some lesions may be composed of bland cells that resemble nevus cells, although mitoses are usually present within the dermal component (Fig. 16–2D). It has been suggested that in epidermotropic melanomas, the epidermis tends to be thinned, and rete ridges at the perimeter of lesions turn inward toward the center of the metastatic deposit. Moreover, there is seldom lateral intraepidermal extension beyond the dermal nodule, although this is not a helpful distinguishing point with reference to primary nodular melanoma.

Amelanotic Melanoma[4]

- ASYMMETRICAL DERMAL NODULE COMPOSED OF ANAPLASTIC CELLS
- ABSENCE OF INTRAEPIDERMAL OR INTRAFOLLICULAR GROWTH
- INTRANUCLEAR PSEUDOINCLUSIONS MAY BE PRESENT
- EARLY MELANOSOMES AND PREMELANOSOMES SEEN BY ELECTRON MICROSCOPY
- S100 AND HMB-45 POSITIVITY

Metastatic amelanotic melanoma presents clinically as a dermal or subcutaneous, skin-colored nodule or nodules of relatively recent onset. At scanning magnification, there is an asymmetrical, well-demarcated tumor nodule within the dermis and subcutaneous fat (Fig. 16–3A). Tumor cells may be anaplastic and are devoid of evidence of melanin synthesis (Fig. 16–3B). As is the case in melanoma metastases, there is a lack of an infiltrative lymphoid response at the perimeter of the tumor nodule, and evidence of epidermal origin is absent. These lesions raise a differential diagnosis that includes metastatic carcinoma, anaplastic lymphoma, and mel-

anoma. The presence of intranuclear pseudoinclusions resulting from small invaginations of cytoplasm into the nuclear membrane is consistent with a diagnosis of melanoma, although it is not specific. Ultrastructural analysis is useful only if early stage melanosomes and premelanosomes are detected, because late-stage melanized organelles, which also may be contained within epidermal cells and follicular mel-

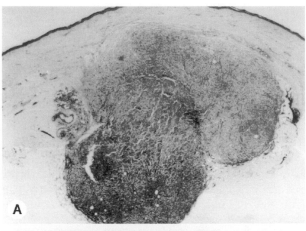

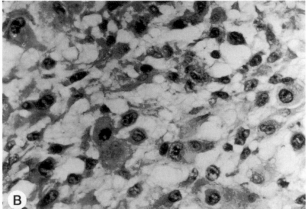

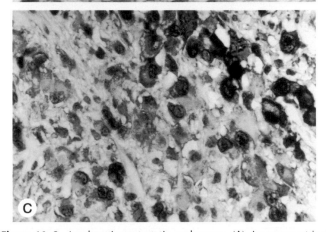

Figure 16–3. Amelanotic metastatic melanoma. (A) An asymmetrical tumor nodule within the deep dermis and subcutis is separated from the epidermal layer by a broad band of superficial and mid-dermal collagen. (B) The tumor cells are malignant in appearance but lack signs of differentiation such as intracellular pigment, intercellular junctions, or glandular differentiation. (C) A panel of immunohistochemical stains reveals that many of the tumor cells strongly express S100 protein, as well as HMB-45 antigen (not shown), confirming the diagnosis of metastatic melanoma, nonepidermotropic type.

anocytes, may be phagocytized by a number of malignant tumors. Immunohistochemistry, however, will generally reveal positivity for S100 protein and variable reactivity for HMB-45 antigen in metastatic melanomas (Fig. 16–3C), facilitating accurate diagnosis. The immunohistochemistry panel should also include antibodies to exclude lymphoma (leukocyte common antigen) and carcinoma (various molecular weight cytokeratins) to serve as negative controls.

Gastrointestinal Malignancies[5, 6]

Gastrointestinal carcinomas that may metastasize to the skin include gastric, intestinal, and pancreatic adenocarcinomas, as well as hepatocellular carcinomas. "Sister Mary Joseph nodule" (Fig. 16–4A) refers to the development of a tumor nodule on umbilical skin as the first sign of an intraabdominal, usually gastrointestinal, adenocarcinoma. Gastrointestinal tumors may retain glandular differentiation with secretion into well-formed lumens (Fig. 16–4B, C), or they may infiltrate skin as single cells with only perinuclear packets of mucin as evidence of cellular origin and differentiation. Signet-ring cells represent cells that are so filled with mucin that the nucleus is markedly compressed to the cell perimeter. These cells are typical of metastatic gastric adenocarcinoma. Occasionally, signet cells may epidermotropically infiltrate into the epidermal layer, mimicking melanoma or extramammary Paget disease. Detection of mucin within metastatic gastrointestinal adenocarcinomas requires knowledge that it is PAS-positive, diastase-resistant sialomucin; this mucin stains with alcian blue at pH 2.5 but not at pH 0.4, indicating its nonsulfated nature, and it is resistant to hyaluronidase.

Breast Carcinoma[7-10]

- MODERATELY DIFFERENTIATED ADENOCARCINOMA
- SUBTLE DEPOSITS WITHIN DERMAL LYMPHATICS ASSOCIATED WITH EDEMA (e.g., INFLAMMATORY CARCINOMA)
- INDIAN-FILE INFILTRATION OF DERMAL COLLAGEN BY SMALL MALIGNANT CELLS (e.g., SMALL CELL/LOBULAR VARIANTS)
- DIFFUSE DERMAL DESMOPLASIA WITH RELATIVELY FEW MALIGNANT CELLS (e.g., CARCINOMA EN CUIRASSE)

Metastatic breast carcinoma may take a number of clinical and histologic forms. *Inflammatory carcinoma* refers to development of warmth, erythema, and induration in skin and soft tissue involved by metastases showing primarily intralymphatic spread. The histology of inflammatory carcinoma consists of diffuse dermal edema and lymphatic ectasia at scanning magnification (Fig. 16–5B). Close scrutiny at higher-power magnification reveals plugs of malignant adenocarcinoma cells within dilated dermal lymphatic channels (Fig. 16–5C). *Carcinoma en cuirasse* is a term that connotes diffuse induration as a result of florid desmoplasia induced by metastatic tumor spread. An even more insidious form of metastatic breast cancer involves diffuse infiltration of dermal collagen by small numbers of tumor cells with inconspicuous but hyperchromatic nuclei and scant cytoplasm (Fig. 16–6A, B). These cells tend to align in single rows between collagen bundles (i.e., "Indian filing"; Fig. 16–6C), in a pattern similar to primary *small cell carcinoma* of the

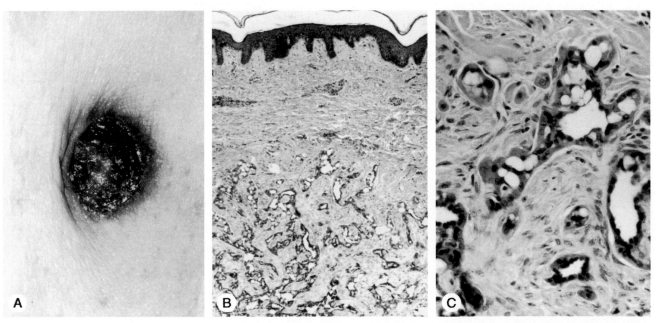

Figure 16–4. Metastatic gastrointestinal carcinoma. (**A**) This ulcerated umbilical nodule was the first sign of internal gastrointestinal malignancy (i.e., "Sister Mary Joseph nodule"). (**B**) Irregular islands of gland-forming epithelium are proliferating within a distinctive fibrous stroma within the mid-dermis to deep dermis. (**C**) The nuclei are hyperchromatic and pleomorphic, and the glandular spaces are irregularly and abortively formed. The patient had pancreatic adenocarcinoma.

plasmic lumina with antibodies to epithelial membrane antigen is a helpful adjunct in identifying such rare atypical cells as adenocarcinoma (Fig. 16–7C). Other more obvious histologic patterns of breast carcinoma involve larger cells exhibiting prominent, moderately differentiated ductular differentiation, as would be evident at the primary tumor site. This

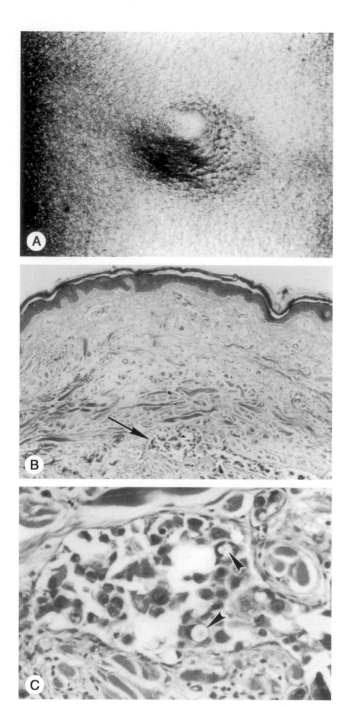

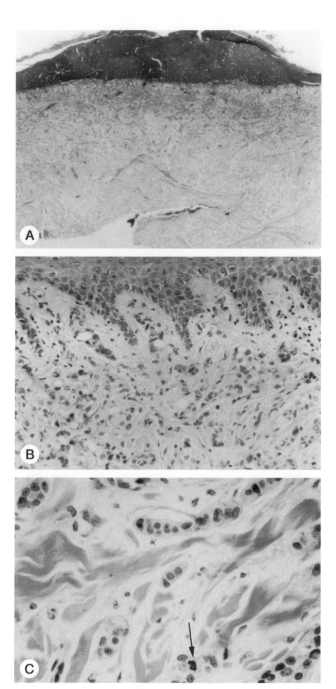

Figure 16–5. Metastatic intralymphatic carcinoma from the breast. (**A**) This metastatic nodule is surrounded by a halo of edematous skin with patulous follicular orifices resembling the skin of an orange (i.e., peau d'orange appearance). (**B**) At low magnification, there is diffuse dermal edema; it may be easy to overlook the plug of tumor cells responsible for these changes (arrow). (**C**) Within this widened lymphatic space, there are malignant cells, some of which show cytoplasmic vacuolization due to mucin (arrowheads). This pattern of local or distant spread has sometimes been called "inflammatory carcinoma."

Figure 16–6. Metastatic small cell adenocarcinoma from the breast. (**A**) This crusted lesion shows only subtle hypercellularity within the superficial dermis. As with most lesions, higher magnification than scanning is needed to insure a correct diagnosis. (**B**) At midrange magnification, small cords of innocuous appearing cells are observed; some are reminiscent of a dermal nevus. (**C**) At high power, the cells are arranged in "Indian-file" configurations and contain oval nuclei with distinctive nucleoli. Occasional mitoses are present (arrow). Collectively, these findings are those of metastatic breast carcinoma of the small cell type, or infiltrating lobular carcinoma.

breast (i.e., infiltrating lobular carcinoma). Variable desmoplasia may be present (Fig. 16–7), and occasional lesions appear to represent only mild, diffuse dermal fibrosis until small numbers of malignant cells are detected at high magnification. Immunohistochemical detection of intracyto-

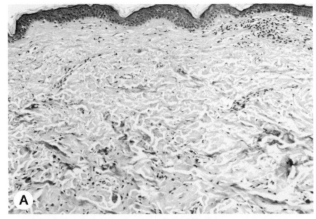

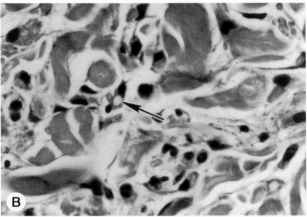

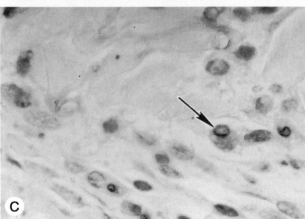

Figure 16–7. Metastatic adenocarcinoma from the breast: sclerosing or interstitial pattern. (**A**) At scanning magnification, there is a vague impression of increased dermal cellularity, particularly in the lower left portion of the panel. (**B**) At high magnification, malignant cells with densely hyperchromatic nuclei and occasional intracytoplasmic vacuoles (arrow) insidiously infiltrate between collagen bundles. The pattern resembles the relation between cells and matrix seen in early granuloma annulare, dermatofibroma, or Kaposi sarcoma. (**C**) Immunohistochemistry for epithelial membrane antigen reveals that the vacuoles represent intracytoplasmic lumena (arrow), confirming the impression of metastatic adenocarcinoma.

pattern may be similar to metastatic adenocarcinoma derived from other sites, such as the lung, colon, rectum, stomach, prostate, pancreas, endometrium, ovaries, and endocervix. A localized form of spread of breast cancer cells occurs in *Paget disease,* in which malignant cells epidermotropically migrate from sites of parenchymal carcinoma to areolar skin (Fig. 16–8). This pattern may mimic pagetoid melanoma or squamous cell carcinoma in situ with an intraepidermal epithelioma pattern. Paget cells are often mucin– and carcinoembryonic antigen–positive, however, and careful search will usually reveal sites of in situ intraductal malignancy within underlying breast parenchyma (see Fig. 16–8B).

Lung Carcinoma[11]

- DIFFUSE DERMAL INFILTRATION BY MALIGNANT CELLS
- CRUSH ARTIFACT MAY BE PROMINENT
- PROMINENT MITOTIC ACTIVITY AND INDIVIDUAL CELL NECROSIS
- ABSENCE OF PERINUCLEAR CYTOKERATIN AGGREGATES IN SMALL CELL VARIANTS

Although adenocarcinoma and squamous cell carcinoma of the lung may mimic dermal metastases from other extracutaneous sites, metastatic *small cell carcinoma* has a characteristic pattern that may be confused with lymphoma and primary neuroendocrine carcinoma. At scanning magnification, there are sheets and coalescent clusters of small, lymphocyte-like cells throughout the superficial and deep dermis (Fig. 16–9A). Crush artifact, in which tumor cells become compressed and smudged on minor trauma, is often a prominent feature of this lesion. At higher magnification, individual cells are observed to contain hyperchromatic, rounded nuclei surrounded by a scant, inconspicuous rim of cytoplasm. Mitotic figures and individual cell necrosis are generally prominent (Fig. 16–9B). Tumor cells are unreactive for leukocyte common antigen, as would be expected in lymphoma, and usually will fail to reveal perinuclear clusters of cytokeratin, as is typical of primary neuroendocrine carcinomas.

Genitourinary Tumors[12, 13]

Genitourinary tumors that may metastasize to the skin include neoplasms originating in the uterus, cervix, vagina, ovaries, bladder, kidneys, and prostate. In general, metastases, to a variable degree, recapitulate changes that characterize the tumors at the primary sites. Although a complete review of all tumors from these sites is beyond the scope of this section, specific illustrative examples are offered. Papillary carcinomas from the ovary may maintain their papillarity within the dermis (Fig. 16–10) and even exhibit psammoma body formation. Metastatic prostate carcinoma may proliferate in the dermis as small islands and nests of malignant basaloid cells but without the typical mucinous stroma of primary basal cell carcinoma, a primary tumor with which it could be confused (Fig. 16–11). Such a tumor, when evaluated with a comprehensive panel of antibodies to define histogenesis, will generally prove to be reactive for prostatic acid phosphatase, confirming it to be a metastasis of prostatic origin. Metastatic renal cell carcinoma may appear as glandular formations of solid aggregates, and the cytoplasm of tumor cells may be either granular as a result of the concentration of mitochondria, or clear as a result of glycogenation

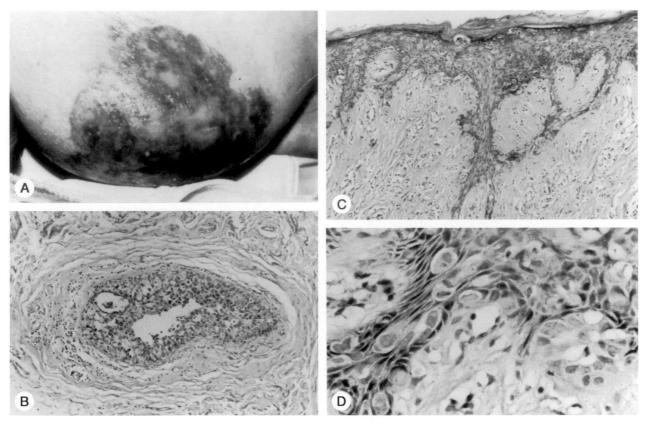

Figure 16–8. Paget disease. (**A**) An eroded, oozing, erythematous plaque affects breast skin. (**B**) A focus of in situ carcinoma within an underlying breast duct. (**C, D**) Similar adenocarcinoma cells are present throughout the overlying epidermal layer.

Figure 16–9. Metastatic lung carcinoma: small cell type. (**A**) Sheets, clusters, and strands of small, lymphocyte-like cells fill the papillary dermis and diffusely infiltrate the reticular dermis. (**B**) Polygonal dark and ovoid pale, small- to intermediate-sized tumor cells fill the papillary dermis but spare the epidermis. There is tumor cell necrosis in the upper half of the field, and a suggestion of molding between several adjacent cells. Mitotic figures *(arrow)* are also observed.

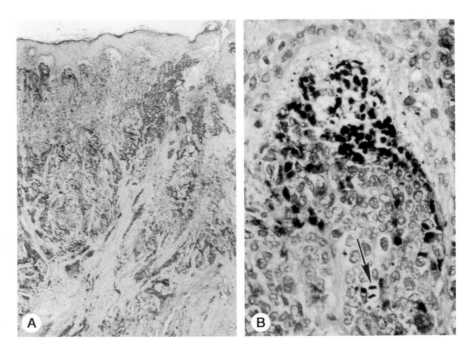

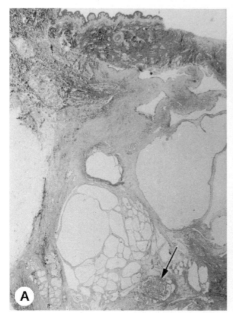

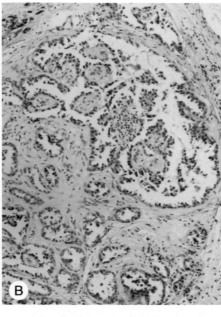

Figure 16–10. Metastatic ovarian papillary serous cystadenocarcinoma. (**A**) At scanning magnification, within the deep dermis there are multiple, variably sized, epithelial-lined cysts, filled with pale fluid or with complex papillary infoldings *(arrow)*. (**B**) An epithelial-lined cystic structure filled with papillary processes, similar to the region in A *(arrow)*, is composed of partially stratified epithelium overlying a fibrovascular core. Epithelial buds also are found within smaller cystic structures infiltrating the dermal stroma.

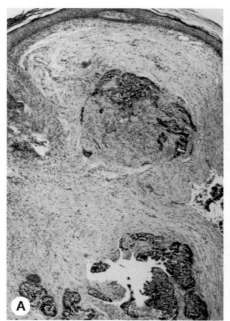

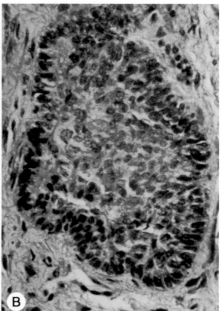

Figure 16–11. Metastatic prostatic adenocarcinoma. (**A**) Irregular basaloid islands are present within a desmoplastic dermal stroma. (**B**) Although some regions demonstrate cribriform growth, this solid nest mimics basal cell carcinoma. Tumor cells are positive for prostatic acid phosphatase by immunohistochemistry.

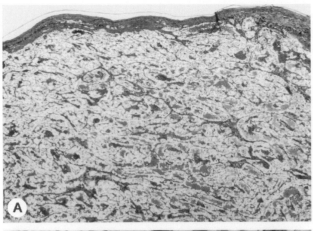

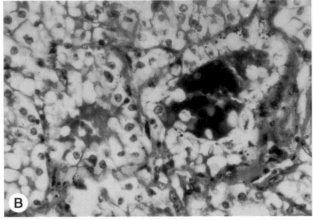

Figure 16–12. Metastatic renal cell carcinoma. (**A**) Clear cells with a vascular stroma are present within the dermis and compress the overlying epidemis. (**B**) Tumor cells form glands and alveolar spaces, contain relatively uniform round-to-oval nuclei with distinct nucleoli, and exhibit a clear, highly glycogenated cytoplasm. Collapsed vessels form thin trabeculae that separate aggregates of tumor cells.

(Fig. 16–12). These tumors are usually highly vascularized, an important clue to the diagnosis of metastatic renal cell carcinoma as opposed to the less vascular malignant nodular hidrademona with clear cells.

DIFFERENTIAL DIAGNOSIS

Poorly differentiated metastases to the dermis may be confused with lymphoma, including nonepidermotropic forms of CTCL and B-cell lymphoma of the large cell type; nodular melanoma; malignant adnexal neoplasms; and poorly differentiated squamous cell carcinoma invading the dermis as a primary tumor. Metastatic small cell carcinoma of the lung may mimic primary neuroendocrine carcinoma and occasionally, variants of basal cell carcinoma. Metastatic adenocarcinoma in general leads to diagnostic confusion with gland-forming appendageal carcinomas, and clear cell–type metastatic renal carcinoma may closely resemble malignant clear cell hidradenoma. Immunohistochemical reagents that may be routinely used to suggest the site of origin of metastatic carcinoma in paraffin-embedded tissue include antibodies for the detection of prostatic acid phosphatase, leukocyte common antigen, human chorionic gonadotrophin, calcitonin, carcinoembryonic antigen, epithelial membrane antigen, alpha-fetoprotein, and HMB-45, among others. In addition, tissue retrieved from formalin-fixed, paraffin-embedded blocks may be extremely helpful for clarification of histogenesis and sites of origin when studied ultrastructurally. Factors integral to adequate preservation of ultrastructure in this setting include rapid formalin fixation of relatively small tissue fragments and re-fixation of deparaffinized, rehydrated tissue in glutaraldehyde and subsequent dehydration and routine processing to generate ultrathin sections.

SELECTED REFERENCES

1. Tidman MJ, MacDonald DM. Cutaneous endometriosis: a histopathologic study. J Am Acad Dermatol 1988;18:373.
2. Steck WD, Helwig EB. Cutaneous endometriosis. JAMA 1965;191:167.
3. Kornberg R, Harris M, Ackerman AB. Epidermotropically metastatic malignant melanoma. Arch Dermatol 1978;114:67.
4. Azar HA, Espinoza CG, Richman AV, et al. "Undifferentiated" large cell malignancies: an ultrastructural and immunocytochemical study. Hum Pathol 1982;13:323.
5. Powell FC, Cooper AJ, Massa MC, et al. Sister Mary Joseph's nodule. J Am Acad Dermatol 1984;10:610.
6. Cawley EP, Hsu YT, Weary PE. The evaluation of neoplastic metastases of the skin. Arch Dermatol 1964;90:262.
7. Pickard C, Callen JP, Blumenreich M. Metastatic carcinoma of the breast. An unusual presentation mimicking cutaneous vasculitis. Cancer 1987;59:1184.
8. Sherry MM, Johnson DH, Page DL, et al. Inflammatory carcinoma of the breast. Am J Med 1985;79:355.
9. Baum EM, Omura EF, Payne RR, et al. Alopecia neoplastica, a rare form of cutaneous metastasis. J Am Acad Dermatol 1981;4:688.
10. Brownstein MH, Helwig EB. Metastatic tumors to the skin. Cancer 1972;29:1298.
11. McPhee PH. Cutaneous metastases. J Cutan Pathol 1985;12:239.
12. Batres E, Knox JM, Wolf JE Jr. Metastatic renal cell carcinoma resembling a pyogenic granuloma. Arch Dermatol 1978;114:1082.
13. Nadji M, Tabei SZ, Castro A, et al. Prostate-specific antigen. Cancer 1981;48:1229.

IV

Pigmentary, Systemic-Metabolic, and Degenerative Disorders

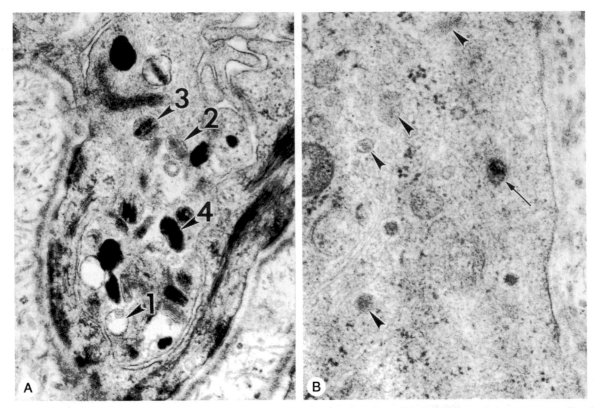

Figure 17–3. Electron microscopy of melanocytes in albinism. (**A**) Normal melanocytes contain complete evolutionary stages of melanosomes, consisting of stage 1 through stage 4 organelles. Stage 1 melanosomes are nonmelanized vesicular structures (1), whereas stage 2 melanosomes have a lattice-like internal structure with minimal melanization (2). Stage 3 melanosomes demonstrate moderate electron density in the lattice, indicating partial melanization (3), whereas stage 4 melanosomes are completely obscured by electron-dense melanin (4). (**B**) In albinism, melanization of melanosomes is partially *(arrow)* or completely *(arrowheads)* diminished due to tyrosinase deficiency.

with the latter form do not. Although the clinical aspects of the disease are generally sufficient to render a diagnosis, biopsy may be performed to confirm the clinical impression, to further define subtype, or to evaluate secondary pathology (e.g., actinic change or skin cancer resulting from defective endogenous protection from ultraviolet light).

Microscopically, biopsy specimens of skin in albinism show normal patterns of basal melanocyte number and distribution; however, as in vitiligo, basal cell layer pigmentation is absent (Fig. 17–2B). By electron microscopy, tyrosinase-negative disease is typified by melanocytes that contain unmelanized type I and II melanosomes (Fig. 17–3). In some melanocytes, it may be difficult to identify melanosomes within the cytoplasm because of the lack of structural definition imparted by tyrosinase-dependent melanization within the delicate internal membraneous lamellae of this organelle (Fig. 17–4). Tyrosinase-positive patients have melanocytes that contain occasional melanized organelles (i.e., type III and IV) in addition to type I and II melanosomes, although the number of melanized organelles is significantly less than the preponderance of these structures in normal controls. Subtyping may also be accomplished by plucking nonpigmented anagen hairs and incubating the melanocyte-containing bulb portion of the hairs in deoxyphenylalanine (DOPA) solution. This procedure results in darkening of the hair bulbs in tyrosinase-positive but not tyrosinase-negative individuals.

Chemical Leukoderma

- HISTOLOGIC ALTERATIONS MIMIC VITILIGO OR ALBINISM
- DIAGNOSIS DEPENDS ON CLINICAL HISTORY AND GROSS PATHOLOGY

Awareness of this relatively common category is essential in the biopsy evaluation of amelanotic and hypomelanotic macules, because it underscores the limitations of routine histology and the importance of clinicopathological correlation. Exogenous chemicals that may produce inhibition of melanin synthesis, toxic destruction of melanocytes, or both include hydroquinone derivative, which is used as an antioxidant in the manufacture of rubber. Typical lesions occur as confetti-like macules which may mimic acrofacial vitiligo on the hands and feet. Permanent depigmentation may result from hydroquinone monobenzylether, which has been employed for cosmetic reasons to alter constitutive skin color. Adhesive plaster contains a hydroquinone derivitive that may result in depigmentation after a single exposure. Close contact with *p-tert*-butylphenol and *p-tert*-pentylphenol in disinfectants may also result in depigmentation. Inhalation and air-borne contact with these agents may trigger systemic effects that result in vitiligo-like changes both at points of contact and at sites presumably shielded from direct exposure. Systemic administration of certain drugs, such as the

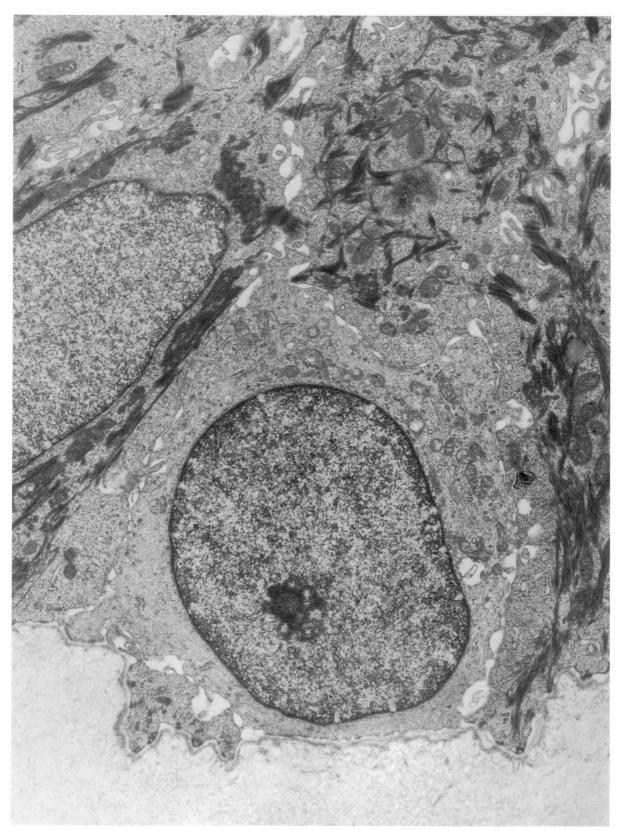

Figure 17–4. Electron micrograph of tyrosinase-negative albinism. A melanocyte within the basal cell layer is entirely devoid of even partially melanized melanosomes.

antimalarial chloroquine, may result in cutaneous pigment loss.

Because the histologic manifestations of such agents can closely mimic changes seen in true vitiligo and related conditions, biopsy interpretation must always consider the possibility of industrial exposure and drug history in formulating a diagnostic opinion in situations of cutaneous depigmentation.

Pityriasis Alba and Postinflammatory Hypopigmentation

- VARIABLE MELANIN PIGMENT INCONTINENCE
- EVIDENCE OF LOW-GRADE OR RESIDUAL DERMATITIS

Pityriasis alba is prototypical of hypopigmentation related to mild inflammation. This disorder occurs predominantly in children and is characterized by macules and patches covered by fine scale, faint erythema, and hypopigmentation (Fig. 17–5A). Lesions frequently occur on the face, and it has been posited that they may be related to impetigo or atopic dermatitis. Other forms of postinflammatory hypopigmentation are commonly seen after a variety of unrelated inflammatory processes in darkly pigmented individuals, who also may hyperpigment as a result of the same stimulus. Chronically sun-exposed skin, which also tends to be inflamed subclinically, may also show small, atrophic, depigmented macules known as *ideopathic guttate hypomelanosis*.

The tendency for inflamed skin to hyperpigment or hypopigment probably depends on the balance between epidermal pigment retention and dermal pigment deposition. Although inflammation is almost always associated with some measure of melanin sequestration within superficial dermal melanophages, the degree of epidermal pigment varies. When epidermal melanin remains normal or increased, underlying melanophages contribute to clinical hyperpigmentation. On the other hand, when epidermal melanin content is markedly diminished due to decreased production by melanocytes or decreased pigment donation to adjacent keratinocytes, the degree of melanin incontinence into the dermis may not be sufficient to compensate, and clinical hypopigmentation results. Accordingly, biopsy specimens of postinflammatory hypopigmentation, including pityriasis alba, generally paradoxically demonstrate melanophages about superficial dermal vessels in the face of a clinical history of hypopigmentation. Careful inspection may also reveal residual foci of lymphocytic infiltration or epidermal changes (e.g., slight spongiosis, parakeratosis) which correlate with the inflammatory stimulus that underlies such pigmentary changes (Fig. 17–5B, C).

Tinea Versicolor[5, 6]

- SHORT, THICK MYCELIA AND SPORES IN STRATUM CORNEUM
- ORGANISMS GENERALLY BASOPHILIC ON HEMATOXYLIN-AND-EOSIN STAIN
- MILD ASSOCIATED SPONGIOTIC DERMATITIS

A fungal infection (tinea) characterized by a change in color (versicolor), tinea versicolor is caused by *Malassezia*

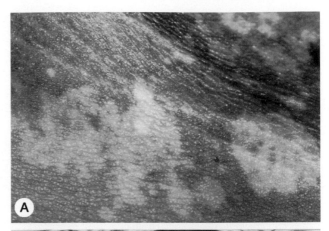
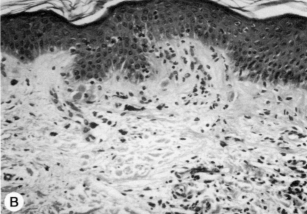
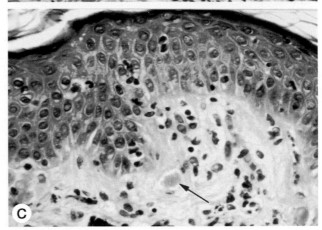

Figure 17–5. Pityriasis alba. (**A**) Numerous coalescent macules show hypopigmentation. (**B, C**) Evidence of an associated inflammatory dermatitis consists of a sparse, nonspecific, superficial, perivascular, lymphocytic infiltrate and zones of colloid body formation indicative of previous interface change (**C**, *arrow*). In some lesions, spongiotic alterations predominate.

furfur, a normal commensal of human skin and hair follicles. Clinically, some patients develop a mild inflammatory reaction to this organism, accompanied by vague erythema, hyperpigmentation, and hypopigmentation, with the latter frequently dominating the clinical picture (Fig. 17–6A). Other patients may develop obstructive inflammatory folliculitis due to *M. furfur* (i.e., pityrosporon folliculitis), and rarely, immunosuppressed individuals receiving hyperalimentation may develop *M. furfur* sepsis. The organism thrives on C12

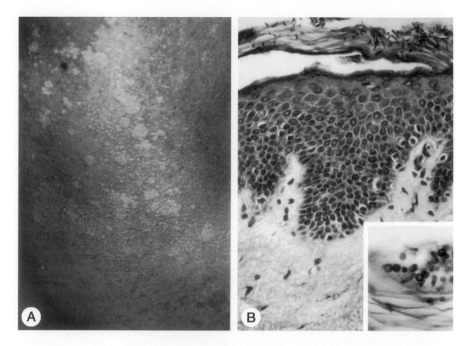

Figure 17–6. Tinea versicolor. (**A**) Multiple hypopigmented macules are present on truncal skin; there is a velvety, adherent scale covering some of these macules. (**B**) A biopsy specimen demonstrates small, basophilic, hyphal organisms within hyperkeratotic scale, even in routine hematoxylin-and-eosin stains. Yeast forms and several short hyphal forms are observed within the scale stained by periodic acid–Schiff *(inset).*

and C24 fatty acids present in human skin and also in lipid-rich intravenous fluids.

Histologically, budding yeast forms and hyphae are usually present in the stratum corneum and, unlike most dermatophytes, are readily apparent in routinely stained material (Fig. 17–6*B*). Hyphae are short, thick mycelia which, with associated rounded yeast forms, have been likened to "spaghetti and meatballs." A mild subacute spongiotic dermatitis may accompany the presence of *M. furfur* in the stratum corneum. In pityrosporon folliculitis, which does not manifest as a pigmentary disorder, there is acute and chronic folliculitis associated with rupture of follicular contents containing predominantly yeast forms into the surrounding perifollicular adventitia.

Hyperpigmentation

Postinflammatory Hyperpigmentation[7]

- MELANIN PIGMENT WITHIN PAPILLARY DERMAL MACROPHAGES
- COLLOID BODIES AND EVIDENCE OF RESIDUAL BASAL CELL LAYER DESTRUCTION

Postinflammatory hyperpigmentation is a common cause of biopsy for evaluation of disordered pigmentation. The best prototype of this condition is perhaps the quiescent phase of a fixed drug eruption. In this disorder, repeated antigenic stimulation results in cytotoxic interface dermatitis, in which the pigment-rich basal cell layer is repeatedly damaged or destroyed. The result is striking loss of epidermal melanin pigment into the superficial dermis, where it is engulfed by perivascular and papillary dermal macrophages. Such zones of pigment deposition may be so striking that they may closely mimic atypical or malignant melanocytic proliferative processes. Even mild interface reactions and noninterface forms of inflammation (e.g., spongiotic dermatitis) may result in postinflammatory hyperpigmentation, particularly in darkly pigmented individuals. Inflammation as-

sociated with scarring, chronic rubbing (Fig. 17–7*A*), and wound healing may produce a similar effect.

Histologic examination routinely reveals melanin-laden histiocytes about superficial vessels and in severe cases,

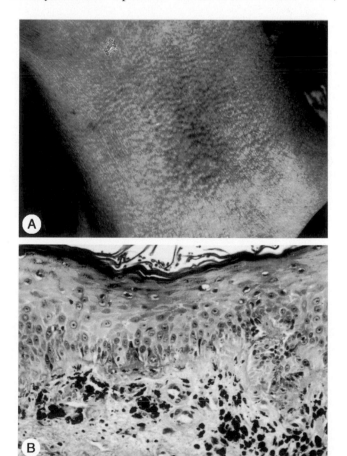

Figure 17–7. Postinflammatory hyperpigmentation. (**A**) Chronic rubbing and a low-grade primary irritant effect to neck skin produced in mottled hyperpigmentation. (**B**) A biopsy specimen reveals numerous brown, melanin-laden macrophages within the superficial dermis.

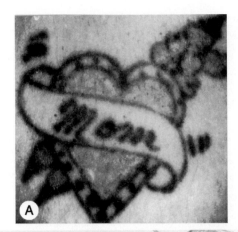

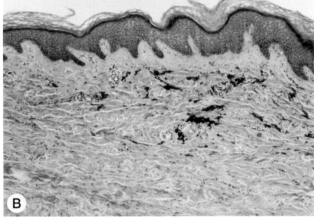

Figure 17–8. Traumatic tattoo. Whether due to unintentional trauma or (**A**) premeditated sentiment, tattoos are often removed for diagnostic or cosmetic purposes. (**B**) The pigment of tattoos, in contrast to that of postinflammatory hyperpigmentation, is black and located within melanophages, which generally involve deep as well as superficial epidermal layers.

within the papillary dermal interstitium (Fig. 17–7*B*). Pigment tends to be finely particulate, brown, and devoid of the tan-green, refractile quality typical of hemosiderin. Special stains for iron will differentiate between hemosiderin and melanin pigment in difficult cases. It should be remembered that in inflammatory disorders in which epidermal damage

and vascular injury coexist (e.g., erythema multiforme), both melanin and hemosiderin may be detected within dermal histiocytes. Traumatic tattoos, both decorative and unintentional, may produce a similar pattern of pigment deposition, although the particles are most often black in histologic sections (Fig. 17–8). Accumulation of heavy metals (e.g., silver) within dermal macrophages generally produces extremely fine brown-black granules within cells that are situated both about small vessels as well as within the adventitia of sweat glands and hair follicles.

Café-au-Lait Macule[8, 9]

- ROUTINE HISTOLOGY UNREVEALING
- GIANT AGGREGATED MELANOSOME-LYSOSOME COMPLEXES WITHIN MELANOCYTES ON ELECTRON MICROSCOPY

While generally associated with neurofibromatosis and other neurocutaneous syndromes, café-au-lait macules are common, occurring in up to 10% of the normal population. They range from less than 1 to 20 cm in diameter, and present as well-defined, circumscribed, uniformly pigmented, tan-brown macules (Fig. 17–9).

The microscopic appearance of the café-au-lait spot is reported to be similar to that of an ephelis or freckle, with increased pigmentation of the basal cell layer with respect to the constitutive pigment normally present in the adjacent, unaffected skin. However, this determination may be difficult without a mirror-image biopsy of normal skin from the same individual, and most lesional biopsy specimens are unrevealing by routine microscopy. Macromelanosomes, representing consolidated melanin-lysosomal complexes which form large, spherical, intracytoplasmic melanin globules, are found in melanocytes of café-au-lait macules (Fig. 17–10). These structures are not entirely specific, however, and they may also be identified in freckles, solar lentigos, and certain nevi. Electron microscopy is not necessary to definitively identify macromelanosomes. Preparation of plastic-embedded tissue and sectioning at 1- to 2-μm intervals yields histologic preparations adequate for resolution of many macromelanosomes by oil immersion microscopy. Search by light microscopy may even enhance sensitivity of detection, because relatively large expanses of the basal cell layer may be surveyed.

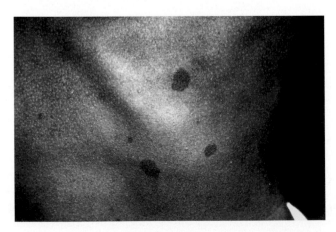

Figure 17–9. Clinical pathology of café-au-lait macules. Multiple coffee stain–like macules are present on the trunk of a patient with neurofibromatosis.

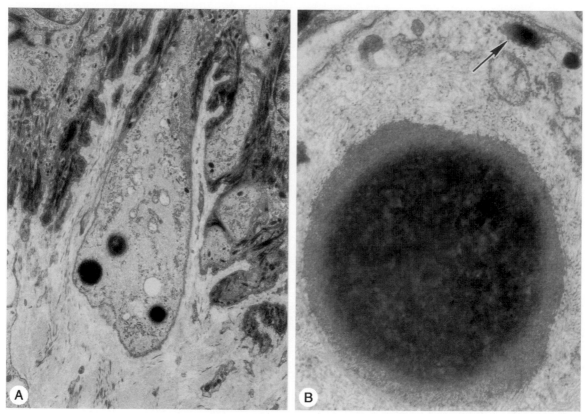

Figure 17–10. Macromelanosomes of café-au-lait macules. The primary microscopic defect in café-au-lait macules is the formation of macromelanosomes. (**A**) Even by scanning or low-power magnification of the ultrastructure, these electron-dense, globoid bodies predominate in the cytoplasm of basal melanocytes. (**B**) Too large to be transferred to adjacent keratinocytes, these bodies are uniformly electron dense and many times greater in volume than normal melanosomes *(arrow)*. Macromelanosomes probably form by condensation of normal melanosomes that are partially degraded by phagolysosomes.

Stasis Dermatitis[10]

- PROLIFERATION OF THICK-WALLED CAPILLARIES WITHIN DERMAL PAPILLAE
- VARIABLE SUPERFICIAL DERMAL EDEMA AND FIBROSIS
- RECENT HEMORRHAGE AND HEMOSIDERIN DEPOSITION
- DERMAL SIDEROPHAGES POSITIVE WITH IRON STAINS
- SECONDARY EPIDERMAL ATROPHY OR HYPERPLASIA WITH HYPERKERATOSIS

Hyperpigmented plaques on the legs (Fig. 17–11A) are not infrequently biopsied, with differential clinical diagnoses that encompass melanocytic proliferative processes, pigmentary purpura, postinflammatory hyperpigmentation, poikiloderma, and superficial pigmented dysplasia or neoplasia (e.g., pigmented actinic keratosis, multicentric pigmented basal cell carcinoma). Localized stasis dermatitis is a frequent cause of confusion (Fig. 17–11A). In addition to variable epidermal atrophy and hyperplasia, dermal vascular proliferation, and dermal edema and fibrosis, which may further complicate the clinical picture, some forms of stasis dermatitis are dominated by hemosiderin deposition within the superficial dermis, accounting for zones of tan-brown pigmentation appreciated in the gross pathology.

Biopsy specimens of localized stasis dermatitis lesions reveal hemosiderin-laden macrophages (i.e., siderophages) about superficial dermal vessels and sometimes diffusely within the papillary dermis (Fig. 17–11D). The following associated features are also generally present in varying degrees: (1) epidermal alterations, consisting of hyperkeratosis with either atrophy or hyperplasia; (2) superficial dermal vascular ectasia and proliferation; (3) superficial dermal edema; and (4) mild dermal fibroplasia (Fig. 17–11B, C). Stasis dermatitis differs from the other common cause of hemosiderin deposition within the superficial dermis, pigmentary purpura, in that the latter has a pericapillary lymphocytic infiltrate within dermal papillae and lacks the aforementioned findings associated with chronic stasis.

Drug-Induced Hyperpigmentation[11-17]

The following disorders are some of the most commonly encountered drug-related forms of cutaneous hyperpigmentation in the United States.

Minocycline-Induced Hyperpigmentation

Patients receiving long-term minocycline therapy for acne vulgaris may develop blue-black hyperpigmentation of the skin, teeth, thyroid gland, cartilage, and bones (Fig. 17–

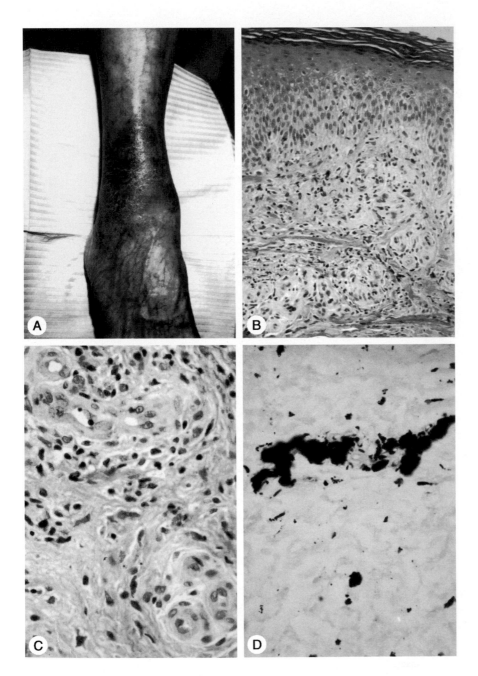

Figure 17–11. Hyperpigmentation due to localized stasis. (**A**) The gross pathology of a lower extremity subjected to chronic stasis change is erythema admixed with zones of brawny, copper-colored hyperpigmentation. (**B, C**) Histologically, there is prominent vascular proliferation and fibrosis within chronically inflamed dermal papillae. (**D**) Stains for iron reveal foci of particulate hemosiderin deposition, which is the result of chronic erythrocyte extravasation from the leaky vessels, which proliferate as a consequence of this condition.

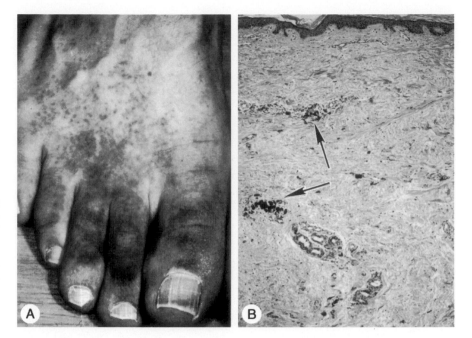

Figure 17–12. Drug-induced hyperpigmentation: Minocycline. (**A**) The distal extremity of this young man shows mottled, confluent, brown macular hyperpigmentation. He had been treated with minocycline for facial acne. (**B**) Histologically, there are pigment-laden macrophages about superficial and deep dermal vessels *(arrows)*. This pigment stains for iron, and the macrophages have been shown to contain elemental iron by energy-dispersive x-ray microanalysis.

12*A*). Histologically, there is hemosiderin within perivascular macrophages of the superficial and deep dermis (Fig. 17–12*B*). Changes that accompany stasis dermatitis or pigmentary purpura, however, are not present. It is believed that siderosomes, composed of lysosomes and iron, form within histiocytes, possibly as a result of initial uptake of a minocycline metabolite that subsequently complexes or chelates circulating iron.

Hyperpigmentation Due to Heavy Metals

These disorders usually result in diffuse, rather than localized, hyperpigmentation and thus are suspected clinically. The three most common metals to be deposited are iron, silver, and gold. Iron may be deposited locally and secondarily, as described previously in association with minocycline administration, or diffusely and primarily, as in *hemochromatosis* and *hemosiderosis*. In hemochromatosis, there is bronze-colored cutaneous hyperpigmentation, diabetes mellitus, cirrhosis, cardiomyopathy, and arthropathy due to idiopathic or genetically determined enhanced intestinal absorption of dietary iron. In hemosiderosis, iron overload, usually due to repeated transfusions or chronic hemolysis, is responsible. Pigmentation due to silver (i.e., *argyria*) results from ingestion of at least 8 g of silver proteinate (Argyrol) or silver arsphenamine (Neo-Silvol), which were used medicinally during the first quarter of the twentieth century. Clinically, the pigment is blue to slate gray, may involve mucosae as well as skin, and is accentuated in sun-exposed areas. Gold-induced hyperpigmentation (i.e., *chrysiasis*) is seen primarily in patients who received gold therapy for the treatment of tuberculosis during the first third of the twentieth century. Clinical features are similar to those described for argyria. Scleral involvement has been reported. Histologically, heavy metal deposits may be differentiated as shown in Table 17–1. Metal deposits within dermal macrophages also have characteristic ultrastructural features (Fig. 17–13), and when analysis is coupled with x-ray dispersive microanalysis, definitive identification of the stored heavy metals is possible.

Table 17–1. DIFFERENTIAL DIAGNOSIS OF HEAVY METAL DEPOSITS

METAL	EPIDERMIS	DERMIS	SPECIAL STUDIES
Iron	Normal melanin in basal and suprabasal keratinocytes	Brown-green granules in perivascular macrophages	Perls iron–positive; siderosomes on electron microscopy
Silver	Normal melanin in basal and suprabasal keratinocytes	Brown-gray granules in macrophages, basement membranes, and elastic fibers	Perls iron–negative; polyhedral granules on electron microscopy; x-ray analysis confirms Ag
Gold	Normal melanin in basal and suprabasal keratinocytes	Black granules in macrophages, basement membranes, and endothelial cells	Perls iron–negative; polyhedral and spindle granules on electron microscopy; x-ray analysis confirms Au

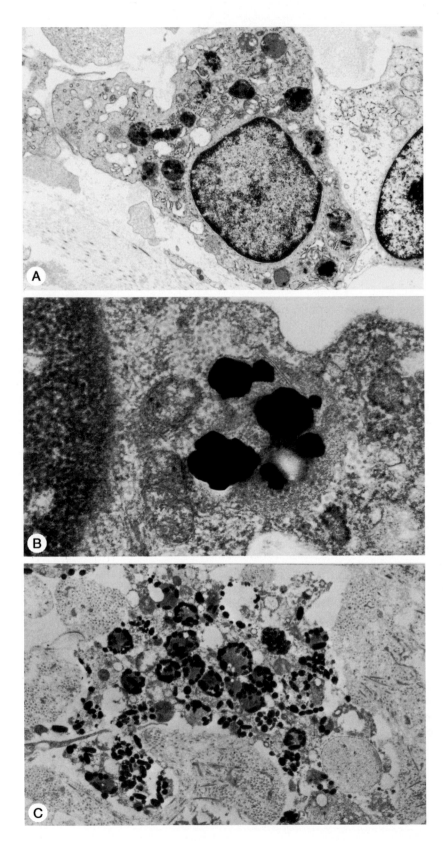

Figure 17–13. Ultrastructure of pigment within dermal macrophages in pigment incontinence. (**A**) Siderosomes (i.e., phagolysosomes containing particulate iron) occurred as a result of minocycline ingestion. (**B**) Argyria occurred is a result of silver ingestion. (**C**) Melanin phagolysomes are a result of postinflammatory hyperpigmentation. Although the electron-dense material within phagosomes is subtly different among these three groups, elemental analysis by x-ray probe methods is sometimes necessary for definitive identification.

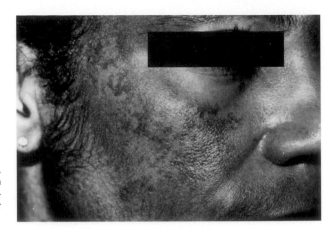

Figure 17–14. Melasma: Hyperpigmentation due to enhanced melanogenesis. The primary defect in this common condition appears to be the result of an enhanced threshold for melanogenesis. This results in increase in both epidermal and dermal melanin pigment deposition. Either epidermal melanin or dermal melanin may predominate in the clinical and histologic picture.

Psoralen-Induced Hyperpigmentation

Psoralens are commonly used along with UVA to induce tanning and to treat certain photosensitive dermatoses. Some perfumes contain oil of bergamot, a psoralen that stimulates epidermal melanin synthesis. Other naturally occurring substances have similar photoenhancing effects, such as buckwheat, lemon peels, carrot tops, and pigweed. All may result in exaggerated tanning due to increased melanin synthesis and transfer at sites of cutaneous contact.

Chlorpromazine-Induced Hyperpigmentation

Phenothiazine-induced hyperpigmentation typically involves sun-exposed areas. Lesions vary from violaceous zones to metallic, blue-gray regions. Because chlorpromazine produces a dechlorinated free radical that binds to melanin and impedes its degradation, there is increased basilar and suprabasilar melanin histologically. Melanin is also present within dermal macrophages about superficial blood vessels.

Contraceptive-Induced Hyperpigmentation

Melasma is a patchy hyperpigmentation of the face, particularly involving the malar skin (Fig. 17–14). This condition may be made worse by sunlight and is associated with pregnancy, excessive ovarian hormone production, and administration of oral contraceptives. Histologic findings consist of increased numbers of melanin granules within basal keratinocytes and, in some cases, dermal pigment deposits. Along with the typical clinical presentation, clinicopathological distinction from other causes of increased melanin synthesis (e.g., chlorpromazine administration) is usually not difficult.

Systemically Induced Hyperpigmentation[18, 19]

Aside from melasma related to pregnancy and ovarian dysfunction, skin changes due to adrenal insufficiency are the most common form of hyperpigmentation induced by endogenous systemic factors. Deficient adrenal cortisol results in diminished feedback inhibition to the pituitary gland, with resultant increases in release of melanocyte-stimulating hormone and adrenocorticotropic hormone. Diffuse clinical hyperpigmentation may be accentuated in areas of trauma and may involve the buccal mucosa. Although there may be a slight increase in intraepidermal melanin and in the number of melanophages in the superficial dermis, the histologic findings are not specific. When systemically induced hyperpigmentation is clinically suspected, confirmation depends on laboratory findings.

DIFFERENTIAL DIAGNOSIS

In cases of cutaneous hyperpigmentation, the explanation is generally found within dermal histiocytes, although occasionally, there may be contributing epidermal factor(s), as is the case in certain forms of melasma and in café-au-lait macules. After pigment is identified in the dermis, special stains will assist in determining whether or not iron is present. Melanin pigment may be bleached away and is generally positive with the Fontana stain, although this is not entirely specific. In cases other than iron heavy metal deposition resulting in hyperpigmentation, elemental analysis using x-ray dispersive microanalysis technology may be required for definitive elemental identification.

In the setting of hypopigmentation, the histologic changes are considerably more subtle and less straightforward. Figure 17–15 is designed to address some of the branch points in the differential diagnosis of this problematic group of disorders.

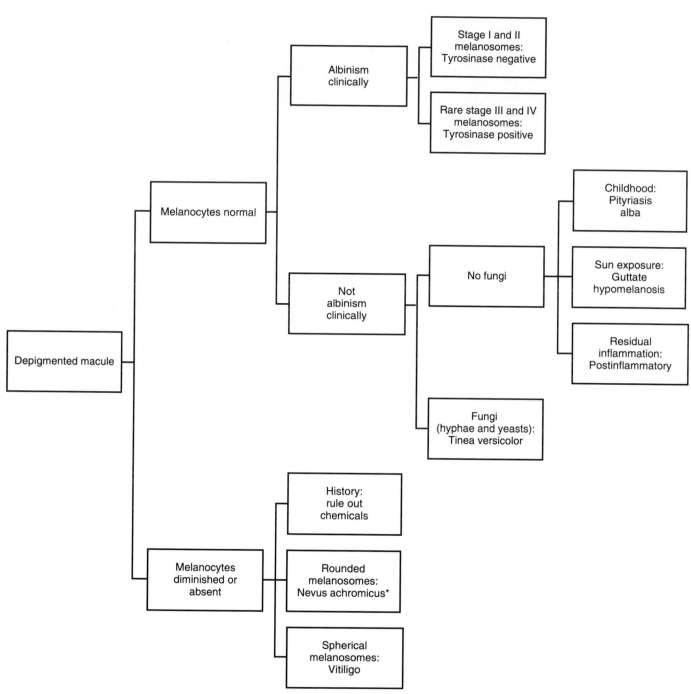

Figure 17–15. Algorithmic approach to differential diagnosis of cutaneous hypopigmentation.

SELECTED REFERENCES

1. Lerner AB. Vitiligo. J Invest Dermatol 1959;32:285.
2. Grimes PE, Ghoneum M, Stockton T. T cell profiles in vitiligo. J Am Acad Dermatol 1986;14:196.
3. Kugelman TP, VanScott EJ. Tyrosinase activity in melanocytes in human vitiligo. J Invest Dermatol 1961;37:73.
4. Quevedo WC, Witkop CJ Jr, Fitzpatrick TB. Albinism. In: Stanbury JB, Wyngaarden JB, Frederickson DS, eds. The Metabolic Basis of Inherited Disease. New York: McGraw-Hill, 1978.
5. Mcginley KJ, Lantis LR, Marples RR. Microbiology of tinea versicolor. Arch Dermatol 1970;102:168.
6. Potter BS, Burgoon CF Jr, Johnson WC. Pityrosporon folliculitis. Arch Dermatol 1973;107:388.
7. Konrad K, Wolff K. Hyperpigmentation: Melanosome size and distribution pattern of melanosomes. Arch Dermatol 1973;107:853.
8. Morris TJ, Johnson WG, Silvers DN. Giant pigment granules in biopsy specimens from café-au-lait spots in neurofibromatosis. Arch Dermatol 1982;118:385.
9. Jimbow K, Szabo G, Fitzpatrick TB, et al. Ultrastructure of giant pigment granules (macromelanosomes) in cutaneous pigmented macules of neurofibromatosis. J Invest Dermatol 1973;61:300.
10. Mali JWH, Kuiper JP, Hamers AA. Acro-angiodermatitis of the foot. Arch Dermatol 1965;92:515.
11. Sato S, Murphy GF, Hernhard JD, et al. Ultrastructural and x-ray microanalytical observations on minocycline-related hyperpigmentation of the skin. J Invest Dermatol 1981;77:264.
12. Ridgway HA, Sonnex TS, Kennedy CTC, et al. Hyperpigmentation associated with oral minocycline. Br J Dermatol 1982;107:95.
13. Gherardi R, Brochard P, Chamek B, et al. Human generalized argyria. Arch Pathol 1984;108:181.
14. Johansson JP, Kanerva L, Niemi KM, et al. Generalized argyria. Clin Exp Dermatol 1982;7:169.
15. Pelachyk JM, Bergfeld WF, McMahon JT. Chrysiasis following gold therapy for rheumatoid arthritis. J Cutan Pathol 1984;11:491.
16. Blois MS Jr. On chlorpromazine binding in vivo. J Invest Dermatol 1965;45:475.
17. Harber LC, Baer RL. Pathogenic mechanisms of drug-induced photosensitivity. J Invest Dermatol 1972;58:605.
18. Clerkin EP, Sayegh S. Melanosis as the initial symptom of Addison's disease. Lahey Clin Found Bull 1966;15:173.
19. Abe K, Nicholson E, Liddle GW, et al. Radioimmunoassay of beta-MSH in human plasma and tissues. J Clin Invest 1967;46:1609.

18

Maturational and Degenerative Disorders

DEFINITIONS AND GENERAL CONSIDERATIONS

The group of largely unrelated conditions discussed in this section are reflective of the more common cutaneous conditions characterized by altered maturation or degeneration of dermal or epidermal elements. Several of the disorders addressed, such as ichthyosis and porokeratosis, present clinically primarily as a result of abnormal formation of the most superficial skin layers. Others, such as anetoderma and keloids, result in gross pathology indicative of the absence or increased deposition of normal dermal constituents. These conditions, although linked together pathogenetically by anomalous development or inability for homeostatic maintenance, are unrelated, and their histologies share little common ground, impeding an algorithmic approach to their diagnosis. Most of these disorders occur commonly enough to produce confusion with a number of other dermatoses and even neoplasms discussed in this text; therefore, it is prudent to be aware of their salient clinicopathological characteristics.

Although conditions such as solar elastosis and keloids may be observed daily in a busy dermatopathology practice, others in this category, such as anetoderma and ichthyosis, are only rarely observed. These are important conditions that are seen from time to time in virtually every practice, however. Therefore, they will be discussed in detail in the main body of this chapter, obviating the need for a special subsection dealing separately with rare disorders.

GROSS PATHOLOGY

The clinical appearance of each of the maturational and degenerative disorders enumerated previously are discussed individually in the text that follows. The gross pathology of each, initially reflected in the pathology requisition that accompanies the biopsy specimen, may be critical for accurate interpretation. Disorders characterized by abnormal epidermal maturation or keratinocyte degeneration may present as diffuse or localized zones of hyperkeratosis or even as blisters or erosions. Accordingly, the differential diagnosis may include causes of chronic spongiotic, cytotoxic, or even vesiculobullous processes. Dermal pathology may result in even more confusing gross pathologic characteristics; however, many of the lesions discussed herein have important clues in the clinical data. For example, site of occurrence (e.g., ear for chondrodermatitis, region of previous trauma for keloid), family history (e.g., Darier disease), and character of lesions (e.g., resembling fish scales, as in ichthyosis) may provide important clues that will direct the dermatopathologist through algorithmic pathways to correct diagnostic assessment.

GENERAL HISTOLOGY AND TEMPORAL EVOLUTION

The majority of disorders discussed in this section are of long duration by the time of biopsy. Accordingly, issues related to temporal evolution are less important in these disorders than they are in cases with conditions that present routinely at various stages of disease progression (e.g., spongiotic dermatitis).

HISTOLOGY OF SPECIFIC DISORDERS

Ichthyoses[1–3]

- LAMELLAR COMPACTION OF ORTHOKERATOTIC SCALE
- ABNORMALITIES OF STRATUM GRANULOSUM

333

The term ichthyosis, derived from the Greek root "ichthy-," meaning fishy, refers to a family of unrelated, genetically inherited conditions that result in coarse, fish-like scales on the body surface (Fig. 18–1A). In keeping with their tendency to be inherited disorders, most of the ichthyoses become apparent around the time of birth or during early childhood. Noninherited forms of ichthyosis, particularly the vulgaris type, may occur in adults in association with lymphoproliferative malignancies and carcinoma. Ichthyosis is often accompanied by hyperkeratosis of the palms and soles, although inherited forms of hyperkeratosis exclusively involving the palms and soles also exist (Fig. 18–1B). The various clinically recognized forms of ichthyosis are listed in Table 18–1.

The general histology of all forms of ichthyosis is extraordinarily subtle, and diagnostic recognition is generally facilitated by clinical suspicion. Common to all forms of this group of disorders is abnormal scale, consisting of deviation from the normal basket-weave pattern to compacted lamellae of slightly increased orthokeratin (Fig. 18–1C, D). In lamellar, X-linked, and congenital ichthyosiform erythroderm, the stratum granulosum is normal to slightly thickened (Fig. 18–1C), whereas in ichthyosis vulgaris and acquired forms, the stratum granulosum is generally thinned or absent. The ichthyosis that accompanies various congenital syndromes, such as Rud, Conradi, Netherton, and Refsum syndromes, is generally diagnosed based on clinical manifestations of ichthyosis in the setting of clinically overt developmental or metabolic anomalies.

The primary abnormality in ichthyosis may reside in defective mechanisms of desquamation, leading to retention of abnormally formed scale. For example, in X-linked ichthyosis, it is known that affected homozygotes demonstrate a deficiency in steroid sulfatase, an enzyme critical to the removal of proadhesive cholesterol sulfate secreted into the intercellular spaces with Odland (membrane-coating) bodies. Abnormal accumulation of nondegraded cholesterol sulfate results in persistent cell-cell adhesion within the stratum corneum, hindering the desquamation process.

Porokeratosis[4-6]

- SHALLOW EPIDERMAL INVAGINATION FILLED WITH KERATIN
- FOCAL ABSENCE OF STRATUM GRANULOSUM
- PARAKERATOTIC COLUMN (CORNOID LAMELLA)

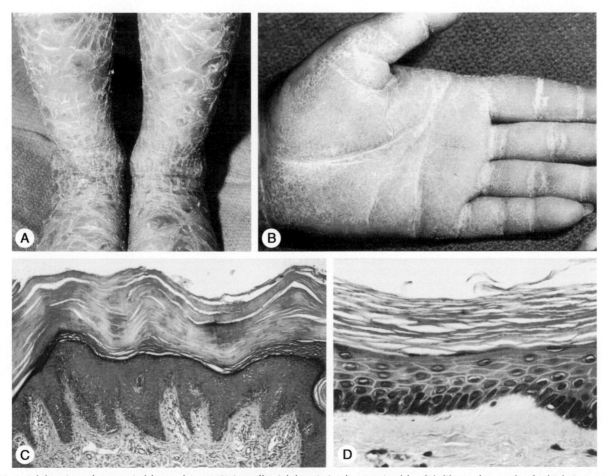

Figure 18–1. Ichthyosis and congenital keratoderma. (**A**) Lamellar ichthyosis is characterized by fish-like scales, each of which is composed of thousands of anomalous stratum corneocytes. (**B**) Palmar keratoderma is an autosomal dominant condition characterized by diffuse hyperkeratosis. Both ichthyosis and keratoderma result from thickening of the stratum corneum. (**C**) Lamellar ichthyosis demonstrates compacted hyperorthokeratotic stratum corneum, which accounts for the plate-like scales observed clinically in **A**. (**D**) Ichthyosis vulgaris is associated with subtle compacted hyperkeratosis (note complete absence of the normal basket-weave pattern) as well as marked thinning of the stratum granulosum.

Table 18–1. CLINICAL CHARACTERISTICS OF ICHTHYOSES

TYPE OF ICHTHYOSIS	INHERITANCE PATTERN	CLINICAL CHARACTERISTICS
Ichthyosis vulgaris	Autosomal dominant	Extensor skin (flexural sparing)
Congenital ichthyosiform erythroderm	Autosomal recessive	Fine white scale with erythroderm; flexural involvement; improves by puberty
Lamellar ichthyosis	Autosomal recessive	Large, plate-like scales wtih faint erythroderm; flexural involvement; ectropion
X-linked ichthyosis	X-linked recessive	Progressive scale abnormality during childhood; flexural involvement; most severe in male patients
Acquired ichthyosis	None	Endocrine disease; malignancy; immunodeficiency; drug-related
Ichthyosis-associated congenital syndromes	Variable	Congenital, developmental, and metabolic defects

Like ichthyosis, porokeratosis has a number of clinical variant forms, all of which share in common the focal production of increased parakeratotic scale from a pore-like invagination (Fig. 18–2A, B). Knowledge of the basic features of these forms is necessary for accurate biopsy interpretation of the relatively straightforward histologic features shared by these diverse clinical entities. Table 18–2 summarizes the salient clinical features of the variants of porokeratosis.

The histopathology of porokeratosis is characteristic, regardless of the clinical setting in which it occurs. The hallmark of the disorder is the *cornoid lamella,* a discrete "leaning tower" of parakeratotic scale that originates from an underlying epidermal dell or shallow invagination (see Fig. 18–2B). The base of the column is bordered by cells of the upper stratum spinosum that give rise to the parakeratotic zone without formation of an intermediate stratum granulosum. Disseminated superficial actinic porokeratosis (DSAP), a condition that is not always disseminated and is not always actinically-induced. It presents clinically as multiple erythematous hyperkeratotic plaques, usually on sun-exposed skin (Fig. 18–3A). In this form of porokeratosis, the cornoid lamellae may lean in the direction of a zone of epidermis showing features of an actinic keratosis (Fig. 18–3B).

It should be remembered that in addition to correlating with a specific disorder, cornoid lamella formation may also be a nonspecific manifestation of secondarily altered epidermal maturation. Accordingly, incidental cornoid lamella formation, as is also the case for epidermolytic hyperkeratosis and focal acantholytic dyskeratosis, may be detected in re-excisions of certain skin tumors and in the setting of unrelated inflammatory dermatitis, making correlation of such findings with gross pathology and clinical history all the more important. Certain epidermal nevi and congenital malformations may show verrucous epidermal hyperplasia predominated by the formation of porokeratotic scale, thus accounting for many of the cases in the variant form of linear porokeratosis.

Acantholytic and Dyskeratotic Disorders[7–9]

- FOCAL HYPERORTHOKERATOSIS
- SUPRABASAL ACANTHOLYSIS
- PRESERVATION OF DERMAL PAPILLAE LINED BY INTACT STRATUM BASALIS
- DYSKERATOSIS OF ACANTHOLYTIC CELLS (CORPS RONDS AND CORPS GRAINS)
- LARGE VERRUCOUS PAPULES (DARIER DISEASE) OR SMALL KERATOTIC FOCI (GROVER DISEASE)

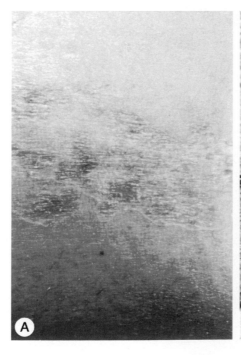
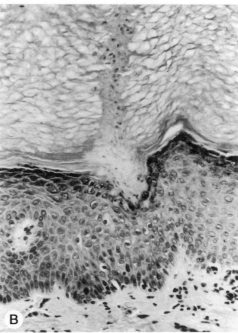

Figure 18–2. Porokeratosis, plaque type. (**A**) Clinically, there is a well-defined plaque surrounded by a hyperkeratotic ridge at its perimeter. (**B**) A biopsy specimen from the edge of a lesion shows a well-developed cornoid lamella typical of this condition. The lamella consists of a discrete tower of parakeratotic scale overlying a small invagination showing focal hypogranulosis.

Table 18–2. CLINICAL VARIANTS OF POROKERATOSIS

CLINICAL TYPE OF POROKERATOSIS	DISTINGUISHING FEATURES
Porokeratosis of Mibelli (plaque-type)	One or several discrete plaques bordered by ridge of scale originating from surface furrow
Punctate porokeratosis	Keratotic plugs on palms and soles
Disseminated actinic porokeratosis	Multiple small plaques defined by peripheral keratotic ridge; often on sun-exposed surfaces; may worsen upon sun exposure
Porokeratosis palmaris et plantaris disseminata	Many small keratotic papules; onset in adolescence and early adulthood; begins on palms and soles, then spreads to other body surfaces
Secondary (linear) porokeratosis	Generalized or segmental involvement within epidermal nevoid malformation

Darier disease and Grover disease, two unrelated disorders, share in common the occurrence of multiple zones of focal acantholytic dyskeratosis and therefore are discussed together in this section. This shared histologic feature is not diagnostically trivial, however, and confusion may result be-

cause large lesions of Grover disease may histologically mimic small papules of Darier disease. Like cornoid lamella formation and epidermolytic hyperkeratosis, focal acantholytic dyskeratosis may indicate either a specific disorder or a secondary alteration in epidermal maturation. Therefore, clinical parameters are very important in accurate histologic interpretation.

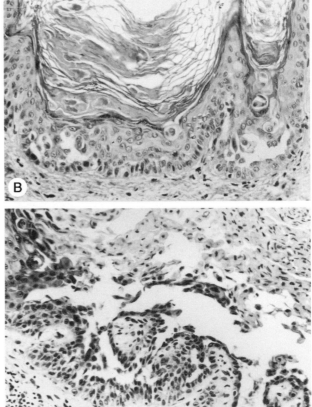

Figure 18–4. Darier disease (keratosis follicularis). (**A**) This crusted, erythematous plaque formed as a consequence of coalescence of multiple hyperkeratotic follicular papules. (**B**) Histology of an early lesion demonstrates small foci of suprabasal acantholysis, verrucous epidermal hyperplasia, and hyperkeratosis. (**C**) A more advanced lesion shows a suprabasal cleft containing rounded acantholytic cells near the base (i.e., corps ronds) and condensed, smaller acantholytic cells near the surface (i.e., corps grains).

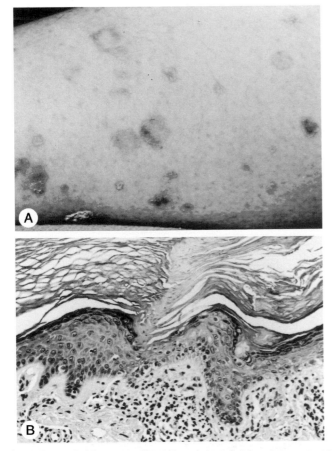

Figure 18–3. Porokeratosis, disseminated superficial actinic type. (**A**) Multiple erythematous hyperkeratotic plaques are present on sun-exposed skin. (**B**) A biopsy specimen from the edge of one of the lesions reveals a cornoid lamella leaning inward toward a zone of epidermal atypia, variable atrophy, and a patchy, superficial, dermal, inflammatory infiltrate.

Typical patients with Darier disease inherit the disorder in an autosomal dominant pattern. The eruption, which is persistent and slowly progressive, consists of multiple hyperkeratotic and crusted papules that coalesce to form verrucous plaques, often with a seborrheic distribution (Fig. 18–4A). Individual papules may show a follicular distribution (hence the alternative term keratosis follicularis), although oral mucosal involvement has also been documented. As is the case in porokeratosis, several clinical variants have been described. These include a hyperkeratotic form, which preferentially involves intertriginous skin; a ''vesiculobullous'' type; and a linear or systematized variant that probably represents epidermal nevi predominated by the reaction pattern of focal acantholytic dyskeratosis. On the other hand, Grover disease, also called transient acantholytic dermatosis, is not inherited and generally affects the truncal skin of middle-aged and older men. The clinical appearance is predominated by small, hyperkeratotic papules (Fig. 18–5A). Lesions are small and pruritic, do not coalesce, and resolve within months to several years. These are all important distinctions from Darier disease.

Both Darier disease and Grover disease demonstrate zones of hyperorthokeratosis associated with focal acantholytic dyskeratosis, a reaction pattern consisting of suprabasal acantholysis and dyskeratosis of the sloughed acantholytic keratinocytes (Figs. 18–4B, C and 18–5B, C). This is in contradistinction with pemphigus vulgaris (see Chap. 5), which shows suprabasal acantholysis without dyskeratosis, an important distinction because some lesions of Darier disease may clinically mimic vesiculobullous disease. The suprabasal acantholysis seen in Darier and most forms of Grover disease leaves the basal cell layer overlying dermal papillae intact and predominantly involves the cells of the lower stratum spinosum. The dyskeratosis typically occurs along a continuum defined at one extreme by large, round acantholytic cells showing early nuclear degeneration in the form of chromatin clumping, perinuclear clear zones (i.e., halos), and slight cytoplasmic eosinophilia; the other extreme of the continuum is defined by small millet seed–shaped acantholytic cells characterized by compact, pyknotic nuclei and dense, eosinophilic cytoplasm (see Fig. 18–4C). The larger cells are commonly referred to as corps ronds and the smaller ones as corps grains.

The scanning magnification of Darier disease and Grover disease is important in distinguishing these two entities histologically. Whereas the former shows verrucous epidermal hyperplasia associated by focal to diffuse well-formed acantholytic dyskeratosis (see Fig. 18–4B), the latter simply demonstrates minute skip areas of focal acantholytic dyskeratosis within an otherwise unremarkable epidermal layer (see Fig. 18–5B). Often, a nonspecific superficial perivascular inflammatory infiltrate containing mononuclear cells and eosinophils is present in Grover disease. The acantholysis of Grover disease is not always as discrete and localized within the lowermost epidermal layers as that seen in Darier disease. For example, certain biopsy specimens may show acantholysis at all levels of the epidermis in Grover disease, whereas others will demonstrate only superficial epidermal acantholysis reminiscent of that seen in pemphigus foliaceous, bullous impetigo, and staphylococcal scalded skin syndrome. Other examples may resemble suprabasal spongiosis more than true acantholysis. All forms, however, show

at least minute foci of hyperkeratosis and acantholysis at scanning magnification that usually correlate with a clinical history of pruritic hyperkeratotic papules of relatively recent onset in older individuals.

In addition to Darier disease, another form of inherited acantholytic dermatosis is *Hailey-Hailey disease*, also known as benign familial pemphigus. Inherited as an autosomal dominant trait, the rarely encountered Hailey-Hailey disease differs from Darier disease in that typical lesions present as recurrent vesicles on an erythematous base, often forming circinate configurations affecting intertriginous skin. Histo-

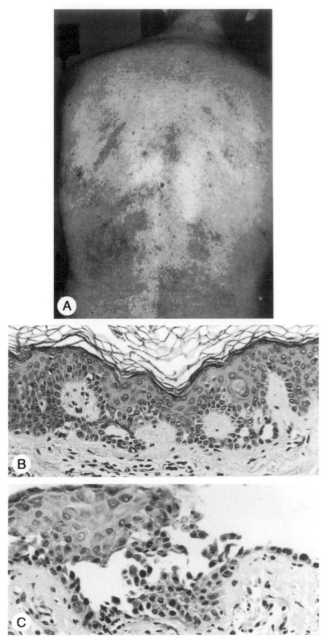

Figure 18–5. Grover disease (transient acantholytic dermatosis). (**A**) The back of this patient is covered by numerous, slightly erythematous, hyperkeratotic papules. (**B**) Early lesions show multiple microscopic foci of suprabasal acantholysis with minimal hyperkeratosis. (**C**) Advanced lesions may have well-developed suprabasal acantholytic clefts, but these are seldom as extensive as those seen in Darier disease and are not accompanied by significant verrucous epidermal hyperplasia.

logically, lesions do not show acantholytic clefts confined to a suprabasal plane, as is the case in Darier disease, but rather show suprabasal acantholysis affecting all epidermal layers to form a "dilapidated-brick-wall" appearance.

Epidermolytic Hyperkeratosis[10, 11]

- DIFFUSE HYPERORTHOKERATOSIS
- VACUOLIZATION OF SUPRABASAL KERATINOCYTES
- OCCASIONAL SLOUGHING OF SUPERFICIAL EPIDERMAL LAYERS
- PROMINENT, ENLARGED KERATOHYALIN GRANULES
- GRANULES RESEMBLING TRICHOHYALIN IN UPPERMOST EPIDERMAL LAYERS

Epidermolytic hyperkeratosis is most commonly encountered as a nonspecific reaction pattern in the setting of scarring and inflammatory cutaneous processes. Occasionally, epidermal nevi are predominated by the pattern of epidermolytic hyperkeratosis in a manner analogous to the sim-ilar phenomena involving cornoid lamella formation and focal acantholytic dyskeratosis. The most profound occurrence of epidermolytic hyperkeratosis, however, is in the setting of bullous congenital ichthyosiform erythroderma, an autosomal dominantly inherited, ichthyosis-like disorder characterized by the onset soon after birth of thick, tan-brown scales involving primarily flexural skin (Fig. 18–6A). Superficial vesicles and bullae resulting from midepidermal lysis also may be observed.

Histologically, at scanning magnification, epidermolytic hyperkeratosis is characterized by lamellar hyperkeratosis and suprabasal keratinocyte cytoplasmic lucency due to lytic vacuolization. Lesions may be widespread, as in the setting of congenital systematized disease, or focal, as in the case of incidental secondary findings (Fig. 18–6B–D). At higher magnification, suprabasal keratinocytes have a shredded appearance, with irregular lytic dissolution and condensation of cytoplasmic elements (Fig. 18–6B). Within the upper epidermal layers, the stratum granulosum contains enlarged, irregularly shaped keratohyalin granules as well as dense eosinophilic granules resembling follicular trichohyalin (see Fig. 18–6D). Although some lesions may, at first glance, resemble the effects of human papillomavirus (HPV), in epider-

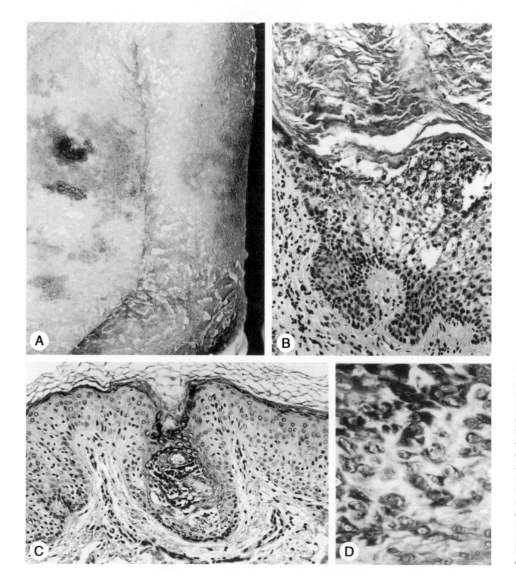

Figure 18–6. Epidermolytic hyperkeratosis. (**A**) The gross pathology consists of marked hyperkeratosis and scaling, particularly in regions of flexural creases. Soon after birth, bullae and vesicles may also be observed. (**B**) Histologically, there is cytoplasmic lysis of cells forming the midepidermis to upper epidermis, coarse keratohyalin granules associated with the formation of eosinophilic trichohyalin granules within the stratum granulosum, and marked overlying hyperkeratosis. (**C**) Focal involvement of a follicular infundibulum by epidermolytic hyperkeratosis. (**D**) High magnification of prominent keratohyaline granules within the the uppermost epidermal layers.

molytic hyperkeratosis, the cytoplasmic lucency is the result of lytic degeneration rather than koilocytotic pallor, and the prominent keratohyalin granules are irregular in shape rather than rounded in contour, as is the case in HPV-induced cytopathic effect.

Localized Superficial Amyloidosis[12, 13]

- PALE PINK GLOBULES INITIALLY WITHIN TIPS OF DERMAL PAPILLAE
- CONGO RED POSITIVITY AND APPLE GREEN BIREFRINGENCE
- SUPERFICIAL DERMAL PIGMENT INCONTINENCE
- EPIDERMIS NORMAL (MACULAR) OR HYPERPLASTIC (LICHENOID)

Localized amyloidosis is clinically divided into three categories: two superficial forms (i.e., macular and lichenoid), and one rarely encountered deep form (i.e., nodular amyloidosis). The more superficial forms appear as variably defined pigmented macules and papules that often affect sites subject to repeated trauma (Fig. 18–7A). The differential clinical features of the more common macular and lichenoid amyloidosis are presented in Table 18–3; nodular amyloidosis is characterized by 1- to 3-cm nodules and plaques in which amyloid light chain protein, deposited locally by plasma cells, diffusely fills and replaces the reticular dermis and subcutaneous fat.

The key histologic finding in superficial forms of amyloidosis is the presence of small, pale pink globules within dermal papillae (Fig. 18–7B). These globules may be present as small, colloid body–like structures at the tips of dermal papillae, or they may totally fill the affected papillae. Although the epidermis tends to be relatively normal in macular clinical variants, verrucous acanthosis is often present in lichenoid variants. Both forms may show variable pigment incontinence within superficial dermal melanophages. Staining with Congo red will reveal positivity within the papillary dermal globules, which are believed to derive from amyloid transformation of cytokeratin protein deposited into the superficial dermis. Examination with polarized light demon-

Table 18–3. DIFFERENTIAL DIAGNOSIS OF MACULAR AND LICHENOID AMYLOIDOSIS

CLINICAL FEATURE	MACULAR	LICHENOID
Pruritus	Present	Intense
Location	Upper back, trunk, extremities	Legs, shins, other sites
Pigmentation	Reticulated	Diffuse brown-red
Texture	Smooth	Verrucous, scaling
Size and shape	Variably defined macules	Discrete, clustered papules
Coalescence	Variable	Often prominent to variably defined plaques
Clinical differential	Postinflammatory hyperpigmentation	Lichen planus, lichen simplex chronicus

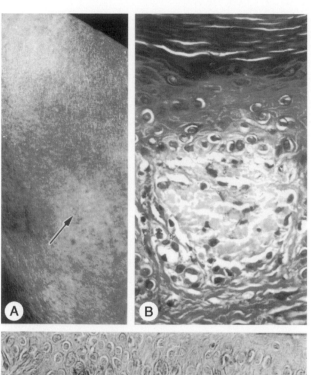

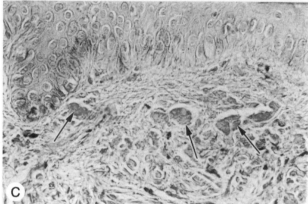

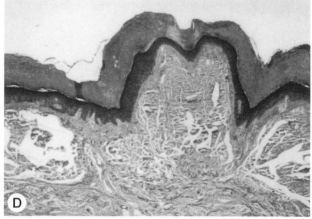

Figure 18–7. Lichenoid amyloidosis. (**A**) Coalescence of small, red-brown papules on the lower extremity has produced an ill-defined, pigmented plaque. There is a central zone of relative sparing where residual papules are still observed *(arrow)*. (**B**) Small, rounded, amyloid deposits are characteristically observed in dermal papillae and within the superficial layers of the papillary dermis. (**C**) Congo red stain reveals dull staining of amyloid deposits *(arrows)* in the superficial dermis. (**D**) Amyloid within the superficial dermis must be distinguished from colloid milium, depicted here; note deposits of amyloid-like material associated with large clefts within the superficial dermis.

strates characteristic apple green birefringence within the congophilic globules. Both superficial and deep forms of localized amyloid differ from colloid, a degenerated from of dermal extracellular matrix (probably elastin) with tinctorial and histochemical properties similar to those of amyloid. Colloid degeneration, unlike amyloid deposition, characteristically shows prominent cleft-like clear spaces throughout the pale homogenous material that displaces and replaces normal dermal elements (Fig. 18–7D).

Lichen Sclerosus[14, 15]

* PAPILLARY DERMAL PALLOR AND HOMOGENIZATION
* SUPERFICIAL DERMAL VASCULAR ECTASIA AND PIGMENT INCONTINENCE
* BASAL CELL LAYER DEGENERATION
* SPARSE LYMPHOPLASMACYTIC INFILTRATE WITHIN THE PAPILLARY DERMIS
* VARIABLE EPIDERMAL ATROPHY AND HYPERKERATOSIS
* FOLLICULAR INFUNDIBULAR KERATOTIC PLUGS

Lichen sclerosus, also discussed in Chapter 22 with regard to its specific effects on anogenital skin, is a relatively common disorder characterized by degenerative alterations within the papillary dermis. The alterations within the extracellular matrix share some qualitative similarities with the deeper dermal alterations observed in scleroderma, a condition discussed in Chapter 19 because of its systemic implications. Clinically, lichen sclerosus may mimic localized scleroderma, or morphea. Extragenital cutaneous lesions usually appear as firm white patches and plaques with variably atrophic overlying epidermis containing patulous follicular ostia filled with cornified material (Fig. 18–8A). Erosions and frank bullae are occasionally encountered and are the result of compromised dermal-epidermal integrity. Although truncal skin is the most common extragenital location, rarely, generalized lesions also may occur.

Early lesions of lichen sclerosus often reveal a superficial, papillary dermal, interstitial, nonangiocentric infiltrate of lymphocytes and plasma cells, associated with pallor and slight homogenization of superficial dermal connective tissue (Fig. 18–8B). At this stage, the epidermis may be unremarkable or even show mild reactive hyperplasia. With chronicity, however, there is progressive sclerosis and hyalinization of the papillary dermal extracellular matrix (Fig. 18–8C, D), accompanied by entrapment of occasional mononuclear inflammatory cells within the altered connective tissue. Vascular ectasia, melanin pigment incontinence, and epidermal atrophy with hyperkeratosis and variable basal cell layer vac-

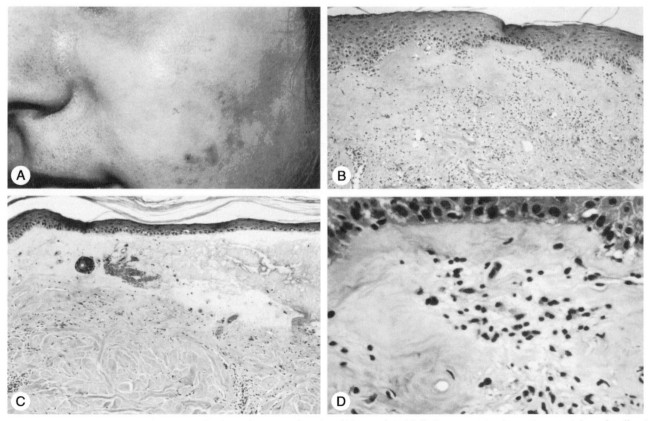

Figure 18–8. Lichen sclerosus. (**A**) An indurated, white plaque involves facial skin. Dilated follicles containing keratotic material are focally visible within this plaque. (**B**) A biopsy specimen from a relatively early lesion reveals pale, hyalinized, superficial dermal collagen associated with a diffuse underlying lymphocytic infiltrate containing occasional plasma cells. (**C**) A biopsy specimen from an advanced lesion reveals marked pallor and hyalinization of the superficial dermis, associated with epidermal atrophy and hyperkeratosis. (**D**) At higher magnification, collections of lymphocytes associated with melanophages are associated with the altered extracellular matrix. Foci suggestive of basal cell vacuolization are present within the overlying basal cell layer.

uolization also may be seen at this late evolutionary stage. Included hair follicles demonstrate follicular infundibular ectasia and keratotic plugging similar to that observed in chronic lesions of lupus erythematosus. Occasional lesions in which deep reticular dermal sclerosis accompanies the aforementioned papillary dermal alterations are regarded as the coexistence of morphea and lichen sclerosus.

Chronic Radiation Dermatitis[16]

- SUPERFICIAL AND DEEP DERMAL SCLEROSIS
- VARIABLE EOSINOPHILIA WITHIN ALTERED DERMAL MATRIX
- VASCULAR ECTASIA AND THROMBOSIS
- ATYPICAL FIBROBLASTS AND ENDOTHELIAL CELLS
- VARIABLE EPIDERMAL ATROPHY AND HYPERPLASIA

Chronic radiation dermatitis is commonly present in biopsy specimens taken adjacent to or from overlying tumor sites included within radiation ports and from lesions arising in previously irradiated skin that is prone to the development of aggressive epithelial malignancies. Clinically, chronic dermatitis resulting from fractional doses of X-radiation or ra-

dium is characterized by epidermal atrophy, telangiectasia, and mottled hyperpigmentation and hypopigmentation, or poikiloderma (Fig. 18–9A). Accordingly, these regions may be confused with poikilodermatous variants of cutaneous T-cell lymphoma, steroid atrophy, or certain connective tissue disorders. Occasionally, regions of ulceration or focal hyperkeratosis are present, prompting biopsy to exclude the development of aggressive carcinoma within the radiation field.

Histologically, there is superficial and mid-dermal sclerosis characterized by irregular hyalinization, variable tinctorial qualities ranging from hypereosinophilia to pallor, and sometimes a patchy, nonspecific lymphocytic inflammatory infiltrate with foci of superficial dermal pigment incontinence. Typically, the abnormal connective tissue extends up to the basal cell layer of the epidermis, without a Grenz zone of unaltered papillary dermal collagen. The epidermal layer is generally diffusely atrophic and shows loss of rete ridges and follicular epithelium (Fig. 18–9B, C). Within the hyalinized dermal matrix are plump, stellate fibroblasts containing enlarged, hyperchromatic nuclei; these features are characteristic of radiation-induced atypia (Fig. 18–9D). Similar atypical features may be observed in nuclei contained within bulging endothelial cells that line ectatic superficial vessels. Acute and remote evidence of intravascular thrombosis also may be observed.

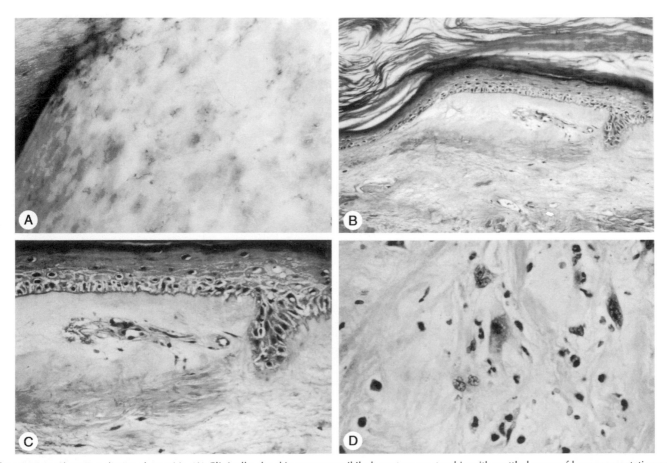

Figure 18–9. Chronic radiation dermatitis. (**A**) Clinically, the skin appears poikilodermatous or atrophic with mottled areas of hyposegmentation and hyperpigmentation and associated telangiectasias. (**B**) At low magnification, the superficial dermis and mid-dermis show variably dense sclerosis and hyalinization associated with epidermal atrophy and hyperkeratosis. (**C, D**) Within the altered collagen are endothelial cells and plump, stellate fibroblasts containing enlarged, hyperchromatic nuclei indicative of radiation effect.

Solar Elastosis

- NODULAR AND COALESCENT AGGREGATES OF BLUE-GRAY MATERIAL WITHIN UPPER DERMIS
- THIN ZONE OF NORMAL PAPILLARY DERMAL CONNECTIVE TISSUE BENEATH BASAL CELL LAYER
- ECTATIC SUPERFICIAL DERMAL VESSELS
- OVERLYING KERATINOCYTE ATYPIA OFTEN PRESENT

Solar elastosis is perhaps the most commonly encountered pathologic condition in biopsy specimens of human skin. Clinically, elastosis is associated with diminished elasticity (i.e., wrinkles), epidermal atrophy, and telangiectasias (Fig. 18–10A, B), and papular and even nodular, flesh-colored, tumor-like lesions that may be sampled to exclude basal cell carcinoma. Histologically, elastosis is characterized by coarse aggregates of basophilic material within the superficial dermis and occasionally within the mid-dermis as a result of expansion of the normal papillary dermis (Fig. 18–10C). Occasionally, elastotic bodies resembling colloid bodies are present within the uppermost papillary dermis. Unlike pale eosinophilic colloid bodies, however, these areas of micronodular elastosis consistently are pale gray in color. Foci showing transitions between abnormal elastic fibers and preexisting normal ones indicate that the process of elastosis is characterized by deposition of enlarged, pale, poorly formed fibers that completely replace the normal elastin network (Fig. 18–10D). These abnormal fibers generally stain less intensely than their normal counterparts with elastic tissue stains (e.g., Verhoeff). The area of dermal elastosis is usually separated from the overlying epidermal layer by a thin zone of unaltered papillary dermal collagen (i.e., Grenz zone). Elastotic regions often contain dilated blood vessels and frequently are associated with epidermal atrophy, basal cell layer atypia, diffuse lentiginous melanocytic hyperplasia, and focal parakeratosis, all sequelae of chronic exposure to ultraviolet light. In cases in which basal cell carcinoma is suspected and only nodular aggregates of elastosis are identified after levels through the specimen block are examined, a diagnosis of "consistent with nodular elastosis" may be rendered and additional local sampling recommended if clinical suspicion of associated epithelial neoplasia persists.

Pseudoxanthoma Elasticum[17]

- ENLARGED, CLUMPED, FRAGMENTED, PALE BLUE FIBERS WITHIN MID-DERMIS AND LOWER DERMIS
- FIBERS POSITIVE FOR ELASTIC TISSUE STAINS AND CALCIUM SALTS
- OCCASIONAL GIANT CELL REACTION TO CALCIFIED FIBERS

Pseudoxanthoma elasticum is a rare disorder that is inherited either as an autosomal dominant or recessive trait and is characterized by formation of abnormal elastic fibers in the skin, retina, and walls of muscular arteries. Skin lesions first appear during early adulthood and are progressive. These lesions consist of soft, yellow papules that coalesce. Clinically, they are associated with wrinkled skin. The groin, axillae, and sides of the neck are preferentially involved, although other surfaces may be affected (Fig. 18–11A). Morbidity and even mortality may result from gastrointestinal hemorrhage and myocardial infarction as a result of arterial involvement at these sites. Retinal involvement is associated with angioid streaks and progressive visual impairment.

The histologic appearance of pseudoxanthoma elasticum is characteristic in established lesions in which altered fibers

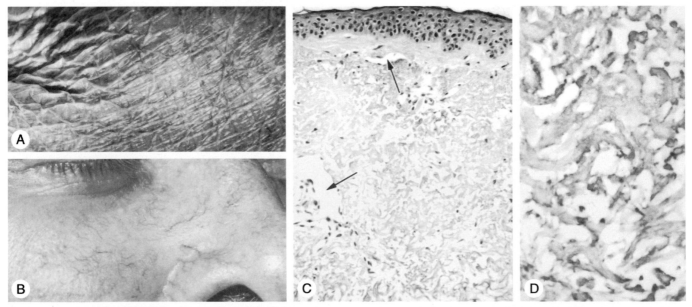

Figure 18–10. Solar elastosis. Chronically sun-damaged, elastotic skin may show premature loss of normal recoil and cohesive properties resulting in (**A**) wrinkles or (**B**) widely dilated blood vessels (i.e., telangiectasias). Histologically, elastosis is characterized by coarse aggregates of basophilic material within the superficial dermis and mid-dermis. Note the associated dilated vessels in **C** *(arrows)* and the comparison in **D** between elastotic fibers *(top)* and relatively normal, smaller fibers *(bottom)*.

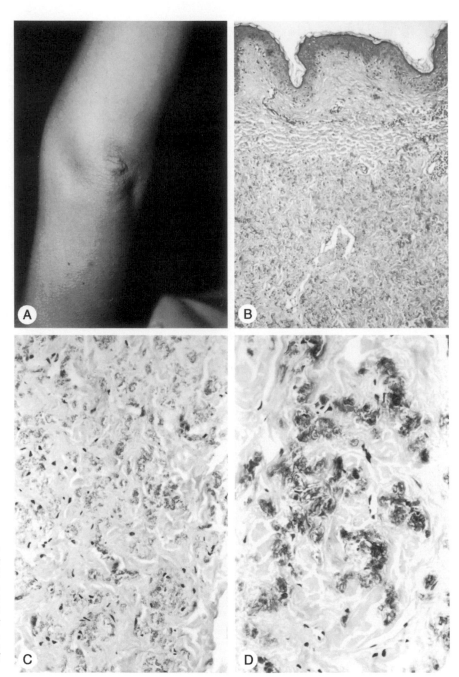

Figure 18–11. Pseudoxanthoma elasticum. (**A**) Coalescent, yellow-tan papules involve the elbow skin. (**B**) At low magnification, the mid-dermis and deep dermis are diffusely infiltrated by clumped, fragmented, markedly abnormal elastic fibers. (**C**) At higher magnification, many of the fibers have a pale purple hue (here dark grey) and a granular quality, which are indicative of early calcification. (**D**) Elastic tissue stain of the abnormal fibers demonstrates the marked clumping and aggregation of the abnormal fibers.

have undergone calcification; earlier lesions may be more subtle, and require elastic tissue stains for evaluation. At scanning magnification (Fig. 18–11B), the mid-dermis and deep dermis are diffusely infiltrated by clumped and fragmented pale blue fibers, which are visible as pink-purple structures because of dystrophic calcification. At higher magnification, individual fibers appear swollen, irregular in contour, and finely granular as a result of associated deposits of calcium salts (Fig. 18–11C). Elastic tissue stains confirm the chemical nature of the abnormal fibers and demonstrate the fibers to be markedly irregular, swollen, and fragmented (Fig. 18–11D). It is probable that this condition results in the

anomalous expression of a gene responsible for elastin synthesis or assembly. Because this condition may require monitoring and intervention which could be lifesaving, it is critical that skin biopsy specimens from patients with covert extracutaneous disease be accurately diagnosed when changes of pseudoxanthoma elasticum are present. Conversely, biopsy specimens from normal-appearing flexural skin or traumatic scars may reveal characteristic histologic changes of pseudoxanthoma elasticum in affected patients with covert cutaneous involvement but with a suspicious history of instability of vascular walls within internal viscera.

Perforating Disorders of Collagen and Elastin[18-21]

- EPIDERMAL HYPERPLASIA
- ELIMINATION OF DERMAL ELEMENTS INTO FOLLICULAR-EPIDERMAL EPITHELIUM
- CONTINUITY OF FOLLICULAR-EPIDERMAL CONTENTS WITH DERMAL MESENCHYME
- VARIABLE INFLAMMATORY RESPONSE

Perforating disorders are a small group of pathogenetically unrelated conditions that share the common feature of abnormal communication between epidermal and dermal elements that normally do not come into contact. The resultant lesions generally are predominated by reactive epidermal and dermal inflammatory changes. Although any condition that can result in transepidermal elimination or perforation (e.g., perforating dermatofibroma) could broadly be included in this category, the present discussion focuses on four conditions.

Elastosis Perforans Serpiginosa

Elastosis perforans serpiginosa is a relatively rare disorder characterized by hyperkeratotic papules generally arranged in arcuate and circinate configurations. Lesions preferentially affect skin of the face, neck, and upper extremities (Figs. 18–12A and 18–13A). Histologically, there is nodular, often endophytic epidermal hyperplasia and hyperkeratosis at sites where altered elastic fibers are extruded upward through perforations, forming either straight (Fig. 18–12B, C) or narrow, winding channels (Fig. 18–13B). The material within the channels consists of basophilic degenerated elastic fibers, cellular debris, and keratin (Fig. 18–12C) and focally stains positively with the Verhoeff reagent (Fig. 18–13C). The dermis at the base of the perforating channel may contain a reactive chronic inflammatory infiltrate, occasionally with a giant cell response. Increased quantities of altered elastic fibers may also be detected within adjacent dermal papillae, suggesting that the basic defect in this condition is the production of increased amounts of superficial dermal elastin, which undergoes reactive transepidermal elimination.

Reactive Perforating Collagenosis

Reactive perforating collagenosis is a rare condition that may show an autosomal recessive pattern of inheritance. It clinically results in umbilicated papules and nodules which are first observed during infancy and childhood at sites of trauma (Fig. 18–14A). An acquired form may also occur in adulthood in association with chronic renal failure and diabetes. Histologically, there is a cup-shaped epidermal depression filled with orthokeratotic scale (Fig. 18–14B). The base of the depression communicates with basophilic, degenerating collagen bundles associated with inflammatory debris (Fig. 18–14C). The basophilic material, which represents degenerating collagen, may also be detected within the cup-shaped invagination as it is eliminated to the epidermal surface. The findings of reactive perforating collagenosis are not dissimilar to those of elastosis perforans serpiginosa; however, in the former condition, basophilic altered collagen is eliminated, whereas in the latter, the eliminated material consists of altered elastic fibers.

Perforating Folliculitis

In perforating folliculitis, inflammatory, noncoalescent, follicular papules with central cornified plugs preferentially

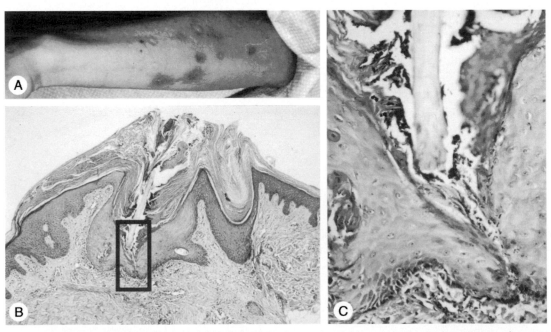

Figure 18–12. Elastosis perforans serpiginosa. (**A**) In this patient, annular lesions formed by grouped hyperkeratotic papules are associated with marked postinflammatory hyperpigmentation. (**B**) There is a broad, follicle-like invagination associated with hyperkeratosis and foci of perforation at the base of the lesion *(enclosed in rectangle)*. (**C**) Transepithelial perforation is associated with extrusion of altered elastic fibers within the underlying dermis. Although a small hair follicle is secondarily entrapped, most lesions were discontinuous with follicular epithelium.

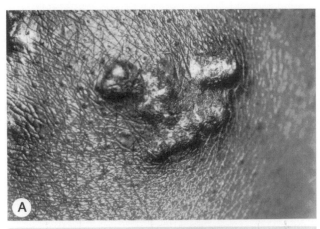

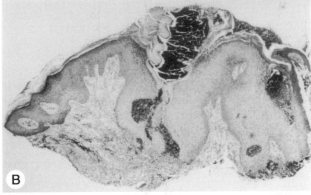

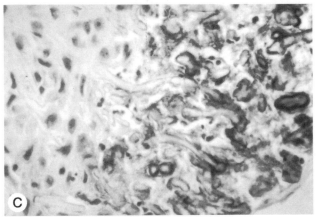

Figure 18–13. Elastosis perforans serpiginosa with elastic tissue stain. (**A**) Annular hyperkeratotic papules may be misdiagnosed as reactive epidermal and dermal alterations unless perforating disorders are considered and appropriate stains obtained. (**B**) Low and (**C**) higher magnification of a lesional biopsy specimen show altered elastic fibers within the hyperplastic epithelium and within the cornified plug being extruded.

affect the extensor surfaces of the extremities and buttocks. Many of the reported cases involve patients with uremia. The primary pathology consists of the formation of follicular infundibular hyperkeratosis, often associated with a distorted, coiled hair shaft. Secondary perforation of the follicular infundibulum results in local extrusion of follicular contents, eliciting an inflammatory reaction and degeneration of the perifollicular extracellular matrix. Occasionally, elastic fibers and basophilic perifollicular debris find their way into the follicle through the site of perforation. Thus, follicular con-

tents may be extruded into the dermis, and basophilic dermal contents and cellular debris may enter the follicle. However, the amount of elastic fibers adjacent to the site of perforation is not increased, and perforation involving interfollicular epidermis does not occur, as is the case in elastosis perforans serpiginosa.

Kyrle Disease

Kyrle disease is a rare condition characterized by generalized follicular and nonfollicular papules containing central keratotic plugs. The papules typically coalesce to form verrucous plaques. Extensor skin of the extremities is most frequently involved, and there is a reported association with diabetes mellitus. The histology of Kyrle disease involves the formation of a broad, shallow epidermal invagination that generally does not show evidence of follicular association. The scale within the invagination is parakeratotic, and the underlying viable epidermis is variably thinned to the point that scale approximates the underlying dermis. It appears that

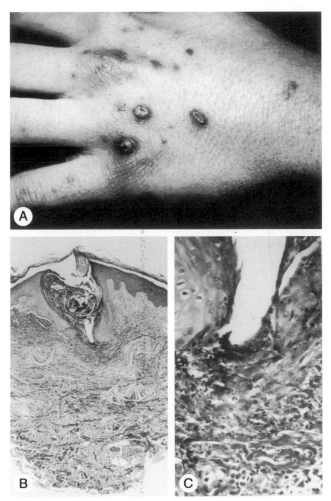

Figure 18–14. Reactive perforating collagenosis. (**A**) Multiple hyperkeratotic papules, some with central umbilications, are present at sites of trauma on the dorsum of the hand. (**B**) At scanning magnification, there is a cup-shaped depression filled with parakeratotic and hyperorthokeratotic scale and inflammatory debris. (**C**) At the base of the depression, there is a site of transepithelial perforation of degenerating basophilic collagen bundles associated with mixed inflammatory cells.

the basal cell layer is unable to keep pace with the rate of overlying epidermal maturation and desquamation. As a result, zones of communication between the keratotic contents of the invagination and the underlying dermis develop, leading to the formation of granulomatous inflammation and basophilic debris that is subsequently transepidermally eliminated into the invagination.

Any disorder leading to chronically inflamed or degenerating dermal connective tissue may show a tendency for transepidermal elimination. Accordingly, granuloma annulare, rheumatoid nodule, necrobiosis lipoidica, pseudoxanthoma elasticum, chondrodermatitis nodularis, lichen nitidus,

and dermatofibroma may show epidermal perforation. An algorithmic approach to diagnosing perforating disorders is suggested in Figure 18–15.

Anetoderma[22]

- LOSS OR ABSENCE OF ELASTIC FIBERS WITHIN SUPERFICIAL AND DEEP DERMIS
- PERIVASCULAR MONONUCLEAR CELL INFLAMMATORY INFILTRATE
- OCCASIONAL INFLAMMATORY CELLS ADHERENT TO ELASTIC FIBERS

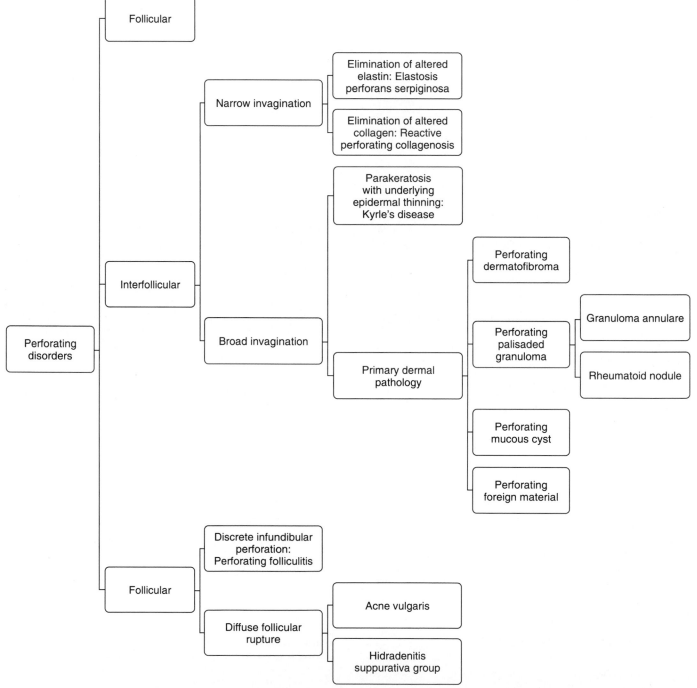

Figure 18–15. Algorithmic diagnostic approach to perforating disorders.

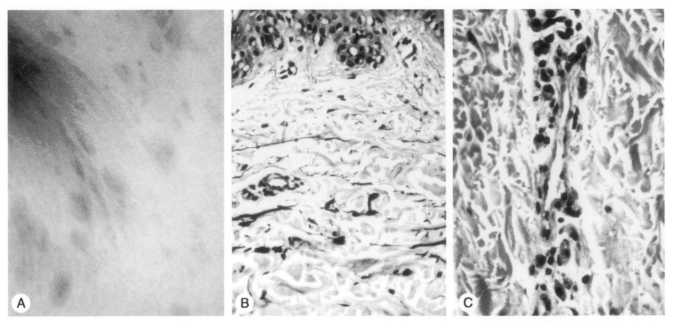

Figure 18–16. Anetoderma. (**A**) Multiple atrophic plaques involve the upper trunk. Palpation yields a hernia-like defect because of diminished elastic recoil. (**B**) Elastic tissue stain reveals markedly attenuated elastic fibers within the superficial dermis and mid-dermis. (**C**) A variable perivascular lymphocytic infiltrate may be present, particularly in early lesions, in which loss of elastic fibers is generally less prominent.

Anetoderma, also called macular atrophy, is an unusual disorder characterized by pale blue-red dermal plaques, most commonly involving truncal skin (Fig. 18–16A). Typically, lesions are best appreciated by palpation; pressure may result in the sensation of loss of supportive dermal elements, or of a hernial orifice. Lesions may progress over time, and new plaques may develop over a several-year period. Some patients have plaques that appear red and inflamed, presumably representing an early evolutionary stage of this cryptic disorder.

Histologically, there is variable loss or even complete absence of superficial and deep dermal elastic fibers (Fig. 18–16B). There may be a superficial and sometimes mid-dermal perivascular inflammatory infiltrate composed of lymphocytes and occasional eosinophils (Fig. 18–16C). Some reports have described apposition of inflammatory cells to elastic fibers, and others have documented a vasculitic component of the inflammatory process. In most lesions, however, the degree of inflammation is slight, and suspicion of a degenerative abnormality in elastic tissue is largely based on the gross pathology. The diagnosis is confirmed by obtaining elastic tissue stains that confirm a reduction in number of elastic fibers and thinning and attenuation of residual fibers (see Fig. 18–16B).

Some forms of anetoderma appear to be acquired as a result of persistent inflammation due to lupus erythematosus, syphilis, or leprosy or related to the administration of certain drugs (e.g., penicillamine). It is probable that these processes are related to elastolysis resulting from inflammatory and metabolic factors that cause decreased elastin synthesis, increased enzymatic degradation, or both.

Dissolution of elastic fibers with associated clinical loss of cutaneous elastic recoil is also seen in the rare condition *cutis laxa*. In this disorder, there is generalized elastolysis, resulting in loose, redundant skin folds (Fig. 18–17A). In-volvement of internal organs may result in pulmonary emphysema, gastrointestinal diverticula, and hernia formation. Interestingly and potentially relevant to the pathogenesis of anetoderma, many cases of acquired cutis laxa are heralded by urticarial and papulovesicular inflammatory skin lesions. Congenital lesions with autosomal recessive and dominant inheritance patterns have also been described. Histologically, there is a decrease in the number of elastic fibers within the superficial and deep dermis. Residual fibers often are centrally thickened and show tapered ends that appear to be melting away as if they are tips of icicles (Fig. 18–17B). Other fibers may have a beaded appearance or persist only as small, nondescript, elastin-positive flecks. The associated inflammatory infiltrate is similar to that seen in inflammatory lesions of anetoderma.

Atrophoderma[23]

- DERMAL THINNING
- SCLERODERMOID ALTERATIONS IN DEEP DERMAL COLLAGEN BUNDLES

Atrophoderma is a poorly understood degenerative disorder of dermal connective tissue characterized by depressed, slightly indurated, slate gray zones occurring in otherwise normal-appearing skin of the trunk and back. Individual lesions may have diameters of up to 10 cm, irregular geographic contours, and characteristically, a "cliff-drop" border best appreciated by side lighting. Histologically, the dermis is 25 to 75% thinner than a mirror-image biopsy of normal contralateral skin. The deep dermis is composed of collagen bundles that are thickened and hyalinized, resulting in decreased intercollagenous spaces. These latter changes qualitatively resemble morphea, a disorder that differs quan-

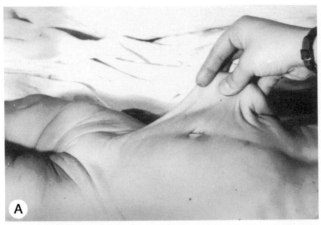

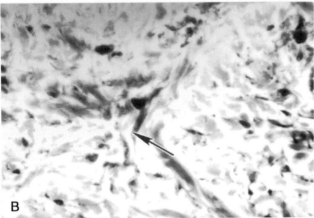

Figure 18–17. Cutis laxa. (**A**) The skin of this patient is loose, pendulous, and without elastic recoil. (**B**) A biopsy specimen reveals diminished numbers of elastic fibers; those that remain often are focally thickened but characteristically taper at the ends *(arrow)*. Small, thin, beaded fibers may also be detected.

titatively from atrophoderma by showing increased rather than diminished net dermal thickness. Controversy exists, however, as to whether atrophoderma represents a variant form of morphea.

Keloid

- DERMAL COLLAGEN REPLACED BY IRREGULAR BUNDLES OF COLLAGEN AND FIBROBLASTS
- HYALINIZED BANDS OF COLLAGEN IMPARTING STRIPED PATTERN
- OVERLYING EPIDERMAL ATROPHY

Keloids are clinically and histologically distinctive, biologically fascinating, epidemiologically common, and pathogenetically poorly understood. Typical lesions occur at sites of trauma, and individuals with darkly pigmented skin are more prone to the development of these tumor-like lesions. Occasional keloids appear spontaneously as linear lesions that particularly involve presternal skin and possibly are related to lines of tension defined by underlying muscle groups. A common site of keloid formation observed in excision

specimens by dermatopathologists is earlobe skin at sites of previous ear piercing (Fig. 18–18*A*).

Histologically, keloids appear to occur along a continuum with hypertrophic scars. Both show superficial and deep dermal replacement by poorly defined bands of collagen and admixed fibroblasts at scanning magnification (Fig. 18–18*B*). At higher magnification, however, keloids display characteristic bands of hyalinized, deeply eosinophilic collagen that produce a pattern often likened to zebra stripes. This histologic appearance is pathognomonic for keloids. Because keloids may be confused with primary mesenchymal neoplasia, they are also discussed in Chapter 15.

Chondrodermatitis[24]

- DERMAL FIBROSIS AND REACTIVE EPIDERMAL HYPERPLASIA INVOLVING EAR SKIN
- DEGENERATION OF CARTILAGE, PERICHONDRAL FIBROSIS, AND DERMAL CHONDROID METAPLASIA
- MIXED INFLAMMATORY INFILTRATE

These common, painful nodules arise as solitary and occasionally multiple lesions on the upper portion of the helix of the ears of older individuals (Fig. 18–19*A*). Men appear to be preferentially affected. Some lesions may be

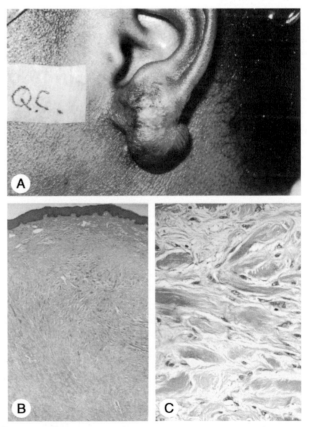

Figure 18–18. Keloid. (**A**) A characteristic location for this lesion, which is caused by abnormal matrix deposition, is the site of earlobe piercing. (**B**) The dermis is replaced by abnormal bundles of collagen, which consist of (**C**) thick, hyalinized bundles of collagen intermingled with loose foci of fibroblastic proliferation.

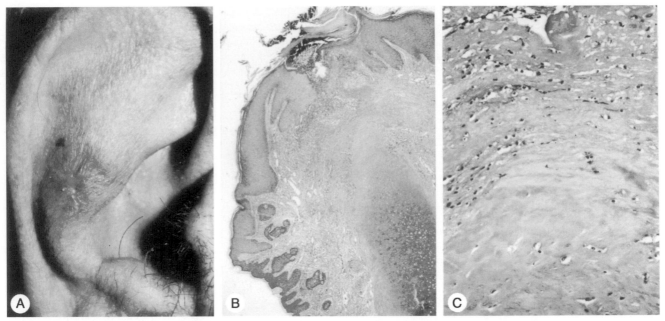

Figure 18–19. Chondrodermatitis. (**A**) A hyperkeratotic nodule with central ulceration on the ear clinically mimics squamous cell carcinoma. (**B**) At scanning magnification, cartilage *(lower right)* gradually merges with the fibrotic and inflamed dermis, which is surmounted by hyperplastic, focally ulcerated epidermis. (**C**) A zone of characteristic hyalinization and chondroid change is present within perichondral connective tissue.

associated with repeated trauma or mechanical pressure, although many cases do not have a definite associated cause. Lesions may ulcerate and clinically mimic squamous and basal cell carcinoma, necessitating biopsy. Histologically, the primary pathology is in the superficial dermis, which shows fibrosis, vascular proliferation, a mixed inflammatory infiltrate, and importantly, zones of chondroid metaplasia (Fig. 18–19B, C). These metaplastic zones are generally in continuity with underlying cartilage demonstrating degenerative alterations and perichondral fibrosis. Metaplastic foci are characterized by hyalinized eosinophilic dermal matrix containing mesenchymal cells isolated within small, round, lacuna-like spaces (Fig. 18–19C). The finding of dermal chrondroid metaplasia at this site is so characteristic as to permit diagnosis in specimens that do not include intact underlying cartilage. The overlying epidermis is generally markedly hyperplastic, focally ulcerated, and devoid of significant dysplasia.

Stasis[25]

- SUPERFICIAL DERMAL CAPILLARY PROLIFERATION FORMING GLOMERULOID TUFTS
- SUPERFICIAL DERMAL EDEMA, FIBROSIS, AND HEMOSIDERIN DEPOSITION
- EPIDERMAL ATROPHY OR ACANTHOSIS
- HYPERKERATOSIS

Stasis dermatitis is described in this section, because it does not represent a form of dermatitis but rather a type of chronic dermal degeneration as a result of altered hydrostatic homeostasis within leg vessels. Because it may be confused with vascular neoplasia and pigmentary disorders, it is also addressed in Chapters 15 and 17, respectively. Clinical lesions of stasis dermatitis are polymorphous, ranging from diffuse, brawny induration (Fig. 18–20A) to localized regions

Figure 18–20. Stasis. (**A**) Brawny, indurated edema of the ankle is present in a patient with chronic venous insufficiency. (**B**) Histologically, there is abnormal deposition of collagen and almost tumoral proliferation of small vessels within the superficial dermis.

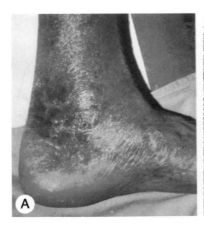

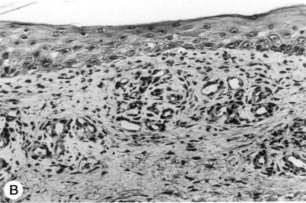

that may be clinically confused with squamous cell carcinoma, infection, Kaposi sarcoma, and dermatitides such as psoriasis and hypertrophic lichen planus.

The essential histologic finding in stasis degeneration is superficial vascular proliferation (Fig. 18–20B). Affected vessels generally form aggregates within the superficial dermis; these aggregates may preferentially involve dermal papillae and progress to resemble capillary tufts within renal glomeruli. The surrounding connective tissue shows variable fibrosis and edema, and perivascular hemorrhage and hemosiderin deposition is common. The overlying epidermis usually shows variable hyperkeratosis, although the characteris-

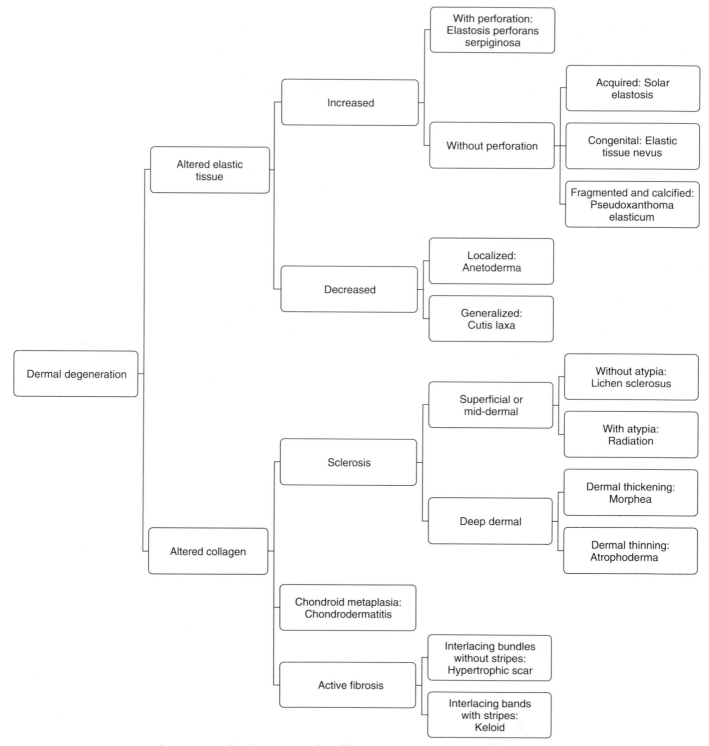

Figure 18–21. Algorithmic approach to differential diagnosis of dermal degeneration.

tic of the viable epidermal layers may range from severe atrophy to reactive hyperplasia with features similar to those of lichen simplex chronicus.

DIFFERENTIAL DIAGNOSIS

There is no single differential diagnosis applicable to the maturational and degenerative disorders described in this chapter. This is because each condition has characteristic and divergent clinical and histologic findings. Within each group, however, there are differential diagnostic branch points. For example, in the setting of ichthyosis, clinical and histologic characteristics (e.g., thickness of the stratum granulosum) are critical in formulating and refining an already difficult and subtle diagnosis. Once recognized based on characteristic histologic findings, different forms of porokeratosis, acantholytic and dyskeratotic disorders, and epidermolytic hyperkeratotic diseases may be further differentiated based on clinical information and gross pathology. In a similar way, each of the dermal deposits and degenerative alterations described have one or more key features that represent algorithmic branch points in differential diagnostic assessment. An algorithmic approach to dermal degenerative changes is summarized in Figure 18–21.

SELECTED REFERENCES

1. Epstein EH, Williams NL, Elias PM. Biochemical abnormalities in the ichthyoses. Curr Probl Dermatol 1987;17:32.
2. Williams ML. The dynamics of desquamation. Lessons to be learned from the ichthyoses. Am J Dermatopathol 1984;6:381.
3. Flint GL, Flam M, Soter NA. Acquired ichthyosis: A sign of nonlymphoproliferative malignant disorder. Arch Dermatol 1975;111:1446.
4. Wade TR, Ackerman AB. Cornoid lamellation. A histologic reaction pattern. Am J Dermatopathol 1980;2:5.
5. Schwartz T, Seiser A, Gschnait F. Disseminated superficial "actinic" porokeratosis. J Am Acad Dermatol 1984;11:724.
6. Himmelstein R, Lynnfield YL. Punctate porokeratosis. Arch Dermatol 1984;120:263.
7. Ackerman AB. Focal acantholytic dyskeratosis. Arch Dermatol 1972;106:702.
8. Ishibashi Y, Kajiwara Y, Andoh I, et al. The nature and pathogenesis of dyskeratosis in Hailey-Hailey's disease and Darier's disease. J Dermatol (Tokyo) 1984;11:335.
9. Chalet M, Grover R, Ackerman AB. Transient acantholytic dermatosis. Arch Dermatol 1977;113:431.
10. McCurdy J, Beare JM. Congenital bullous ichthyosiform erythroderma. Br J Dermatol 1967;79:294.
11. Mehregan AH. Epidermolytic hyperkeratosis. J Cutan Pathol 1978;5:76.
12. Brownstein MH, Hashimoto K, Greenwald G. Biphasic amyloidosis: Link between macular and lichenoid forms. Br J Dermatol 1973;88:25.
13. Masu S, Hosokawa M, Seiji M. Amyloid in localized cutaneous amyloidosis: Immunofluorescence studies with anti-keratin antiserum. Acta Derm Venereol (Stockh) 1981;61:381.
14. Uitto J, Santa Cruz DJ, Bauer EA, et al. Morphea and lichen sclerosus et atrophicus. J Am Acad Dermatol 1980;3:271.
15. Di Silverio A, Serri F. Generalized bullous and hemorrhagic lichen sclerosus and satrophicus. Br J Dermatol 1975;93:215.
16. Young EM Jr, Barr RJ. Sclerosing dermatosis. J Cutan Pathol 1985;12:426.
17. Lebwohl M, Phelps RG, Yannuzzi L, et al. Diagnosis of pseudoxanthoma elasticum by scar biopsy in patients without characteristic skin lesions. New Engl J Med 1987;317:347.
18. Beck HI, Brandrup F, Hagdrup HK, et al. Adult-acquired reactive perforating collagenosis. J Cutan Pathol 1988;15:124.
19. Burkhart CG. Perforating folliculitis. Int J Dermatol 1981;20:597.
20. Patterson JW. The perforating disorders. J Am Acad Dermatol 1984;10:561.
21. Mehregan AH. Elastosis perforans serpiginosa. Arch Dermatol 1968;97:381.
22. Kossard S, Kronman KR, Dicken CH, et al. Inflammatory macular atrophy: Immunofluorescent and ultrastructural findings. J Am Acad Dermatol 1979;1:325.
23. Brownstein MH, Rabinowitz AD. The invisible dermatoses. J Am Acad Dermatol 1983;8:579.
24. Goette DK. Chondrodermatitis nodularis chronica helicis: A perforating necrobiotic granuloma. J Am Acad Dermatol 1980;2:148.

19

Dermatopathology of Systemic Disease

DEFINITIONS AND GENERAL CONSIDERATIONS

This chapter considers the more common disorders that relate to cutaneous manifestations of systemic disease. Skin biopsy specimens in such settings may potentially reveal life-threatening yet covert metabolic, endocrine, or neoplastic disorders. The dermatopathology of systemic disease could by itself easily be the subject of a book or monograph; therefore, discussion in this text is restricted to those conditions that occasionally present in routine practice or fall within the limits of routine differential diagnostic considerations.

Some manifestations of systemic disease are discussed in detail in chapters that emphasize their primary histologic patterns (e.g., lupus erythematosus in Chap. 6). These conditions may be mentioned briefly in this chapter for purposes of completeness, but detailed discussions are not reiterated.

GROSS PATHOLOGY

The gross pathology of cutaneous changes in systemic disease is extraordinarily diverse. Variations in cutaneous color and pigmentation may result from endocrine disturbances or vascular lesions, as in the mottled livedo pattern that usually affects skin of the lower extremities after cholesterol emboli. Connective tissue diseases may produce maculopapular, poikilodermatous, hyperkeratotic, sclerotic, or purpuric lesions, and accordingly, they are often confusing mimics of other conditions. On the other hand, certain disorders result in highly characteristic lesions; this is the case in necrolytic migratory erythema associated with glucagonoma and in xanthelasma, which may be an indicator of hyperlipoproteinemia in some individuals. As has been the case in the preceding chapters, careful clinicopathologic correlation is essential in accurate diagnostic recognition of systemic conditions. Moreover, close communication between the clinician and the dermatopathologist is particularly important in diagnosing cutaneous disorders related to systemic disease, because the most precise and focused metabolic, serologic, and internal work-up may depend in part on this interaction.

GENERAL HISTOLOGY AND TEMPORAL EVOLUTION

Just as the clinical appearance of systemic disorders affecting the skin may be extremely diverse, the histology also is extraordinarily polymorphous. Dermal sclerosis, dermal-epidermal blisters, pigmentary abnormalities, verrucous epidermal hyperplasias, tumor-like deposits, and vasculitic lesions all are discussed in this chapter. Some of these disorders could appropriately be placed in other chapters according to their histologic patterns; however, they are detailed here in the hope that reference to this chapter may facilitate recognition of certain systemic diseases based on the skin biopsy specimen—further evidence of the critical importance of the dermatopathologist in the care of some systemically ill patients.

With regard to temporal evolution of skin disorders related to systemic disease, it is not possible to deal with each group of conditions in view of the complexity and scope of their clinical and histologic diversity. However, it is possible to take a prototypical example of a skin disease resulting from a systemic condition and provide an example of the diagnostic importance of understanding the evolutionary steps of disease progression. For example, progressive systemic sclerosis, or scleroderma, begins as subtle alterations within the deep reticular collagen at the interface between dermis and subcutaneous fat. The early inflammation and sclerosis that occur at that site are belied by normal-appearing superficial dermis and epidermis that may predominate in a small biopsy specimen. As the disease becomes more advanced, the sclerotic and inflammatory alterations move upward, replacing dermal collagen in a wave-like manner, and downward, replacing subcutaneous fat in a similar fashion. Progressive entrapment of adnexal epithelium results in its atrophy and eventual disappearance. As the advancing front of altered dermal connective tissue approaches the epidermis, loss of rete ridges, diffuse thinning of the viable epidermal layers, and hyperkeratosis may ensue. Accordingly, the early and late lesions may appear quite dissimilar, and without thorough knowledge of the various evolutionary patterns, diagnosis may be difficult or impossible. The same is true for other forms of cutaneous disease related to systemic pathology, and these issues are taken into consideration individually in the following sections.

HISTOLOGY OF SPECIFIC DISORDERS

Scleroderma[1-4]

- DEEP DERMAL SCLEROSIS PROGRESSING TO SUPERFICIAL DERMAL AND SUBCUTANEOUS SCLEROSIS
- THICKENING OF SEPTA WITHIN SUBCUTIS
- PROGRESSIVE ADNEXAL AND EPIDERMAL ATROPHY
- ENLARGEMENT, PALLOR, AND HOMOGENIZATION OF AFFECTED COLLAGEN BUNDLES
- DEEP LYMPHOPLASMACYTIC ANGIOCENTRIC INFILTRATES

The most common cutaneous manifestations of connective tissue disease encountered in general dermatopathology practice include lupus erythematosus (see Chaps. 2 and 6), scleroderma and eosinophilic fasciitis, and rheumatoid arthritis (see Chap. 9). This section focuses on the cutaneous manifestations of systemic scleroderma (i.e., progressive systemic sclerosis) and its deep inflammatory counterpart, eosinophilic fasciitis, and briefly considers the differential diagnosis of deep lymphocytic venulitis, which may be seen in connective tissue diseases, including inflammatory scleroderma and rheumatoid arthritis.

The typical clinical history that accompanies a biopsy specimen of suspected systemic sclerosis is that of ill-defined induration, often first observed on the skin of the distal extremities or the face (i.e., acrosclerosis) and associated with Raynaud syndrome. Some patients may present with primarily truncal involvement from the outset. Some isolated plaques may have a discrete violaceous hue about a centrifugally expanding perimeter, although such findings are more commonly seen in localized scleroderma without systemic involvement, or morphea (Fig. 19–1A). Patients may complain of dysphagia and show signs of malabsorption as a result of esophageal and intestinal involvement, respectively. Pulmonary fibrosis may result in dyspnea or right-sided heart failure, and renal involvement may be associated with rapidly progressive hypertension and azotemia. A clinical variant of systemic scleroderma is referred to as the CREST syndrome, and consists of calcinosis cutis (C), Raynaud phenomenon (R), esophageal involvement (E), sclerodactyly (S), and telangiectasia (T).

At scanning magnification, biopsy specimens, which must include full-thickness dermis and a portion of underlying subcutis, are often squared-off rather than trapezoidal as a result of the diffuse replacement of the normally elastic dermis by abnormal connective tissue. The dermal thickness may appear markedly increased as a result of downward replacement of subcutaneous tissue by altered collagen (Fig. 19–1B). A helpful indicator of this feature in advanced lesions is the location of entrapped eccrine coils, which normally demarcate the junction between reticular dermis and subcutis. Extension of altered collagen down widened subcutaneous septa may also be observed. At higher magnification (Fig. 19–1C), collagen bundles are thickened and pale, and they display a homogeneous rather than a finely fibrillar quality. Spaces that normally separate adjacent collagen bundles are attenuated. Angiocentric cuffs of lymphocytes and plasma cells associated with thickening of vessel walls and endothelial cell hypertrophy and apparent degeneration (i.e., lymphocytic vasculitis) are commonly observed in the deep dermis (Fig. 19–1C). Inflammation may also show an interstitial pattern among altered collagen bundles. Dermal eccrine coils and neurovascular bundles are no longer surrounded by a cuff of loose adventitial connective tissue as in normal skin; rather, they are entrapped within the altered sclerotic dermal matrix (Fig. 19–1D). In very advanced lesions, all adnexal structures are absent, and the epidermis is diffusely atrophic.

Eosinophilic fasciitis is an unusual variant of scleroderma characterized by acute onset of painful, firm, swollen regions, usually affecting the skin of one or several extremities. Occasionally, there are surface irregularities in these regions, suggesting variable fibrosis and tethering of skin to underlying fascial planes. The majority of affected individuals also have peripheral blood eosinophilia and hypergammaglobulinemia. Internal disease involving viscera, however, is unusual. Histologic evaluation, which requires wide, deep surgical excision, reveals abnormal collagen, primarily within the lowermost reticular dermis, within widened septa of the subcutaneous fat, and involving the underlying fascia (Fig. 19–2A). Qualitatively, the altered collagen within the subcutaneous septa, replacing the fat lobules, and within the fascia is similar to that observed in ordinary scleroderma, although most of the reticular dermis is spared. The inflammatory infiltrate in eosinophilic cellulitis may be brisk and is composed of lymphocytes, occasional plasma cells, and often but not invariably, eosinophils in perivascular and interstitial array (Fig. 19–2B). Skeletal muscle, if present, may also show infiltration by inflammatory cells and foci of fibrous replacement. The similarities between systemic scleroderma and eosinophilic fasciitis have prompted some dermatopathologists to suggest the name morphea profunda for the latter condition, although it should be remembered that the two disorders have distinct clinical presentations and well-defined histologic differences.

The dermal and subcutaneous fibrotic thickening that may occur in scleroderma must be differentiated from a disorder termed *scleredema*, which at first glance may appear to show similar histologic changes. Scleredema is characterized by the abrupt onset of thickening of facial, neck, and upper

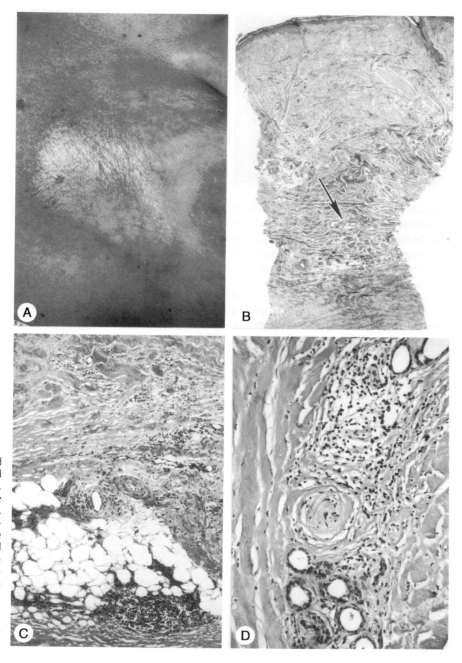

Figure 19–1. Scleroderma. (**A**) An indurated plaque is anchored to the underlying fascia and covered by a glistening, atrophic epidermal layer. There is a violaceous hue at the perimeter of the lesion, where it has been expanding centrifugally. (**B**) At scanning magnification, the biopsy specimen shows a markedly thickened dermis. Eccrine coils are atrophic and appear to be entrapped within the thickened deep dermal collagen bundles *(arrow)*. (**C**) Higher magnification reveals sclerotic, thickened, hyalinized collagen bundles infiltrating and replacing subcutaneous adipose tissue. Angiocentric cuffs of lymphocytes and plasma cells are focally observed at the base of the panel. (**D**) Entrapped eccrine coils and a dermal nerve twig. Note the pale, thickened collagen bundles.

is noteworthy (Fig. 19–5B). A potentially related and more common condition with similar vascular alterations is *pretibial pigmented patches*, which are oval, well-defined, slightly depressed macules that involve skin of the shins in about one fifth of all diabetics. Histologic examination discloses vascular alterations similar to those seen in bullosis diabeticorum, perivascular hemosiderin deposition, and absence of epidermal degenerative changes.

Thyrotoxicosis[7–9]

- MUCIN DEPOSITION IN MID-DERMIS AND DEEP DERMIS
- EMPTY SPACES WITHIN MUCIN DEPOSITS
- STELLATE CELLS WITHIN MUCIN
- FIBROBLASTS NOT INCREASED

There are a number of endocrine disorders that affect the skin, many of which are rare, have indistinct histologic patterns, and are seldom biopsied. A good example is the diffuse hyperpigmentation that accompanies Addison disease. However, a relatively common disorder occasionally queried on pathology requisitions is the dermal mucinosis associated with hyperthyroidism (i.e., *pretibial myxedema*). These lesions occur on the anterior aspects of the legs as yellow, multinodular plaques with prominent follicular ostia (Fig. 19–6A). Lesions are usually associated with thyrotoxicosis, although they occasionally occur in euthyroid and even hypothyroid individuals. Histologically, scanning magnification reveals coalescent aggregates of pale blue-gray mucin primarily situated in the mid-dermis to deep dermis (Fig. 19–6B). At higher magnification (Fig. 19–6C), mucin is detected as thin, beaded strands separated by clear spaces resulting from retraction that occurs during tissue processing. Although the number of fibroblasts is not increased, stellate mesenchymal cells (i.e., muciblasts) may be identified within the dermal mucin.

It is important to differentiate pretibial myxedema from another form of dermal mucinosis, *lichen myxedematosus.* This condition is characterized by multiple, grouped, noncoalescent papules that preferentially affect skin of the face and upper extremities. When accompanied by induration and erythema of the involved skin, the condition is referred to as *scleromyxedema.* Unlike pretibial myxedema, lichen myxedematosus shows mucinous infiltration primarily in the superficial dermis rather than the mid-dermis and deep dermis (Fig. 19–7A). There is also a proliferation of benign fibroblasts within the foci of mucinosis (Fig. 19–7B), a feature that is most pronounced in the clinical variant called scleromyxedema. Nearly all patients with lichen myxedematosus and scleromyxedema have a circulating, highly basic, nonmyeloma, monoclonal IgG paraprotein, which in some individuals is associated with plasma cell hyperplasia in the bone marrow. The potential relation between this paraprotein and the production of superficial dermal mucin remains to be elucidated.

In addition to cutaneous manifestations of thyroid disease, other common endocrine manifestations in skin are predominated by lesions resulting from excessive steroid hormone stimulation. Glucocorticoids may be overproduced endogenously, as is the case in Cushing syndrome, or result

from iatrogenic administration internally or even topically. The gross pathology is so typical that biopsy is seldom required. The two most common presentations are *striae distentiae* and *steroid-induced acne.* Striae distentiae consist of erythematous, slightly depressed streaks (Fig. 19–8A), and steroid acne is manifested by multiple comedones that typically are synchronized at the same stage of clinical evolution (Fig. 19–8B). In these and most other forms of endocrine-induced cutaneous disease, the gross pathology is sufficient for generation of a presumptive diagnosis. Generalized myxedema due to hypothyroidism is seldom biopsied and usually fails to show striking abnormalities.

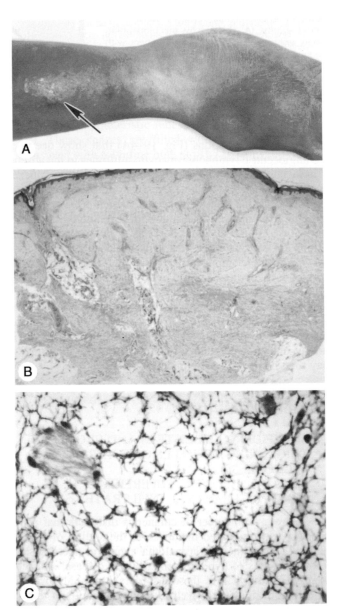

Figure 19–6. Pretibial myxedema: Thyrotoxicosis. (**A**) Nodular, yellow, waxy plaques with follicular prominence *(arrow)* are present on the anterior tibial skin of this patient, who has severe hyperthyroidism. (**B**) At scanning magnification, there is striking dermal thickening due to mucin deposition, which extends into the mid-dermis to deep dermis. (**C**) At high magnification, the mucin widely separates adjacent collagen bundles and appears as fine, branching strands.

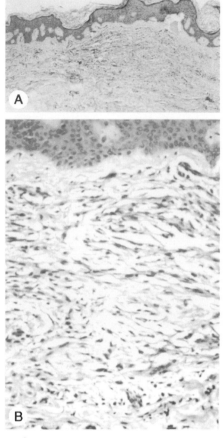

Figure 19–7. Lichen myxedematosus. (**A**) Associated with paraproteinemia, this disorder has large quantities of mucin in the upper dermis to mid-dermis. (**B**) However, unlike in pretibial myxedema, there is prominent associated proliferation of fibroblasts within the mucinous deposits in lichen myxedematosus.

Porphyria[10–12]

- SUBEPIDERMAL, NONINFLAMMATORY BLISTER
- EOSINOPHILIC, PERIODIC ACID–SCHIFF-POSITIVE DEPOSITS AROUND BLOOD VESSELS
- HOMOGENEOUS MANTLES OF IgG AND ALBUMEN AROUND AFFECTED VESSELS ON DIRECT IMMUNOFLUORESCENCE

There are a number of different forms of porphyria as defined according to clinical and biochemical parameters. These include erythropoietic porphyria, erythropoietic protophorphyria, porphyria variegata, porphyria cutanea tarda, acute intermittent porphyria, hepatoerythrocytic porphyria, and hereditary coproporphyria. Acute intermittent porphyria is the only form of porphyria that does not produce skin lesions. The most common form of porphyria seen by the dermatopathologist is the sporadic type of porphyria cutanea tarda, a disorder in which only the hepatic activity of uroporphyrinogen is decreased. Clinical lesions usually result when liver function is further compromised, as is the case in chronic alcoholics.

Clinically, sporadic porphyria cutanea tarda presents as blisters, shallow erosions, and scars occurring on sun-ex-

posed skin such as the face or the dorsae of the hands (Fig. 19–9A). At scanning magnification, there is a well-formed subepidermal blister with relative absence of associated dermal inflammation (Fig. 19–9B); porphyria and inherited forms of epidermolysis bullosa are the two noninflammatory subepidermal blisters. At higher magnification, small superficial vessels have characteristic hyalinized thickening of their walls (Fig. 19–9C). PAS stain reveals the affected vessels to be variably positive, and direct immunofluorescence of fresh-frozen tissue sections demonstrates glassy thickening of microvessels, which contain IgG, albumin, and occasionally C_3 within their thickened outer mantles (see Chap. 2). This immunofluorescence pattern is quite characteristic of porphyria and may be of assistance in separating this entity from others with subepidermal blisters associated with thickened superficial dermal microvessels, such as diabetic bullae.

Storage Diseases[13, 14]

- ROUTINE HISTOLOGY USUALLY NONSPECIFIC
- CYTOPLASMIC INCLUSIONS IN DERMAL CELLS OR ADNEXAL EPITHELIUM ON TRANSMISSION ELECTRON MICROSCOPY

Diagnostic work-up to exclude various storage disorders in infants and young children often involves skin biopsy

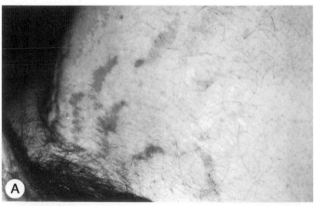

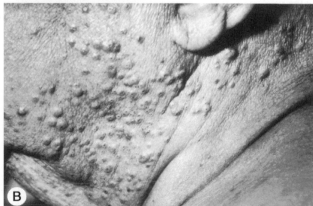

Figure 19–8. Gross pathological manifestations of glucocorticoid overproduction. (**A**) Striae distentia consist of erythematous, slightly depressed streaks, which show altered collagen bundles in biopsy specimens. (**B**) Steroid acne. Note that all lesions are synchronized with regard to evolutionary stage. Both of these manifestations are generally diagnosed based on clinical appearance alone.

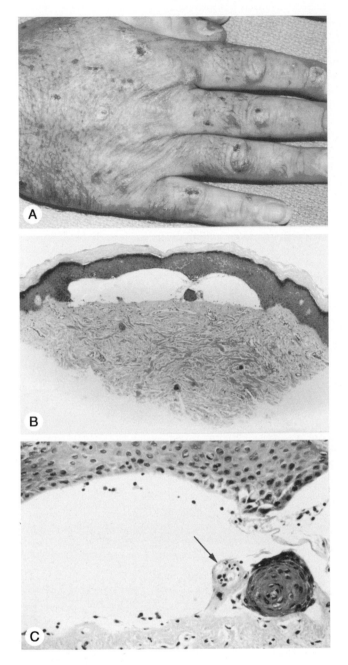

Figure 19–9. Porphyria cutanea tarda. (**A**) Small blisters and shallow erosions occur after sun exposure. (**B**) Scanning magnification reveals a noninflammatory subepidermal blister. (**C**) The blister base contains a rigid papilla *(arrow)* containing vessels with thickened walls. The walls are composed of glassy pink material which stains for albumin and immunoglobulin by direct immunofluorescence (see Chap. 2).

because of accessibility. However, routine histology is frequently noncontributory, and ultrastructural examination is required for detection of cytoplasmic storage deposits (Fig. 19–10A, B). Intracytoplasmic deposits may take the form of lipofuscin (i.e., fingerprint profiles), lipid vacuoles, lysosomes containing tubular structures, and laminated inclusions with defined periodicity. However, it may be difficult to differentiate lipid inclusions and autophagic vacuoles from true storage products, and the absence of positive findings does not exclude disease in view of the sampling problems inherent in electron microscopy and the tendency of skin in some forms of widespread storage disease to be unrevealing (e.g., Niemann-Pick disease).

Extracutaneous Malignancy[15, 16]

A number of markers for extracutaneous malignancy, such as the explosive onset of seborrheic keratoses, are discussed in other chapters (see Chap. 11). In this section, *acanthosis nigricans* and *necrolytic migratory erythema* are briefly addressed, because they represent intriguing and informative lesions of potential interest to the practicing dermatopathologist. Acanthosis nigricans consists of papillomatous brown plaques that generally affect intertriginous skin (Fig. 19–11A). Histologically, there is undulant papillomatosis formed by interdigitation between slightly hyperplastic epidermis and enlarged dermal papillae (Fig. 19–11B). The

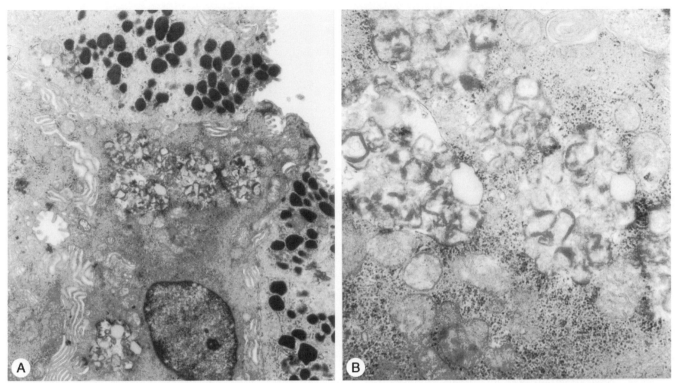

Figure 19–10. Storage disease: Lipofuscinosis. (**A**) Electron micrograph of the secretory portion of a dermal sweat gland shows collections of cytosomes near the apical portion of a lumenal cell. (**B**) At higher magnification (×20,000), these inclusions have fingerprint profiles compatible with lipofuscinosis. Although skin biopsy may occasionally be useful for ultrastructural detection of abnormal deposits in various metabolic storage disorders, the routine histology is seldom abnormal or informative.

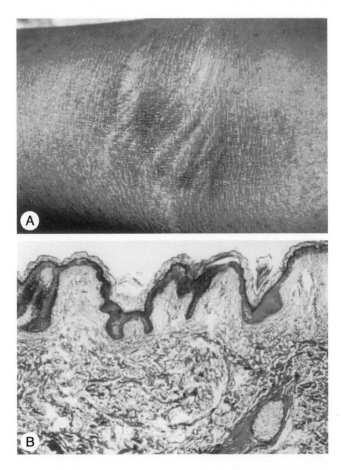

Figure 19–11. Early acanthosis nigricans. (**A**) A potential harbinger of internal malignancy or endocrine (e.g., pituitary) dysfunction, this disorder manifests as slightly verrucous, hyperpigmented plaques, often involving flexural and intertriginous skin. (**B**) Histologically, there is papillomatous epidermal and superficial dermal hyperplasia.

surface is covered by hyperorthokeratotic scale, and there generally is a diffuse increase in melanin pigment distributed within the cytoplasm of basal keratinocytes. Acanthosis nigricans may be idiopathic, inherited, associated with endocrine abnormalities, or a marker of internal malignancy. In the latter case, acanthosis nigricans may be associated with gastric carcinoma and Hodgkin and non-Hodgkin lymphoma, among other internal neoplasms, and skin lesions may be the first presenting sign of disease. It is believed that production of epidermal growth factors by tumor cells may be responsible for the development of acanthosis nigricans in the setting of malignancy.

Necrolytic migratory erythema, on the other hand, is an even more specific marker for internal neoplasia than acanthosis nigricans. Clinical lesions consist of cyclic, erythematous patches that become vesicular and edematous centrally. Skin of the legs and perioral and perineal regions is preferentially affected. Histologically, early lesions show edema and necrosis of the most superficial epidermal layers (i.e., upper one third). The clinical and histologic picture correlates with the presence of an alpha cell tumor of the pancreas (i.e., glucagonoma). Similar cutaneous histology may also be seen in certain vitamin-, mineral-, and essential amino acid–deficiency states, and it is now believed that the pathogenesis of lesions may involve hypoaminoacidemia as a result of excessive glucagon production.

Advanced Atherosclerosis[17, 18]

- INTIMAL PROLIFERATION AND LUMINAL OBLITERATION OF SMALL- TO MEDIUM-SIZED DERMAL ARTERIES
- DYSTROPHIC CALCIFICATION OF ARTERIAL WALLS
- INTRALUMINAL THROMBOEMBOLI CONTAINING CHOLESTEROL CLEFTS

Little is written in standard dermatopathology texts concerning the common event of severe atherosclerosis. In the skin, arterial ulcers, trophic alterations in acral skin and nails, livedo patterns of erythema, frank purpura, and zones of dermal atrophy and scarring are likely to be the result of at least focal occlusive atherosclerotic changes. The pattern of livedo reticularis is perhaps the best indicator of acute or chronic arterial insufficiency, although certain relatively young individuals devoid of significant vascular pathology may also show a similar pattern. Livedo reticularis refers to pink-blue, mottled, net-like discoloration, often involving skin of the lower extremities (Fig. 19–12A). Histologically, deep dermal arteries may show intimal proliferation with variable luminal obliteration, and occasionally, associated thrombus formation (Fig. 19–12B, C). Similar clinical lesions may occur acutely after insertion of a catheter into an aorta lined by friable atherosclerotic plaques. The resultant shower of cholesterol emboli produces microthrombi within cutaneous arterioles and arteries. These microthrombi characteristically contain crescent-shaped clear spaces indicative of cholesterol crystals. Emboli to the kidneys may result in

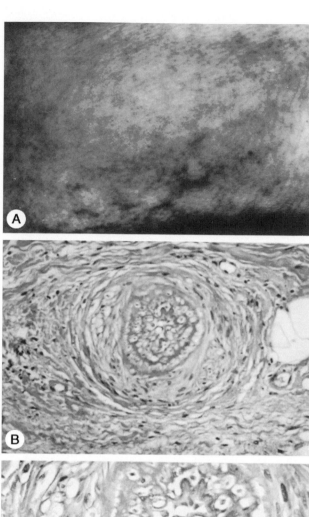

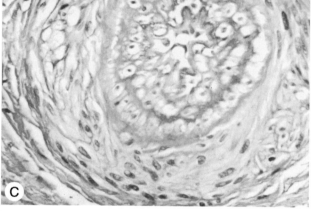

Figure 19–12. Systemic vascular disease: Livedo reticularis. (**A**) Net-like, mottled erythema of the lower extremity is typical of the clinical appearance of livedo reticularis. (**B, C**) In this case, obliterative intimal hyperplasia of medium-sized vessels was responsible. In other patients, thromboembolic disease may result in a similar pattern, particularly in the case of atheromatous emboli to the lower extremities.

the classic picture of acute renal failure associated with recent-onset, lower-extremity livedo reticularis. In this situation, a skin biopsy specimen may be extremely revealing with respect to the nature of life-threatening visceral dysfunction.

Hyperuricemia[19]

- AGGREGATES OF NEEDLE-SHAPED URATE CRYSTALS WITHIN DERMIS
- CRYSTALS TIGHTLY PACKED IN SHEAVES
- BIREFRINGENCE OF CRYSTALS ON POLAROSCOPY
- CRYSTALLINE AGGREGATES SURROUNDED BY FIBROSIS AND GRANULOMATOUS INFLAMMATION

Hyperuricemia refers to elevated blood levels of uric acid as a result of either increased metabolic production or decreased excretion. The clinical sequelae include bouts of painful arthritis and nodular deposits or urate crystals in skin and soft tissue (i.e., tophi). Most of the deposits involve skin overlying the elbows, finger and toe joints, and the helix of the ear (Fig. 19–13A). Tophi represent an additional disorder in which transepidermal elimination may take place (see Chap. 18).

Histologically, uric acid deposits are best appreciated in alcohol-fixed tissue specimens. At scanning magnification, there are coalescent nodules containing delicate, tightly-packed, needle-shaped, tan-brown crystals within the deep dermis and subcutaneous tissue (Fig. 19–13B). On closer inspection, the packed aggregates of crystals appear to form bundles or sheaves enclosed by mantles of fibrous tissue containing granulomatous foci replete with foreign-body–type giant cells (Fig. 19–13C). Examination of the crystals under polarized light reveals them to be characteristically doubly refractile (Fig. 19–13D). The possibility of gout should be entertained in formalin-fixed tissue in which similar stromal features are associated with entrapped aggregates of pale amorphous material, representing the destroyed

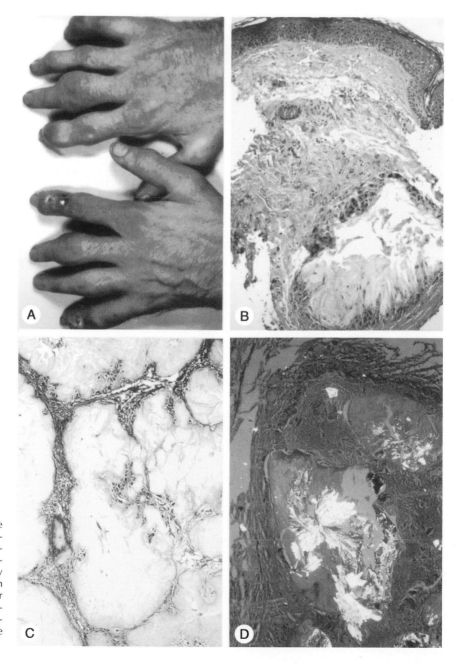

Figure 19–13. Hyperuricemia with tophi. (**A**) The proximal and distal interphalangeal joints are deformed by urate deposits (i.e., tophi). (**B, C**) In alcohol-fixed material, urate deposits are seen as aggregates of thin, needle-shaped crystals surrounded by a foreign-body giant cell response and fibrosis within the deep dermis. In **C,** the crystals are relatively clear and separated by trabeculae containing inflammatory cells. (**D**) Examination by polarization microscopy reveals characteristic birefringence in these otherwise nondescript regions.

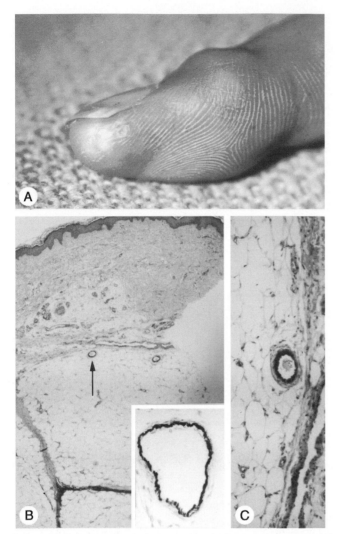

necrosis. An excellent example of dystrophic calcification occurs at sites of enzymatic fat necrosis in pancreatic disease (see Chap. 10), where saponified fat attracts calcium salts to the site of necrosis. Dystrophic calcification is often referred to as calcinosis cutis. Some examples are idiopathic, whereas others are associated with scleroderma, dermatomyositis, and rarely, lupus erythematosus. Clinically, dystrophic calcinosis cutis presents as a firm subcutaneous nodule with relatively normal overlying skin (Fig. 19–14A).

Metastatic calcinosis cutis, on the other hand, is the result of hypercalcemia due to primary and secondary hyperparathyroidism, excessive intake of calcium-containing substances or vitamin D, or destruction of bone due to carcinoma or infection. Both visceral and cutaneous calcinosis may be observed. Clinical lesions may appear as whitish papules, nodules, and small plaques. Histologically, a characteristic finding is mural calcification of arteries and arterioles within the dermis and subcutis (Fig. 19–14B, C). This pattern is especially suggestive of secondary hyperparathyroidism associated with renal failure. In other examples, particulate or nodular aggregates of calcium salts may be deposited in the dermis and subcutis. Although deposits characteristically appear as deep blue particles in routine stains, confirmation of their calcium content may be established with the von Kossa stain (see Fig. 19–14B, inset).

Figure 19–14. Dystrophic and metastatic calcification. (**A**) Firm, calcified dermal and subcutaneous nodules in a patient with scleroderma. This phenomenon is likely to result from dystrophic calcification of abnormal matrix elements. (**B**) Metastatic calcification of normal vessel walls in a patient with hypercalcemia due to hyperparathyroidism. The majority of involved vessels *(arrow)* are in the subcutaneous fat. Von Kossa stain for calcium confirms the nature of the deposit *(inset)*. (**C**) Higher magnification of an involved vessel; note the deposits in the vessel wall, indicating calcium salts.

residua of uric acid crystals. If gout is suspected, formalin fixative should be avoided and an alcohol-based fixative such as Carnoy solution substituted in its place.

Hypercalcemia[20]

- DEEP BLUE DEPOSITS IN DERMIS AND SUBCUTIS
- INVOLVEMENT OF VESSEL WALLS CONTAINING ELASTIC TISSUE
- GRANULOMATOUS RESPONSE TO LARGER DEPOSITS

Deposits of calcium within the dermis are either dystrophic or metastatic. Dystrophic deposits are not associated with hypercalcemia but rather with tissue degeneration and

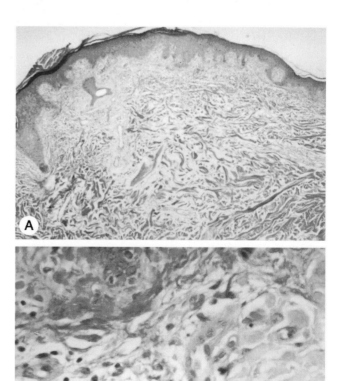

Figure 19–15. Systemic amyloidosis. (**A**) At scanning magnification, the epidermis is slightly hyperplastic, but definite pathology is difficult to detect. (**B**) Careful scrutiny at higher magnification reveals pale pink aggregates of amyloid *(arrow)* about superficial and deep dermal vessels and around adnexae. Amyloid restricted to dermal papillae, as is the case in lichenoid amyloidosis, is not detected.

Systemic Amyloidosis[21, 22]

- HOMOGENEOUS, PALE, EOSINOPHILIC DEPOSITS IN VESSEL WALLS
- DEPOSITS INVOLVE PERIADNEXAL ADVENTITIA
- PERIVASCULAR HEMORRHAGE
- AMYLOID DEPOSITION ABOUT ADIPOCYTES (AMYLOID RINGS)

Primary systemic amyloidosis is a fatal disease that is associated with often widespread infiltration of mesenchymal elements of skin and internal viscera. The condition is caused by plasma cell dyscrasia in the bone marrow, with overproduction of lambda light chains which in turn are transformed to the beta-pleated–sheet molecular structure of amyloid. Amyloid is deposited in muscle, in vessel walls, and about nerves in numerous organs, resulting in vascular compromise (i.e., myocardial insufficiency and infarction) and gastrointestinal bleeding. In the skin, waxy, hemorrhagic plaques or sites of traumatic purpura about the eyes and face may be observed. Plaques resembling morphea have also been described, and occasional lesions show bulla formation. Tongue involvement leading to macroglossia occurs in slightly less than one fifth of affected individuals.

Histologically, early lesions may be subtle, defying diagnostic assignment at scanning or intermediate magnification (Fig. 19–15A). On closer inspection, however, pale, eosinophilic, homogeneous deposits may be detected in vessel walls and in the vicinity of adnexal structures (Fig. 19–15B). As in localized forms of amyloidosis (see Chap. 18), the deposits are Congo red–positive and exhibit characteristic apple green birefringence when viewed with polarized light. Perivascular hemorrhage and sites of hemosiderin deposition are also commonly identified. Infiltration of the subcutaneous fat may produce an amyloid mesh that surrounds individual adipocytes, producing "amyloid rings." Advanced disease may result in nodular replacement of dermal collagen by aggregates of amorphous, pale amyloid disrupted by prominent crack-like fissures which may give rise to dermal blisters.

Hyperlipoproteinemia[23–25]

- DERMAL INFILTRATION BY FOAMY HISTIOCYTES
- CYTOPLASMIC VACUOLES INDENT NUCLEAR CONTOURS OF HISTIOCYTES

Although the histopathology of cutaneous xanthomas is relatively straightforward, the clinical implications of various clinicopathological entities are considerably more complex. There are six forms of hyperlipoproteinemia relevant to cutaneous pathology; each form is defined by the nature of the lipid abnormality in the serum. There are five clinical types of xanthoma: eruptive, tuberous, tendinous, and plane xanthomas and xanthelasmata. Table 19–1 provides an overview of the associations that exist between the biochemical groups and the clinical types of lesions.

Of the clinical variants of xanthomas, eruptive lesions are yellow papules that typically involve skin of the buttocks and posterior thighs. Tuberous xanthomas are plaques in-

Table 19–1. RELATION BETWEEN TYPE OF HYPERLIPOPROTEINEMIA AND CLINICAL TYPES OF XANTHOMA

BIOCHEMICAL ABNORMALITY	CLINICAL LESIONS
Type I: lipoprotein lipase deficiency (increased chylomicrons)	Eruptive
Type IIA: familial hypercholesterolemia	Tuberous, tendinous, and plane; xanthelasmata
Type IIB: mildly increased cholesterol and triglycerides; low density and very low density	Eruptive, tuberous, and tendinous
Type III: markedly increased cholesterol and triglycerides; low density and very low density	All 5 types of clinical lesions may occur
Type IV: primarily elevated triglycerides	Eruptive and tuberous
Type V: mixture of types I and IV	Eruptive

volving buttock, knee, elbow, and finger skin. Tendinous xanthomas infiltrate the Achilles tendon as well as tendons of the digits. Plane xanthomas affect skin folds such as the palmar creases. Xanthelasmata involve eyelid and periorbital skin.

Histologically, xanthomas all share the feature of dermal infiltration by pale, foamy histiocytes, sometimes clustered in loose, coalescent aggregates (Fig. 19–16A). On closer inspection, individual cells contain uniform round vacuoles that indent and scallop the nuclear contour (Fig. 19–16B), a

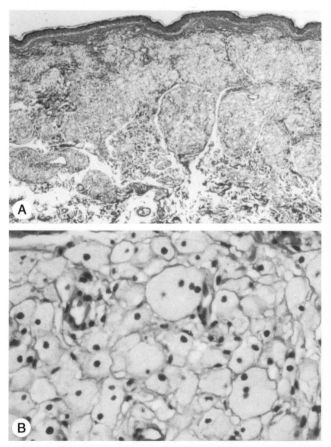

Figure 19–16. Xanthelasma. (**A**) There are nodular aggregates of foam cells in the superficial dermis and mid-dermis. (**B**) The cells have small, centrally located nuclei and abundant cytoplasm filled with small lipid vacuoles.

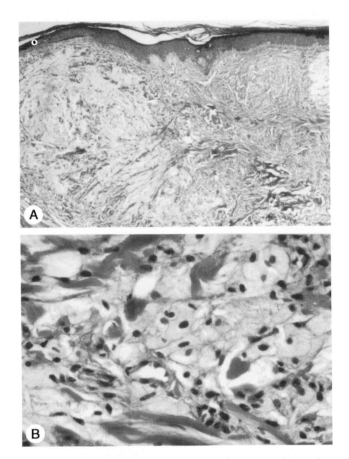

Figure 19–17. Tuberous xanthoma. (**A**) This relatively late lesion shows poorly aggregated clusters of lipidized histiocytes admixed with fibroblasts. (**B**) At higher magnification, the characteristic cytoplasmic vacuoles are apparent.

feature helpful in distinguishing lipid vacuoles from other forms of cytoplasmic vacuolization. Older lesions, particularly those of tuberous and tendonous xanthomas, may show an admixture of fibroblasts within the foam cell infiltrate (Fig. 19–17). Eruptive xanthomas frequently show a spectrum of vacuolated and relatively nonvacuolated histiocytes.

Rare Disorders

- NECROBIOTIC XANTHOGRANULOMA WITH PROTEINEMIA[26]
- LIPOID PROTEINOSIS (HYALINOSIS CUTIS ET MUCOSAE)[27]
- OCHRONOSIS[28]

Necrobiotic xanthogranuloma with paraproteinemia is a rare cutaneous manifestation associated with systemic disease which has received considerable recent attention. This condition presents clinically as indurated nodules and plaques involving truncal skin. Plaques are often covered by an atrophic epidermis, display telangiectasia, and may show focal ulceration. Periorbital and facial papules and plaques have also been described. Histologically, there is pale pink material (referred to as hyalin necrobiosis) within the superficial and deep dermis associated with granulomatous inflammation. The inflammatory infiltrate focally contains Touton

and foreign-body–type giant cells and may be associated with cholesterol clefts within the adjacent amorphous deposits. Serum evaluation usually reveals an associated light chain monoclonal gammopathy, and some of the affected individuals have overt multiple myeloma.

An equally rare and unusual disorder is *lipoid proteinosis*. This condition is inherited as an autosomal recessive trait and is characterized by cutaneous and mucosal (including laryngeal) deposition of hyalinized glycoproteins. Affected skin acquires a pebbly, pig skin–like appearance. Dysphonia may develop as a result of buccal and lingual infiltration, and some affected individuals also develop seizures. Histologically, there is deposition of eosinophilic hyaline in superficial vessel walls, which leads to characteristic encasement of vessels and adnexal epithelium within a hyalinized mantle (Fig. 19–18). The overlying epidermis often shows papillomatous hyperplasia. The deposits are PAS-positive and diastase-resistant. Autopsies of affected patients have revealed widespread hyaline deposits, and there may be cerebral involvement. Current evidence suggest that patients have an inherited defect resulting in increased fibroblast synthesis of noncollagenous proteins.

Finally, *ochronosis* is the abnormal accumulation of homogentisic acid in connective tissue, including joint cartilage, tendons and ligaments, sclerae, and skin. This defect is

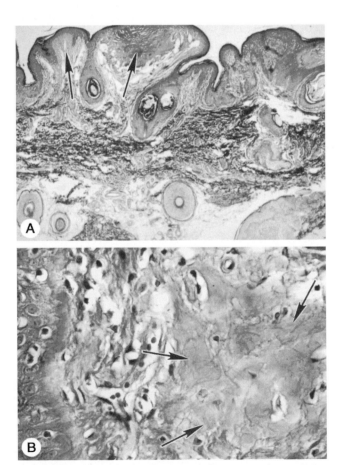

Figure 19–18. Lipoid proteinosis. (**A**) At low magnification, there is epidermal papillomatosis overlying deposits of hyaline-like material (*arrows*). (**B**) At higher magnification, this material consists of pale pink aggregates that are PAS-positive and diastase-resistant (*arrows*). Occasionally the material forms a mantle about blood vessels and adnexal epithelium.

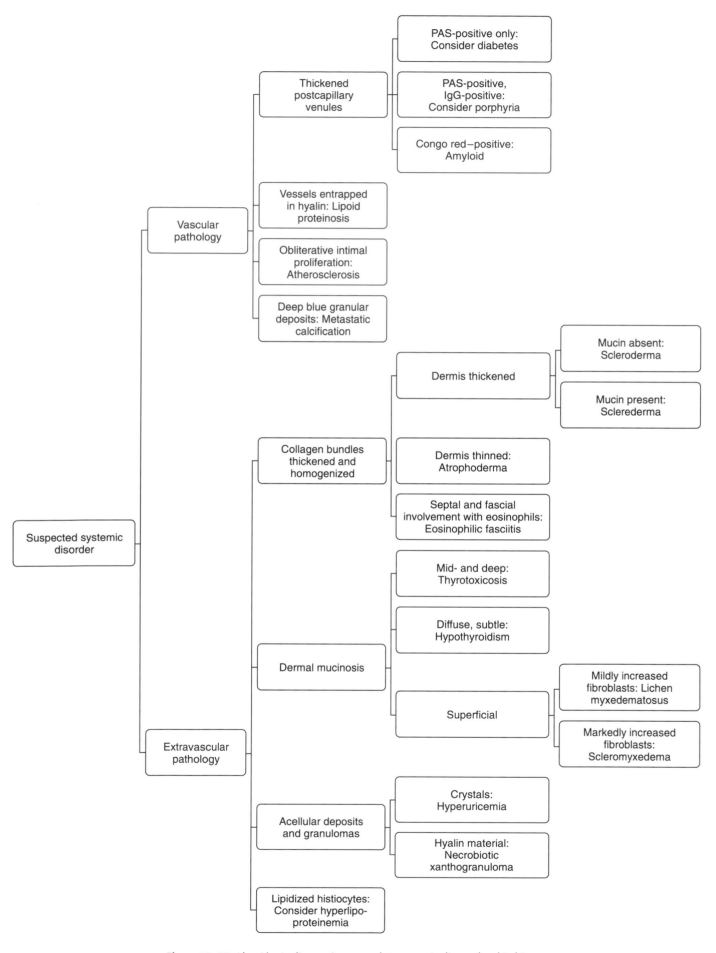

Figure 19–19. Algorithmic diagnostic approach to systemic disease by skin biopsy.

20
Dermatopathology of Hair

Christine Jaworsky

Hair is the end-product of an actively growing and cycling population of terminally differentiated cutaneous structures. Although the structure of hair is known, its exact function in humans is uncertain. It may provide protection from the environment, enhance tactile senses, and contribute to thermoregulation. For the most part, however, it seems to have cosmetic value as an adornment, as evidenced by the extensive demand for products that can stimulate hair growth and for procedures that minimize the appearance of hair loss.

STRUCTURE AND ANATOMIC VARIATIONS[1]

The structure of hair is generally the same throughout the body. The major components of hair are the outer root sheath, inner root sheath, hair shaft, and follicular bulb (Figs. 20–1 through 20–3). The outer root sheath is a modified extension of the epidermis that descends from the skin surface to the most deeply placed portion of the hair follicle, the bulb. The bulb is composed of the follicular papilla, a specialized condensation of connective tissue and vasculature, and follicular matrix keratinocytes. The follicular matrix contains germinative cells, which produce the inner root sheath and the hair shaft, which is centrally placed within the follicular canal. The outer root sheath forms an envelope that surrounds the inner root sheath and the hair shaft. The entire follicular unit is surrounded by a delicate mantle of fibrous tissue which holds an elaborate network of arterioles, venules, cutaneous nerves and resident perivascular mast cells,

monocytes, and T lymphocytes. The adventitial sheath is most easily seen in microscopic sections as a delicate band of fibrovascular tissue surrounding an anagen hair (see Fig. 20–3A) or as a collapsed tract trailing behind a telogen hair (see Fig. 20–3B). When a hair begins the anagen phase of its growth cycle, it descends through this tract into subcutaneous adipose tissue, where it normally resides for several years. The integrity of this support network in the adventitial sheath is crucial to normal functioning of the follicular unit. Interruption of the cycle, inflammation, or entrapment of hair in thickened collagen will likely compromise normal cycling and hair growth.

Although the structure of hair is similar throughout the body, its caliber and density vary among anatomic sites. For example, the scalp and body of the neonate are covered by small-caliber, miniature follicles with little or no pigment, known as vellus hairs. These hairs are eventually replaced by larger-caliber hairs, which are well-endowed with pigment, known as terminal hairs. In adults, vellus hairs can still be found in limited areas, such as the forehead, ears, and in women, the face. Knowing the normal distribution of hair throughout the body can provide clues to diagnosis. For example, finding vellus hairs in large number in a scalp biopsy of a man would suggest a diagnosis of male pattern baldness, or androgenetic alopecia.

HAIR CYCLING AND REGULATION[2–5]

A normal scalp has an average of 100,000 hairs, each of which cycles through three phases of growth (Table 20–

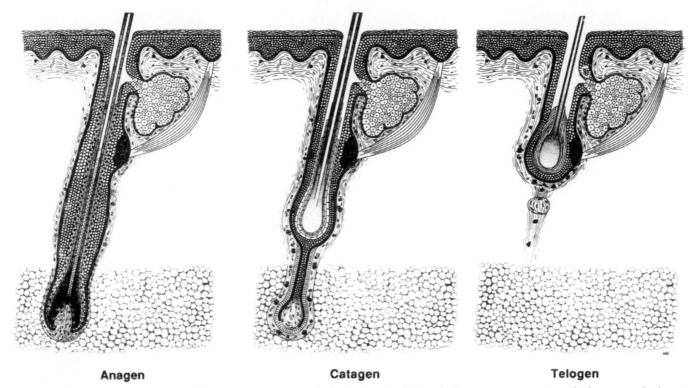

Anagen   **Catagen**   **Telogen**

Figure 20–1. Schematic representation of the major components of a hair and of the hair cycle (i.e., anagen, catagen, and telogen growth phases). (Courtesy of Michael Ioffreda, M.D.)

1). Approximately 85 to 90% of these hairs are actively growing (i.e., anagen), 1 to 2% are in transition from growing to resting phase (i.e., catagen), and 10 to 15% are in resting phase (i.e., telogen; see Figs. 20–1 and 20–2). Under normal circumstances, nearly 100 hairs are shed daily as they finish the growth cycle in telogen phase. In a scalp biopsy specimen, the growth phase of hair can be estimated by the location of the hair papilla: anagen hair has its papilla deeply placed within the subcutaneous adipose tissue (see Fig. 20–2A); catagen hair has its papilla located near the dermal-subcutaneous junction (see Fig. 20–2B); and telogen hair has its papilla within the reticular dermis (see Fig. 20–2C).

Two anatomic sites of the follicular unit are of particular interest in understanding hair cycling and inflammatory alopecias: the follicular papilla and the follicular bulge (see Fig. 20–1). It was once thought that cells that regulated hair growth and hair cycling resided in the follicular bulb, or more specifically, the hair matrix. More recent research indicates that the regulatory cells, known as follicular stem cells,

reside in a bulge in the follicular epithelium just below the junction of the follicle and its sebaceous duct. Follicular stem cells at this site appear to trigger a telogen hair follicle to restart anagen phase and the synthesis of a new hair shaft. Thus, the control site of hair growth is physically separate from the site of synthesis. This separation of function may provide clues to the pathophysiology of inflammatory alopecias. Inflammatory infiltrates centered around the follicular bulb, as in alopecia areata, produce a temporary loss of hair. Regeneration of the hair shaft often follows. By contrast, infiltrates around the follicular infundibular epithelium, as seen in lupus erythematosus, may injure the stem cells. If the injury is of sufficient severity or duration, it could result in irreparable damage to a hair follicle and loss of its regenerative capabilities. Permanent alopecia is often the result of lupus erythematosus in hair-bearing sites. Thus, the location of inflammatory infiltrates in alopecias may be indicators for estimating the outcome of hair loss.

GENERAL CLINICAL CONSIDERATIONS AND GROSS PATHOLOGY

Clinically, the threshold for perception of hair loss is strikingly variable from one individual to the next. One person may complain of excess loss when a few hairs are noticed in daily brushing, whereas another may dismiss pronounced shedding. In some individuals, hair loss is immediately apparent, whereas in others it is barely noticeable unless compared with earlier photographs. To a certain

Table 20–1. BASIC STATISTICS OF SCALP HAIR

CHARACTERISTIC	NORMAL VALUES
Number	100,000 hairs
Average shed	100 hairs/day
Rate of growth	0.35 mm/day, average of 2 mm/week, or 1 cm month
Cycling	
Anagen	1000 days (2–6 years); 85–90% of hair
Catagen	10 days (2–3 weeks); 1–2% of hair
Telogen	100 days (3 months); 10–15% of hair

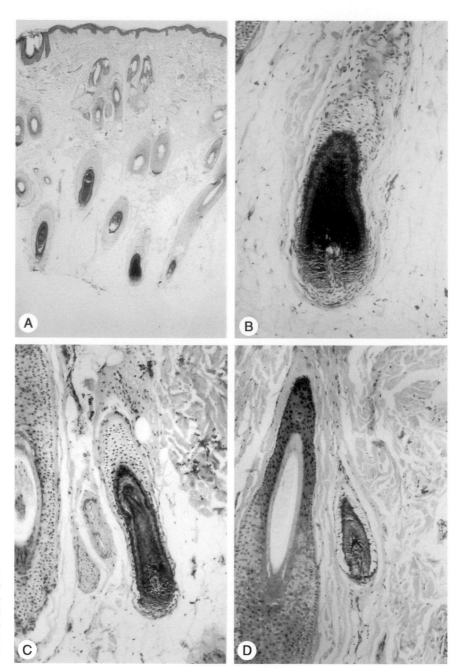

Figure 20–2. Phases of the normal hair cycle. **(A)** Normal hair density on the scalp. **(B)** Anagen hair in sections: The papilla is embedded deep in the subcutaneous adipose tissue. **(C)** Hair in transition to catagen growth phase: The hair papilla ascends to the dermal-subcutaneous junction. **(D)** Telogen hair in sections have their papillae entirely within dermal stroma.

degree, the texture and color of hair alter the perception of hair loss. For example, curly hair masks areas of thinning much more efficiently than straight hair. In a similar manner, thinning is less apparent when there is less contrast between scalp skin color and hair color (i.e., thinning in a fair-skinned individual with blonde hair is less noticeable than it is in a fair-skinned individual with black hair).

Once the diagnosis of alopecia is made, many different factors must be evaluated to determine its cause. Evaluations include an estimate of the duration of the loss, assessment of the general health and hormonal status of the patient, and family history of hair loss. Equally important considerations are the distribution of hair loss (scalp, body, or both), localization (discrete areas versus diffuse loss), associated symp-

toms (e.g., pruritus, burning), and signs (erythema, scaling, induration and discharge).

Initial diagnostic tests may include a hair pluck (i.e., extracting a small group of hairs to examine under the microscope), potassium hydroxide preparations to exclude fungal infection, hair culture, blood tests, and scalp biopsy. The utility of a scalp biopsy depends on the nature of the presenting complaint and the findings on physical examination. An adequate scalp biopsy specimen is at least a 4 mm punch biopsy that includes subcutaneous fat, which is where follicular bulbs of anagen follicles can be evaluated.

Two different methods of studying scalp biopsy specimens have been advocated in the literature. One is the customary vertical section, which is oriented with the epidermal

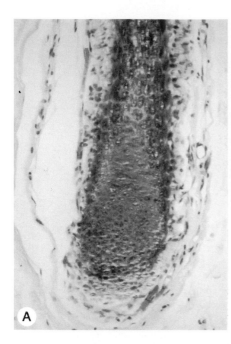
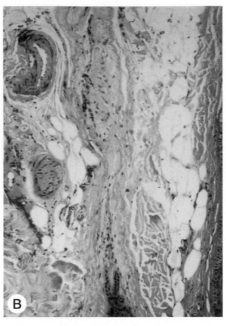

Figure 20–3. Perifollicular adventitial sheath. **(A)** This delicate fibrovascular envelope surrounding the hair follicle carries a complex vascular network and resident mononuclear cells and mast cells. **(B)** Collapsed adventitial sheath appears as a fibrous streamer left behind in the path of a hair in telogen growth phase.

surface at one pole and subcutaneous fat at the opposite pole. The other is the horizontal section, which allows examination of tissue planes parallel to the epidermal surface and shows folliculosebaceous units at various levels in different sections. Because conventional vertical sections are most frequently used, and special expertise is necessary to interpret horizontal sections, the material presented in this chapter is illustrated with vertical sections.

HISTOLOGY OF SPECIFIC DISORDERS

Hair Breakage and Fragility

When history or physical examination show that there is breakage of hair shafts, diagnostic considerations include improper care, overprocessing, traumatic alopecia, tinea capitis, exposure to systemic toxins (e.g., chemotherapeutic agents), and hair shaft abnormalities. Often, the patient history clarifies the cause. For example, patients with hair shaft defects often note fragility of hair early in life and may have short hair on the scalp as well as elsewhere on the body. Patients with exogenous causes of alopecia often have a recent history of chemical application or drug ingestion. In instances in which the history or initial evaluation fail to provide adequate information, scalp biopsy specimens can be of value in establishing the cause (Table 20–2).

Hair Shaft Abnormalities[6, 7]

A variety of hair shaft abnormalities may cause fragility and breakage of hair. The most common abnormalities in-

Table 20–2. HAIR BREAKAGE

DISORDER	CAUSES	SPECIFIC AGENTS	CLINICAL APPEARANCE	HISTOLOGY
Hair shaft abnormalities	Trichorrhexis nodosa Trichorrhexis invaginata Pili torti Monilethrix		Fragile, broken hair with or without alopecia	Paint brushes on end Bamboo hair Twisted hair Beaded hair
Improper care, overprocessing	Improperly applied chemicals and physical agents	Permanent wave solutions, curling irons	Burns, ulcers anywhere on scalp	Epithelial and/or dermal necrosis, mixed inflammation
Traumatically induced alopecia	Excess tension in styling	Curlers and curling irons	Receding hairlines, widened parts	Hair casts, perifollicular hemorrhage, pigment incontinence, variable scarring
	Trichotillomania	Self-inflicted	Irregular patches of complete hair loss	
Tinea capitis	Ectothrix	Microsporum audouinii, ferruginium, canis, distortum	Erythematous patches and/or plaques with hair loss	Spores and/or hyphae penetrate outer layers of hair shaft
	Endothrix	Trichophyton tonsurans, violaceum, schönleinii	Broken hair at follicular ostia, black dots	Spores and/or hyphae penetrate cortex
Chemotherapy-induced	Antimetabolites	Methotrexate, 5-fluorouracil, 6-mercaptopurine	80–90% hairs break off 1–3 weeks after chemotherapy	All hair broken at similar length
	Alkylating agents	Nitrogen mustard, Leukeran, Cytoxan		
	Other	Actinomycin D, vinblastine, colchicine		

clude trichorrhexis nodosa, trichorrhexis invaginata, pili torti, and monilethrix. The syndrome associations of these disorders are beyond the scope of this chapter but are well discussed elsewhere.

Trichorrhexis Nodosa

- SPLAYING OF THE CORTEX AT MULTIPLE SITES ALONG THE LENGTH OF THE HAIR SHAFT

The most common hair shaft abnormality is trichorrhexis nodosa, which roughly translated means ruptured hair with node-like changes. This defect occurs in a sporadic or familial form; it may be either acquired or congenital. Characteristically, patients notice that their hair breaks off at a short distance from the scalp. In addition, hair may have a beaded appearance which may be confused clinically with nit infestation (Fig. 20–4A). Patients with the congenital form of this hair shaft disorder may have other ectodermal defects or be mentally retarded in association with an inborn error of metabolism (e.g., arginosuccinic aciduria).

Microscopic examination shows splaying of the hair cortex along the length of the hair shaft, which mimics the appearance of the bristles of two paint brushes pushed into each other (Fig. 20–4B). Similar changes at the distal ends of hair usually indicate weathering of hair and are not diagnostic of trichorrhexis nodosa.

Trichorrhexis Invaginata

- INVAGINATIONS ALONG THE LENGTH OF THE HAIR SHAFT WITH A BALL-AND-SOCKET ARRANGEMENT

Trichorrhexis invaginata, another hair shaft defect associated with hair fragility, appears early in life and may affect all body hair. Clinically affected patients have lusterless, short hair that breaks easily, especially in areas of friction.

Microscopically, abnormal invaginations along the

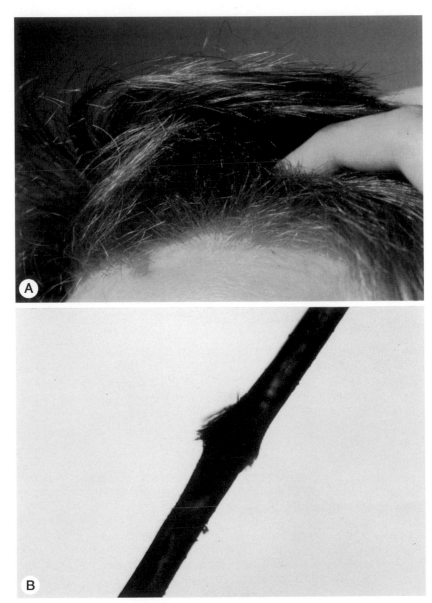

Figure 20–4. Trichorrhexis nodosa. **(A)** Clinical appearance of scalp hair in a patient with trichorrhexis nodosa. Note the beaded appearance of the hair shafts. **(B)** Along the hair shaft, there are zones of splaying of the hair cortex, similar to two paint brushes being pushed together at their bristle ends.

length of the hair shaft mimic the appearance of bamboo (Fig. 20–5A). The nodes or invaginations have a ball-and-socket arrangement, with the socket located proximal to the hair bulb.

Pili Torti

- TWISTS OF THE HAIR SHAFT AT IRREGULAR INTERVALS

Pili torti, or twisted hair, is usually noticeable by the age of 2 years as abnormally brittle and fragile hair, which breaks easily and is therefore short. This hair shaft defect occurs in several autosomal dominant forms with associated ectodermal defects, including auditory deficits and mental deficiency. It may occur also in an X-linked recessive form associated with a defect in copper metabolism (i.e., Menke kinky-hair syndrome), which eventuates in death by 3 years of age.

Microscopically, pili torti hair shafts are flat and have clusters of several twists along the shaft length distributed in irregular intervals (Fig. 20–5B). If there is doubt regarding the diagnosis, scanning electron microscopy can be used to show abnormal overlapping of the cuticle as compared with normal hair.

Monilethrix

- ALTERNATING SWELLINGS AND CONSTRICTIONS AT REGULAR INTERVALS ALONG THE LENGTH OF THE HAIR SHAFT

Monilethrix, or beaded hair, can also be a cause of hair breakage. The hair of the face, axilla, pubis, and extremities can be affected and appear brittle and lusterless. The scalp may appear bald because of hair breakage.

Histologically, the hair appears to undulate. There are alternating swellings and constrictions along the length of the hair shaft at intervals of approximately 0.7 to 1.0 mm (Fig. 20–5C). The swellings contain a medulla, whereas the constrictions do not; thus, the constrictions are the points of weakness and breakage.

Processing[8]

- EPITHELIAL NECROSIS WITH OR WITHOUT DERMAL NECROSIS
- IF EXTENSIVE, ULCERATION MAY BE PRESENT
- NEUTROPHILS IN ADJACENT STROMA
- LATE: GRANULATION TISSUE IF DERMAL INJURY OCCURRED
- SUPPORTIVE HISTORY AND CLINICAL APPEARANCE

The application of chemical agents (e.g., hair dyes, permanent solutions, straightening solutions) or physical agents (e.g., hot combs, curling irons, hot oils) to the scalp may result in injury and breakage of hair shafts. Burns or sharply localized erythema delimited by the hairline are characteristic findings that indicate overprocessing or improper hair-styling habits. The history usually includes burning or stinging sensations when the chemical was applied. Hair fragility or scalp

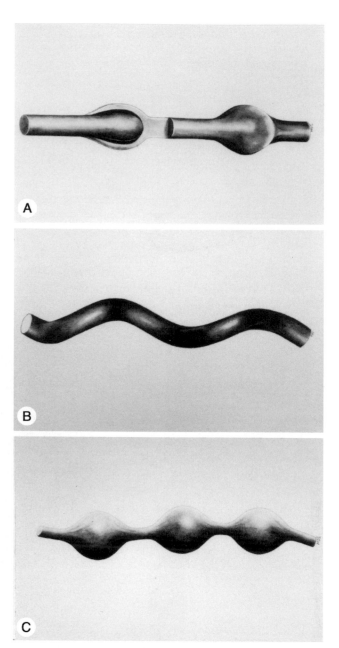

Figure 20–5. Abnormalities of the hair shaft. **(A)** Trichorrhexis invaginata: Hairs have invaginations along their shafts which have the appearance of a ball-and-socket. **(B)** Pili torti: Multiple twists at irregular intervals occur along the hair shaft. **(C)** Monilethrix: Hair shafts have a beaded appearance. (Courtesy of Michael Ioffreda, M.D.)

damage are closely related in time to the application of the chemical or physical agent.

Because the history usually confirms clinical suspicions, biopsies are done only on rare occasions. In such instances, biopsy specimens show nonspecific changes such as epithelial and dermal necrosis with ulcer formation. Neutrophilic inflammatory infiltrates can be found in intact epithelium and adjacent stroma when irritation or ulceration has occurred. Late changes may include granulation tissue, scar formation, or both. The extent, depth, and chronicity of injury determine whether or not hair can regenerate.

Traction Alopecia and Trichotillomania[9–12]

- TRICHOMALACIA: CORKSCREW HAIR SHAFTS AND PIGMENT CASTS WITHIN FOLLICULAR CANALS
- HEMOSIDERIN DEPOSITS FROM PERIFOLLICULAR HEMORRHAGE
- MELANIN INCONTINENCE
- VARIABLE PERIFOLLICULAR FIBROSIS

Traumatically induced alopecias include traction alopecia and trichotillomania. These two disorders can usually be separated clinically by the distribution of hair breakage or loss.

Traction alopecia results from chronic styling maneuvers that place excess tension on the hair shaft. Avulsion of hair shafts by this means eventuates in pronounced shortening of hair shafts closest to the site of greatest tension and lesser shortening in areas of lesser tension. Application of chronic tension, as in tight curling or braiding, results in clinically apparent gradients within widened parts and recession of the frontoparietal, postauricular, or occipital hairlines (Fig. 20–6A, B). The chronic downward pull of excessively long hair causes recession of the frontal hairline. Traction alopecia is seen almost exclusively in female patients. Even when patients are made aware that their practices are causing the hair loss, they often fail to modify these deeply ingrained habits.

Trichotillomania is self-inflicted avulsion of hair in patients with psychologic disturbances. This condition is independent of styling procedures. These manipulations result in patches of broken hairshafts in areas with partial or complete hair loss. Bizarre patterns of hair loss in the scalp should arouse suspicion of trichotillomania.

Early in the course of both of these processes, clinical

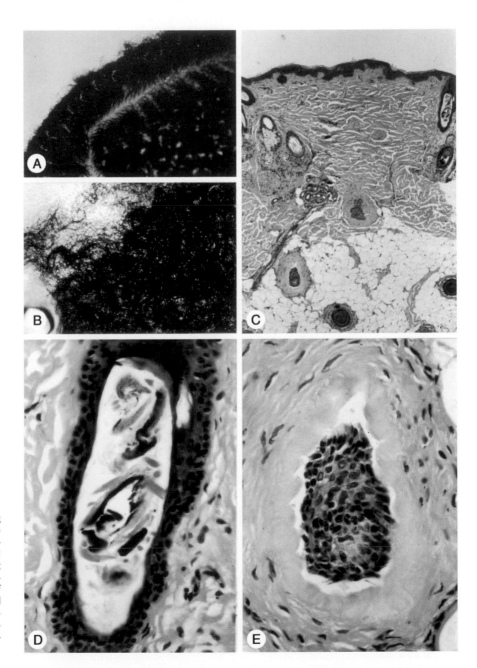

Figure 20–6. Traumatic alopecia. **(A)** Widening of parts occurs as a result of chronic tension. **(B)** The marginal hairline recedes: Greatest shortening of hair shafts occurs at the point of maximal tension (occiput to the right in this recumbent patient, anterior hairline in the upper left of photograph). **(C)** There is prominent thickening of perifollicular adventitial sheaths and an isolated hair cast in a follicular infundibulum. **(D)** Corkscrew hair and hair cast are located in the follicular infundibulum. **(E)** Fibrosis of the perifollicular sheath.

diagnostic considerations may include androgenetic alopecia, fungal infection, or alopecia areata. In such cases, scalp biopsy is useful not only to exclude these possibilities but also to confirm suspicions of trauma.

Histologic findings in traumatically induced alopecias include corkscrew hairs and pigment casts in follicular canals (Fig. 20–6C, D). These changes are known as trichomalacia (i.e., sick hairs), and they occur on the basis of applied tension; as the hair shaft breaks along its length, the unavulsed lower half recoils within the canal and assumes a contorted appearance. The mechanical stresses cause clumping of melanin in the traumatized shaft. Perifollicular hemorrhage or hemosiderin deposition occur from avulsion of the hair shaft. Melanin incontinence and perifollicular fibrosis may be seen as well (Fig. 20–6E).

Although extraction of hair shafts alone will not cause permanent hair loss, repeated trauma to the hair bulb and inflammation of the surrounding stroma causes local aberrations, which over time result in the inability to regenerate a normal hair follicle. Thus, with chronicity, both traction alopecia and trichotillomania may result in complete loss of follicular structures and reticular dermal fibrosis, which are indicative of permanent alopecia.

Fungal Infections[13–16]

- PERIFOLLICULAR INFLAMMATORY INFILTRATES, USUALLY WITH A NEUTROPHILIC COMPONENT OF VARIABLE INTENSITY
- EXAMINE STRATUM CORNEUM AND HAIR SHAFTS CAREFULLY FOR SPORES AND HYPHAE

Broken hair shafts are often found with fungal infections of the scalp. Fungi weaken the structural integrity of hair shafts as they grow within them. If the fungi invade the hair medulla, they cause the hair to break as it exits onto the scalp, giving the appearance of black dots studding the affected surface. This finding is a clinical clue to endothrix fungal infection, in which Trichophyton tonsurans and Trichophyton violaceum are common culprits. Fungi may also invade the outer layers of the hair shaft (i.e., ectothrix infection). The affected areas may be only slightly scaly and erythematous or studded with pustules and abundant scale. The degree of hair loss is variable. Clinical diagnostic maneuvers may include a Wood light examination, because some fungi will fluoresce; potassium hydroxide preparation of affected hair shafts; hair culture; and scalp biopsy.

Microscopically, the presence of infection is usually heralded by neutrophils adjacent to or within affected hair follicles: they may form sparse collections or coalesce to form abscesses. Usually, there is an admixture of lymphocytes and histiocytes. Plasma cells usually indicate chronicity of infection. Careful scrutiny of the hair shafts and stratum corneum will usually disclose the presence of fungal elements. A helpful maneuver is to lower the position of the substage condenser of the microscope to increase refractility in the tissue and allow identification of fungi within these structures. Fungal stains (e.g., periodic acid–Schiff or silver stains) are used to confirm the diagnosis of fungal infection. Localizing spores to the outer cuticle or medulla may suggest

a narrower spectrum of fungal organisms (i.e., ectothrix versus endothrix); however, for specific identification of the causative organism, culture is essential.

Cytotoxic Drugs[17–19]

- SHAFT CONSTRICTIONS AT SAME LEVEL OF NEARLY ALL HAIRS

Exposure to chemotherapeutic agents, particularly antimetabolites and alkylating agents, may induce breakage of 80 to 90% of hairs 1 to 3 weeks after a therapeutic cycle. Breakage of hairs at similar lengths indicates a synchronized arrest in the growth cycle of all of the involved hairs, and widespread distribution suggests a systemic insult. These changes are reversible with discontinuation of the drugs.

The temporal relation of profound hairloss to medication intake usually makes the cause of this alopecia obvious. Biopsies in these instances are rarely performed. Constrictions of the hair shaft at the same level of nearly all hair shafts indicate a synchronous injury to the hair follicles.

Folliculitis

Folliculitis is a generic term that refers to inflammation of the hair follicle but does not ascribe a cause. Folliculitis may be caused by infectious agents such as bacteria, fungi, spirochetes, or viruses. Folliculitis also may arise on a noninfectious basis, as in eosinophilic pustular folliculitis, follicular mucinosis, and folliculitis decalvans.

Bacterial Folliculitis[20]

- ACUTE: NEUTROPHILIC INFLAMMATORY INFILTRATES IN AND AROUND HAIR FOLLICLES
- CHRONIC: LYMPHOCYTES AND PLASMA CELLS ADMIXED; PERIFOLLICULAR FIBROSIS
- INFLAMMATION BELOW THE LEVEL OF SEBACEOUS DUCT FREQUENTLY RESULTS IN INABILITY OF HAIR TO REGENERATE

Discrete, 1 to 5-mm pustules surrounding a central hair are characteristic of bacterial folliculitis. Culture of the purulent material usually yields Staphylococcus aureus. Hot, tender nodules (i.e., furuncles) occur when the infection descends deep into the hair follicle. Large, hot, tender nodules with discharge from several hair follicles (i.e., carbuncles) may be accompanied by systemic symptoms such as fever. Permanent hair loss may result from furuncles and carbuncles but does not occur as a result of superficial folliculitis.

Microscopically, bacterial folliculitis shows a subcorneal pustule in the ostium of a hair follicle. There may be disruption of follicular epithelium and perifollicular fibrosis (Fig. 20–7A, B). Bacterial stains may disclose the presence of gram-positive cocci surrounded by neutrophils, but they are not always revealing. Culture of the purulent material is optimal to establish a bacterial role in folliculitis. The deeper the inflammation in follicular epithelium, in particular beneath the attachment of the sebaceous gland to the follicular epithelium, the greater the likelihood of permanent hair loss.

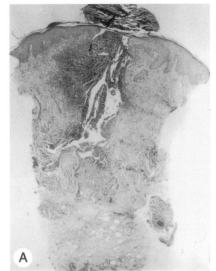

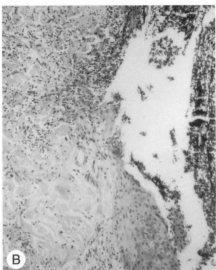

Figure 20–7. Furuncle. **(A)** A dermal abscess surrounds a disrupted hair follicle along its length. **(B)** An intense, neutrophilic, inflammatory infiltrate completely disrupts portions of the follicular epithelium.

Fungal Folliculitis[21]

Patchy zones of hair loss with scaling should arouse suspicion of the possibility of fungal infection (Fig. 20–8A). Fungal growth in the hairs weakens them and causes breakage (see Breakage and Fragility). The degree of grossly appreciable erythema varies with the host response to infection and is extremely variable. An intense inflammatory response is seen in kerion, in which there are perifollicular pustules accompanied by boggy induration of the scalp. This process frequently leads to grossly appreciable scarring and permanent alopecia.

Ectothrix or Endothrix Infection

- BUDDING YEASTS AND/OR BRANCHING HYPHAE IN OR SURROUNDING HAIR SHAFTS
- VARIABLE INFLAMMATORY INFILTRATES, USUALLY WITH A NEUTROPHILIC COMPONENT
- PERIFOLLICULAR FIBROSIS IN LATE LESIONS WHERE INFLAMMATION WAS INTENSE

Budding spores and septate or branching hyphae in hair shafts are the histologic hallmark of fungal infection of hair (Fig. 20–8B). Dermatophyte organisms are found in the keratinized portion of the hair shaft; they do not grow in living tissue. The presence of neutrophilic aggregates or abscesses surrounding the follicular epithelium should trigger a search for infectious organisms, which includes special stains for fungi (Fig. 20–9A, B). With chronicity, the infiltrates will be admixed with lymphocytes, histiocytes, and plasma cells. If the follicular epithelium ruptures, multinucleated giant cells can be found around affected hair follicles as well. Perifollic-

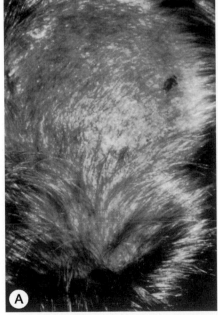

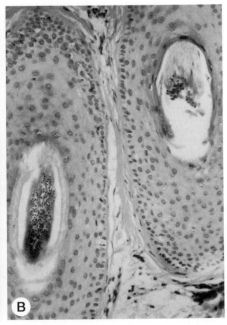

Figure 20–8. Tinea capitis. **(A)** Pronounced breakage and hair loss have resulted from fungal infection. The erythema and scaling seen here may be absent in some cases. **(B)** There are large numbers of basophilic spores in hair shafts, with only sparse dermal inflammatory infiltrates.

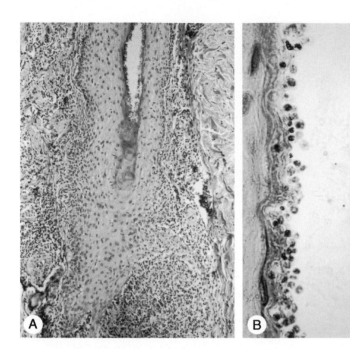

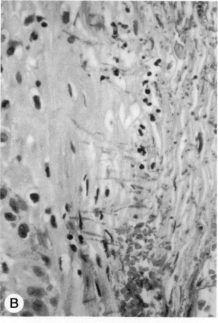

Figure 20–9. Inflammatory tinea capitis. (A) The perifollicular abscess is composed of large numbers of neutrophils. (B) Higher magnification of A shows large numbers of spores in the follicular canal.

ular fibrosis frequently ensues when inflammation is intense and disrupts the follicular epithelium. Although in general, *Trichophyton* species cause endothrix infection (Fig. 20–10A), both *Trichophyton* and *Microsporum* species can cause ectothrix infection (Fig. 20–10B). Definitive identification of the causative organism relies on culture.

Pityrosporum Folliculitis

- FOLLICULAR OSTIA WITH CLUSTERS OR CHAINS OF BASOPHILIC SINGLE-BUDDING YEAST FORMS

Single-budding *Pityrosporum* yeasts are approximately 2 to 4 mm in diameter and are commonly found in clusters and chains in follicular ostia and the adjacent stratum corneum. These organisms may occasionally cause inflammation of the follicular epithelium, known as *Pityrosporum* folliculitis. The lack of hyphae, presence of single buds, and location of organisms in ostia and periosteal stratum corneum are clues to this diagnosis. The yeast is easily visible in routine sections as a basophilic structure that stands out on the background of eosinophilic stratum corneum. Fungal stains will highlight the presence of the yeast. To exclude the possibility of *Candida* folliculitis, culture of the affected area is optimal.

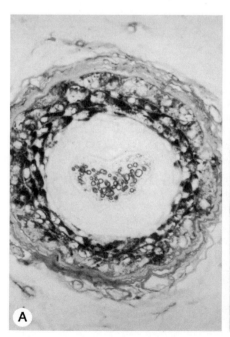

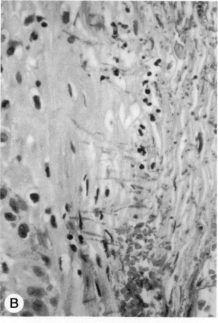

Figure 20–10. Endothrix and ectothrix infection. (A) In endothrix infection, spores are found in the center of the hair shaft (periodic acid–Schiff stain). (B) In ectothrix infection, branching hyphae can be seen traversing follicular epithelium and entering adjacent dermal stroma (hematoxylin and eosin stain).

Syphilitic Alopecia[22, 23]

- LYMPHOPLASMACYTIC INFLAMMATORY INFILTRATE WITH VARIABLE HISTIOCYTIC COMPONENT
- COMMONLY INFILTRATES INVOLVE THE EPIDERMIS AND HAIR FOLLICLES (LICHENOID); PERIVASCULAR INFILTRATE MAY OR MAY NOT HAVE AN INTERSTITIAL COMPONENT

Although hair loss associated with syphilis infection may be diffuse and generalized (e.g., scalp, face, axillae, pubis), more characteristically, syphilis produces ill-defined patches of partial alopecia that gives the scalp a moth-eaten appearance. This usually occurs in the secondary stage of infection, when other cutaneous lesions, such as ham-colored macules on the palms and soles and split papules around facial orifices, may be apparent as well. At this stage of infection, serologic tests are usually positive for syphilis. Alopecia may also accompany the tertiary stage of syphilis.

The composition and architecture of the inflammatory infiltrate provide important diagnostic clues in making the diagnosis of syphilis (Fig. 20–11A, B). The constant participation of plasma cells and involvement of blood vessels, nerves, and epithelia (i.e., epidermis and hair follicles) should prompt suspicion of treponemal infection. Occasionally, the infiltrate may have an admixture of epithelioid histiocytes and multinucleated giant cells, which gives the infiltrate a granulomatous appearance. Nonetheless, plasma cell participation and lichenoid distribution of the infiltrate should trigger a search for spirochetes with silver stains (e.g., Dieterle stains) and confirmation of the diagnosis with serologic studies.

Viral Folliculitis[24, 25]

Herpes Simplex and Herpes Zoster

- EARLY: KERATINOCYTES PALE, WITH WINDBLOWN APPEARANCE
- MULTINUCLEATION OF KERATINOCYTES, OCCASIONALLY EOSINOPHILIC CYTOPLASMIC INCLUSIONS
- INTRAEPIDERMAL VESICLE FORMATION
- LATE: EPITHELIAL AND DERMAL NECROSIS
- INFLAMMATION EXTENDS DEEPER INTO THE DERMIS IN HERPES ZOSTER THAN IN HERPES SIMPLEX
- HERPES ZOSTER ALSO SHOWS PERINEURAL INFLAMMATION AND A LYMPHOCYTIC VASCULITIS

Although herpes infection is not commonly thought of as a follicular process, the earliest microscopic changes of infection are often seen in the follicular epithelium. Clinically, both herpes simplex and zoster may be presaged by pain or tingling at the site of the eruption. Early lesions appear as small groups of vesicles on erythematous bases. Most often, these lesions have a localized distribution; on occasion (e.g., in atopic dermatitis or an immunocompromised host), they may have a generalized pattern. Herpes zoster characteristically arises as a painful vesicular eruption with a dermatomal distribution. Scrapings of intact vesicles (i.e., Tzanck smear) will often show multinucleated keratinocytes with nuclear molding, indicative of herpes virus infection.

The earliest change of herpetic infection is a windblown appearance of keratinocytes of the follicular epithelium and adjacent epidermis (Fig. 20–12A, B). Keratinocytes become pale and slightly disordered, whereas their nuclear membranes become thickened. Subsequently, keratinocytes become multinucleated and show molding of one nucleus against the other, as if they were being compressed by a limiting outer rim. Occasionally, cells contain small, pink, eosinophilic inclusions as well. As more cells are affected by viral infection, keratinocytes lose cohesiveness and form blisters. After necrosis of keratinocytes ensues, viral cytopathic changes become difficult to find. In herpes zoster infection, the inflammation is intense, and it extends deeper into the reticular dermis than that of herpes simplex infection. In

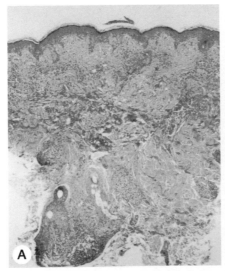
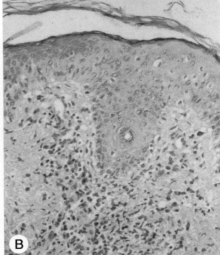

Figure 20–11. Secondary syphilis. **(A)** Low magnification shows a perivascular, perifollicular, lichenoid inflammatory infiltrate. **(B)** High magnification discloses a lymphoplasmacytic infiltrate with occasional histiocytes that infiltrates epithelium. Special stains revealed the presence of spirochetes.

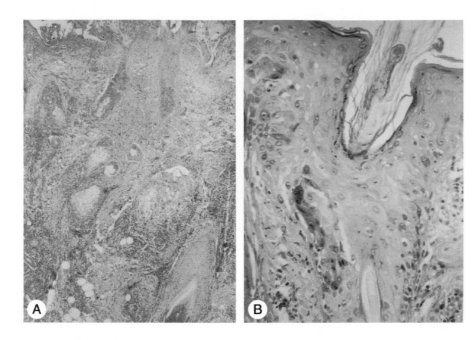

Figure 20–12. Herpes zoster of the scalp. **(A)** There are broad zones of epidermal and superficial follicular necrosis. Note the depth of the inflammatory infiltrate. **(B)** Follicular keratinocytes acquire a windblown, disarrayed appearance. Note the early formation of multinucleated keratinocytes with nuclear molding. These changes are characteristic of the herpes virus cytopathic effect.

addition, perineural inflammation is frequent and may account for the symptom of pain that often accompanies herpes zoster infection. In addition, extravasation of erythrocytes can be noted around vessels inflamed by lymphocytes.

Molluscum Contagiosum

- EOSINOPHILIC, HOMOGENEOUS, UNIFORMLY OVOID BODIES WITHIN KERATINOCYTES
- BASOPHILIC, OVOID BODIES IN THE STRATUM CORNEUM

- HOST RESPONSE VARIABLE: NONE TO SO INTENSE THAT THE INCLUSIONS ARE OBSCURED

Molluscum contagiosum (see Chap. 11) is a common infection that causes the formation of discrete, flesh-colored, 2- to 5-mm papules that have a sunken or umbilicated center. These lesions can occur anywhere on the body by inoculation from another infected site. In patients with underlying eczema, generalized eruptions may occur. In children, lesions are commonly found on the face, trunk, and extremities. In

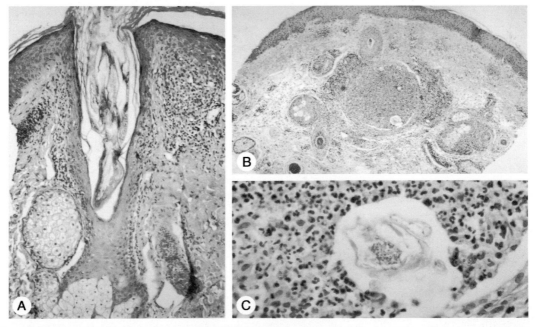

Figure 20–13. *Demodex folliculorum.* **(A)** The mite is embedded head-first into an ectatic follicular orifice. **(B)** A dermal abscess is produced at the level of a follicular infundibulum. **(C)** Higher magnification of Figure 20–15B shows the abscess abutting remnant follicular epithelium and surrounding a *Demodex* organism.

young adults, the lesions are commonly found in the genital area and arise as a result of sexual contact. The infection is frequently self-limited. This condition may be more difficult to control or eradicate when the host has an underlying immunologic deficit or is undergoing immunosuppressive therapy.

Frequently, the follicular epithelium appears hyperplastic and seems to form a central cystic cavity. Keratinocytes are distended by homogenous, uniformly ovoid, eosinophilic bodies rimmed by the compressed, more basophilic, keratinocytic cytoplasm and nucleus. As the molluscum bodies are extruded into the stratum corneum, they appear as basophilic, ovoid bodies, which stand out against the background of the eosinophilic stratum corneum. Follicular epithelium may rupture from the infection. At this stage, the diagnostic viral inclusions are more difficult to find because they are located in a sea of inflammatory cells in the dermis.

Parasitic Folliculitis[26]

Demodex *Folliculitis*

- ELONGATED BASOPHILIC ORGANISMS WITH INTERNAL STRUCTURE, INDIVIDUALLY OR IN LONGITUDINAL CLUSTERS, IN THE FOLLICULAR INFUNDIBULUM OR FOLLICULO-SEBACEOUS JUNCTION

Demodex organisms commonly colonize postpubertal skin, particularly where sebaceous glands are prominent. The organism is a saprophyte and rarely causes clinical disorders. Its role in adult acne, or rosacea, and perioral dermatitis has been speculative. *Demodex* folliculitis has also been reported in patients with acquired immunodeficiency syndrome (AIDS).

There are two varieties of *Demodex* organisms: *Demodex folliculorum* and *Demodex brevis*. The first organism is larger and is found in the follicular openings. The latter organism is smaller and is found in the junction between the sebaceous duct and follicular epithelium. The mite has a thick, somewhat corrugated outer cuticle and discernible internal organs (Fig. 20–13A). It is commonly found on the face in dilated pores where sebaceous glands are plentiful. Occasionally, abscesses may surround the mites and result in follicular rupture (Fig. 20–13B, C). Identifying the organism does not necessarily imply a pathogenic role, because it is a common inhabitant of the face of postpubertal patients.

Eosinophilic Pustular Folliculitis[27, 28]

- SPONGIOSIS OF THE FOLLICULAR INFUNDIBULUM WITH OR WITHOUT EPITHELIAL DISRUPTION
- MIXED MONONUCLEAR INFLAMMATORY INFILTRATE WITH EOSINOPHILS
- SPECIAL STAINS NEGATIVE FOR FUNGAL INFECTION

Typically, eosinophilic pustular folliculitis presents as 1- to 3-mm, pruritic, perifollicular papules or pustules on erythematous bases on the face and upper torso of young individuals (Fig. 20–14A). Eosinophilia in the peripheral blood of up to 40% has been reported in a large percentage

of affected individuals. Although this condition was originally described in healthy patients, it is currently also seen in patients with AIDS. The cause of eosinophilic pustular folliculitis is not yet known.

Microscopic changes of eosinophilic pustular folliculitis include spongiosis of the infundibulum and isthmus of the hair follicle and an accompanying lymphohistiocytic inflammatory infiltrate with eosinophils (Fig. 20–14B). Follicular rupture may occur (Fig. 20–14C). An inflammatory infiltrate of similar composition is present in the adjacent dermal stroma. Because fungal infections may show similar findings, exclusion of this possibility with special stains is essential in establishing the correct diagnosis.

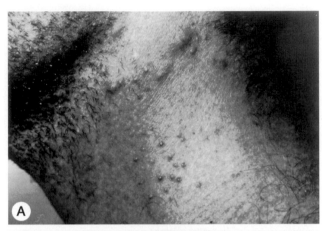

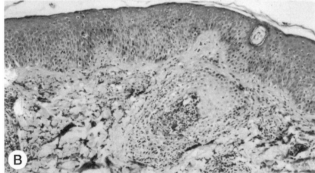

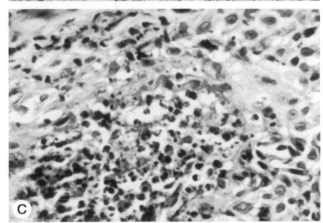

Figure 20–14. Eosinophilic pustular folliculitis. **(A)** Erythematous perifollicular papules are seen on the neck and beard area. **(B)** Discrete zones of inflammation are concentrated around hair follicles. **(C)** Follicular epithelium is disrupted by collections of eosinophils admixed with rare lymphocytes. Special stains are negative for fungal elements.

Follicular Mucinosis[29-31]

- FOLLICULAR EPITHELIUM AND/OR SEBACEOUS GLANDS DISTENDED BY MUCOPOLYSACCHARIDE DEPOSITS
- MONONUCLEAR INFLAMMATORY INFILTRATE WITH VARIABLE NUMBERS OF EOSINOPHILS
- IF MONONUCLEAR ATYPIA PRESENT, MAY BE ASSOCIATED WITH LYMPHOMA
- MUCIN STAINS HELP DISTINGUISH FOLLICULAR MUCINOSIS FROM FOLLICULAR ECZEMA

The clinical spectrum of follicular mucinosis is broad. Lesions may occur as erythematous follicular papules or as confluent zones forming indurated erythematous plaques (Fig. 20–15A). They may be evanescent, mimicking urticaria, or disturbingly stable. If lesions are accompanied by hair loss, the process is termed alopecia mucinosa. The most common anatomic sites of involvement are the scalp and face, followed by the upper torso. Follicular mucinosis has been observed in children as well as in adults. Although it can be seen in association with various lymphomas, its relation to these neoplasms is uncertain. In the absence of lymphoma, follicular mucinosis has a benign, although at times protracted, course.

The histologic hallmark of follicular mucinosis is expansion of the follicular epithelium and sebaceous glands by deposits of mucopolysaccharides between epithelial cells (Fig. 20–15B, C). Inflammatory infiltrates composed of lymphocytes, histiocytes, and eosinophils are present in affected epithelia as well as in the surrounding dermal stroma. The possibility of an associated lymphoproliferative disorder should be considered if there is atypia of mononuclear cells. Some studies suggest that the presence of eosinophils may herald a more benign outcome. Absence of hair shafts may be indicative of alopecia mucinosa; however, this possibility is best ascertained by the gross pathology.

The histologic differential diagnosis of follicular mucinosis includes follicular eczema, which shows spongiosis rather than mucin deposition in the follicular epithelium. Mucin stains, such as an alcian blue, can be helpful in confirming the presence of mucin if there is doubt on routine sections. Follicular mucinosis, best regarded as a reaction pattern of follicular epithelium, is not alone predictive of the eventual outcome.

Folliculitis Decalvans[32, 33]

- EARLY: INFILTRATION OF FOLLICULAR INFUNDIBULUM BY COLLECTIONS OF NEUTROPHILS
- INTERMEDIATE: LYMPHOCYTES AND HISTIOCYTES OBSCURE THE NEUTROPHILIC COMPONENT; GIANT CELLS MAY OR MAY NOT BE PRESENT
- LATE: PERIFOLLICULAR FIBROSIS
- EVENTUATES IN COMPLETE DESTRUCTION OF FOLLICULAR UNIT AND REPLACEMENT BY SCAR

Folliculitis decalvans is an inflammatory alopecia that most often affects adults. It begins as grouped follicular pus-

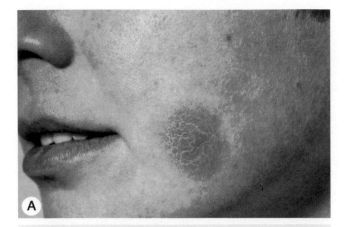

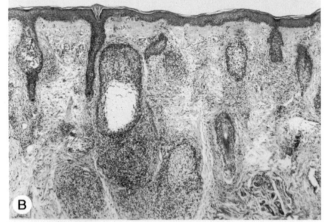

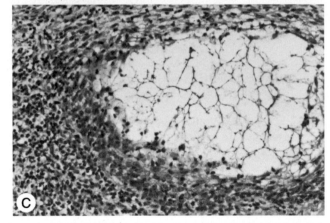

Figure 20–15. Follicular mucinosis. **(A)** A discrete plaque of erythema and crusting is present on the cheek of a young woman. **(B)** Hair follicles and sebaceous glands have a reticulated appearance. They are surrounded by inflammatory infiltrates. **(C)** The reticulated pattern of follicular and sebaceous epithelium is caused by deposition of mucopolysaccharides (i.e., mucin) between epithelial cells. Mucin forms cyst-like cavities in these areas. (Central follicle from **B** turned 90° to the right.)

tules that crust and leave behind areas of scarring and permanent hair loss (Fig. 20–16A). It is best classified with the nonreversible alopecias but is noted in this section because it begins with discrete follicular pustules. Although bacteria have been found in the pustules, their role in the pathogenesis of this disorder is in doubt, because administration of antibiotics does not bring about complete resolution.

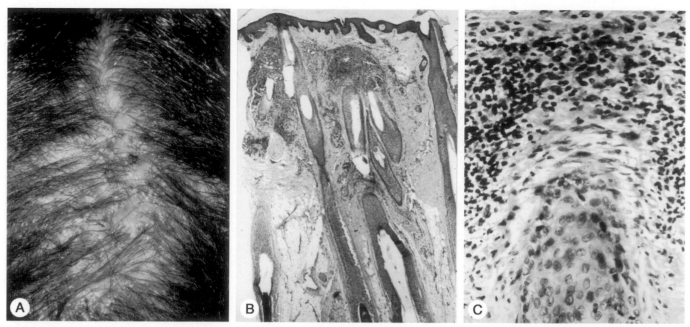

Figure 20–16. Folliculitis decalvans. **(A)** Perifollicular pustules and crusting surround intact hair follicles. There is a background of erythema and a localized decrease in hair density. **(B)** Dense inflammation is present about the superficial portions of hair follicles. **(C)** Advanced lesions show perifollicular fibrosis and lymphoplasmacytic infiltrates enmeshed in scar.

Microscopically, the follicular ostium is surrounded and infiltrated by neutrophils in pustular lesions. With persistence, the infiltrate acquires a mononuclear component (i.e., lymphocytes and histiocytes) and may acquire an admixture of giant cells. Late lesions show perifollicular fibrosis and replacement of follicular units by scar (Fig. 20–16B, C). Because the histology does not show pathognomonic changes, the diagnosis of folliculitis decalvans is arrived at through clinicopathologic correlation.

Reversible Alopecia

Entities considered in this section are disorders in which hair loss is temporary and usually does not eventuate in permanent hair loss. Either these processes do not have a significant inflammatory component, or the inflammatory infiltrate does not damage follicular stem cells. As a group, these alopecias do not show fibrosis of perifollicular sheaths or interfollicular dermis (Table 20–3).

Table 20–3. REVERSIBLE ALOPECIA

DISORDER	CAUSES	SPECIFIC AGENTS	CLINICAL APPEARANCE	HISTOLOGY
Telogen effluvium	Parturition, stress, fever, anesthesia, surgery, psoriasis, crash diet		Diffuse thinning of scalp hair; loss in excess of 200 hairs/day	Early: >20% of hairs in telogen Late: Rare or no telogen hairs (all anagen)
	Drugs	Coumadin, allopurinol, probenecid, lithium carbonate, β-blockers, vitamin A, thiourea, others		
Alopecia areata	Unknown trigger; immune-mediated process		Coin-like areas of hair loss; may have total scalp hair loss and loss elsewhere on the body	Lymphocytic infiltrates around follicular papillae (active lesions)
Alopecia mucinosa	Unknown		Erythematous, boggy plaques with hair loss on head and neck more than trunk	Follicular sheaths expanded by mucin and lymphocytic infiltrate
Infections	Syphilitic alopecia	*Treponema pallidum*	Moth-eaten appearance of scalp hair	Lymphoplasmacytic infiltrates in and around hair follicles; may have interface alterations as well
	Fungal	See Table 20–1	Erythematous patches or plaques with or without black dots at surface	Organisms in or around hair shafts

Telogen Effluvium[34–36]

- EARLY: GREATER THAN 20% OF HAIR FOLLICLES IN TELOGEN PHASE
- LATE: RARE OR ABSENT TELOGEN PHASE HAIR FOLLICLES

The most common cause of transient alopecia is telogen effluvium, which is caused by the premature conversion of anagen follicles into telogen follicles. This results in increased shedding of hair, often in excess of 200 hairs per day. Hair loss may be localized, for example, at a site of prolonged pressure (e.g., occiput during prolonged surgery). More often, however, it is diffuse. Numerous causes for telogen effluvium have been reported and include those listed in Table 20–3. It is important to recognize this process, because it is self-limited, and patient reassurance is all that is necessary. Normal growth resumes after the inciting cause is removed.

Histologic examination early in the course of the disorder shows increased numbers of hair follicles in telogen phase as compared to those in anagen phase (>20%). Occasionally, increased numbers of catagen follicles and empty follicular tracts may be observed as well. Because patients often seek attention after the shedding or thinning is established (i.e., late in the course of the disorder), biopsy specimens at that point in time show a rarity or lack of telogen hairs, and nearly all hairs present are anagen hairs.

Alopecia Areata[37–39]

- EARLY: INTENSE LYMPHOCYTIC INFLAMMATORY INFILTRATE AROUND ANAGEN FOLLICULAR PAPILLAE
- INTERMEDIATE TO LATE: CONVERSION OF ANAGEN FOLLICLES TO CATAGEN AND TELOGEN; INFLAMMATION LESS PROMINENT

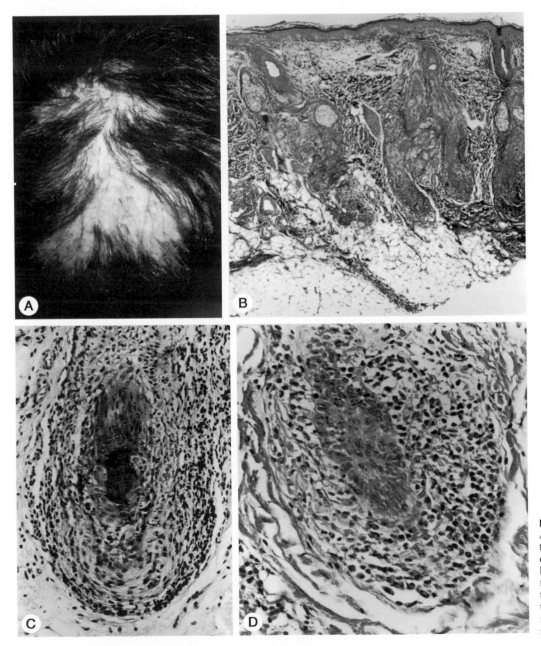

Figure 20–17. Alopecia areata. **(A)** Areas of hair loss, within which there are hair shafts with tapered ends known as exclamation-point hairs. **(B)** Intense inflammatory infiltrates as seen around multiple follicular papillae. **(C, D)** The intense lymphocytic infiltrate surrounds a hair papilla, mimicking a swarm of bees.

Alopecia areata is thought to be an immunologically mediated disorder in which hair follicles and nails are the target organs. This disorder can affect persons of any age and involve any hair-bearing surface. In the scalp, alopecia areata is most commonly detected as circular, coin-like zones of complete hair loss (Fig. 20–17A). Along the periphery of these areas, there may be broken hairs that have normal distal diameters with proximal constrictions, mimicking exclamation points. The hair loss also may be noted in the eyebrows, bearded area, trunk, and extremities. The complete loss of scalp hair is known as alopecia totalis. Alopecia universalis indicates total loss of body hair. Another manifestation of alopecia areata is pigment loss, or poliosis, in which patches of hair have completely lost their pigment and are white. Nail pitting may be seen in all or a few nails.

Alopecia areata has a higher incidence in patients affected with Down syndrome, in patients with an atopic background (e.g., hayfever, asthma, eczema), and in patients with other autoimmune disorders (e.g., diabetes, vitiligo, Hashimoto thyroiditis). The outcome of alopecia areata often relates to the age at onset and extent of involvement. Limited involvement in postpubertal patients often results in complete regrowth. Alopecia areata may recur in an unpredictable fashion throughout life.

Histologically, early lesions are the most informative. Finding an intense lymphocytic inflammatory infiltrate (i.e., swarm of bees) around anagen hair papillae is the histologic hallmark of alopecia areata (Fig. 20–17B–D). Midstage lesions show conversion of anagen follicles into catagen and telogen phases in increased numbers. Late lesions show miniaturization of terminal hairs and a paucity of anagen hair follicles. This process has been termed an anagen effluvium by some observers.

Alopecia Mucinosa[40, 41]

- MULTIPLE HAIR FOLLICLES IN A SECTION WITH CHANGES OF FOLLICULAR MUCINOSIS
- INFILTRATES OF LYMPHOCYTES AND EOSINOPHILS OF VARYING INTENSITY
- LOSS OF HAIR SHAFT MAY BE APPARENT ON ROUTINE SECTIONS

Indurated erythematous plaques devoid of hair are characteristic of alopecia mucinosa. They are most commonly found on the head, neck, and upper torso. In most instances, alopecia mucinosa has a benign, self-limited course, particularly in young patients and in those with few lesions. Usually, hair regrows in previously affected sites. In various studies, up to 30% of patients with alopecia mucinosa have had prior or concurrent diagnoses of cutaneous T-cell lymphoma and, more rarely, Hodgkin disease or other lymphomas.

Histologically, multiple hair follicles show infiltration of follicular epithelium by mucin, lymphocytes, histiocytes, and eosinophils. Some studies suggest that extension of the inflammatory infiltrate into the overlying epidermis, cytologic atypia of mononuclear cells, and lack of eosinophils in the infiltrate are indicative of the presence of cutaneous T-cell lymphoma. If an associated T-cell dyscrasia is suspected by routine histology, confirmation with cell marker analysis or gene rearrangement studies and close clinical examination of the patient for visceral disease are warranted.

Alopecia Secondary to Infection

Alopecia secondary to infectious agents is usually reversible in its early phases. If the inflammatory infiltrate incites significant damage to the follicular epithelium and causes perifollicular fibrosis, normal regeneration of hair may be impaired. Specific agents have been addressed in the section on folliculitis.

Irreversible Alopecia

Various processes may eventuate in permanent hair loss. They are summarized in Table 20–4.

Table 20–4. IRREVERSIBLE ALOPECIA

DISORDER	CAUSES	LOCATION	CLINICAL APPEARANCE	HISTOLOGY
Androgenic alopecia	Multifactorial: heredity, hormonal target site sensitivity	Scalp	Men: Loss in temporal angles; recession of frontal hairline Women: Gradual diffuse thinning of crown	Inflammation at folliculo-sebaceous junction; slow miniaturization of hair follicles
Acne keloidalis	Curvature of hair shaft, mechanical irritation	Posterior neck; may involve beard	Follicular skin-colored papules; variable inflammation; may form plaques	Fibrosis and inflammation (acute and chronic); isolated hair shafts without epithelium
Lupus erythematosus	Autoimmune disease, unknown trigger	Scalp, face, other sun-exposed sites	Alopecic plaques with follicular plugs, variable erythema and scarring	Follicular plugging; band-like infiltrate of lymphocytes in superficial dermis; mucinous stroma; late follicular dropout
Lichen planopilaris	Unknown	Scalp, axillae, pubic area	Red-to-violaceous perifollicular papules and hair loss	Lichenoid infiltrates along dermal-epidermal and follicular junctions
Morphea	Unknown	Frontal scalp, often extends onto face	Bound-down, white, hairless plaque with or without erythema	Sclerotic reticular dermal collagen bundles with or without inflammation; loss of hair follicles
Pseudopelade	Preceding inflammatory process	Scalp	Shiny, white, atrophic areas with hair loss	Complete loss of hair follicles; remnant hair tracts

Androgenetic Alopecia[42–46]

- REPLACEMENT OF TERMINAL HAIRS BY VELLUS HAIRS; FOCAL IN EARLY STAGES, DIFFUSE LATE
- MONONUCLEAR INFLAMMATORY INFILTRATES AROUND THE FOLLICULO-SEBACEOUS JUNCTION

Androgenetic alopecia is hormonally driven hair loss in genetically predisposed individuals, commonly referred to as male pattern baldness. The clinical expression of androgenetic alopecia is influenced by many elements, such as hereditary factors, hormones, and target site sensitivity. Undoubtedly, many other factors are as yet unknown.

In men, the process begins with recession of the frontal hairline and increased loss in the temporal angles. This may be accompanied by hair loss at the vertex as well. Progression of androgenetic alopecia is variable. It may extend to involve much of the frontal and parietal scalp but characteristically does not involve the occipital fringe. In women, the pattern is usually not as striking as in men; it generally consists of diffuse thinning at the crown with variable regression of the frontal hairline and temporal angles (Fig. 20–18A). Although common in postmenopausal women, the finding of premature androgenetic alopecia in prepubertal boys or premenopausal women should trigger a search for a source of an underlying hormonal imbalance.

Morphologically, the changes of androgenetic alopecia can be subtle and vary with the stage at sampling. In the early phases, there is a mononuclear inflammatory infiltrate centered about the junction of the follicular infundibulum and its accompanying sebaceous duct. As the process progresses, occasional terminal hair follicles become replaced by vellus or rudimentary anagen hair follicles (Fig. 20–18B, C). During this stage, fibrous streamers are conspicuous in the dermis, because hair follicles entering telogen phase are more prominent. Areas of established androgenetic alopecia show pronounced miniaturization of hair follicles and complete zones of replacement of terminal hair by vellus hair. In this setting, sebaceous glands may appear to be more prominent, and inflammatory infiltrates are minimal. If inflammatory cells near the follicular bulge damage follicular stem cells, normal regeneration of hair follicles would be impeded. Of interest, recent ultrastructural findings indicate that with progression of androgenetic alopecia, perifollicular fibrous sheaths become thickened. This alteration of the normally delicate envelope surrounding the hair follicle may impede the normal descent of the hair follicle as it cycles and there-

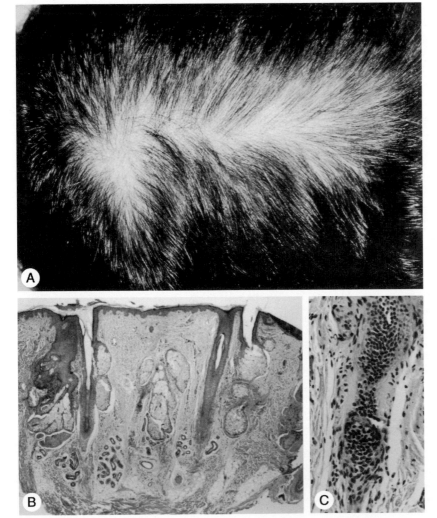

Figure 20–18. Androgenic alopecia. **(A)** Thinning of the crown has occurred in an adult woman. **(B)** Two terminal anagen hair follicles are present. Centrally, there are mature sebaceous glands around a miniaturized hair follicle. **(C)** There is marked diminution of the caliber of a telogen hair follicle and thickening of the perifollicular sheath.

fore alter normal hair growth. This morphologic change may explain the irreversible nature of hair loss after it becomes established.

Acne Keloidalis[47–49]

- HAIR SHAFTS DEVOID OF FOLLICULAR EPITHELIUM ENTRAPPED WITHIN THE DERMIS
- VARIABLE MIXED INFLAMMATORY INFILTRATES OF NEUTROPHILS AND MONONUCLEAR CELLS
- CHRONIC LESIONS SHOW LARGE NUMBERS OF PLASMA CELLS AND PROMINENT FIBROSIS

Acne keloidalis, sometimes referred to as dermatitis papillaris capillitii, occurs in patients with tightly curled hair. Although it most often occurs in those of African descent, Caucasians may be affected as well. Lesions most commonly occur at the nape of the neck and appear as perifollicular, flesh-colored, dome-shaped papules (Fig. 20–19A). Frequently, they are arranged in a linear pattern within the skin creases. The degree of inflammation is variable; quiescent lesions may appear to have none, whereas others may discharge abundant purulent material. Lesions are thought to form as the distal end of a curved hair embeds itself into the dermis and incites stromal inflammation and perifollicular fibrosis. The process is frequently relentless and requires surgical excision for treatment. A similar process that occurs in the bearded area is known as pseudofolliculitis barbae.

The histology of acne keloidalis varies with the stage of the lesion at biopsy. Early lesions show a hair shaft embedded in the dermis, frequently surrounded by neutrophils. Later lesions show an admixture of mononuclear and giant cells surrounding the hair shaft. The hair shaft provides a continuous stimulus for inflammation in the stroma and induces stromal fibrosis, which correlates with the clinically apparent dome-shaped scar. The histology of this process in the beard area is similar in that dome-shaped papules may display inflammation and fibrosis surrounding hair shafts. Alternatively, the inflammatory infiltrates may form deep-seated aggregates around hair shafts that are no longer surrounded by normal follicular epithelium (Fig. 20–19B, C).

Lupus Erythematosus[50, 51]

- EARLY: EFFACEMENT OF THE RETE RIDGE PATTERN OF THE EPIDERMIS AND FOCAL NECROSIS OF BASILAR KERATINOCYTES
- LYMPHOCYTES AND PLASMA CELLS ALONG THE DERMAL-EPIDERMAL JUNCTION, SURROUNDING BLOOD VESSELS, HAIR FOLLICLES, AND ECCRINE DUCTS
- ESTABLISHED LESIONS: THICKENING OF THE BASEMENT MEMBRANE (OFTEN MORE APPARENT WITH PERIODIC ACID–SCHIFF STAINS)
- FOLLICULAR PLUGGING
- INTERSTITIAL MUCIN DEPOSITION

Lupus erythematosus may produce discrete zones of hair loss or diffuse thinning of scalp hair. It rarely affects the scalp without affecting other cutaneous or extracutaneous sites. Discoid lupus erythematosus localized to the head and neck region has an overall better prognosis than generalized discoid lupus, as well as less tendency to evolve into systemic lupus erythematosus.

Discoid lupus erythematosus appears as well-demarcated, erythematous, scaly plaques (Fig. 20–20A). Long-standing lesions are studded with comedonal plugs, which are the result of perifollicular fibrosis and retraction of follicular ostia. Scarring is often apparent in the center of the lesion and is grossly appreciated as areas of hypopigmentation with complete loss of hair follicles. Other areas may show hyperpigmentation. Examination of the remainder of

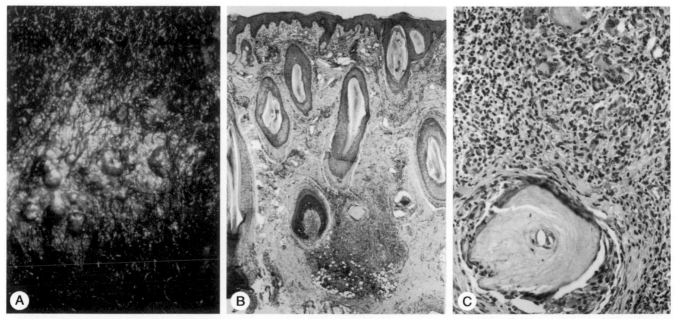

Figure 20–19. Acne keloidalis and pseudofolliculitis barbae. **(A)** Acne keloidalis: Firm, flesh-colored, perifollicular papules stud the nape of the neck. **(B)** Pseudofolliculitis barbae: A biopsy specimen from the beard area shows a focus of intense inflammation in the deep dermis. **(C)** Higher magnification of **B** shows a granulomatous infiltrate surrounding a hair shaft with an attached remnant of follicular epithelium.

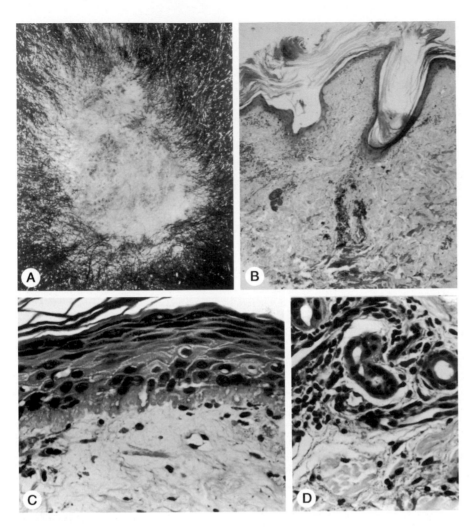

Figure 20–20. Lupus erythematosus alopecia. **(A)** Multiple patches of hair loss are present in the scalp. Many show prominent erythema; centrally, the white areas correlate with zones of scarring. **(B)** There is prominent follicular ectasia and plugging. The undulating rete ridge pattern of the epidermis is lost, and hyperkeratosis is present. **(C)** There is prominent thickening and tortuosity of the basement membrane. The dermis contains abundant mucin. **(D)** A lymphoplasmacytic inflammatory infiltrate commonly surrounds eccrine glands in the deep dermal stroma.

the skin, detailed inquiry and workup of systemic complaints, and correlation with serologic studies are essential in evaluating such patients.

The early histologic changes of discoid lupus erythematosus consist of perivascular inflammatory infiltrates of lymphocytes and plasma cells that approximate the dermal-epidermal junction, follicular epithelium, and eccrine glands. At the dermal-epidermal interface, the infiltrate is associated with subepidermal vacuolization and necrosis of individual basilar keratinocytes. Similar changes can be discerned along dermal-follicular junctions. As the cytotoxic injury becomes established, immunoreactants are deposited in the basement membrane zone of the dermal-epidermal junction and follicular-dermal junction. These deposits are detected with immunofluorescence or immunohistochemical stains directed against C_3, IgG, IgM, or IgA. Finding these deposits in basement membranes in lesional and nonlesional skin are reported as positive lupus band tests. These deposits are associated with noticeable thickening and tortuosity of basement membranes in routine sections. In addition, careful examination of the dermal stroma frequently reveals the presence of thin strands of faintly basophilic material between collagen bundles, indicating interstitial deposition of mucopolysaccharides. Papillary dermal hemorrhage may occasionally be seen as well.

In long-standing lesions, the epidermis loses its undulating rete ridge pattern and is surmounted by compact hyperorthokeratotic scale. Perifollicular fibrosis results in ectasia and plugging of follicular ostia (Fig. 20–20B). With chronicity, there is striking thickening of the basement membrane zone and prominent mucin deposition (Fig. 20–20C). In established lesions of discoid lupus erythematosus, a constant finding is the presence of lymphocytes and plasma cells about eccrine apparatus within the deep dermis (Fig. 20–20D). Pigment incontinence from damage to basilar epithelial cells can be appreciated as collections of melanophages in the papillary dermis. Without early intervention, these changes lead to irreversible loss of viable hair follicles and permanent alopecia.

Lichen Planopilaris[52-54]

- EARLY: MONONUCLEAR INFILTRATE HUGGING THE UPPER ONE HALF OF FOLLICULAR EPITHELIUM WITH OR WITHOUT NECROSIS OF INDIVIDUAL KERATINOCYTES
- MONONUCLEAR INFLAMMATORY INFILTRATE BENEATH EFFACED DERMAL-EPIDERMAL JUNCTION
- LATE: FOLLICULAR ECTASIA AND PLUGGING OF OSTIA
- PERIFOLLICULAR FIBROSIS

Lichen planopilaris, or follicular lichen planus, affects hair-bearing surfaces including the scalp, trunk, extremities, and intertriginous areas such as the axillae. On the scalp, lichen planopilaris appears as areas of hair loss within which intact hair follicles are surrounded by red-to-violaceous papules. Areas of involvement tend to slowly enlarge, leaving behind scarring and permanent hair loss. Finding lesions of lichen planopilaris should trigger a careful search for evidence of lichen planus of glaborous skin or mucosa, because these lesions often coexist.

Microscopically, a band-like lymphocytic inflammatory infiltrate hugs the upper half of hair follicles and extends to involve adjacent interfollicular epithelium (Fig. 20–21A–C). Features that help to distinguish lichen planopilaris from lupus erythematosus are the lack of thickening and tortuosity of the basement membrane and lack of inflammation around eccrine coils in the former (Fig. 20–21C, D). Individual necrotic basilar keratinocytes may be seen along the upper portion of the follicular epithelia. Late changes include plugging of ectatic follicular ostia with compact orthokeratin and perifollicular fibrosis. Inflammation of the upper half of the hair follicle may result in injury to stem cells, which in concert with perifollicular fibrosis could explain the permanent nature of the hair loss. Eventually, all viable follicles are lost, and only residual fibrous tracts remain. This endstage is known as pseudopelade.

Morphea[55, 56]

- EARLY: LYMPHOPLASMACYTIC INFLAMMATORY INFILTRATES DEEP IN THE DERMIS AT THE DERMAL-SUBCUTANEOUS JUNCTION
- LATE: REDUCED NUMBERS OF HAIR FOLLICLES, THICKENING AND HOMOGENIZATION OF DERMAL COLLAGEN BUNDLES, LOSS OF ADIPOCYTES WHICH WOULD NORMALLY SURROUND DEEPLY-PLACED ECCRINE COILS

Morphea, or localized scleroderma, may affect the central forehead and extend into the scalp in a linear configuration mimicking a blow to the head with a sabre, hence the name en coup de sabre. This form of morphea often occurs in young children as erythematous-to-violaceous patches which evolve into indurated plaques. As the process becomes established, alopecia ensues. This form of morphea may cause skin to be bound down to underlying bone, which restricts normal growth and causes bone deformities.

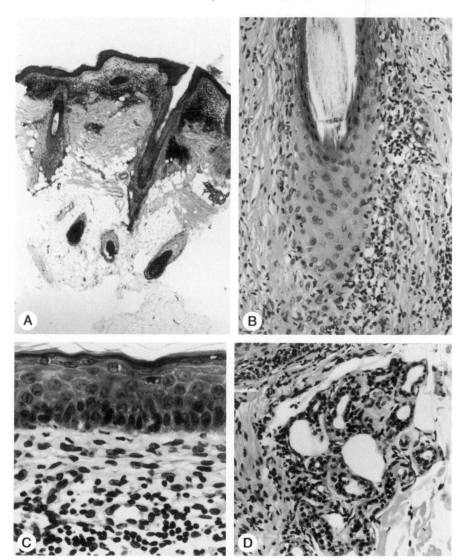

Figure 20–21. Lichen planopilaris. **(A, B)** A band-like infiltrate surrounds the upper half of a hair follicle and extends along adjacent interfollicular epithelium. **(C)** Interfollicular epithelium shows loss of the rete ridge pattern but no thickening of the basement membrane as in lupus erythematosus. **(D)** In contrast to lupus erythematosus, eccrine glands are free of inflammation.

The histology of en coup de sabre is that of morphea: lymphoplasmacytic inflammatory infiltrates are present at the dermal-subcutaneous junction and are associated with decreased cellularity and thickening of dermal collagen bundles. As this process continues, eccrine glands become entrapped in thick collagen bundles and are eventually obliterated. Follicular loss may occur on the basis of vascular compromise and stromal fibrosis rather than as a result of direct assault on follicular apparatus. Late lesions show replacement of normal-caliber collagen bundles by thick homogenous acellular bundles. Appendageal structures are conspicuously absent. Remnant follicular fibrous tracts may appear to interrupt the arrangement of collagen bundles. The histology at this stage is that of pseudopelade.

Pseudopelade[57, 58]

- SEVERE DIMINUTION IN THE NUMBER OF INTACT HAIR FOLLICLES; SOMETIMES NONE LEFT
- FIBROUS TRACTS MARK SITES OF PREVIOUSLY CYCLING HAIR FOLLICLES

The literature on pseudopelade is fraught with confusion. Some dermatopathologists reserve this term for the end-stage of various permanent alopecias (e.g., lupus erythematosus, lichen planopilaris, morphea), whereas others consider

it to be an idiopathic scarring alopecia. Idiopathic, however, only implies that the cause of the problem may not be recognized. Pseudopelade is clinically characterized by areas of complete hair loss on the scalp interrupted by zones of apparently normal hair growth. The alopecic areas are nonscaly and devoid of inflammation.

Microscopic examination of the alopecic zones shows a severe decrease in number or complete absence of hair follicles (Fig. 20–22A). Only fibrous tracts remain as indicators of previously cycling hair follicles (Fig. 20–22B). Sampling of hair-bearing areas has variably shown changes of lupus, lichen planopilaris, or morphea, which suggests that pseudopelade is related to these disorders.

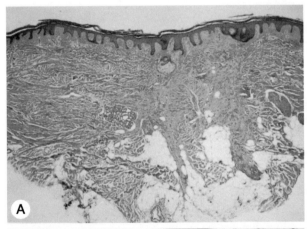

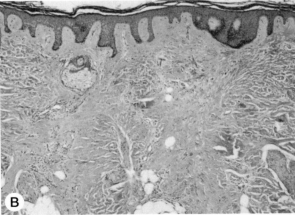

Figure 20–22. Pseudopelade. **(A)** Complete loss of hair follicles has occurred. Only follicular tracts remain as indicators of previously cycling hairs at this site. **(B)** Rare appendages (i.e., a sebaceous gland and pilar muscle) surround fibrotic tracts. Note the absence of inflammation.

SELECTED REFERENCES

1. Pinkus H. Anatomy and histology of skin. In: Graham JH, Johnson WC, Helwig EB, eds. Dermal Pathology. Hagerstown: Harper & Row, 1972:1.
2. Kligman AM. The human hair cycle. J Invest Dermatol 1959;33:307.
3. Cotsarelis G, Sun T-T, Lavker RM. Label-retaining cells reside in the bulge area of the pilosebaceous unit: Implications for follicular stem cells, hair cycle, and skin carcinogenesis. Cell 1990;61:1329.
4. Lavker RM, Miller S, Wilson C, et al. Hair follicle stem cells: Their location, role in the hair cycle, and involvement in skin tumor formation. J Invest Dermatol 1993;101:16S.
5. Jaworsky C, Kligman AM, Murphy GF. Characterization of inflammatory infiltrates in male patter alopecia: Implications for pathogenesis. Br J Dermatol 1992;127:239.
6. Stroud JD. Hair-shaft anomalies. Dermatol Clin 1987;5:581.
7. Whiting DA. Structural abnormalities of the hair shaft. J Am Acad Dermatol 1987;16:1.
8. Bulengo-Ransby SM, Bergfeld WF. Chemical and traumatic alopecia from thioglycolate in a black woman: A case report with unusual clinical and histologic findings. Cutis 1992;49:99.
9. Scott DA. Disorders of the hair and scalp in blacks. Dermatol Clin 1988;6:387.
10. Monk BE, Neill SM, du Vivier A. Fashion causes traction alopecia. Practitioner 1986;230:401.
11. Dean JT, Nelson E, Moss L. Pathologic hair-pulling: A review of the literature and case reports. Compr Psychiatry 1992;33:84.
12. Muller SA: Trichotillomania. Dermatol Clin 1987;5:595.
13. Shelley WB, Shelley ED, Burmeister V. The infected hairs of tinea capitis due to *Microsporum canis*: Demonstration of uniqueness of the hair cuticle by scanning electron microscopy. J Am Acad Dermatol 1987;16:354.
14. Grigoriu D, Delacretaz J. Mixed dermatophytic infection of the hairy scalp. Dermatologica 1982;164:407.
15. Vanbreuseghem R. Moder classification of dermatophytes. Dermatologica 1977;155:1.
16. Gaisin A, Holzwanger JM, Leyden JJ. Endothrix tinea capitis in Philadelphia. Int J Dermatol 1977;16:188.
17. Patratii VK, Kokoshchuk GI, Bukharovich AM, Bezrukov LA. Chemical intoxication syndrome in children with diffuse alopecia. Pediatriia 1991;12:52.
18. Brodin MB. Drug-related alopecia. Dermatol Clin 1987;5:571.
19. Bronner AK, Hood AF. Cutaneous complications of chemotherapeutic agents. J Am Acad Dermatol 1983;9:645.
20. Pinkus H. Furuncle. J Cutan Pathol 1979;6:517.
21. Stephens CJ, Hay RJ, Black MM. Fungal kerion—total scalp involvement due to *Microsporum canis* infection. Clin Exp Dermatol 1989;14:442.
22. Lee JY, Hsu ML. Alopecia syphilitica, a simulator of alopecia areata: Histopathology and differential diagnosis. J Cutan Pathol 1991;18:87.
23. Kennedy C. Syphilis presenting as hair loss. Br Med J 1976;2:854.
24. Moriyama K, Imayama S, Mohri S, et al. Localization of herpes simplex virus type 1 in sebaceous glands of mice. Arch Virol 1992;123:13.
25. Muraki R, Baba T, Iwasaki T, et al. Immunohistochemical study of skin lesions in herpes zoster. Virchows Arch A Pathol Anat Histopathol 1992;420:71.

26. Ashack RJ, Frost ML, Norins AL. Papular pruritic eruption of *Demodex* folliculitis in patients with acquired immunodeficiency syndrome. J Am Acad Dermatol 1989;21:306.

27. Camacho Martinez F. Eosinophilic pustular folliculitis. J Am Acad Dermatol 1987;17:686.

28. Takematsu H, Nakamura K, Igarashi M, Tagami H. Eosinophilic pustular folliculitis. Report of two cases with a review of the Japanese literature. Arch Dermatol 1985;121:917.

29. Mehregan DA, Gibson Le, Muller SA. Follicular mucinosis: Histopathologic review of 33 cases. Mayo Clin Proc 1991;66:387.

30. Gibson LE, Muller SA, Leiferman KM, Peters MS. Follicular mucinosis: Clinical and histopathologic study. J Am Acad Dermatol 1989;20:441.

31. Hempstead RW, Ackerman AB. Follicular mucinosis. A reaction pattern in follicular epithelium. Am J Dermatopathol 1985;7:245.

32. Abeck D, Korting HC, Braun-Falco O. Folliculitis decalvans. Long-lasting response to combined therapy with fusidic acid and zinc. Acta Derm Venereol (Stockh) 1992;72:143.

33. Scribner MD. Folliculitis decalvans. Arch Dermatol 1971;104:451.

34. Headington, JT. Telogen effluvium: New concepts and review. Arch Dermatol 1993;129:356.

35. Spencer LV, Callen JP. Hair loss in systemic disease. Dermatol Clin 1987;5:565.

36. Desai SP, Roaf ER. Telogen effluvium after anesthesia and surgery. Anesth Analg 1984;63:83.

37. Fiedler VC. Alopecia areata. A review of therapy, efficacy, safety, and mechanism (editorial). Arch Dermatol 1992;128:1519.

38. Perret CM, Steijlen PM, Happle R. Alopecia areata. Pathogenesis and topical immunotherapy. Int J Dermatol 1990;29:83.

39. Mitchell AJ, Balle MR. Alopecia areata. Dermatol Clin 1987;5:553.

40. Sentis HJ, Willemze R, Scheffer E. Alopecia mucinosa progressing into mycosis fungoides. A long-term follow-up study of two patients. Am J Dermatopathol 1988;10:478.

41. Raznatovskii IM, Moshkalova IA. Alopecia mucinosa and skin lymphoma. Vestn Dermatol Venerol 1987;5:35.

42. Sawaya ME, Hordinsky MK. Advances in alopecia areata and androgenetic alopecia. Adv Dermatol 1992;7:211.

43. Brodland DG, Muller SA. Androgenetic alopecia (common baldness). Cutis 1991;47:173.

44. Olsen EA, Buller TA, Weiner S, Delong ER. Natural history of androgenetic alopecia. Clin Exp Dermatol 1990;15:34.

45. Headington JT. Androgenetic alopecia, trichotrophic substances, and histologic studies of the human scalp. Clin Dermatol 1988;6:188.

46. DeVillez RL, ed. Androgenetic Alopecia: From Empiricism to Knowledge. Philadelphia: JB Lippincott, 1988.

47. Herzberg AJ, Dinehart SM, Kerns BJ, Pollack SV. Acne keloidalis. Transverse microscopy, immunohistochemistry, and electron microscopy. Am J Dermatopathol 1990;12:109.

48. Dinehart SM, Herzberg AJ, Kerns BJ, Pollack SV. Acne keloidalis: A review. J Dermatol Surg Oncol 1989;15:642.

49. Cosman B, Wolff M. Acne keloidalis. Plast Reconstr Surg 1972;50:25.

50. Wilson CL, Burge SM, Dean D, Dawber RP. Scarring alopecia in discoid lupus erythematosus. Br J Dermatol 1992;126:307.

51. Wysenbeek AJ, Leibovici L, Amit M, Weinberger A. Alopecia in systemic lupus erythematosus. Relation to disease manifestations. J Rheumatol 1991;18:1185.

52. Mehregan DA, Van Hale HM, Muller SA. Lichen planopilaris: Clinical and pathologic study of forty-five patients. J Am Acad Dermatol 1992;27:935.

53. Matta M, Kibbi AG, Khattar J, et al. Lichen planopilaris: A clinicopathologic study. J Am Acad Dermatol 1990;22:594.

54. Waldorf DS. Lichen planopilaris. Histopathologic study of disease. Progression to scarring alopecia. Arch Dermatol 1966;93:684.

55. Antonelli JR. Morphea: A localized scleroderma, with en coup de sabre. Compendium 1992;13:722.

56. David J, Wilson J, Woo P. Scleroderma 'en coup de sabre.' Ann Rheum Dis 1991;50:260.

57. Dawber R. What is pseudopelade? Clin Exp Dermatol 1992;17:305.

58. Braun-Falco O, Imai S, Schmoeckel C, et al. Pseudopelade of Brocq. Dermatologica 1986;172:18.

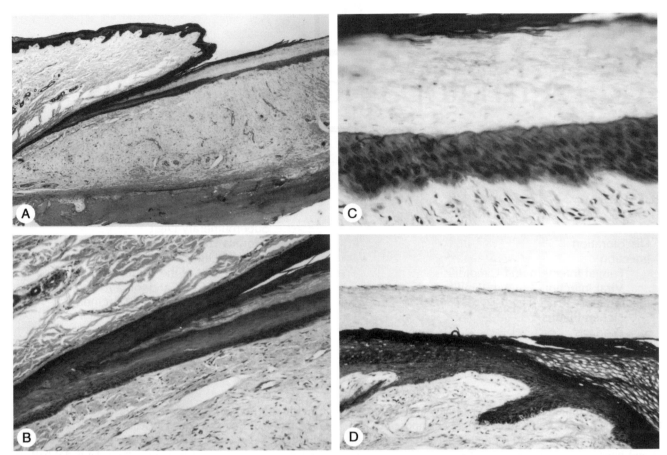

Figure 21–1. Normal anatomy of the nail plate, bed, and matrix. **(A)** Panoramic view of a normal nail. The nail plate exits from beneath the proximal nail fold. Beneath the nail plate is the nail matrix proximally, and nail bed distally. Bone is present at the deep portion of the specimen *(bottom).* **(B)** Synthesis of the nail plate occurs in the area of the proximal nail fold and nail matrix. **(C)** The nail bed is seen with its undulating dermal-epithelial junction and overlying nail plate. **(D)** The hyponychium is the place where the nail plate meets the stratum corneum at the distal end of the nail. Subungual keratotic debris collects in the hyponychium in pathologic states.

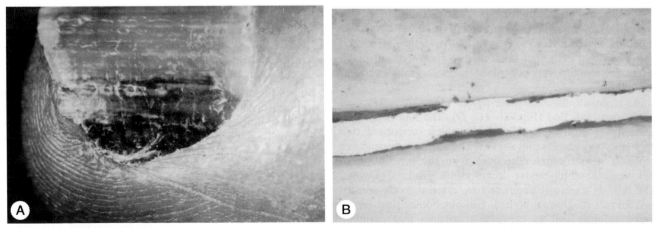

Figure 21–2. Manifestations of nail trauma. **(A)** Subungual hemorrhage: a pigmented band on the lateral edge of the great toe nail. **(B)** The removed nail plate shows a split in the plate which contains erythrocytes; Prussian blue stain confirms the presence of iron (hemosiderin) in the nail plate from prior hemorrhage.

sume the appearance of discrete, linear, red-brown streaks or large ovoid areas of discoloration (Fig. 21–2A). If the injury was severe, hemorrhage may separate the nail plate from the nail bed, resulting in onycholysis. In most instances, the history will provides clues that lead to the diagnosis. Alternatively, observing migration of the pigment toward the distal end of the nail plate over time will confirm the diagnosis. Occasionally, when there is no known history of trauma, and the pigment in the nail plate is dark brown, a biopsy is done to exclude the possibility of malignant melanoma.

Microscopically, there is a localized collection of extravasated erythrocytes in (Fig. 21–2B) or beneath the nail plate if the hemorrhage is recent. If the injury is remote, collections of hemosiderin may be found at these sites. If there is doubt as to the type of pigment present, Prussian blue stains can confirm the presence of iron in the affected areas.

Discoloration[2]

- COLLECTIONS OF PIGMENT IN THE NAIL PLATE, NAIL BED, OR DERMIS

Pigmentary changes of the nails are seen in endocrine disorders (e.g., acromegaly, adrenal insufficiency) and metabolic diseases (e.g., porphyria cutanea tarda) and with drug ingestion. The latter is the most common cause. The list of medications associated with nail discoloration is extensive. The most common discoloration produced is blue to blue-grey and is caused by drugs such as quinacrine, zidovudine, phenolphthalein, heavy metals (e.g., silver in argyria, arsenic, copper in Wilson disease), and phenothiazines. Occasionally, yellow-gold discoloration can occur with ingestion of tetracycline or lithium. Rarely, red discoloration can be seen with demethylchlortetracycline. Antineoplastic or cytotoxic agents usually produce brown to brown-black discoloration.

The color change of the nails usually correlates temporally with ingestion of the medication and careful questioning of the patient can obviate the need for a biopsy. If biopsy is performed, the specimens show deposition of fine to coarsely granular pigment in the nail plate, the nail bed, or the stroma in macrophages. The pigment may represent localized collections of the drug, drug metabolites, melanin, or combinations of these. Routine histology will permit detection, but not definitive identification, of the pigment deposits.

Infection[3, 4]

Fungal Infection and Candidiasis

- BRANCHING AND/OR SEPTATE HYPHAE, BUDDING YEAST FORMS IN THE NAIL PLATE
- VARIABLE INFILTRATE OF NEUTROPHILS AND/OR MONONUCLEAR CELLS

Individuals who immerse their hands in water for prolonged periods of time become predisposed to infections of the nail plates and surrounding soft tissues by fungi and yeast because of maceration. Invasion of the nail plate by *Candida albicans* can occur in this setting as well as in chronic mucocutaneous candidiasis syndromes and acrodermatitis enteropathica. Dermatophytes such as *Trichophyton rubrum* or

Trichophyton mentagrophytes commonly affect nails, particularly toenails in individuals who wear occlusive footwear for prolonged periods of time. In these instances, the organisms invade from the nail folds or stratum corneum of the hyponychium and extend into the nail plate. Once they grow within the plate, they become difficult to eradicate.

In either setting, the nail plate becomes friable, opaque and yellowish brown and has an irregular surface (Fig. 21–3A). Subungual debris may be collected onto a slide, pre-

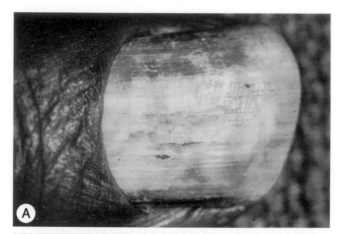

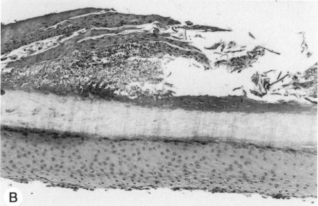

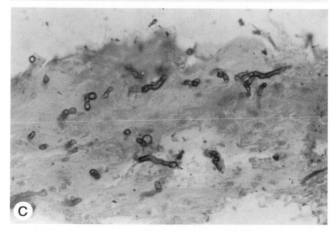

Figure 21–3. Onychomycosis. **(A)** An opaque nail plate has ridging of the surface and yellow discoloration laterally. **(B)** The nail bed and attached nail plate show erosion and inflammation of the superficial nail plate and prominent layering of neutrophilic cell aggregates within a parakeratotic nail plate. **(C)** Periodic acid–Schiff stain highlights the presence of septate branching hyphae of a *Dermatophyte* organism in the nail plate.

treated with potassium hydroxide to dissolve keratin, and examined under the microscope to disclose the presence of yeast or fungi. Occasionally, a portion of the nail plate may be sent for microscopic examination or culture.

A clue to this diagnosis is the presence of abundant parakeratosis and an inflammatory infiltrate of neutrophils or mononuclear cells in the nail plate (Fig. 21–3B). If candidal invasion of the nail plate occurs, budding yeast forms and hyphae can be found by staining the nail with periodic acid–Schiff (PAS) reagent or Gomori–methenamine silver. With these stains, dermatophytes are seen as elongate hyphae with branching or septation (Fig. 21–3C). Culture is usually necessary for definitive identification of the causative organism.

Viral Infection: Human Papillomavirus

- EPITHELIUM HAS A PAPILLOMATOUS ARCHITECTURE
- SCALE WITH PARAKERATOTIC COLUMNS WITH OR WITHOUT HEMORRHAGE OVER PAPILLARY TIPS
- WIDELY ECTATIC BLOOD VESSELS IN ELONGATE PAPILLAE
- WITH RECENT INFECTION, PERINUCLEAR HALOS AND VARIABLY SIZED KERATOHYALINE GRANULES IN GRANULAR CELL LAYER

Verrucae may occur at the proximal and lateral nail folds and on the hyponychium (Fig. 21–4A). They have irregular, rough, keratotic surfaces and may have superimposed foci of pinpoint bleeding or fissuring. As warts grow, they may cause nail deformities by encroaching on the nail matrix or by lifting the nail plate. Periungual and subungual verrucae are difficult to eradicate.

Histologically, the changes are similar to those of verrucae on other glaborous sites. The epidermis has a papillom-

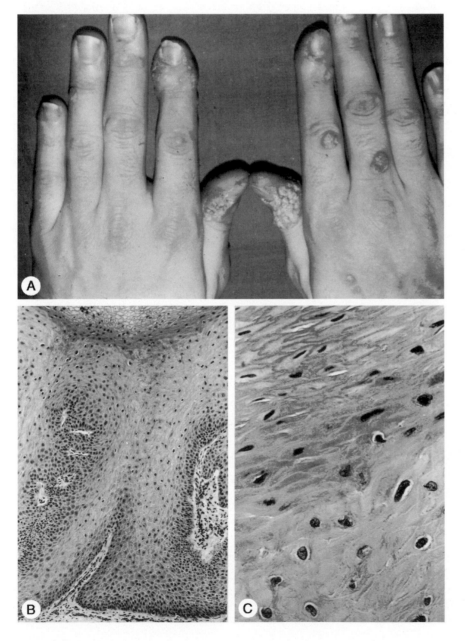

Figure 21–4. Verruca vulgaris of the fingers and nails. **(A)** Multiple verrucous scaly nodules on slightly erythematous bases are present around the nails and on the knuckles. **(B)** The epidermis shows acanthosis and papillomatosis, and the dermis contains widely dilated blood vessels. **(C)** In the stratum granulosum, there are halos about keratinocyte nuclei and variably sized keratohyalin granules, which are papillomavirus cytopathic changes.

atous architecture surmounted by alternating columns of orthokeratotic and parakeratotic scale (Fig. 21–4B). Often, hemorrhage may be seen in the scale overlying papillary tips. The papillary dermal stroma contains widely ectatic blood vessels and inflammatory infiltrates of varying intensity.

If the wart has grown relatively recently, keratinocytes of the stratum granulosum will show perinuclear halos and variably sized keratohyaline granules, which are papillomavirus cytopathic changes (Fig. 21–4C). Staining with papillomavirus immunoperoxidase stains shows intranuclear positivity for viral proteins. In long-standing warts, characteristic cytopathic changes are no longer apparent, but the overall architecture is the same as that in early lesions.

Inflammatory Processes

Lichen Planus[5]

- TAGGING OF BASILAR KERATINOCYTES OF THE NAIL BED BY LYMPHOCYTES
- NECROSIS OF INDIVIDUAL BASILAR KERATINOCYTES
- MAY BE EFFACEMENT OF THE DERMAL-EPITHELIAL JUNCTION

A small fraction of patients with lichen planus (approximately 10%) have discernible changes in their nails. It is possible to have nail involvement without evidence of cutaneous disease elsewhere. One or all of the nails may be altered. The changes vary from periungual violaceous papules in the nail bed or fold to pitting and grooving in the nail (Fig. 21–5A). Loss of nails with scarring may produce a permanent cosmetic defect. A pterygium may form if the nail plate is thinned to the point where the nail bed can adhere to the nail fold.

The histology of active lesions is that of lichen planus: a lymphocytic infiltrate tags the dermal-epithelial junction and causes necrosis of individual keratinocytes (Fig. 21–5B, C). If the inflammation is intense, the undulating contour of the dermal-epithelial junction may be lost.

Psoriasis[6–8]

- PARAKERATOTIC FOCI IN THE NAIL PLATE WITH INTERVENING ZONES OF ORTHOKERATIN
- NAIL MATRIX WITH NEUTROPHILS

Patients with psoriasis frequently have nail changes (approximately 10–50%). These changes may be clues to diagnosis if the characteristic erythematous scaly plaques are absent elsewhere on the body. The nails are commonly pitted and ridged, producing a rough surface. If pitting occurs along the lower surface of the nail plate, greasy-appearing spots (i.e., oil spots) can be seen in the nail plate. Abnormal keratinization of the nail bed results in the formation of subungual keratotic debris, which in turn may cause lifting of the nail plate distally (i.e., onycholysis). Inflammation of the nail matrix can produce nail dystrophy (Fig. 21–6A). In pustular psoriasis, pustules arise under the nail plate, causing destruction and loss of the nail plate. There is a high degree of correlation between nail changes and psoriatic arthritis of the distal interphalangeal joints.

Histologically, nail pits are foci of loose parakeratin on the dorsum of the nail plate. They form as a result of intermittent inflammation in the proximal nail fold. The loose parakeratotic cells desquamate easily, leaving behind small dells in the surface of the nail. Sections of nail plate may also show collections of neutrophils in the parakeratotic foci, similar to psoriatic lesions on glaborous skin (Fig. 21–6B, C). Nail plate dystrophy correlates with extensive parakera-

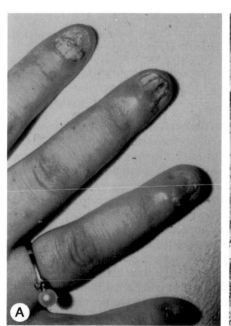
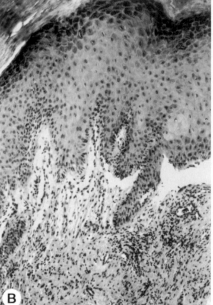
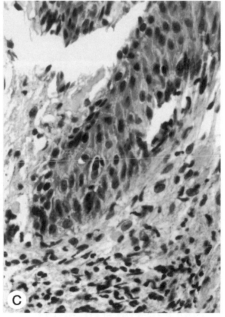

Figure 21–5. Lichen planus of the nails. **(A)** Marked dystrophy of the nail plate and pterygium formation are present. **(B)** There is focal separation of the nail bed epithelium from the dermis and an inflammatory infiltrate in the dermal stroma. **(C)** Lymphocytes tag the basilar layer of the nail bed. Focal basilar keratinocyte necrosis can be seen. These changes are similar to those of lichen planus located elsewhere on the skin.

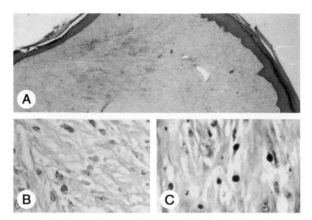

Figure 21–10. Infantile digital fibromatosis. **(A)** A large exophytic nodule is surrounded by an epithelial collarette (top of lesion to the right). **(B)** In the stroma, there is a proliferation of fibroblast-like cells with intracytoplasmic, eosinophilic inclusion bodies. **(C)** These inclusion bodies are easily discerned with Masson trichrome stain.

Infantile Digital Fibromatosis[17, 18]

- INTERLACING FASCICLES OF FIBROBLASTS IN A DENSE DERMAL STROMA
- CHARACTERISTIC SMALL, ROUND, EOSINOPHILIC PERINUCLEAR INCLUSIONS IN THE CYTOPLASM OF FIBROBLASTIC CELLS

This disorder is characterized by multiple, well-circumscribed, firm, erythematous nodules on the dorsal and lateral aspects of the digits in infants and children. Lesions frequently recur despite surgical excision. These neoplasms can cause joint deformities and compromise joint mobility. They are thought to be hamartomas of myofibroblasts.

The dermis contains poorly defined, nodular collections of fibroblasts arranged in fascicles seen in various planes of section. The most characteristic finding is the presence of small, round, eosinophilic inclusions in the cytoplasm of the proliferating cells adjacent to their nuclei (Fig. 21–10). These inclusions stain positively with trichrome or phospotungstic acid and hematoxylin (PTAH). Immunohistochemically, these inclusions have been found to contain actin, which suggests that infantile digital fibromatosis is a neoplasm of myofibroblastic cells.

Myxoid Cyst of the Digit[19, 20]

- COLLECTIONS OF MUCIN IN THE DERMIS
- CONSPICUOUS ABSENCE OF A SURROUNDING EPITHELIAL WALL

A myxoid cyst of the digit is not a cyst in the classic sense of an epithelial-lined cavity, but it is a dermal collection of mucopolysaccharides. This lesion is thought to represent a degenerative change in connective tissue rather than an extension of the synovium outside of the joint cavity. A myxoid cyst grossly appears as a flesh-colored to reddish, dome-shaped, soft nodule, most often located close to the proximal nail fold. The cyst may exude a thick, clear, odorless fluid. If the lesion impinges on the nail matrix, it produces a localized depression that runs from the proximal nail fold to the distal edge of the nail plate (Fig. 21–11A).

Microscopically, the dermis contains collections of stringy, granular-appearing, basophilic material representing mucopolysaccharide deposits in the dermal stroma; the dermis also contains stellate-shaped fibroblasts (Fig. 21–11A, B). These aggregates are not surrounded by a synovial or epithelial lining. Special stains such as alcian blue confirm the nature of this material. Occasionally, if a superficial biopsy is taken, the only clue to an underlying myxoid cyst is the presence of pooled mucin that has been eliminated into the stratum corneum.

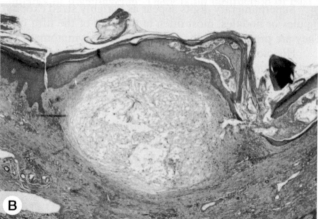

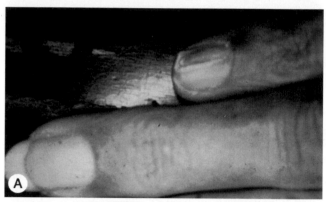

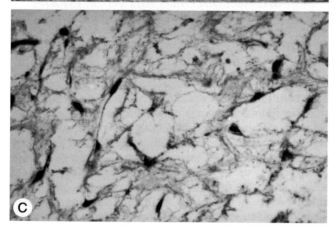

Figure 21–11. Digital myxoid cyst. **(A)** An erythematous, dome-shaped nodule is present at the base of the nail on the fifth digit. The longitudinal groove in the nail plate occurred because the cyst impinges on the nail matrix. **(B)** A large, nodular collection of basophilic material expands the dermal stroma. Mucin is eliminated through the epidermis and into the stratum corneum. **(C)** Dermal deposits of stringy, granular, basophilic material characteristic of mucin are separated by stellate fibroblasts.

Squamous Cell Carcinoma in Situ[21–24]

- FULL-THICKNESS ATYPIA OF KERATINOCYTES
- SUPERFICIALLY PLACED MITOTIC FIGURES, MANY ABNORMAL
- PARAKERATOTIC SCALE COMMON

Squamous cell carcinoma-in-situ may present as a periungual erythematous or pigmented lesion. The surface may be hyperkeratotic or eroded. This disorder commonly affects the fingers, particularly the thumbs, and most often arises in patients older than the age of 50 years. Although disease progression is slow, invasive squamous cell carcinoma may arise in this neoplasm; therefore, biopsy sampling of the most infiltrated area is essential. Because squamous cell carcinoma-in-situ may proliferate under the nail plate, nail avulsion is necessary to ensure removal of the entire lesion.

The histology of squamous cell carcinoma-in-situ at this site is the same as that elsewhere on the skin; there is atypia of keratinocytes at all levels of the epidermis, often associated with the formation of parakeratotic scale. Mitotic figures, including abnormal ones, are often seen in superficial epithelial layers. It is important to thoroughly sample the lesion to exclude the possibility of an invasive component in this neoplasm.

Invasive Squamous Cell Carcinoma[25–28]

- ATYPICAL KERATINOCYTES INVADE THE DERMAL STROMA INDIVIDUALLY AND IN NESTS
- INDIVIDUAL CELL KERATINIZATION IN WELL-DIFFERENTIATED FORMS
- VARIABLE HOST RESPONSE ALONG THE BASE

Similar to squamous cell carcinoma-in-situ at this site, invasive squamous cell carcinoma affects the fingers more than the toes, in particular the thumb and index finger. Individuals whose fingers were exposed to radiation are at risk for developing this tumor. The presenting signs and symptoms vary from localized pain and swelling to ulceration and destruction of the nail plate. Bony invasion occurs rarely and late in the course of the disease. The inflammatory changes associated with this neoplasm may mask the true nature of the process and delay biopsy and treatment.

Invasive squamous cell carcinoma shows invasion of the dermal stroma by keratinocytes with variable degrees of differentiation. If the neoplasm is well-differentiated and has pushing borders, it is called verrucous carcinoma. The keratinization of atypical neoplastic cells is a clue to their lineage. If keratinization is not apparent, and the infiltration of atypical cells is deep, immunohistochemical stains for keratin may be helpful in defining the nature and delineating the extent of the tumor.

Lentigines and Nevi

- LENTIGINES: INCREASED NUMBERS OF MELANOCYTES IN A HYPERPLASTIC EPITHELIUM
- NEVI: NEVOMELANOCYTES IN NESTS AT TIPS OF RETE RIDGES

- LACK OF SIGNIFICANT INTER-RETE MELANOCYTIC PROLIFERATION
- LACK OF INFLAMMATION IN THE DERMIS

Linear brown to black bands along the length of the nail plate often herald the presence of a melanocytic process in the nail bed or nail matrix (Fig. 21–12A). These lesions are more common in individuals with more constitutive pigmentation, such as patients of Asian or African descent. Because lentigines, nevi, and melanomas may have similar clinical presentations, biopsy or excision of these lesions is important to accurately diagnose the cause of pigmented bands of the nails.

As with lentigines at other anatomic sites, in the fingers and toes, there are increased numbers of individually disposed melanocytes without nest formation along the dermal-epithelial junction. Occasionally, melanophages may be found in the subjacent stroma (Fig. 21–12B). The epithelium may be hyperplastic and may show basilar hyperpigmentation.

Nevi show nesting of melanocytes, normally among the tips of rete ridges. Nested melanocytes are relatively uniform in size and shape and lack nuclear pleomorphism. Although there may be occasional individual basilar melanocytes between rete ridges, these are few. Some nevi (i.e., compound nevi) may also show a dermal component, which is arranged in nests and strands. Dermal melanocytes usually acquire smaller cytoplasmic contours as they descend deeper into the stroma. Lack of melanocytic atypia, mitotic activity, necro-

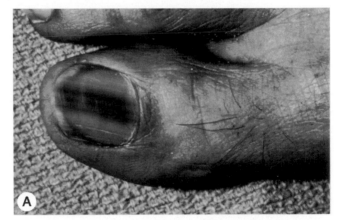

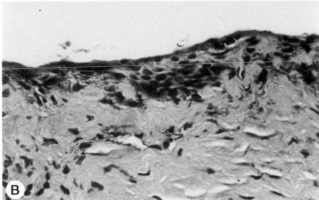

Figure 21–12. Lentigo of nail bed. **(A)** A pigmented band in the nail of the great toe represents a lentigo of the nail bed. **(B)** The basilar layer of nail bed epithelium shows increased numbers of melanocytes. There are melanophages in the superficial dermal stroma.

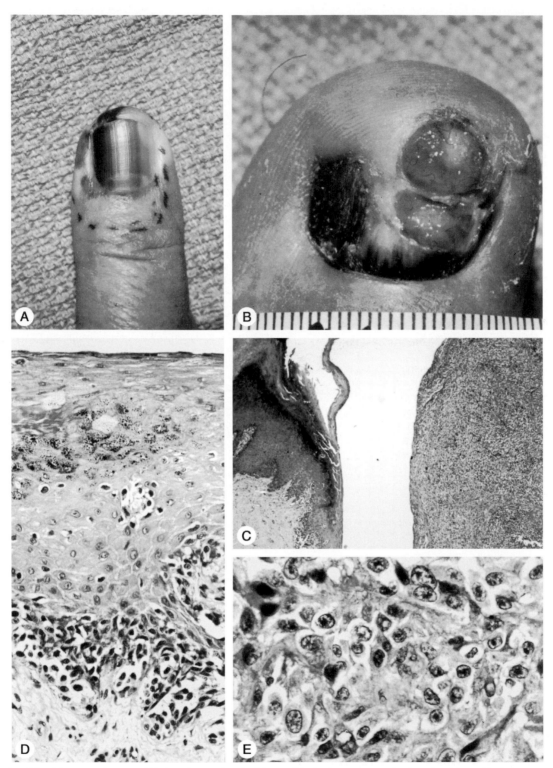

Figure 21–13. Acral lentiginous melanoma. **(A)** A variegate band of brown-black pigment runs the length of the nail plate. Note the spillage of pigment on to the proximal and lateral nail folds. **(B)** There is complete loss of the nail plate. The nail bed is black. Centrally, there are two exophytic nodules representing the vertical growth phase. (Courtesy of the Pigmented Lesion Group at the University of Pennsylvania.) **(C)** Scanning magnification shows a continuous proliferation of melanocytes along the basilar layer of the nail bed (*left*; radial growth phase) and a large exophytic nodule (*right*; vertical growth phase). **(D)** Pleomorphic melanocytes grow in a continuous fashion along the basilar layer of epithelium with little tendency for upward growth of individual cells. **(E)** Cells of the vertical growth phase display a high degree of cytologic pleomorphism, abundant mitotic activity, and minimal pigment in their cytoplasms.

sis, and inflammation distinguish acral nevi from acral melanoma.

Acral Lentiginous Melanoma

- NEARLY CONTINUOUS PROLIFERATION OF MELANOCYTES WITH OR WITHOUT NESTING ALONG ELONGATE RETE RIDGES
- UPWARD INTRAEPITHELIAL MELANOCYTIC MIGRATION MUCH LESS COMMON THAN IN SUPERFICIAL SPREADING MELANOMA
- USUALLY, A MONONUCLEAR HOST RESPONSE PRESENT IN THE DERMIS
- VERTICAL GROWTH PHASE, IF PRESENT, FORMS A NODULE OF ATYPICAL CELLS IN THE DERMIS OR ILL-DEFINED FASCICLES OF SPINDLE CELLS WHICH MAY SURROUND AND INFILTRATE NERVES

Malignant melanoma of the nail area is uncommon. This type of melanoma is seen with higher frequency in individuals of African descent (15–20%) than in Caucasians (2–3%). The actual incidence, however, is similar in both races, because Caucasians develop melanoma at other sites more often than patients of African descent. Most acral lentiginous melanomas are found on the thumbs and great toes in individuals older than 50 years of age.

The early clinical changes are usually subtle; an asymptomatic localized discoloration of the nail bed or periungual tissues may go unnoticed until it becomes traumatized. The lesion may have a regular or irregular border in the nail plate, bed, or matrix. A band of brown-black pigment may extend the length of the nail. If the pigmentation spreads to the nail fold or surrounding skin (i.e., Hutchinson sign) it is a highly valuable clue to the diagnosis of melanoma at this site (Fig. 21–13A). The presence of a nodule in association with discoloration or erosion of the nail plate is indicative of an invasive growth phase (Fig. 21–13B). A significant percentage of these lesions are amelanotic and are therefore perceived as inflammatory or reactive processes, which can cause significant delays in diagnosis. Surgical excision or amputation are the treatments of choice. The extent of the procedure depends upon the growth phase of the lesion and the depth of tumor invasion.

Microscopically, there are increased numbers of melanocytes proliferating in a continuous pattern along the dermal-epithelial interface (Fig. 21–13C, D). The cells grow in a dyshesive manner, focally forming loose nests which appear to separate the dermal-epidermal junction. There is only a slight tendency to individual melanocytic upward growth as is characteristically seen in superficial spreading melanoma. A lymphocytic infiltrate is usually present in the dermis in a band-like configuration and is a valuable clue to the abnormal melanocytic process. Invasion of the dermis is seen as individual cells or small clusters of abnormal melanocytes dropping down into the inflamed stroma. The vertical growth phase may evolve as a single dominant dermal nodule (Fig. 21–13E) or as spindle cells of the type seen in desmoplastic melanomas. In the latter type, neurotropism may be prominent. The prognosis varies with the presence of the vertical growth phase, the depth of invasion, the host response, and the adequacy of treatment.

SELECTED REFERENCES

1. Omura EP. Histopathology of the nail. Dermatol Clin 1985;3:531.
2. Pfister R. Color changes in the nails in medical diagnosis: Black-brown and other discolorations. Fortschr Med 1982;100:795.
3. Haneke E. Fungal infections of the nail. Semin Dermatol 1991;10:41.
4. English MP. Nails and fungi. Br J Dermatol 1976;94:697.
5. Alkiewicz J, Nowak Z. Clinical aspects and histology of lichen planus ruber of the nails. Arch Klin Exp Dermatol 1970;238:346.
6. Achten G, Parent D. The normal and pathologic nail. Int J Dermatol 1983;22:556.
7. Norton LA. Nail disorders. A review. J Am Acad Dermatol 1980;2:451.
8. Farber EM, Nail L. Nail psoriasis. Cutis 1992;50:174.
9. Tosti A, Fanti PA, Morelli R, Bardazzi F. Trachyonychia associated with alopecia areata: A clinical and pathologic study. J Am Acad Dermatol 1991;25:266.
10. Fanti PA, Tosti A. Histologic aspects of dystrophy of the 20 nails associated with alopecia areata. G Ital Dermatol Venereol 1988;123:533.
11. Laporte M, Andre J, Stouffs-Vanhoof F, Achten G. Nail changes in alopecia areata: Light and electron microscopy. Arch Dermatol Res 1988;280(Suppl):85.
12. Mortimer PS, Dawber RP. Dermatologic diseases of the nail unit other than psoriasis and lichen planus. Dermatol Clin 1985;3:401.
13. Kint A, Baran R, De-Keyser H. Acquired (digital) fibrokeratoma. J Am Acad Dermatol 1985;12:816.
14. Cahn RL. Acquired periungual fibrokeratoma. A rare benign tumor previously described as the garlic-clove fibroma. Arch Dermatol 1977;113:1564.
15. Kouskoukis CE. Subungual glomus tumor: A clinico-pathological study. J Dermatol Surg Oncol 1983;9:294.
16. Rettig AC, Strickland JW. Glomus tumor of the digits. J Hand Surg [Am] 1977;2:261.
17. Mukai M, Torikata C, Iri H, et al. Immunohistochemical identification of aggregated actin filaments in formalin-fixed, paraffin-embedded sections. I. A study of infantile digital fibromatosis by a new pretreatment. Am J Surg Pathol 1992;16:110.
18. Choi KC, Hashimoto K, Setoyama M, et al. Infantile digital fibromatosis. Immunohistochemical and immunoelectron microscopic studies. J Cutan Pathol 1990;17:225.
19. Miller PK, Roenigk RK, Amadio PC. Focal mucinosis (myxoid cyst). Surgical therapy. J Dermatol Surg Oncol 1992;18:716.
20. Sonnex TS. Digital myxoid cysts: A review. Cutis 1986;37:89.
21. Kouskoukis C-E, Scher RK, Kopf AW. Squamous-cell carcinoma of the nail bed. J Dermatol Surg Oncol 1982;8:853.
22. Guitart J, Bergfeld WF, Tuthill RJ, et al. Squamous cell carcinoma of the nail bed: A clinicopathological study of 12 cases. Br J Dermatol 1990;123:215.
23. Lumpkin LR III, Rosen T, Tschen JA. Subungual squamal cell carcinoma. J Am Acad Dermatol 1984;11:735.
24. Hazelrigg DE, Renne JW. Squamous-cell carcinoma of the nail bed. J Dermatol Surg Oncol 1982;8:200.
25. Wells KE, Reintgen DS, Cruse CW. The current management and prognosis of acral lentiginous melanoma. Ann Plast Surg 1992;28:100.
26. Gutman M, Klausner JM, Inbar M, et al. Acral (volar-subungual) melanoma. Br J Surg 1985;72:610.
27. Sondergaard K. Histological type and biological behavior of primary cutaneous malignant melanoma. An analysis of 86 cases located on socalled acral regions as plantar, palmar, and sub-/parungual areas. Virchows Arch A Pathol Anat Histopathol 1983;401:333.
28. Coleman WP III, Loria PR, Reed RJ, Krementz ET. Acral lentiginous melanoma. Arch Dermatol 1980;116:773.

22
Dermatopathology of Anogenital Skin

Suzanne M. Jacques and W. Dwayne Lawrence

DEFINITIONS AND GENERAL CONSIDERATIONS[1, 2]

Anogenital skin, especially the skin of the vulva, is prone to affliction with a variety of lesions that rarely affect other skin areas, probably because of local environmental factors. Clothing contributes to the unusual environment of anogenital skin by trapping heat and restricting air circulation; this creates a moist environment with an increased hydrophilic state of the stratum corneum. The absorptive power of the skin is dependent on its state of hydration; therefore, the comparatively wet anogenital area is far more absorptive of extrinsic, often irritating substances than is extragenital skin. The apposition of anogenital skin folds, particularly in obese people, leads to skin friction and consequent chronic irritation in a mucosa that is inherently easily irritated. All these factors lead to an environment conducive to the growth of bacteria and fungi. Because many sexually transmitted organisms also affect the anogenital skin, diagnostic confusion concerning otherwise distinctive histopathologic entities may result from both a gross and microscopic perspective because of the superimposed changes of sexually transmitted diseases and local environmental factors.

The skin of the labia majora is identical to extragenital skin. Hair follicles are present on the lateral aspects of the labia majora, but are absent on the medial aspects. Because squamous vulvar intraepithelial neoplasia (VIN), Paget cells, and melanoma cells may extend into the hair sheath and its associated pilosebaceous unit, these structures must be encompassed in any treatment modality for VIN; consequently, excision or ablation of lesions must be of sufficient depth (at least 3–4 mm) to insure the destruction of these cells. Hart line is the demarcation between the skin and mucous membrane of the vulva. This line extends in a curvilinear fashion, starting anteriorly from the medial aspect of the labia majora, extending to the most inferiorposterior aspect of the labia minora, and ending posteriorly at the vaginal fourchette. Sebaceous glands are present medial and posterior to the labia minora at the junction with Hart line; these open directly onto the epithelial surface, resulting in small, pale yellow elevations known as Fordyce spots. The vulvar epithelium contains melanocytes, and increased pigmentation may result from hormonal influences. Langerhans cells and Merkel cells are present in the vulva, as in other skin sites.

The vulvar vestibule is that portion of the vulva demarcated by the clitoris anteriorly, fourchette posteriorly, labia minora anterolaterally, and Hart line posterolaterally. The skin in this area is of endodermal origin, unlike the remainder of genital skin, which is of ectodermal origin. The squamous epithelium of the vestibule is predominantly nonkeratinized, whereas that of the labia minora, fourchette, and prepuce is thinly keratinized. In women of reproductive age, the squamous epithelium is well glycogenated in this area. The high moisture content of the anogenital skin may affect the appearance of dermatoses; in particular, scaling may be much less obvious.

The mucous membrane of the glans penis is composed of nonglycogenated, stratified, squamous epithelium, which is keratinized in circumcised men and nonkeratinized in uncircumcised men. Lamina propria and the corpus spongiosum lie beneath the epidermis; normal skin adnexal structures are not present in the glans. The outer surface of the foreskin has a dermis containing a few sebaceous and sweat glands. The inner surface of the foreskin is lined by a mucosa identical to that of the glans. The epidermis of the penile shaft is thin and minimally keratinized. Few sebaceous and sweat glands are present, and hair follicles are present in the proximal portion. As in the vulva, the skin is relatively hyperpigmented. Perianal skin is keratinized and contains sweat glands, apocrine glands, sebaceous glands, and hair follicles.

Most dermatologic conditions affecting extragenital skin can also affect anogenital skin. Herpesvirus infection and specific dermatoses such as psoriasis and lichen planus are discussed in detail elsewhere in this book and are not repeated in this chapter. Benign melanocytic lesions such as freckles and nevi, as well as adnexal tumors, are identical grossly and microscopically in anogenital and extragenital skin; of the adnexal tumors, the most common is the papillary hidradenoma, a benign eccrine tumor seen most frequently in the vulva. The lesions discussed in this chapter are restricted to those characteristically found in anogenital skin or those that have a prognosis or presentation altered by their location in this area. Additionally, this chapter reflects the fact that the preponderance of non-neoplastic and infectious lesions as well as intraepithelial neoplasia and invasive carcinomas that afflict the anogenital skin affect women.

HISTOLOGY OF SPECIFIC DISORDERS

Non-neoplastic Epithelial Disorders[3, 4]

Non-neoplastic epithelial disorders (NNEDs), or vulvar dystrophies, are commonly encountered lesions of female anogenital skin, particularly in the vulva. They represent a major component of clinically recognized white lesions, formerly referred to as leukoplakia. The nomenclature of these disorders has been confusing, because these conditions fall within the realms of both gynecology and dermatology, and each specialty, including pathology, has developed its own terminology. The following discussion uses the classification developed by the nomenclature committees of the International Society for the Study of Vulvar Disease (ISSVD) and the International Society of Gynecological Pathologists (ISGP, Table 22–1). This classification scheme recognizes the categories of lichen sclerosus, squamous cell hyperplasia, and other dermatoses. One of the many previous classifications employed the categories of hyperplastic dystrophy and mixed dystrophy and included such lesions with concurrent presence or absence of atypia as subcategories (Table 22–2). In the newest classification, the term hyperplastic dystrophy has been dropped and replaced with squamous cell hyperplasia. Similarly, the term mixed dystrophy, which referred primarily to lichen sclerosus with foci of squamous cell hyperplasia, has been eliminated. Lichen sclerosus and squamous cell hyperplasia coexist in about 15% of NNEDs, and the current recommendation is to report both diagnoses separately. Both categories of squamous cell hyperplasia and lichen sclerosus exclude lesions with atypia; the latter should be placed in the appropriate category of VIN. Lesions that have the characteristic histopathologic features of specific, well-defined dermatoses (e.g., lichen simplex chronicus) or

Table 22–1. NON-NEOPLASTIC EPITHELIAL DISORDERS OF SKIN AND MUCOSA

I. Lichen sclerosus
II. Squamous cell hyperplasia, not otherwise specified
III. Other dermatoses

ISGP, International Society of Gynecological Pathologists; and ISSVD, International Society for the Study of Vulvar Diseases, 1990.

From Lawrence WD: Non-neoplastic epithelial disorders of the vulva (vulvar dystrophies): Historical and current perspectives. In: Rosen PP, Fechner RE, eds. Pathology Annual, part II, vol. 28. Norwalk, CT: Appleton & Lange, 1993:23–51.

Table 22–2. VULVAR DYSTROPHIES

I. Hyperplastic dystrophy
A. Without atypia
B. With atypia
II. Lichen sclerosus
III. Mixed dystrophy (lichen sclerosus with foci of epithelial hyperplasia)
A. Without atypia
B. With atypia

ISSVD, International Society for the Study of Vulvar Diseases, 1975.

From Lawrence WD: Non-neoplastic epithelial disorders of the vulva (vulvar dystrophies): Historical and current perspectives. In: Rosen PP, Fechner RE, eds. Pathology Annual, part II, vol. 28. Norwalk, CT: Appleton & Lange, 1993:23–51.

papulosquamous disorders (e.g., seborrheic dermatitis, lichen planus) should be classified as such and excluded from the category of squamous cell hyperplasia.

Lichen Sclerosus[3, 4]

- WHITE MACROPAPULES THAT COALESCE
- FREQUENTLY MULTIFOCAL AND SYMMETRICALLY BILATERAL
- THIN EPIDERMIS WITH LOSS OF RETE PEGS
- SUBEPIDERMAL HOMOGENEOUS COLLAGENOUS OR HYALINIZED ZONE
- LYMPHOCYTIC INFILTRATE BENEATH THE SUBEPIDERMAL HOMOGENEOUS ZONE
- ABSENCE OF ATYPIA

Lichen sclerosus may affect the skin of the trunk or extremities of people of either gender, but it is most common in the vulva. When it involves the penile foreskin or glans, this disorder is known as balanitis xerotica obliterans. Lichen sclerosus most frequently affects postmenopausal women, but it may be found in any age group, including children. It is the most common cause of vulvar leukoplakia and accounts for 30 to 40% of NNEDs. The most frequent presenting symptom is pruritus.

Lesions of lichen sclerosus are commonly multiple and bilateral so that extension to the perianal skin, inner buttocks, and thighs may result in a characteristic butterfly or figure-of-eight pattern (Fig. 22–1A). Involvement of extragenital skin is more prone to occur in children.

Lichen sclerosus has more distinctive gross and microscopic characteristics than does squamous cell hyperplasia. Irregular, white macropapules coalesce to form plaques, which may progress until normal skin folds are destroyed. Adhesions, comedo-like plugs, and in early cases, edema of the clitoral foreskin may help distinguish lichen sclerosus from other white vulvar lesions. In late-stage cases, the labia majora and minora and clitoris may be completely obliterated. Severe shrinkage and contraction may cause the vaginal introitus to become very small, a process previously referred to as kraurosis, although this term is a misnomer, because kraurosis is derived from the Greek word meaning brittle. The skin becomes pale, shiny, and wrinkled, and assumes an appearance that has been likened to parchment or cigarette paper.

Microscopically, advanced lichen sclerosus is characterized by a thin epidermis with decreased number of layers

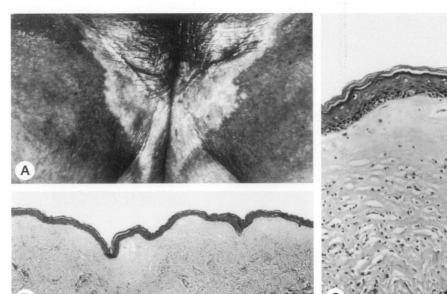

Figure 22–1. Lichen sclerosus. **(A)** This whitish plaque has a characteristic bilaterally symmetrical pattern (i.e., butterfly pattern). **(B)** At scanning magnification, there is epidermal atrophy with loss of rete ridges and a pale band of hyalinized collagen within the superficial dermis. **(C)** The hypocellular zone of hyalinization is better appreciated at higher magnification; note the absence of cellular atypia in the overlying epidermis. **(A** from Deppe G, Lawrence WD: Vulvar dystrophy and neoplasia. In: Gusberg SB, Deppe G, Shingleton HM, eds. Female Genital Cancer. New York, Churchill Livingstone, 1988: 223–251.)

and loss of rete pegs. Hyperkeratosis is frequently present. A diminution in the number of melanocytes may contribute to the whiteness of the lesion. Perhaps the most characteristic feature, however, is a subepithelial, paucicellular, homogeneous zone that appears collagenous or hyalinized (Fig. 22–1B). A variably-sized band of lymphocytes often lies directly beneath this zone. Additional features sometimes include follicular plugging and focal hydropic degeneration and edema in the basal layer, which may progress to subepidermal bullae, causing confusion with the bullous dermatoses. Foci of squamous cell hyperplasia may be present, possibly as a reaction to scratching. Rubbing and scratching may also produce acute inflammation, ulceration, and extravasation of red blood cells in the dermis. Squamous atypia is absent, and mitoses are rare to absent (Fig. 22–1C).

The pathogenesis of lichen sclerosus is not well understood. The metabolic activity in the squamous epithelium may be increased, indicating that although thin, the epithelium is not necessarily atrophic. For this reason, the previously applied suffix et atrophicus was dropped. Elastic fibers, possibly secondary to increased levels of a recently isolated elastase-type protease found in vulvar fibroblasts, as well as fibronectin and collagen types I and III are decreased in quantity in the dermis. Hyaluronic acid is also decreased, and the resulting alterations in dermal hydration and electrolyte balance have been considered to be contributors to the pathogenesis of lichen sclerosus. Other possible etiologies include autoimmune and hormonal mechanisms. In general, women with lichen sclerosus have a higher incidence of autoimmune-related disorders and an increased occurrence of organ-specific antibodies. Patients with lichen sclerosus have been shown to have low serum levels of androstenedione, testosterone, and dihydrotestosterone, suggesting a decreased activity of 5-alpha-reductase, the enzyme found in the skin that converts free testosterone to the active form of dihydrotestosterone. Accordingly, the lesion may show good response to the local application of testosterone ointment, and patients with low serum levels of the aforementioned hormones showed normal or elevated serum levels after topical testosterone treatment. Lichen sclerosus is not considered premalignant, but it may be associated with squamous cell carcinoma.

Squamous Cell Hyperplasia[3, 4]

- ACANTHOSIS WITH ELONGATION OF RETE PEGS
- PROMINENT HYPERKERATOSIS
- PROMINENT GRANULAR LAYER FREQUENTLY PRESENT
- SQUAMOUS MATURATION WITH NO MITOSES ABOVE THE BASAL LAYER
- CHRONIC DERMAL INFLAMMATION, SOMETIMES MARKED
- ABSENCE OF CELLULAR ATYPIA

Squamous cell hyperplasia (SCH) usually represents a hyperplastic response of vulvar skin to intrinsic or extrinsic irritation. The lesion has been implicated as accounting for approximately one half of the NNEDs; however, since the recent transfer of lichen simplex chronicus from the SCH category to the category of other dermatoses, its actual incidence may be found to be much lower. SCH has no racial predilection. It occurs in patients with a wide range of ages but is most common in the fourth and fifth decades of life. Patients typically present with pruritus. Clinical examination reveals well-delineated, elevated, pink, red, or white lesions. The lesions may appear white if there is marked hyperkeratosis or pink to red if lesser degrees of hyperkeratosis are present. Decreased amounts of melanin may also contribute to the pallor of squamous cell hyperplasia. Isolated lesions are more common with squamous cell hyperplasia than with lichen sclerosus; however, lesions may also be bilateral and symmetrical and involve the labia majora, outer aspects of the labia minora and posterior commissure, interlabial sulci, and clitoral hood. Ulceration and edema may follow persistent scratching and lichenification. Thickening of skin with

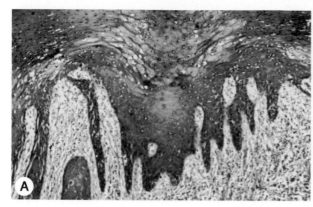

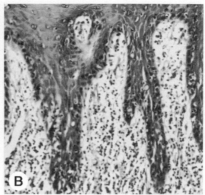

Figure 22–2. Squamous cell hyperplasia. **(A)** There is marked irregular elongation of rete ridges in association with hyperkeratosis and parakeratosis. **(B)** The dermis contains a nonspecific inflammatory infiltrate composed of lymphocytes and plasma cells; dysplasia is not present within the hyperplastic epidermal layer.

accentuation of normal markings secondary to chronic rubbing or scratching is often present.

Microscopically, squamous cell hyperplasia is characterized by acanthosis, hyperkeratosis, and elongated clubbed or pointed rete pegs (Fig. 22–2A). The granular layer is frequently prominent. A dermal lymphocytic infiltrate, sometimes accompanied by plasma cells, may be prominent. Parakeratosis sometimes may be present; because this feature is more commonly seen with human papillomavirus (HPV)–associated lesions, a careful search to exclude nuclear atypia is warranted. Papillomatosis, another feature associated with HPV infection, is absent in squamous cell hyperplasia. The squamous epithelium shows normal maturation with small, uniform, round-to-oval nuclei (Fig. 22–2B). Nucleoli are occasionally prominent. Mitoses normally are not seen above the basal layer.

Squamous cell hyperplasia often responds well to the topical application of steroids and antipruritics. Patients with concurrent squamous cell hyperplasia and lichen sclerosus, formerly referred to as mixed dystrophy, frequently show good response to topical steroids followed by standard therapy for lichen sclerosus (i.e., topical testosterone ointment). However, in rare patients, severe and persistent symptoms may necessitate surgery.

Condyloma Acuminatum[5]

- PAPILLARY OR VERRUCOUS MASS
- MAY BE SESSILE OR ARISE FROM A STALK
- ACANTHOSIS WITH PARAKERATOSIS, AND IN SOME CASES, HYPERKERATOSIS
- PAPILLARY FRONDS SUPPORTED BY A CENTRAL FIBROVASCULAR CORE
- KOILOCYTE IS CHARACTERISTIC CELL
- FEATURES OF DYSPLASIA ARE ABSENT

Condyloma acuminatum, or venereal warts, are distinctive lesions characteristically found on anogenital skin. They are usually caused by venereal transmission of HPV types 6 and 11, serotypes of HPV not found in most extragenital warts. Condyloma acuminatum generally presents as a warty mass but is otherwise asymptomatic. The incidence of condyloma acuminatum is increasing, and although this condition is most common in the third decade of life, it may affect any age group, even children. Occurrence of condy-

loma acuminatum in children should arouse the suspicion of sexual abuse. The lesion has no gender predilection and may be found anywhere on the anogenital skin. Multiple sites of involvement are usual. Condyloma acuminatum appears to have a predilection for the perianal skin of homosexual men. In women, involvement of the vulva is most common. The predilection for multifocality of the lesions necessitates not only a complete examination of the anogenital skin, but also of the lower genital tract in women. Concomitant lesions of the cervix and vagina are relatively common; therefore, a complete gynecologic examination should include a cervical smear for cytology and, if indicated, colposcopic examination of the lower female genital tract. The anogenital region of the patient's sexual partner should also be examined. The growth of condylomata acuminata may be exacerbated during pregnancy or in immunosuppressed individuals.

Diagnosis is frequently possible based solely on the clinical appearance of the lesions. Grossly, condyloma acuminatum is papillary or verrucous (Fig. 22–3A), particularly in the vulva and vagina, where 80% of the lesions are exophytic. They may arise from a stalk or be large, sessile confluent masses. In some cases, the lesions are so small that they may either be missed with the unaided eye or be difficult to characterize. In those lesions with an atypical gross appearance, the differential diagnosis includes entities such as acrochordons, seborrheic keratoses, hemorrhoids, VIN, squamous cell carcinoma, and, if large, verrucous carcinoma. Except in the latter case, the diagnosis is usually easily made after biopsy and microscopic examination.

Microscopically, condyloma acuminatum is characterized by acanthosis and papillomatosis (Fig. 22–3B). The papillary fronds surround a central fibrovascular stroma that extends to the tips of the papillae. Parakeratosis is usually present and may be accompanied by hyperkeratosis. The dermal-epidermal junction is sharply demarcated, and the rete pegs are elongated and narrow. The degree of dermal inflammation is variable. The characteristic and virtually pathognomonic cell of condyloma acuminatum is the koilocyte; when strictly defined, koilocytosis is considered to be the cytologic hallmark of HPV infection. Numerous mitoses may be present in the typical condyloma, but enlarged, hyperchromatic, parabasal nuclei and the presence of abnormal mitoses indicate concurrent dysplasia within the condyloma acuminatum.

Koilocytes have wrinkled, popcorn-like, small-to-moderately-enlarged, single or multiple nuclei surrounded by a

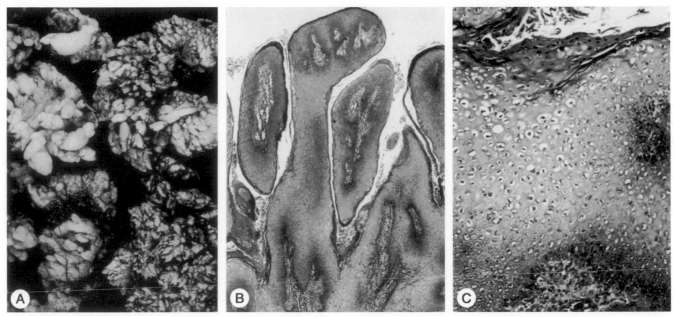

Figure 22–3. Condyloma acuminatum. **(A)** These multiple cauliflower-like, endophytic lesions were surgically removed from the vulva. **(B)** At scanning magnification, papillary fronds formed by delicate fibrovascular cores covered by acanthotic epithelium are seen. **(C)** Higher magnification demonstrates superficial koilocytes with irregular nuclear contours and characteristic perinuclear clear spaces.

relatively large, abundant clear space (Fig. 22–3C). The surrounding cleared area within the cytoplasm imparts the appearance of a perinuclear halo to the cell. Koilocytosis is not limited to condyloma acuminatum but may also be seen in dysplasia and invasive squamous cell carcinoma. Ultrastructurally, the koilocytotic nuclei have irregular, convoluted outlines and clumped chromatin. The perinuclear clear zone is virtually devoid of organelles. Viral particles are dispersed throughout or aggregated within some of the nuclei, especially the pyknotic ones.

In some cases, condyloma acuminatum will regress spontaneously. For those patients seeking medical intervention, a variety of therapies have been used, but none of these has yielded a perfect success rate. Some of the more commonly used treatment modalities have included podophyllin application, carbon dioxide laser therapy, and cryotherapy. The treatment failures may be the result of the persistence of HPV in surrounding tissues that appear grossly and microscopically normal. Previous treatment by these modalities may induce histopathologic changes that cause confusion in the microscopic examination of a resected specimen. This is particularly true of podophyllin-engendered nuclear atypia in the form of enlargement, hyperchromatism, and pyknosis, often with dispersed chromosomes and numerous mitoses arrested in metaphase; the latter have been designated as podophyllin cells and should not be confused with true VIN. These effects disappear after about 2 weeks; therefore, allowance should be made for resolution prior to biopsy. For this reason, knowledge of previous therapy is mandatory when examining these lesions, and this information should be shared with the pathologist prior to microscopic examination.

Giant condylomata, or Buschke-Lowenstein tumors, were first described on the penis as an exophytic, cauliflower-like mass that resembled a large condyloma but exhibited locally aggressive growth; however, they were subsequently reported to afflict vulvar and perianal skin as well as other anogenital tissues. They probably are identical to verrucous carcinoma; therefore, the terms giant condyloma and Buschke-Lowenstein tumor should be discarded. Admittedly, a large condyloma acuminatum may be difficult to differentiate on gross examination from a verrucous carcinoma; however, the former contain central fibrovascular cores that extend to the tips of the papillae, a feature not found in verrucous carcinoma. Additionally, the papillae of the condyloma acuminatum do not penetrate below the plane of the adjacent dermal-epidermal junction, as do the bulbous, pushing cellular borders of verrucous carcinoma.

Vulvar Intraepithelial Neoplasia, Squamous Type[4, 6–9]

- ENLARGED, VARIABLY SIZED, HYPERCHROMATIC NUCLEI BEGINNING IN THE PARABASAL LAYERS
- MITOSES ABOVE THE BASAL LAYER, FREQUENTLY ATYPICAL
- CELLULAR CROWDING
- INCREASED NUCLEAR-CYTOPLASMIC RATIO
- LOSS OF NORMAL MATURATION
- PARAKERATOSIS AND HYPERKERATOSIS FREQUENTLY PRESENT
- KOILOCYTES MAY BE PRESENT, BUT ARE USUALLY LIMITED TO THE MORE SUPERFICIAL LAYERS

Preinvasive intraepithelial lesions of the squamous epithelium frequently involve anogenital skin, particularly the vulva. All of these lesions have some degree of squamous atypia and a certain, but variable, level of risk of progressing to invasive squamous cell carcinoma. Most preinvasive intra-epithelial lesions are relatively indolent, particularly in young women; however, the exact rate of malignant progression is difficult to determine because most lesions are medically treated after diagnosis.

As with condyloma acuminatum, many of the intraepi-thelial lesions are associated with HPV, and the type of HPV appears to affect both the morphologic expression and sub-sequent biologic course. Premalignant vulvar lesions are most commonly associated with HPV type 16, whereas typi-cal condyloma acuminatum is often associated with HPV types 6 and 11.

The classification of vulvar diseases used in this section was affirmed in 1990 by the ISSVD and the ISGYP (Table 22–3). Premalignant squamous lesions have been classified under the general category of VIN, further allowing for three subdivisions, I, II, and III, which correspond to mild dyspla-sia, moderate dysplasia, and severe dysplasia or carcinoma in situ, respectively. VIN III, which encompasses a full-thickness intraepithelial neoplasia, is identical histologically to Bowen disease and erythroplasia of Queyrat; these terms were previously used to describe these lesions in the extra-genital and genital skin; the latter term was restricted to lesions occurring on the penis.

Clinically, VIN may occur in persons of any age, but it is most commonly encountered in young women in the third and fourth decades of life. The usual presenting symptom is pruritus. Less common complaints include pain, burning, dis-colored areas, or a mass. Many lesions are asymptomatic and are detected incidentally during routine physical examina-tion. Although VIN may be present anywhere on the vulvar skin, the fourchette and perineum are most commonly in-volved; in these regions, VIN appears as well-delineated, slightly elevated, and usually roughened lesions. The lesions may vary in color and may be red, pink, white, tan, gray, or black (Fig. 22–4A). A hyperkeratotic lesion appears white. Pigmentation, if present, may be complete or partial, and is sometimes limited to the periphery of the lesion. Redness is caused by dilated capillaries extending up through the pa-pillae and lying close to the surface. Ulceration and indura-tion should raise the suspicion of invasive squamous cell carcinoma. Biopsy and microscopic examination are neces-sary for diagnosis; because of the frequent multifocality and the intralesional and interlesional histologic variability of VIN, taking multiple biopsy specimens is advisable.

Microscopically, VIN is characterized by enlarged, var-iably sized, hyperchromatic nuclei beginning in the parabasal region. Additional characteristics include varying degrees of deficiency or loss of normal squamous epithelial maturation,

cellular crowding, increased nuclear-cytoplasmic ratio, and mitoses above the parabasal layer, including abnormal mi-toses in many cases. Parakeratosis, hyperkeratosis, multinu-cleation, and dyskeratosis are frequent findings. Involvement of skin appendages by VIN is common. Koilocytes are fewer in number than in typical condylomata acuminata, and are generally confined to the superficial layers. The small pyk-notic nuclei of the koilocytes in condylomata acuminata are replaced by larger, irregularly shaped nuclei with coarsely clumped chromatin, histologic findings often indicative of aneuploidy. Areas of usual condyloma may be seen merging with areas of VIN; however, a diagnosis of VIN is made only if the parabasal cells show significant hyperchromasia or enlargement and sufficient mitoses are present. Otherwise, the lesions should be placed in other, more appropriate cate-gories, such as squamous cell hyperplasia, inflammatory squamous atypia, or condyloma acuminatum.

Lesions are placed in the VIN I category (i.e., mild dysplasia) when nuclear hyperchromasia is present, but the cellular disarray and mitoses, usually including abnormal mitoses, are confined to the lower one third or so of the epithelium (Fig. 22–4B). VIN II (i.e., moderate dysplasia) encompasses lesions in which these same changes are seen involving up to the lower two-thirds of the epithelium. In VIN III (i.e., severe dysplasia or carcinoma in situ), these findings involve more than the lower two thirds of the epithe-lium; the term carcinoma in situ is generally applied to full-thickness or nearly full-thickness lesions (Fig. 22–4C, D). VIN III has been further classified as a differentiated type if the cells have prominent eosinophilic cytoplasm with keratin pearl-like changes, usually in the lower one third of the epithelium. The nuclei have prominent nucleoli, and vesicu-lar rather than coarsely clumped chromatin and some matu-ration may be seen in the superficial layers. The concomitant occurrence of koilocytosis does not change the diagnosis or grading of VIN; rather, a statement of these changes should be included in the diagnosis.

In some VIN lesions, few or numerous dyskeratotic or corps rond–type cells within the squamous epithelium may exhibit a pagetoid appearance, being characterized by cells with clear or pale cytoplasm; however, their lack of intracel-lular mucin excludes the diagnosis of Paget disease. Bowen-oid papulosis, or multicentric pigmented Bowen disease, is a term that has been applied to a subset of VIN with a fairly distinctive clinical appearance. It presents as multiple dis-crete, often pigmented (i.e., red-brown to violaceous) papules on the anogenital skin. The lesions are seen in the vulvar skin and the penile glans and shaft, predominantly in young patients. Few of these lesions appear to progress to invasive squamous cell carcinoma, and some of the cases of squamous atypia and VIN that were reported to regress spontaneously following vulvar biopsy probably represented bowenoid pap-ulosis. Although histologically, they are more closely akin to VIN III lesions, the degree of atypia may be somewhat less than is usually associated with VIN III and, only rarely does the clinician who took the biopsy suspect a high-grade VIN lesion.

Bowenoid dysplasia is a term that has been applied to lesions with a clinical presentation similar to bowenoid pap-ulosis but with less than full-thickness epithelial disarray. A considerable overlap, however, exists among bowenoid pap-ulosis, bowenoid dysplasia, and VIN. The presence of en-

Table 22–3. CLASSIFICATION OF VULVAR INTRAEPITHELIAL NEOPLASIA (VIN), SQUAMOUS TYPE

VIN I	Mild dysplasia
VIN II	Moderate dysplasia
VIN III	Severe dysplasia or carcinoma in situ

ISGP, International Society of Gynecological Pathologists; and ISSVD, International Society for the Study of Vulvar Diseases, 1990.

From Lawrence WD: Non-neoplastic epithelial disorders of the vulva (vulvar dystrophies): Historical and current perspectives. In: Rosen PP, Fechner RE, eds. Pathology Annual, part II, vol. 28. Norwalk, CT: Appleton & Lange, 1993:23–51.

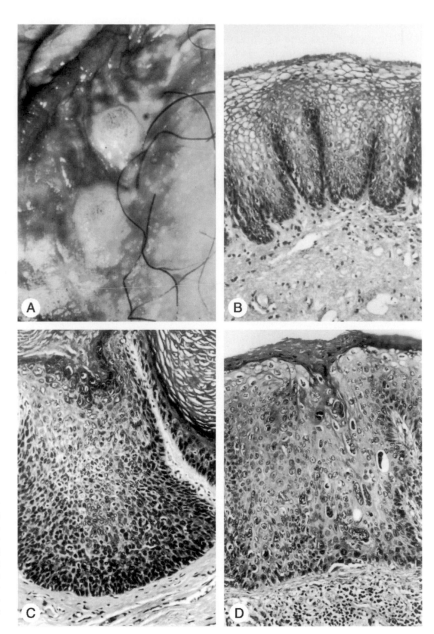

Figure 22–4. Vulvar intraepithelial neoplasia. **(A)** Roughened, red-to-white lesions are present on the vulva and in the vaginal introitus. Central white areas with punctate surface characteristics have been accentuated by the use of topical acetic acid. **(B)** Whereas VIN I (i.e., mild dysplasia) consists of dysplasia affecting cells confined to the lowermost one third of the epithelial layer, **(C, D)** VIN III (i.e., severe dysplasia). **C** contains small uniform cells with a high nuclear/cytoplasmic ratio and coarsely clumped chromatin. **D** shows multiple large multinucleated cells.

larged nuclei and multinucleation in the first two lesions suggests aneuploidy and therefore a precancerous potential, as in VIN. Invasive squamous cell carcinoma has been reported adjacent to lesions with histopathologic features identical to bowenoid papulosis. VIN is not only also found in young patients but is sometimes multifocal and pigmented; furthermore, both lesions are associated with the highly oncogenic HPV type 16. For these reasons, it is not clear whether bowenoid papulosis is a distinctive clinicopathologic entity; therefore, neither the ISSVD nor the ISGYP recommends the use of the terms bowenoid papulosis or bowenoid dysplasia for either clinical or pathologic use.

The clinical diagnosis of VIN may be aided by the use of a magnifying glass or colposcope; however, abnormal vascular patterns are less evident in vulvar lesions than in cervical lesions. Washing with 3 to 5% acetic acid accentuates white plaques, which may exhibit mosaic or punctate patterns (Fig. 22–4A). Toluidine blue stain has been used to delineate these lesions; however, both the false-positive and false-negative rates with its use are relatively high. The diagnosis of VIN necessitates examination of the perianal skin, anal canal, and lower genital tract, including a cervicovaginal smear for cytology. Often, evidence of HPV infection may be found on the penile shaft, glans, or in the distal urethra of male sexual partners of patients with VIN. Histologically, these lesions are frequently flat rather than exophytic and may exhibit only mild acanthosis with no or only subtle koilocytosis.

Although some VIN lesions regress spontaneously, all should be treated, because they carry some risk of developing into invasive squamous cell carcinoma. This is particularly true in older women, who appear to be at greater risk of developing invasive carcinoma. By various specialized techniques, the pathologist can determine which HPV serotypes are present. This information, however, cannot be the only means used to determine the therapeutic approach, even though an association exists between the HPV type, lesional morphology, and risk of progression. Histologic variability in a single lesion may be marked, and more than one HPV type may be present in a single patient or even in a single lesion. Furthermore, invasive squamous cell carcinoma apparently may arise from lesions with less than full thickness VIN or even from otherwise typical NNEDs, suggesting that it originates from malignant basal-layer clones.

Treatment modalities for VIN include carbon dioxide laser therapy and wide local excision with free surgical margins. Even with adequate therapy, VIN has a high recurrence rate, which possibly is secondary to the presence of HPV in adjacent squamous mucosa that appears normal by light microscopic examination.

Vulvar Squamous Cell Carcinoma[6, 7, 9–12]

- EXOPHYTIC OR ENDOPHYTIC MASSES, FREQUENTLY BULKY OR FUNGATING
- USUALLY WELL TO MODERATELY DIFFERENTIATED
- MAY BE ASSOCIATED WITH HPV CHANGES OR VULVAR INTRAEPITHELIAL NEOPLASIA
- HISTOLOGIC FEATURES SIMILAR TO THOSE OF SQUAMOUS CELL CARCINOMA FOUND IN EXTRAGENITAL SKIN

Invasive squamous cell carcinoma of the anogenital skin is a relatively uncommon neoplasm that occurs most frequently in the vulva. Squamous cell carcinoma of the vulva accounts for up to 8% of female genital tract malignancies and up to 95% of vulvar malignancies. Although the histology of this lesion is similar to that of squamous cell carcinoma in extragenital cutaneous sites, several factors involved in the examination of the vulvar specimen warrant special consideration. These factors encompass etiology and pathogenesis, including the relation of invasive squamous cell carcinoma to HPV, and factors involved in staging the neoplasm, especially determination of the depth of invasion.

Vulvar squamous cell carcinoma is generally a disease of postmenopausal women. Most patients are older than 60 years of age at the time of diagnosis; however, the disease occasionally may also affect young women. Pruritus is the most common presenting symptom; others include bleeding, pain, or a mass. In some patients, metastatic disease is the first manifestation, for example, when a lump representing metastases to lymph nodes appears in the inguinal area. As with other vulvar diseases, a long delay between the onset of symptoms and the seeking of medical attention is typical; this is reflected by the fact that more than two thirds of vulvar squamous carcinomas are larger than 2 cm in diameter when resected.

Grossly, vulvar and other anogenital squamous cell carcinomas have a variable appearance. Approximately two thirds are exophytic masses, and roughly another one third are endophytic. Many are bulky, fungating masses; however, nodular, polypoid, plaque-like, or verrucous lesions may also be seen, and concomitant ulceration may be present (Fig. 22–5A, B). Approximately two thirds of these lesions are unilateral, and the other one third occupy a central location; the latter category is important, because these lesions may result in bilateral lymph node metastases.

The most frequent sites of involvement of invasive squamous cell carcinoma are the labia minora and labia majora, especially the upper labia majora, whereas involvement of the fourchette and clitoris is less common. Some researchers have suggested that clitoral cancers may have a greater propensity for pelvic node metastases because of the direct lymphatic drainage to that site, but this hypothesis is currently unproved.

On microscopic examination, most vulvar squamous cell carcinomas are well or moderately differentiated, and most display keratin formation (Fig. 22–5C, D). Three patterns of stromal invasion have been defined: one characterized by a pushing or broad invasive front and large nests of malignant cells; one designated as a stellate, spray, or diffuse pattern, characterized by small nests or cords of invading malignant cells; and one comprised of a mixture of the first two patterns. Some workers have found the diffuse pattern to be associated with an increased risk of lymph node metastases, although others have eschewed this concept. Increasing depth of invasion and the presence of vascular space invasion correspond to a higher rate of lymph node metastases. Other possible but yet controversial predictors of metastatic potential include histologic grade, a confluent growth pattern of invasion (i.e., anastamosing strands of invading tumor), tumor thickness, and surface diameter of the carcinoma.

Determination of the depth of invasion is particularly important when examining vulvar squamous cell carcinomas. The entity of microinvasive carcinoma was created to separate a group of small, superficially invasive vulvar carcinomas with virtually no risk of lymph node metastases from the category of overtly invasive squamous cell carcinoma, so that radical surgery and lymph node dissection could be avoided. Considerable controversy surrounds this concept, including lack of agreement as to the maximum allowable depth of invasion to avoid radical surgery and the point from which the depth of invasion should be measured. The ISSVD does not recommend use of the term microinvasive squamous cell carcinoma; instead, this group recognizes a subset of Stage I squamous cell carcinoma, Stage Ia squamous carcinoma, defined as a "single lesion measuring 2 cm or less in diameter and with a depth of invasion of 1 mm or less. Patients with more than one site of invasion are not included in this definition." Furthermore, the ISSVD recommends that the depth of invasion be measured "as the distance from the epithelial-stromal junction of the adjacent, most superficial dermal papillae to the deepest point of invasion of tumor."

Tumor thickness is defined as the distance from the surface of the carcinoma, or the granular layer if keratin is present, to the deepest point of invasion. The diameter of the tumor includes only invasive carcinoma, not adjacent carcinoma in situ. The pathology report should always detail the method used to determine depth of invasion.

A relatively recent report documented nodal metastases in a case of vulvar squamous carcinoma that invaded only 0.8 mm; therefore, most investigators have begun to doubt the validity of the entity of vulvar microinvasive squamous cancer. In contrast to cervical microinvasive carcinoma, the vulvar counterpart appears to be a more capricious tumor with a greater penchant for vascular space invasion and nodal

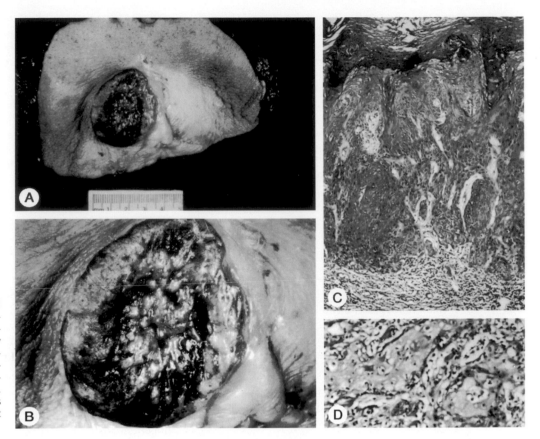

Figure 22–5. Vulvar squamous cell carcinoma. **(A, B)** A large, ulcerated lesion is present in a vulvectomy specimen. **(C)** Moderately well-differentiated invasive carcinoma with anastomosing, finger-like extensions into underlying inflamed connective tissue is seen. **(D)** Nonkeratinizing, invasive nests of vulvar carcinoma are seen at higher magnification.

metastases. The finding of lymph node metastases is a critical factor in evaluating the prognosis of these patients. The Federation Internationale de Gynecologie et Obstetrique (FIGO) staging system defines Stages I and II as those lesions confined to the vulva with no suspicious groin nodes; in Stage I, the tumor diameter is smaller than or equal to 2 cm, and in Stage II, the tumor diameter is larger than 2 cm. Lesions of any size with suspicious groin nodes are classified as Stage III, as are lesions that extend beyond the vulva without grossly positive nodes. Stage IV encompasses lesions of any size with grossly positive nodes; lesions involving the rectal mucosa, bladder, urethra, or bone; and lesions with distant or palpable deep pelvic metastases. Spread of invasive squamous cell carcinoma occurs through the lymphatics to the regional lymph nodes; the 5-year survival drops markedly when inguinal lymph node metastases are present.

Vulvar carcinoma may arise from more than one type of precursor lesion. Although some squamous cell carcinomas clearly progress from HPV-related vulvar intraepithelial neoplasia, others appear unrelated to HPV. The mean age of patients with VIN has decreased, whereas the mean age of patients with invasive squamous carcinoma has remained the same, creating a wider age gap between the two groups. VIN in older women is more frequently associated with invasive carcinoma than it is in younger women; however, several of the reported cases of VIN associated with invasive carcinoma occurred in young, immunosuppressed patients. This may be the result of biologic differences in these patients, or the age of the patient may somehow play a direct but as yet unexplained role in the integrity of the immune system. Heavy cigarette smoking appears to represent another cofactor in

the genesis of HPV-related squamous lesions of the female lower genital tract.

Two thirds of vulvar squamous cell carcinomas develop in the absence of full-thickness VIN, which suggests that invasion may stem directly from malignant clones in the basal layer. Lichen sclerosus and squamous cell hyperplasia are also frequently seen adjacent to squamous cell carcinoma, but the relation among these entities is unclear. All of these lesions may be responses to irritation of anogenital skin superimposed with oncogenic factors in squamous cancer. In the absence of associated squamous atypia, however, NNEDs have a very low progression rate to squamous cancer, particularly when the patient is medically treated and followed closely with biopsies when appropriate.

Verrucous Carcinoma[13–16]

- GRAY-TO-WHITE, BULKY, PAPILLARY MASS
- COMPOSED OF BLAND-APPEARING SQUAMOUS CELLS
- ATYPIA AND MITOSES CONFINED TO BASAL AND PARABASAL LAYERS
- PAPILLARY FRONDS COVERED BY THICK PARAKERATOTIC AND HYPERKERATOTIC LAYERS WITHOUT A CENTRAL FIBROVASCULAR STALK
- CHRONIC INFLAMMATORY CELL INFILTRATE IN ADJACENT STROMA
- BULBOUS EXPANSION OF RETE PEGS WITH APPEARANCE OF COMPRESSION, RATHER THAN INVASION, OF UNDERLYING STRUCTURES

Verrucous carcinoma is a distinct, rare type of squamous cell carcinoma that was originally reported in oral mucosa and since has been described in many locations, including anogenital skin. The vulva is the most frequent site of anogenital verrucous carcinoma, but this lesion may be encountered, although rarely, in the penis and perianal skin. Vulvar verrucous carcinoma most frequently affects postmenopausal women; the peak incidence is in the sixth and seventh decades of life. The most common presenting symptoms are pruritus, a long-standing cauliflower-like mass, or both.

On gross examination, verrucous carcinoma is a gray-to-white, bulky, papillary mass that is usually large and encroaches on contiguous structures. On cut section, the lesion has an easily observed rounded, pushing, but well-demarcated deep margin, giving the appearance of compression, rather than invasion, of the underlying tissue (Fig. 22–6A). The surface of the neoplasm may be ulcerated, and associated infection may lead to induration of the surrounding tissue; consequent reactive lymphadenopathy of groin lymph nodes may engender the clinical and pathologic suspicion of metastatic carcinoma.

Microscopically, verrucous carcinoma is an extremely well-differentiated carcinoma composed of relatively bland-appearing squamous cells with well-preserved polarity. The surface of the tumor is papillary, and the papillary fronds are covered with thick, parakeratotic and hyperkeratotic superficial layers. The well-demarcated deep margin is composed of rounded, bulky rete pegs and well-differentiated squamous cells that extend into the underlying dermis (Fig. 22–6B). The adjacent stroma contains a prominent chronic inflammatory cell infiltrate. The neoplastic cells have abundant eosinophilic cytoplasm with well-defined cell boundaries and a low nuclear-cytoplasmic ratio. Squamous pearls are usually absent. Cellular atypia and mitoses, when present, are minimal and are confined to the basal and parabasal layers (Fig. 22–6C).

The diagnosis of verrucous carcinoma is frequently difficult to establish and may require multiple biopsies. An adequate biopsy specimen must include not only the superficial papillary portion of the neoplasm but also the bulbous, well-demarcated deep margin. The differential diagnosis usually includes condyloma acuminatum and well-differentiated, exophytic, squamous cell carcinoma with a verrucous growth pattern. Ordinary, well-differentiated squamous cell carcinoma may resemble verrucous carcinoma if only the superficial layers are biopsied. In contrast to verrucous carcinoma, however, overt squamous cell carcinoma shows irregular invasion at its epithelial-stromal junction and contains cells with markedly atypical, hyperchromatic or vesicular nuclei

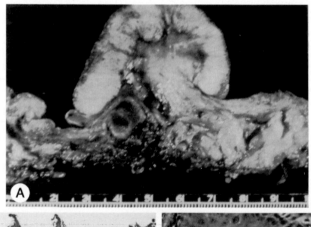

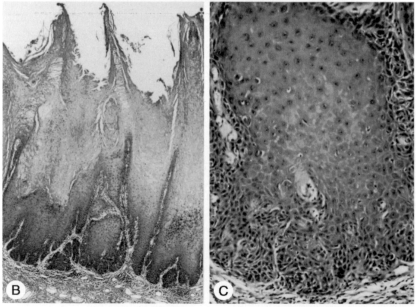

Figure 22–6. Verrucous carcinoma. **(A)** On cross section, this bulky, exophytic tumor has a well-defined inferior border, which appears to compress the underlying stroma rather than to invade it. **(B)** Histologically, the lower border is composed of rounded, bulky rete pegs that extend into the underlying stroma. **(C)** The cells of the verrucous carcinoma are well differentiated with uniform nuclei, a low nuclear/cytoplasmic ratio, and rare mitoses. (A From Deppe G, Lawrence WD: Vulvar dystrophy and neoplasia. In: Gusberg SB, Deppe G, Shingleton HM, eds. Female Genital Cancer. New York, Churchill Livingstone, 1988: 223–251.)

with irregularly clumped chromatin, prominent nucleoli, and often, brisk mitotic activity. Similarly, papillary squamous cell carcinoma in situ contains severely atypical cells and mitotic figures that are often abnormal.

Condyloma acuminatum differs from verrucous carcinoma in that the papillary fronds of the first lesion contain a connective tissue core in the deep as well as the superficial portions of the lesion. Koilocytotic cells may be present in both entities, particularly in the superficial layers. Condyloma acuminatum lacks the bulbous, pushing deep margin of verrucous carcinoma, again illustrating the need for an adequate biopsy specimen that encompasses the epithelial-stromal junction. It is incumbent on the clinician who sends the biopsy specimen to include, along with the clinical history, a clinical description of the tumor and its dimensions.

Treatment of verrucous carcinoma consists of surgical excision; the extent of the surgery depends on the size of the lesion. Wide surgical excision with adequate resection margins results in a good survival rate. The lesion will recur if inadequately excised, and with recurrence, the survival rate decreases. Lymph node dissection is not routine in vulvar verrucous carcinoma because lymph node metastases are not commonly associated with this entity. Radiation has been purported to increase the risk of recurrence as well as induce a more anaplastic malignancy; however, some investigators feel that there is a lack of objective evidence to support this argument.

Paget Disease[16–19]

- MOIST, ERYTHEMATOUS, MAP-LIKE AREAS WITH INTERVENING WHITE AREAS OF HYPERKERATOSIS
- MALIGNANT CELLS (I.E., PAGET CELLS) SCATTERED THROUGHOUT THE EPIDERMIS SINGLY OR IN SMALL CLUSTERS
- INVOLVEMENT OF ADNEXAL STRUCTURES IN THE DERMIS COMMON
- PAGET CELLS HAVE ABUNDANT PALE-TO-CLEAR CYTOPLASM THAT STAINS POSITIVELY WITH MUCICARMINE AND PERIODIC ACID–SCHIFF REAGENT
- NUCLEI FREQUENTLY ECCENTRIC AND MAY SHOW HYPERCHROMATISM AND PLEOMORPHISM
- MITOSES UNCOMMON
- PAGET CELLS FREQUENTLY EXTEND INTO GROSSLY UNREMARKABLE EPIDERMIS
- CAREFUL SEARCH FOR AREAS OF INVASION IS IMPORTANT

Paget disease is a nonsquamous type of vulvar intraepithelial neoplasia. Extramammary Paget disease is rare and accounts for less than 5% of vulvar neoplasms. It affects both men and women and occurs in apocrine gland–bearing skin in areas such as the axillae, umbilicus, and anogenital region. However, extramammary Paget disease occurs most frequently in the vulva, usually affecting postmenopausal Caucasian women in the sixth and seventh decades of life. A high degree of association of extramammary Paget disease with concurrent or prior cancer has been documented. Although these malignancies are most commonly of the female genital tract or breast, other sites have included the rectum, skin, and urinary bladder.

Pruritus is the most common presenting symptom; other symptoms include burning, pain, and irritation. As with other vulvar diseases, the patient frequently endures these symptoms for months or years before seeking medical attention. The average duration of symptoms prior to seeking medical attention in patients with vulvar Paget disease is longer than 3 years.

Grossly, the involved areas of vulva have moist, erythematous, well-demarcated, map-like lesions that most typi-

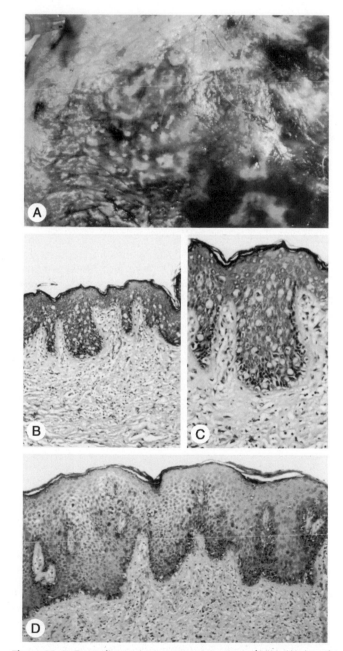

Figure 22–7. Paget disease is a nonsquamous type of VIN. **(A)** A moist, map-like region on the labia is composed of erythema with interposed islands of tan-white hyperkeratosis. **(B)** Pale-staining Paget cells are present as single cells and as small clusters within the epidermal layer. **(C)** Some of these cells have a signet-ring quality to their cytoplasm, with nuclei compressed at the cell periphery. **(D)** Mucicarmine staining reveals that many of the cells contain intracytoplasmic mucin.

cally comprise between 1 and 10 cm of labia majora. Ulceration may be present, and bleeding occurs easily in response to touch. Interspersed white scaly areas usually represent hyperkeratosis (Fig. 22–7A) and may lend a red-and-white, speckled appearance on gross examination. An unusual degree of induration or a palpable mass may herald an underlying invasive cancer.

Microscopically, Paget cells infiltrate the full-thickness epidermis singly and in small clusters, but they are most prominent in the parabasal layers (Fig. 22–7B). The Paget cells are large and polygonal, with abundant pale staining and occasionally, vacuolated cytoplasm. The nuclei are ovoid and may be hyperchromatic, but more frequently they contain finely distributed chromatin with small nucleoli. Signet ring–type cells are occasionally seen (Fig. 22–7C). Intercellular bridges between the Paget cells and adjacent keratinocytes may be seen, and mitotic figures are infrequent. In some cases, clusters of Paget cells may appear to form acinar-type structures. In some cases, a minor component of small basaloid cells with hyperchromatic nuclei and high nuclear-cytoplasmic ratio may be seen in basal and parabasal layers surrounding nests of more typical Paget cells. These cells may represent poorly differentiated Paget cell precursors. Hyperkeratosis and dermal inflammation are also frequent features of Paget disease.

By ultrastructural techniques, the extramammary Paget cells have been shown to be mucin-secreting adenocarcinoma cells. Although the findings are inconclusive regarding the cell of origin, they do indicate that Paget cells have some features of sweat gland cells. The abundant cytoplasm contains mucinogen granules and a prominent Golgi complex. The nucleus is convoluted and often peripherally located and has a prominent nucleolus.

The Paget cells stain positively with mucicarmine and with the periodic acid–Schiff (PAS) reagent, both before and after diastase digestion (Fig. 22–7D). The most important differential diagnosis to be considered in conjunction with vulvar Paget disease is malignant melanoma; the aforementioned stains can be used to differentiate Paget cells from vulvar melanomas. Although some reports have described Paget cells that contain intracytoplasmic melanin granules, these are felt to have been phagocytized by the Paget cells rather than synthesized by them. Furthermore, the presence of intracytoplasmic mucin rules out the possibility of superficial spreading melanoma.

Carcinoembryonic antigen (CEA) is present in Paget cells, as well as in normal eccrine and apocrine glands and ducts. CEA is absent in malignant melanomas and squamous carcinomas.

Most cases of vulvar Paget disease are intraepithelial, with involvement limited to the epidermis and pilary complex. Involvement of the eccrine and apocrine glands is seen in approximately one fourth of all cases, but the phenomenon is still considered to be in situ as long as the Paget cells are confined to the epithelium and have not broken through the basement membrane. Paget disease remains in situ for a long period of time before invading the dermis, and patients with only intraepithelial involvement have a good prognosis, provided they receive appropriate therapy.

In contrast, dermal invasion signifies a poor prognosis, and the disease is frequently widespread at the time of such a diagnosis. It is of the utmost importance to exclude invasion by careful examination of many tissue sections because determination of therapy and prognosis depend on the presence or absence of dermal invasion. The duration of symptoms appears to correlate well with the histologic level of epithelial-stromal involvement. A review of the literature showed that the duration of symptoms was 2.1 years when the Paget disease was limited to the epithelium and pilary complex, 3.9 years when it also involved the sweat glands, and 6.4 years when dermal invasion was present.

The risk of recurrence is similar for all levels of histologic involvement, because Paget disease is multicentric and diffuse with irregular borders, and Paget cells may be demonstrated microscopically in normal-appearing epidermis quite distant from what grossly appears to be the edge of the lesion. Consequently, one fourth to one third of patients treated only with local excision are plagued by multiple recurrences after surgery. Modified radical vulvectomy yields a greater than 90% cure rate in cases of intraepithelial (i.e., noninvasive) Paget disease. Invasive Paget disease is treated with radical vulvectomy and bilateral inguinal lymphadenectomy. Given the frequent association of extramammary Paget disease with other carcinomas, a thorough clinical history and appropriate workup, particularly of the breast and remaining urogenital tract, is in order.

The origin of the Paget cell remains a point of controversy. One theory maintains that Paget cells originate from an underlying adenocarcinoma with subsequent migration or metastasis of the cells into the epidermis. This theory is supported by (1) their tendency to arise in tissues rich in apocrine and sweat glands; (2) their morphology; (3) their similarity to apocrine cells; and (4) the similarity of extramammary Paget disease to Paget disease of the breast. In the breast, however, Paget disease is virtually always accompanied by an underlying adenocarcinoma, whereas an underlying adenocarcinoma is found in only approximately one third of all patients with vulvar Paget disease.

Another theory maintains that the Paget cells have a multifocal origin and arise from the stratum germinativum, which is multipotential and gives rise to the basal layer of the squamous epithelium, pilary complex, and apocrine and eccrine glands. This theory is supported by the natural history of Paget disease, with its long in situ phase and apparently simultaneous and multifocal involvement of the epidermis, pilary complex, and sweat glands.

Malignant Melanoma[20–22]

- SUPERFICIAL SPREADING, NODULAR, OR ACRAL LENTIGINOUS TYPE
- OCCURS ON THE CLITORIS, LABIA MINORA, OR LABIA MAJORA
- GROSS AND HISTOLOGIC FEATURES OF VULVAR MELANOMAS ARE SIMILAR TO THOSE OF EXTRAGENITAL CUTANEOUS MELANOMAS
- PROGNOSIS CORRELATES BEST WITH TUMOR THICKNESS

Vulvar melanomas represent 3 to 5% of all melanomas in women and 8 to 10% of malignant vulvar neoplasms. These lesions are the second most frequently encountered vulvar malignancy; however, they represent a distant second

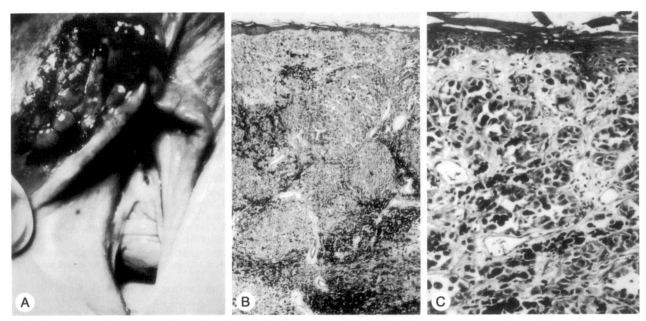

Figure 22–8. Vulvar malignant melanoma. **(A)** This deeply pigmented vulvar tumor shows both macular areas of brown-black discoloration corresponding to the radial growth phase and nodular regions of vertical growth phase. **(B)** The vertical growth phase is characterized by expansile, nodular growth of cells, ranging from relatively nonpigmented cells to zones of heavily pigmented cells and melanophages. **(C)** On higher magnification, the tumor cells in this field are predominantly epithelioid and contain obvious cytoplasmic melanin. The overlying epithelium retains lentiginous growth of malignant cells, residua of the radial growth phase that gave rise to this metastasizing subepithelial component.

to squamous cell carcinoma. Vulvar melanoma is primarily a disease of postmenopausal Caucasian women, but women of other races and even adolescents may be affected. The most common presenting symptoms are an enlarging vulvar mass, bleeding, or pruritus. Although melanomas can occur on the clitoris, labia minora, or labia majora, some workers have found that involvement of the first two locations is most common (Fig. 22–8A). A significant delay between the onset of symptoms and the time the patient consults a physician is common.

The histologic features and the differential diagnoses of vulvar melanomas are similar to those of cutaneous melanomas; therefore, they are not repeated in this section. The prognostic indicators and treatment of vulvar melanomas, however, vary somewhat from those involving extragenital sites. The relatively small number of cases in most series of vulvar melanomas hampers evaluation of the prognostic indicators, which are well defined for extragenital cutaneous melanomas but cannot necessarily be applied to vulvar melanomas. However, the most important prognostic indicators appear to be the thickness of the melanoma and its clinical stage. In most series, the maximum tumor thickness correlated more closely with survival than did the FIGO stage. Using the FIGO system, a Stage I melanoma is defined as a tumor smaller than or equal to 2 cm in maximum dimension with clinically negative nodes; Stage II encompasses melanomas larger than 2 cm in maximum dimension with clinically negative nodes; Stage III applies to melanomas with extension to the urethra, vagina, perineum, or anus or with clinically positive nodes; and Stage IV refers to melanomas that infiltrate the bladder or rectal mucosa, that are fixed to bone, or that have distant metastases.

The Clark level of invasion is more difficult to assess in the vulvar squamous mucosa because of the absence of a

well-defined papillary dermis, but it can be more easily determined in the skin of the labia majora. For this reason, the Breslow determination of tumor thickness is more useful than the Clark level in evaluating vulvar melanomas. Hyperkeratosis is usually absent, and the granular layer is poorly defined; therefore, the Breslow measurement is determined by gauging the distance between the superior and deep tumor margins at the tumor's thickest point. Measurement in areas of ulceration should be avoided if possible. Tumor thickness appears to correlate better with survival than does the clinical staging. A good prognosis is seen for Clark level I or II lesions or those lesions with a thickness of less than 1.5 mm. In one study, no recurrence of melanoma was noted in patients who had a depth of invasion of less than 0.76 mm, whereas two thirds of those with invasion deeper than 1.25 mm experienced recurrence of disease.

Vulvar melanomas may be classified as superficial spreading, nodular, or acral lentiginous types. Acral lentiginous melanomas characteristically occur on the palms, soles, fingernails, and toenails. These lesions are composed of atypical dendritic melanocytes, and they frequently also have marked desmoplasia and epithelioid hyperplasia. Acral lentiginous and nodular melanomas have a poorer prognosis than do superficial spreading melanomas, although nodular melanoma is the least common type in anogenital skin; the difference in prognosis appears to be directly related to the generally greater tumor thickness of the first two types (Fig. 22–8B). Superficial spreading and nodular melanomas can be composed predominantly of epithelioid or spindled types of cells or they can have a mixed pattern (Fig. 22–8C); however, the cell type does not appear to be a significant prognostic factor.

The histopathologic differential diagnosis of vulvar melanomas, particularly of the amelanotic or paucimelanotic

lesions. Acute or short-term lesions may result from superficial or deep laceration of the mucosa (Fig. 23–1A) due to a range of causes. The following are the important features of acute lesions:

- FULL-THICKNESS BREACH OF THE EPITHELIUM AND SUPERFICIAL LAMINA PROPRIA
- DISCRETE MARGINS
- POSSIBLE INVOLVEMENT OF UNDERLYING MUSCLE (WITH INCREASED SCARRING ON HEALING) OR PERIOSTEUM, DEPENDING ON SITE AND EXTENT OF LESION
- PROMINENT LOCAL EDEMA
- NO INCREASE IN LESION SIZE FOLLOWING INITIAL TRAUMA AND EDEMA, UNLESS PATIENT SUFFERS FROM RECURRENT APHTHOUS ULCERATION
- RAPID HEALING WITHIN 3 TO 10 DAYS

Histologically, acute lesions are unremarkable and constitute the archetype of nonspecific oral ulceration. Major features are

- CIRCUMSCRIBED BREAK IN THE EPITHELIUM
- SUPERFICIAL FIBRINOUS EXUDATE THAT IN SOME LESIONS MAY FORM A MAJOR PART OF TISSUE TAGS AS THE LESIONS HEAL
- SUPERFICIAL POLYMORPHONUCLEAR LEUKOCYTIC INFILTRATE
- LOW LEVEL OF CELLULARITY AT DEEPER LEVELS
- SMALL NUMBERS OF LYMPHOCYTES AND MACROPHAGES
- EARLY INGROWTH OF EPITHELIUM UNDER THE SURFACE EXUDATE

More extensive acute lesions may result from chemical burns (e.g., acetylsalicylic acid, phenol, silver nitrate, trichloracetic acid) or from careless use of dental cotton rolls, which can injure large areas of mucosa during removal. Clinically, extensive acute lesions appear as superficial erosions that do not have the pot shape of the smaller discrete lesions. Nonetheless these lesions generally heal rapidly and the histology does not differ from smaller acute lesions.

Complications caused by extensive acute lesions include

1. Loss of normal surface contour
2. Cicatrix formation
3. Mucocele or mucous extravasation phenomenon
4. Post-traumatic melanosis
5. Increased susceptibility to future trauma at the site

Recurrent traumatic lesions should be differentiated from the group of traumatic lesions as a whole. This can be done most satisfactorily on an etiological basis:

1. Dental or dental appliance trauma
2. Dental arch malalignment
3. Factitial injuries which are habitual and so may have a psychogenic component (morsicatio buccarum)

Clearly, recurrent traumatic lesions are more likely to result in chronic ulceration. These lesions must be classified carefully, because there is potential overlap with specific disease conditions such as pemphigoid, erosive lichen planus,

and malignant lesions. As a group, recurrent traumatic lesions have a number of common features:

- TEND TO BE MORE EXTENSIVE THAN ACUTE LESIONS
- APPEAR SUPERFICIAL
- OFTEN INVOLVE THE LATERAL LINGUAL MARGINS (FIG. 23–1B)
- FREQUENTLY DIFFICULT TO RESOLVE
- FREQUENTLY DIFFICULT TO ISOLATE AN ACCEPTABLE ETIOLOGY, BECAUSE LESIONS MAY NOT BEHAVE AS EXPECTED FOLLOWING REMOVAL OF APPARENT LOCAL DENTAL OR OTHER IRRITATIONS
- LESIONS WITH SPECIFIC ETIOLOGY SUCH AS DENTURE FLANGE TRAUMA DO RESPOND RAPIDLY
- MANY ARE ASSOCIATED WITH SIGNIFICANT SURROUNDING ERYTHEMA
- LESION BASE MAY FEEL SLIGHTLY INDURATED
- REACTIVITY OF SURROUNDING TISSUES MAY RESULT IN PERIPHERAL KERATOSIS, SEEN FREQUENTLY ON THE TONGUE, OR FIBROEPITHELIAL HYPERPLASIA, SUCH AS THAT WHICH OCCURS IN ASSOCIATION WITH DENTURE INJURIES AND LIP OR CHEEK BITING

The histology of chronic or recurrent lesions is unremarkable, but several important points arise:

- EPITHELIAL REACTIVITY MIMICS DYSPLASIA
- LOW LEVEL OF CELLULAR ACTIVITY
- LACK OF EVIDENCE OF HEALING

A number of chronic or recurrent lesions require an aggressive approach to encourage healing, particularly when they involve the lateral lingual margins. Treatment may include the following measures:

1. Removal of all local irritations
2. Restoration of edentulous sectors
3. Use of a soft guard over the mandibular teeth during sleeping
4. Topical glucocorticosteroid preparation
5. Intralesional corticosteroid injection (rare)
6. Biopsy to exclude malignancy if lesions persist

After resolution of the ulcerative component, there frequently are residual tissue changes that persist over periods of several months to years. These residual tissue changes include the following:

- RESIDUAL KERATOSIS
- DEPAPILLATION
- CICATRIX FORMATION
- OCCASIONAL ERYTHEMA THAT MAY PROGRESS TO ULCERATION
- LINEAR SCARRING THAT SEEMS TO PREDISPOSE TO FURTHER BREAKDOWN

Recurrent Aphthous Stomatitis[1, 2]

In contradistinction to traumatic lesions, recurrent aphthous stomatitis (RAS) represents a specific disease en-

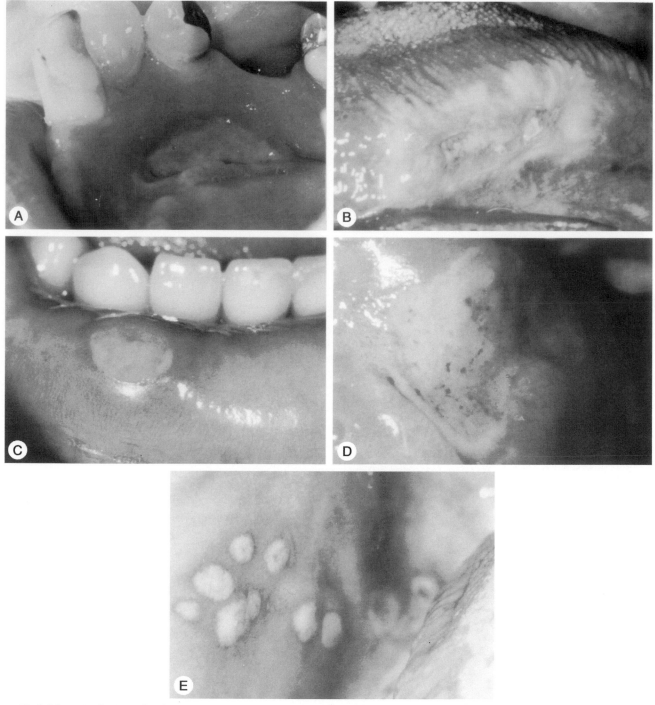

Figure 23–1. Ulcerative lesions of oral mucosa. **(A)** A traumatic ulcer on the lingual aspect of the mandible was caused by a denture flange. **(B)** A chronically traumatized zone on the lateral lingual margin shows central linear ulceration and surrounding hyperkeratosis. **(C)** A minor aphthous ulcer is present on the lower lip. The lesion is less than 1 cm in diameter and typically circular. **(D)** A major aphthous ulcer of the buccal mucosa, which was present for 4 months prior to treatment. **(E)** Nonvesicular, cluster-pattern, herpetiform, aphthous ulcerations.

tity, and excluding dental caries and periodontal diseases, it is the most frequently occurring oral disease. RAS can be defined as a recurrent, nonvesicular, ulcerative disease characterized by the formation of discrete, painful lesions of the nonkeratinized oral mucosa. Typically, the ulcers are round or elliptical lesions that occur singly or in small numbers. Each lesion is discrete, with a deep base covered by a white-

grey slough and surrounded by an edematous and, in the early and painful part of the ulcerative phase, an erythematous margin that gradually contracts as the lesions become fully established and subsequently enter a healing phase.

The clinical considerations with respect to RAS are important, because these lesions are biopsied infrequently. The classification divides RAS into four subtypes:

1. Minor aphthous ulceration—lesions smaller than 1 cm in diameter that heal in 1 to 2 weeks without scarring (Fig. 23–1C)

2. Major aphthous ulceration—lesions smaller than 1 cm in diameter that heal over several weeks to months with scarring (Fig. 23–1D)

3. Herpetiform aphthous ulceration—multiple, small (1–3mm), nonvesicular, cluster-pattern lesions that heal in 1 to 2 weeks and are particularly sensitive to a tetracycline HCl mouthwash (Fig. 23–1E)

4. Behçet syndrome—involves mainly oral and genital ulcerations with ocular and skin lesions and a range of systemic manifestations

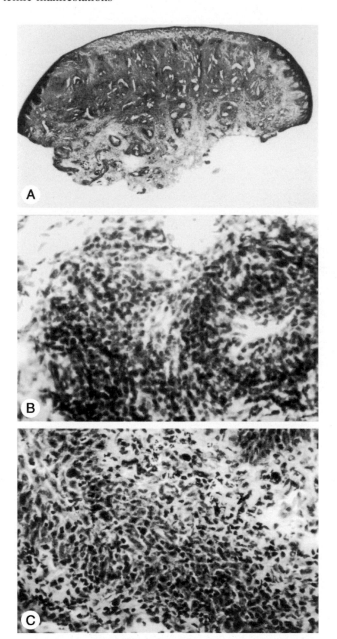

Figure 23–2. Histopathology of recurrent aphthous stomatitis. **(A)** An excisional biopsy specimen of a minor aphthous lesion shows a central surface defect and intense cellularity with deeper, focal, perivascular cell aggregations. **(B)** High-power magnification of the perivascular cell clusters in aphthous lesions. **(C)** The epithelium in aphthous lesions is infiltrated with large numbers of lymphocytes that, in the ulcerative phase, are predominantly CD8-positive.

A number of etiologic agents have been associated with RAS, but at present, no specific cause has been identified. Bacterial and viral infections have been investigated most closely and discarded as causative agents, although recurrent evidence to support a role for HSV has emerged from studies using cDNA probes with specificity for the HSV genome. Currently, an immunopathogenesis based on cell-mediated destruction of oral epithelial targets is accepted as an etiology for RAS, but the initiating mechanisms remain obscure.

The histology of minor aphthous lesions (Fig. 23–2) has been documented extensively, and although many features tend to be nonspecific, there are a number of findings that indicate a recurring sequence of events central to their pathogenesis and are useful in diagnosis. The initial event in preulcerative lesions is the influx of CD4+ T lymphocytes from small vessels in the lamina propria (see Fig. 23–2B). These form small perivascular aggregates, migrate to the basement membrane zone, and subsequently move intraepithelially (see Fig. 23–2C). At this stage, epithelial cells in the area of presumptive ulcer formation become HLA-DR and HLA-A–, -B–, and -C–positive, allowing direct interaction with CD4+ and CD8+ T cells, respectively. Two histopathologic features are of importance at this stage. The subepithelial infiltrate is a primary event; secondly, epithelial disintegration occurs from the basal layer of the epithelium toward the surface. The subsurface epithelium undergoes T-cell–mediated lysis; this is coincident with a large influx of CD8+ cells, which form significant deeper perivascular aggregations and intense infiltrates at both the subepithelial and intraepithelial levels. The ulcerative phase commences with the loss of surface epithelium, and it is only with the appearance of the fibrinopurulent membrane covering the surface that large numbers of polymorphonuclear leukocytes become obvious. The ulcerative phase is also marked by a loss of CD1a+ intraepithelial Langerhans cells. The healing phase commences with the appearance of granulation tissue subjacent to the surface exudate and the proliferation of epithelium across the defect. There is also a reversal in the dominant cell type present; CD4+ T cells displace the CD8+ cells.

These patterns are not as discrete in major as in minor aphthous lesions, because inevitably, major aphthous lesions have been present for a considerable period prior to biopsy. With more extensive surface involvement and more deeply penetrating ulcers, the cellular infiltrates tend to be dominated by polymorphonuclear leukocytes (PMNs).

Erosive and Vesiculoulcerative Disease

Lichen Planus[3–7]

Oral lichen planus is a relatively common disorder that affects as much as 2% of the general population. This condition occupies an important place in both oral medicine and dermatology for several reasons. Oral lesions of lichen planus, although often preceding the appearance of cutaneous lesions by weeks to months, frequently occur without accompanying skin or genital lesions. Conversely, patients with cutaneous lesions display oral mucosal involvement so frequently that lichen planus is probably the most common dermatologic disease with oral mucosal lesions. In comparison with their cutaneous counterparts, oral lesions of lichen planus are more resistant to therapy and are less likely to undergo spontaneous remission.

Lesions of oral lichen planus may be classified into a variety of types:

1. Papular: small white-grey papules
2. Linear: fine white striae
3. Reticular: lacy, reticular plaques (Fig. 23–3A)
4. Atrophic: poorly defined, smooth, erythematous areas
5. Erosive: superficial erosion on a reticular or atrophic background (Fig. 23–3B)
6. Bullous: vesicles that subsequently rupture (Fig. 23–3C)
7. Hyperplastic: elevated white lesions that resemble hyperkeratotic plaques
8. Annular: discrete lesions usually found on the tongue

Peripheral Wickham striae are a feature of most but not all lesions of oral lichen planus. Reticular and papular lesions occur most frequently; however, they are usually asymptomatic. Atrophic, erosive, and bullous variants can cause considerable oral discomfort. Lesions are most frequently distributed on the buccal mucosa and tongue, although other regions, such as the gingivae and palate, may also be affected.

Several lines of evidence indicate that oral lichen planus is a cell-mediated immune reaction with cytotoxicity directed against mucosal epithelial cells as a final common pathway. The similarity between lesions of oral lichen planus and graft-versus-host disease at both the clinical and microscopic level attest to the contribution of lymphocyte-mediated cytotoxic responses in this disorder. Both local and systemic factors that are either associated with the disease or appear causally related have been identified. Local factors include trauma, viral infection, and certain dental restorative materials. Systemic factors include certain drugs (e.g., nonsteroidal antiinflammatory agents, antihypertensives, psychotrophic agents) and stress or anxiety neurosis. These diverse agents may precipitate the condition by altering lymphocyte traffic into the oral mucosa by perturbing the mast cell–endothelial cell network in mucosa of susceptible patients. These individuals display a number of subtle alterations in peripheral blood lymphocyte number and function, including altered CD4 lymphocyte subsets. Whether these changes are causally related to certain human leukocyte antigen (HLA) types that occur at higher frequency in these patients is unclear.

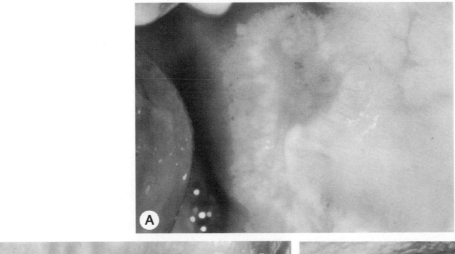

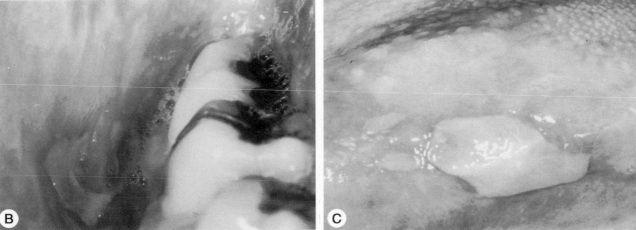

Figure 23–3. Clinical variants of oral lichen planus. **(A)** A lesion of lichen planus is present on the buccal mucosa. The central atrophic zone is surrounded by radiating linear and reticular striae. The parotid papilla is at the upper pole of the lesion. **(B)** Reticular Wickham striae on the posterior buccal mucosa run through the reflection of the buccal sulcus and onto the gingiva. Erosive areas in this site are frequent and may be associated with adjacent amalgam restorations. **(C)** A bullous lesion on the lateral lingual margin is present in a patient with drug-related lichen planus. There is marked peripheral depapillation and small annular lesions on the dorsum.

The following are characteristic histopathologic features of oral lichen planus (Fig. 23–4A, B):

EPITHELIUM
  Superficial layers: Hyperparakeratosis
    Acanthosis, frequently alternating with atrophic sectors
  Deeper layers: Intraepithelial lymphocytes
    Apoptotic bodies in basal layers (e.g., hyaline, colloid, Civatte bodies)
    Liquefaction degeneration of basal cells
    Obliteration of basement membrane
LAMINA PROPRIA
  Band-like subepithelial lymphohistiocytic infiltrate restricted to the superficial lamina propria
  Perivascular lymphocytic aggregations; in some cases, lichenoid vasculitis
  Colloid bodies (i.e., apoptotic bodies)

Microscopically, these lesions are often similar to cutaneous lesions, however saw-tooth rete ridges are less frequently observed. Nonspecific lichenoid stomatitis and drug-related lesions are similar to lesions of oral lichen planus; but they do not show the tight band-like inflammatory infiltrate. This infiltrate tends to extend deeply into the tissues and contains plasma cells as well as the lymphohistiocytic component. Lichenoid dysplasia, which is a separate entity from oral lichen planus, closely resembles the latter in general architecture; however, dysplastic changes can be recognized in mucosal keratinocytes (Fig. 23–4C, D).

Immunohistochemistal staining for involucrin provides a valuable means of further distinguishing between these two entities. In lichen planus, basal and spinous cells display strong involucrin reactivity, whereas a patchy checkerboard pattern of reactivity occurs in lichenoid dysplasia because of nonreactive basal cells and variably reactive spinous cells. Immunofluorescence microscopy is a useful adjunct in the diagnosis of lichen planus as colloid bodies, which nonspecifically take up immunoglobulin (particularly IgM) and produce a characteristic pattern. There is fibrinogen and C_3 deposition at the level of the basement membrane zone. Lichen planus per se is overdiagnosed and, with stringent criteria, should be separated from related lichenoid lesions.

Treatment of oral lichen planus lesions is often difficult. Unlike their cutaneous counterparts, the oral lesions do not show a strong tendency to resolve spontaneously. Corticosteroids, either applied locally or injected into lesions, remain the mainstay of therapy. Psoralen ultraviolet light A (PUVA) therapy and systemic retinoid treatment are occasionally of value. Topical cyclosporine in the form of rinses has been shown to be effective. When exacerbating factors have been identified, these can be dealt with directly. For example, dental restorations responsible for traumatic or galvanic effects can be modified or replaced, and alternative medications can be adopted in patients who have drug-related

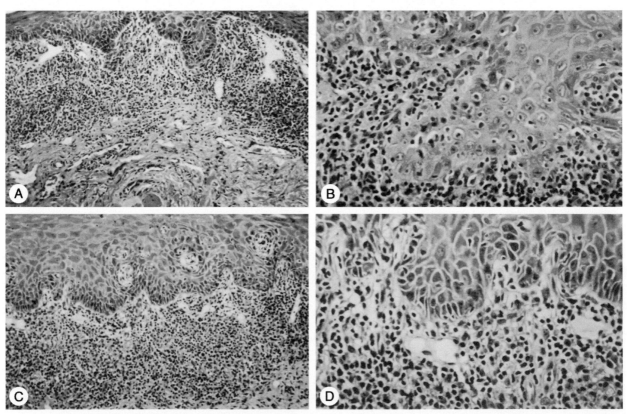

Figure 23–4. Histopathology of oral lichen planus. **(A)** Lichen planus shows the characteristic juxtaepithelial, lymphohistiocytic infiltrate below an acanthotic, parakeratinized epithelium. **(B)** Higher magnification shows intraepithelial lymphocytes, disruption of the basal cells, and the presence of intraepithelial, eosinophilic, apoptotic bodies. **(C, D)** In lichenoid dysplasia, the typical histologic features are combined with epithelial dysplasia. Hyperchromaticity, anisonucleosus, and drop-shaped rete pegs are present.

lichenoid lesions. Because exacerbations frequently correspond to periods of emotional stress, attempts to reduce stress levels in affected individuals may be of benefit.

Lupus Erythematosus[8]

Oral lesions are reported in 20 to 50% of patients with both systemic lupus erythematosus (SLE) and discoid lupus erythematosus (DLE). The cutaneous manifestations of both conditions follow a variable course; therefore, it is likely that oral lesions will present as isolated and often initial lesions.

The oral lesions of DLE typically involve the buccal mucosa and frequently appear lichenoid or as a less complex leukoplakia. They characteristically are described as being surrounded by a keratotic rim with radiating keratotic striae (Fig. 23–5A). The central area is depressed and atrophic and contains a number of small keratotic papules and telangiectases. Scarring is an important but not consistently present sign, often seen on the posterior buccal mucosa and retromolar areas, and may be exacerbated by coincident trauma. Similar lesions occur on the lips; malignant transformation of these neoplasms is a significant clinical problem (Fig. 23–5B). As with many conditions, tongue lesions are less specific and produce depapillation, fissuring, scarring, and ulceration.

The oral lesions of SLE may be similar to those of DLE, but those of SLE tend to be more extensive and ulcerative. The acute phase is entirely nonspecific, with widespread erosions involving most oral surfaces.

The histologic confirmation of the diagnosis is important mainly because many cases of clinical lichen planus actually represent DLE. The following are major features of oral lesions of lupus erythematosus:

- PARAKERATOSIS OR HYPERKERATOSIS
- KERATOTIC PLUGGING
- RETE PEG ATROPHY
- PSEUDOEPITHELIOMATOUS HYPERPLASIA
- LIQUEFACTION DEGENERATION OF BASAL CELLS
- PERIVASCULAR LYMPHOCYTE AGGREGATIONS
- DEGENERATION OF COLLAGEN, PARTICULARLY IMMEDIATELY SUBJACENT TO THE EPITHELIUM
- DEEP, MIXED, INFLAMMATORY CELL INFILTRATE
- THICKENING OF BASEMENT MEMBRANE ZONE, SEEN AS AN EOSINOPHILIC OR PERIODIC ACID–SCHIFF (PAS)-POSITIVE BAND (FIG. 23–5C, D)
- SPECKLED PATTERN OF IMMUNOGLOBULIN DEPOSITION IN THE BASEMENT MEMBRANE ZONE
- DEPOSITS OF IMMUNOGLOBULINS AND COMPLEMENT IN THE BASEMENT MEMBRANE ZONE IN DLE- AND SLE-INVOLVED ORAL MUCOSA OR IN NORMAL ORAL MUCOSA IN SLE

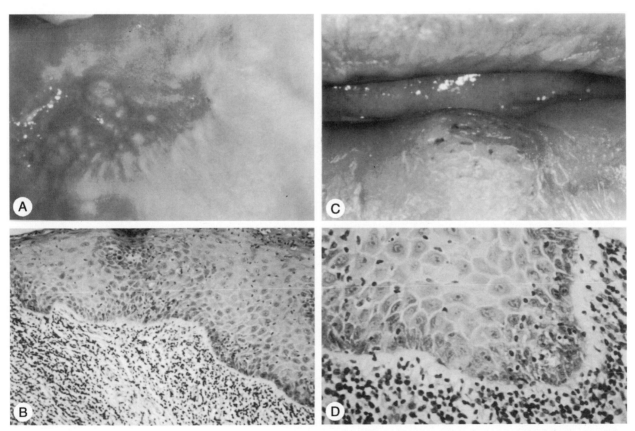

Figure 23–5. Clinical and histologic features of oral lesions of lupus erythematosus. **(A)** A discoid lupus erythematosus (DLE) lesion is present on the buccal mucosa. The central, depressed, atrophic zone contains keratotic papules and telangiectases. The margin shows radiating striae. **(C)** Squamous cell carcinoma is present on the vermilion border of the lower lip in a patient with DLE. **(B, D)** DLE produces parakeratosis with plugging, a mixed inflammatory infiltrate, and thickening of the basement membrane zone.

Many of the features of SLE and DLE are nonspecific and present routinely in lichenoid lesions. Five criteria have been identified to aid in distinguishing lupus erythematosus lesions from lichen planus and leukoplakias.

1. Hyperkeratosis with keratotic plugs
2. Atrophy of the rete processes
3. Deep inflammatory infiltrate
4. Edema in the lamina propria
5. Thick-patchy or continuous PAS-positive deposits juxtaepithelially

These criteria should be supplemented by direct immunofluorescent demonstration of immunoglobulin and complement deposits to make a definitive diagnosis of lupus erythematosus.

Cicatricial Pemphigoid[9, 10]

As distinct from bullous pemphigoid and pemphigus, cicatricial pemphigoid is a chronic bullous dermatosis that may involve the mouth, eyes, and genitalia. The mouth is invariably involved, and this condition manifests as a chronic desquamative gingivitis (Fig. 23–6A) or vesiculobullous eruptions (Fig. 23–6B). The desquamative gingivitis is characterized by extensive involvement of the free and attached gingiva and adjacent alveolar mucosa. The tissues are fragile, show a positive Nikolsky sign, and are usually intensely erythematous, with focal or widespread superficial erosions.

Unlike erosive lichen planus, cicatrical pemphigoid does not produce the characteristic keratotic striae on the papillae or peripheral to the erosive zones.

Definitive diagnosis by biopsy is important because of the possible involvement of other mucosal surfaces, particularly the conjunctiva. Conjunctival involvement commences as a conjunctivitis and the subsequent development of fibrous adhesions between the palpebral and bulbar conjunctiva. The scarring and symblepharon cause entropion, and keratinization may result in blindness.

The histology of cicatrical pemphigoid (Fig. 23–6C, D) shows the following characteristics:

- SEPARATION OF EPITHELIUM FROM UNDERLYING LAMINA PROPRIA AT THE LEVEL OF THE BASEMENT MEMBRANE ZONE
- SUBEPITHELIAL BULLAE
- MIXED, NONSPECIFIC, MONONUCLEAR INFLAMMATORY INFILTRATE OF LYMPHOCYTES, PLASMA CELLS, AND LESS FREQUENTLY, EOSINOPHILS
- NO EVIDENCE OF ACANTHOLYSIS
- BASAL EPITHELIAL LAYER REMAINS INTACT

Definitive diagnosis must be made on the basis of the direct immunofluorescent examination of the tissues; details of this type of examination are presented in Table 23–1. Circulating anti–basement membrane zone antibodies are present in some patients, but these are neither consistent nor

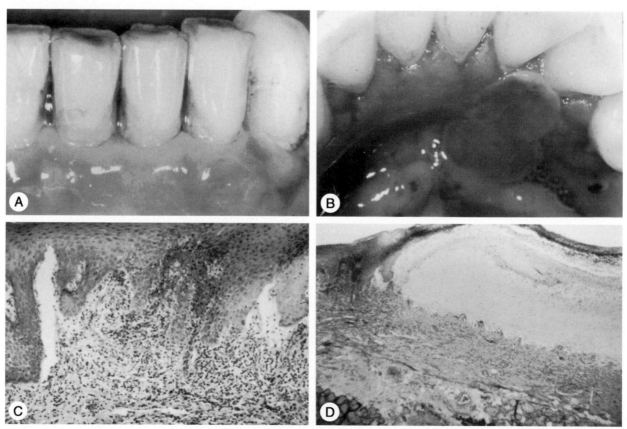

Figure 23–6. Oral mucosal pemphigoid. **(A)** Typical gingival appearance in active cicatricial pemphigoid. There is superficial erosion of an intensely erythematous gingiva with moderate local pain. **(B)** A bulla is present on the lingual aspect of the lower anterior teeth in a pemphigoid patient. The bulla was caused by local trauma during a dental prophylaxis procedure. **(C, D)** Cicatricial pemphigoid demonstrates the characteristic separation of the epithelium from the lamina propria at the basement membrane zone, forming a subepithelial bulla.

Table 23–1. IMMUNOFLUORESCENCE DIAGNOSIS OF EROSIVE AND VESICULOULCERATIVE CONDITIONS

TYPE OF IMMUNO-FLUORESENCE	BULLOUS PEMPHIGOID	CICATRICIAL PEMPHIGOID	LINEAR IgA BULLOUS DERMATOSIS	PEMPHIGUS VULGARIS	LICHEN PLANUS	DISCOID LUPUS ERYTHEMATOSUS	DERMATITIS HERPETI-FORMIS
Direct	Linear IgG and C3 deposits at BMZ of perilesional tissues	Linear IgG and C3 deposits at BMZ of perilesional tissues; IgA often present	Linear IgA deposits at BMZ	Intercellular epithelial IgG deposits in chicken-wire pattern	Fibrinogen deposits at BMZ but not highly specific; IgM in apoptotic bodies	Ig and C deposits at BMZ	Granular IgA deposits in dermal papillae
Indirect	Variably positive for anti-BMZ antibodies	Usually negative	Usually negative	Positive	Negative	Negative	Antigluten and antiendomysial antibodies

BMZ, basement membrane zone; C, complement.

disease phase related. There are numerous other direct immunofluorescent patterns present in many of these conditions, but they do not contribute consistently or specifically to a definitive diagnosis. Immunostaining can establish a definitive diagnosis in both pemphigus vulgaris and bullous pemphigoid, but in other conditions, it is simply an important aid to be used in conjunction with routine histology.

Desquamative Gingivitis

Although desquamative gingivitis can be a manifestation of numerous vesiculobullous conditions, the great majority of cases represent either erosive lichen planus or cicatricial pemphigoid, and diagnosis is not usually difficult. The most critical component in cases that do not show the reticular keratotic striae of lichen planus is obtaining a satisfactory biopsy specimen with an intact dermal-epidermal junction. This is largely a matter of correct site selection (i.e., peripheral to the erosions or bullae) and careful handling of the tissue to ensure preservation of the epithelium.

Lichen Planus Pemphigoides[11, 12]

Lichen planus with a bullous component can be divided into bullous lichen planus (i.e., lichen planus vesiculosis), in which vesicles are superimposed on typical lichen planus lesions, and lichen planus pemphigoides (LPP), in which bullae appear on both involved and uninvolved skin and mucosal sites. Current evidence based on the differing properties and distribution of the bullous pemphigoid (BP) and LPP antigens suggests that LPP is a distinct entity and does not merely accompany lichen planus and BP. However, diagnosis relies on the presence of histologic and immunofluorescence features consistent with both lichen planus and BP.

Plasma Cell Gingivitis[13]

Plasma cell gingivitis describes an unusual but distinctive gingivitis or gingivostomatitis. Classically, there is an intense erythema, with slight edema of the free and attached gingivae and, in some cases, associated cheilitis, glossitis, and buccal mucositis. Mild eosinophilia is the only reported abnormal laboratory value. The majority of cases have been regarded as allergic gingivostomatitis, and when an allergen such as chewing gum, toothpaste, or food is identified, full resolution is rapid, and there is no recurrence.

The histology consists of a variable epithelial hyperplasia and a dense connective tissue infiltrate that is predominantly composed of plasma cells (Fig. 23–7). An association between psoriasis and plasma cell gingivitis has been suggested because of the psoriasiform appearance of some lesions, but as in the case of geographic tongue, this hypothesis has not been sustainable.

Fibroepithelial Hyperplasias[14, 15]

The oral and labial mucosae are frequent sites of non-neoplastic, reactive, fibroepithelial hyperplasias. These hyperplasias are associated with local irritation and therefore may appear on the lower lip adjacent to protruding teeth, on the lateral lingual margins, and on the buccal mucosa (Fig. 23–8A), frequently in association with an edentulous space (i.e., the polyp may fit neatly between adjacent teeth). This type of lesion is also seen in the reflection of the labial and buccal sulci beneath or overlying the flanges of overextended or ill-fitting dentures; in this chapter, these are referred to as denture hyperplasias.

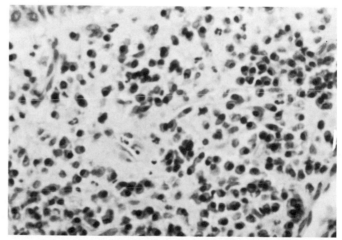

Figure 23–7. Plasma cell gingivitis. Large numbers of plasma cells are present in a vascular lamina propria.

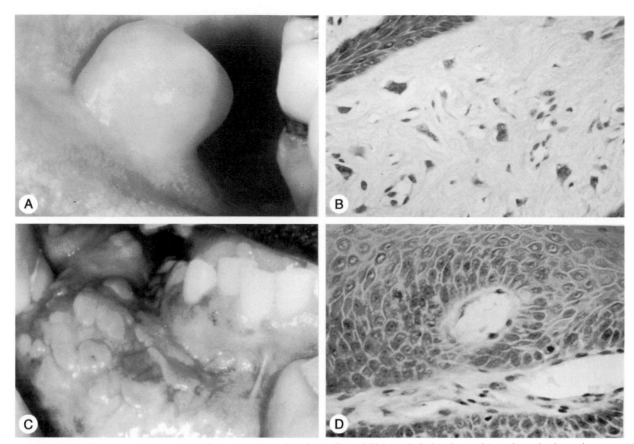

Figure 23–8. Fibroepithelial hyperplasias. **(A)** A firm, smooth-surfaced uninflamed fibroepithelial polyp is located on the buccal mucosa. These lesions are usually caused by local dental trauma. **(B)** Some reactive hyperplastic polyps have large stellate and multinucleated cells in a loosely textured fibrous tissue band immediately subjacent to the epithelium. These polyps have been termed giant cell fibromas. **(C)** Numerous flattened papules are present on the inner aspect of the lower lip in an aboriginal patient with Heck disease. **(D)** Mitosoid bodies in an acanthotic epithelium are typical of Heck disease.

Histologically, this group of lesions is unremarkable. It is important to note that true fibromas, including odontogenic lesions, are very rare in oral tissues. The term irritational fibroma is used frequently but, strictly speaking, is incorrect. Two histologic variants are noteworthy. Some lesions contain areas of myxomatous degeneration but do not constitute a true myxoma. In some fibroepithelial polyps, the subepithelial zone contains a more loosely textured, almost myxoid ground substance that contains large stellate fibroblasts (Fig. 23–8B); these have been referred to as giant cell fibromas. Neither of these variations has any known clinical significance.

Multiple Fibroepithelial Hyperplasias

Rarely, multiple papular or polypoid lesions occur on the oral mucosa, and it is important that these conditions are diagnosed correctly rather than as multiple polyposis or papillomatosis. The differential diagnosis includes the following conditions:

1. Focal epithelial hyperplasia or Heck disease
2. Multiple fibroepithelial hyperplasias
3. Multiple papillomas
4. Multiple oral fibromas (i.e., tuberous sclerosis)

5. Sipple syndrome or multiple mucosal neuromas syndrome
6. Multiple irritational fibromas, or factitial lesions

In multiple fibroepithelial hyperplasias, there are numerous, small, smooth-surfaced, fibroepithelial hyperplastic polyps involving much if not all of the oral and lingual mucosa. The histology of the lesions is unremarkable. An acanthotic epithelium showing rete peg elongation overlies an uninflamed fibrous tissue with no other peculiar features. This histologic picture should not be confused with Heck disease.

Heck Disease

Focal epithelial hyperplasia (FEH), or Heck disease, shows either discrete or confluent, soft polyps or papules (Fig. 23–8C) that occur particularly on the lips and tongue but may involve any oral surface. Most cases are seen in particular ethnic groups; there are only occasional reports of FEH in Caucasians. These lesions are described in Native Americans, Libyans, Swedes, and Australian aborigines as pink, flattened lesions that may disappear when the adjacent mucosa is stretched.

Histologically (Fig. 23–8D), there is a hyperplastic epithelium showing acanthosis and rete peg elongation overlying a normal lamina propria. The epithelium contains mitosoid bodies, or FEH cells, which are large, clear, epithelial cells containing mitosis-like nuclear formations. A number of other reported features, such as dyskeratosis and focal cellular necrosis, have not been consistent in the recent literature.

DNA probe studies have shown that FEH is a papillomavirus infection; papillomavirus types 13 and 32 have been reported. Treatment of FEH and multiple fibroepithelial hyperplasias is empirical; some cases of FEH undergo spontaneous remission.

Papillary and Verrucous Lesions[16]

Papillary lesions are seen frequently on the oral mucosa, and the most frequently represented is the benign squamous papilloma. The papilloma is a papillomavirus lesion that varies considerably in clinical presentation. Most lesions are small, pedunculated or sessile masses (Fig. 23–9A) occurring at any site but frequently located on the palate, tongue, lips, and gingivae. The surface of the lesion is typically papillary, and most are diagnosed clinically on the basis of this feature. Occasionally, lesions reach several centimeters in diameter.

The histology of these lesions (Fig. 23–9B, C) shows a thickened, acanthotic epithelium that is thrown into a series of surface folds. Each papillomatous projection is supported by one or more thin, usually highly vascular connective tissue cores. Mitotic activity and occasional dyskeratotic cells may be noted, but the epithelium is otherwise unremarkable. The presence of parakeratin and keratin is variable.

Papillary and verrucous lesions are treated by simple local excision, and the recurrence rate is extremely low. This group of lesions does not possess any of the aggressive characteristics or the high recurrence rate of nasal or laryngeal papillomas. These lesions should also not be confused with the oral inverted ductal papilloma, which originates in the ducts of minor mucous salivary glands. Condyloma acuminata should be considered in any diagnosis within this group; a list of conditions that should be considered in the differential diagnosis is presented in Table 23–2. The term oral florid papillomatosis is seen occasionally in the literature, but because its usage is inexact, it is no longer an acceptable diagnostic category, although it may be useful clinically in some cases.

Verruciform Xanthoma

Verruciform xanthoma is an uncommon lesion that manifests as an isolated asymptomatic and usually papillary lesion of the oral mucosa. The surface coloration and appearance vary from verrucous to flattened and depend on the variable presence of parakeratin, which to some extent may be site dependent.

Histologically (Fig. 23–9D), the lesion is distinctive,

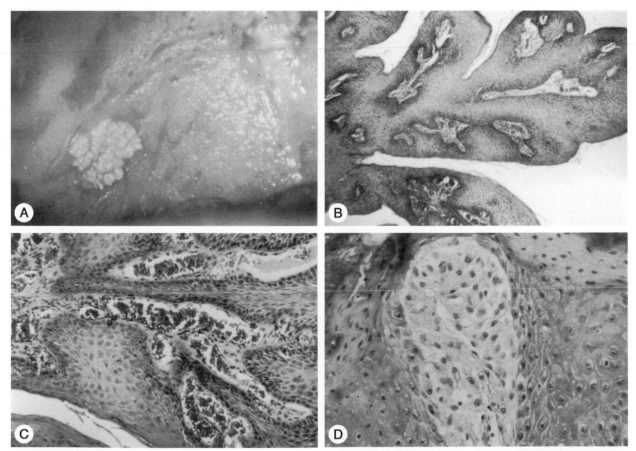

Figure 23–9. Papillary lesions. **(A)** A flattened sessile papilloma with heavy hyperkeratosis of the surface projections is present on the lateral aspect of the posterior hard palate. **(B, C)** This squamous papilloma consists of finger-like projections of acanthotic epithelium supported by thin, highly vascular connective tissues cores. **(D)** In verruciform xanthoma, typical large, clear xanthoma cells fill the clefts between epithelial rete pegs.

Table 23–2. DIFFERENTIAL DIAGNOSIS OF PAPILLARY AND VERRUCOUS LESIONS

UNIFOCAL	MULTIFOCAL
Squamous papilloma	Squamous papilloma
Verruca vulgaris	Verrucae
Condyloma acuminata	Condylomata
Verruciform xanthoma	Squamous cell carcinoma
Keratoacanthoma	Verrucous carcinoma and leukoplakia
Squamous cell carcinoma	Papillary hyperplasia (palate)
Ductal papillomas (simple, inverted, sialadenoma papilliferum)	Focal epithelial hyperplasia
	Keratosis follicularis (Darier-White disease)
	Acanthosis nigricans
	Multiple hamartoma syndrome (Cowden syndrome)
	Focal dermal hypoplasia syndrome (Goltz-Gorlin syndrome)

with a surface topography that may be verrucous, papillary, or flattened with variable parakeratin plugging. The rete pegs are elongated, often in a particularly regular manner, and are supported by connective tissue cores. These cores contain considerable numbers of large, swollen foam cells. The xanthoma cells are confined to the papillae, and subjacent activity is minimal. The foam cells are fat-laden macrophages, but no further information is available regarding their etiology.

The verruciform xanthoma does not recur following conservative excision and is unassociated with any systemic condition. Differential diagnosis from the histology is clearcut, but it is unlikely the lesion would be diagnosed correctly clinically. Extraoral cases have been reported on the vulva, but again these were isolated and without any systemic component.

Lesions of the Tongue and Buccal Mucosa

Median Rhomboid Glossitis

Median rhomboid glossitis (MRG), or central papillary atrophy of the tongue, is a condition seen almost exclusively in adults as a result of a chronic focal candidal infection. This condition originally was regarded as a developmental abnormality, and although this may account for a very small percentage of cases, MRG is now regarded generally as fungal in origin. This condition is more frequent in diabetics.

Clinically, the lesion is a discrete, reddened patch with an irregular outline and variable surface topography located immediately anterior to the foramen caecum (Fig. 23–10A). The appearance of the lesion is a result of filiform depapillation, and it occasionally is misinterpreted as a malignancy.

Histologically (Fig. 23–10B), MRG has the following characteristics:

- HYPERPARAKERATOSIS
- ACANTHOSIS AND RETE PEG ELONGATION
- PSEUDOEPITHELIOMATOUS HYPERPLASIA
- HYALINIZATION WITHIN SUBJACENT MUSCULATURE
- MIXED INFLAMMATORY INFILTRATE
- VARIABLE PRESENCE OF PAS-POSITIVE FUNGAL HYPHAE IN THE UPPER LAYERS OF THE EPITHELIUM.

MRG is diagnosed easily on the basis of the clinical appearance and is biopsied only occasionally. The histology is distinguishable from other lingual pathology, in particular, dysplastic or anaplastic lesions, granular cell tumor, and the lingual thyroid nodule.

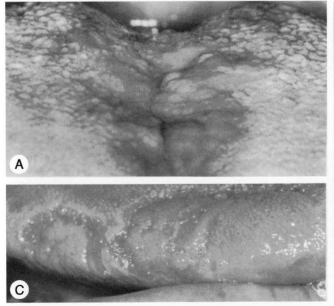
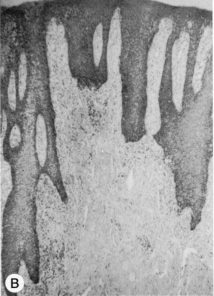

Figure 23–10. Lesions of the tongue. **(A)** Median rhomboid glossitis shows a central depapillated zone with some surface irregularity immediately anterior to the foramen caecum on the dorsum of the tongue. **(B)** Median rhomboid glossitis is histologically unremarkable but often shows pseudoepitheliomatous hyperplasia with hyalinization in the subjacent tissues. **(C)** Typical circinate lesions of benign migratory glossitis. A depressed area shows papillary atrophy and is surrounded by a raised, white border.

Benign Migratory Glossitis

Benign migratory glossitis, also known as geographic tongue or erythema migrans, is a condition of unknown etiology and appears for variable periods at any age, although many patients have the condition for life. It manifests as erythematous, depapillated zones on the dorsum and lateral lingual margins surrounded by a slightly raised yellowish border (Fig. 23–10C). Numerous associations have been made with other dermatoses, in particular, psoriasis, based on the similar histologic picture, but these associations have not been sustained. There is a suggested association with zinc deficiency and atopy, but this has not been our experience.

Histologically, benign migratory glossitis has the following characteristics:

- CENTRAL DEPAPILLATION
- MARGINAL HYPERKERATOSIS
- FOCAL POLYMORPHONUCLEAR LEUKOCYTE ACCUMULATIONS SIMILAR TO THOSE SEEN IN PSORIASIS WITH MICROABSCESS FORMATION
- LAMINA PROPRIA CONTAINS A MIXED INFILTRATE

The psoriasiform lesions include psoriasis, Reiter syndrome, benign migratory glossitis, and ectopic geographic tongue. The interrelations among these conditions seem obscure but because they have similar histologic and occasionally clinical features, they should be included in the differential diagnosis.

Hairy Leukoplakia[17, 18]

Oral hairy leukoplakia (OHL) is an important oral manifestation of human immunodeficiency virus (HIV) infection and is highly predictive for the development of acquired immunodeficiency syndrome (AIDS) within 3 years. Early studies indicated that OHL may be a papillomavirus infection (hence the term oral condyloma planus), but the Epstein-Barr virus is implicated clearly as the trigger for this proliferative epithelial condition. Occasional cases have been reported in HIV-negative patients, but all have been patients with immunosuppressive conditions.

Clinically, OHL manifests as slightly raised, poorly demarcated, keratotic lesions on the lateral and ventral surfaces of the tongue. Typically, the lesions have a corrugated or hairy surface and in many patients carry a significant candidal surface load. The intensity of the lesions varies from faint translucent areas to heavy opaque plaques. The lesions of OHL are treated locally if symptomatic, but they usually will recur after completion of the treatment.

The histologic features of OHL are typical of a squamoproliferative lesion, but OHL lesions are characterized by intranuclear inclusions that are considered diagnostic. The following are histologic features of OHL:

- SURFACE KERATIN PROJECTIONS, OFTEN HAIR-LIKE
- VARIABLE PRESENCE OF CANDIDA
- PARAKERATOSIS AND ACANTHOSIS

- BALLOONING OF CELLS IN ACANTHOUS LAYER
- NUCLEAR PYKNOSIS AND PERINUCLEAR HALOS; KOILOCYTOTIC ATYPIA IS CHARACTERISTIC IN ALL CASES
- INTRANUCLEAR HERPETIC-TYPE INCLUSIONS

Orofacial Granulomatosis[19]

Orofacial granulomatosis (OFG) is a chronic condition that is frequently of unknown etiology and is characterized by noncaseating granulomatous lesions that involve the lips and oral tissues.

OFG encompasses the following disorders, but it may exist as an independent condition:

1. Melkersson-Rosenthal syndrome, which consists of recurrent facial swelling, VII-nerve paralysis, and fissured tongue
2. Cheilitis granulomatosa, or Miescher syndrome
3. Sarcoidosis
4. Crohn disease

Most recent interest in OFG has centered on possible allergic causes. A number of patients, including children have responded well to allergen identification, particularly with foodstuffs, and elimination diets. These procedures should form part of the workup of OFG patients.

Oral Crohn disease has numerous manifestations:

- FACIAL OR LABIAL SWELLING (FIG. 23–11A)
- ANGULAR CHEILITIS AND LIP FISSURES
- MUCOSAL TAGS AND COBBLESTONING
- HYPERPLASTIC GINGIVAL LESIONS (FIG. 23–11B)
- ORAL ULCERATIONS
- PERSISTENT LYMPHADENOPATHY

Histologically (Fig. 23–11C), lesions of OFG show lymphedema of the lamina propria and, generally, small numbers of discrete, noncaseating granulomas. These granulomas consist of ill-defined collections of epithelioid cells, histiocytes, lymphocytes, and usually multinucleated giant cells. Dilated lymphatic vessels are also usually seen.

Treatment of OFG depends on etiology but frequently involves local or systemic steroid therapy and treatment of any particular associated diseases. Some cases appear to resolve after a period of years; this occurrence is more frequent in younger patients.

Fordyce Granules

Fordyce granules (Fig. 23–12A) are small, yellow spots that generally appear in clusters in about 80% of the population. They appear most frequently on the posterior buccal mucosae, inner aspect of the lips, and to a lesser extent, on other oral surfaces.

Histologically (Fig. 23–12B), Fordyce granules are normal sebaceous glands that open directly onto the mucosal surface through a short duct. There are no associated follicles or other skin adnexia. Fordyce granules do not represent a pathologic condition, but they occasionally are biopsied because of their whitish or yellowish appearance.

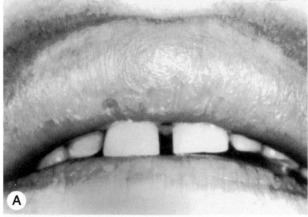

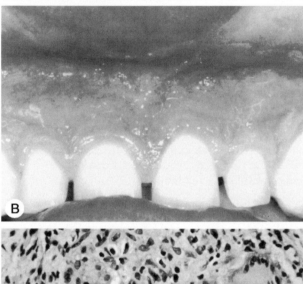

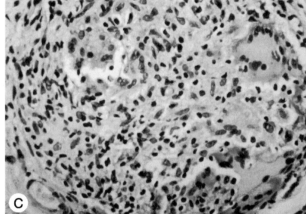

Figure 23–11. Crohn disease and orofacial granulomatosis. **(A)** Enlargement of the upper lip in a patient with Crohn disease. **(B)** Hyperplastic gingival lesions are present in a patient with oral Crohn disease. This patient also had cobblestoning of the buccal mucosa and recurrent ulcerations. **(C)** The discrete, noncaseating granuloma of orofacial granulomatosis contains small numbers of epitheloid cells and multinucleated giant cells.

Submucous Fibrosis[20]

Submucous fibrosis is a chronic condition with progressive stiffness of the oral mucosa, causing trismus and difficulty with oral and facial movements. Most reported cases are from the Indian subcontinent. The etiology is uncertain, but there is strong evidence to implicate chili peppers, and one component has been shown to produce similar mucosal changes in laboratory animals. Vitamin B, protein deficiency,

and the use of "Pam," composed of betel leaf, areca nut, tobacco, and slaked lime, have also been proposed as causative agents.

The onset of submucous fibrosis is gradual and occurs over a period of years as a burning sensation associated with eating spiced food. This sensation is followed in some cases by vesicle formation, ulceration with hypersalivation, and loss of taste acuity. The appearance of a symmetrical blanching of the palate, faucial pillars, buccal mucosa, and to a lesser extent, tongue and lips, is a significant sign. Fibrous bands develop subepithelially and produce a marked change in soft tissue texture and mobility, causing the patient considerable difficulty. The similarity of submucous fibrosis to systemic sclerosis is noteworthy, and the clinical signs of soft tissue immobility with a distorted, board-like texture and difficulty with speech, mastication, and deglutination are parallel to scleroderma.

The histologic features mirror the stage of the condition:

- JUXTA-EPITHELIAL INFLAMMATORY INFILTRATE
- FIBROBLASTIC RESPONSE IN LAMINA PROPRIA
- SUBEPITHELIAL HYALINIZATION
- INCREASING FIBROSIS WITH CONSTRICTION AND EVENTUAL OBLITERATION OF VASCULATURE
- EPITHELIAL ATROPHY WITH LOSS OF RETE PEGS
- POSSIBILITY OF SUBSEQUENT DYSPLASIA AND NEOPLASTIC CHANGE

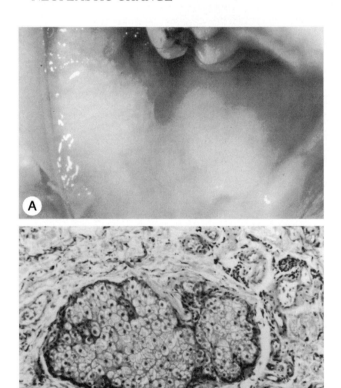

Figure 23–12. Fordyce granules. **(A)** Numerous small, whitish yellow, subepithelial sebaceous glands comprise Fordyce granules. **(B)** Histologically, Fordyce granules show a normal sebaceous gland structure without other associated skin adnexae.

Laboratory studies show an elevated erythrocyte sedimentation rate and in some cases, a normocytic anemia accompanied by eosinophilia and gammaglobulinemia.

Treatment is symptomatic and consists of surgical release of tissues and grafting. Submucosal glucocorticosteroid injections may be helpful in the short term, but most cases continue to be progressive. The most significant feature of submucous fibrosis is its proven role as a premalignant condition.

White Sponge Nevus

White sponge nevus, also known as congenital leukokeratosis or Cannon disease, although an uncommon condition, is the most frequently encountered of the genodermatoses in the oral cavity. Transmitted as an autosomal dominant condition with irregular penetrance and variable expressivity, patients invariably have affected family members, and the diagnosis is usually not difficult.

Clinically, the buccal mucosae and lateral lingual margins are involved most frequently and carry a thickened, irregular, white folded surface (Fig. 23–13A) that reflects an altered pattern of cell maturation involving tonofibril distribution. The change in surface texture may be present at birth

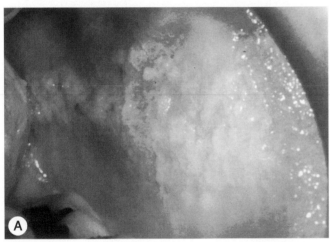

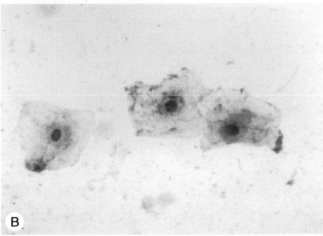

Figure 23–13. White sponge nevus. **(A)** This white sponge nevus involves the buccal mucosa and lateral lingual margins and has a thickened, irregular, white, folded surface. **(B)** A Papanicolaou-stained smear from a white sponge nevus shows the characteristic perinuclear halo.

but in almost all cases has reached its maximum extent by adolescence. Some patients report a cyclical build up of surface irregularity that is shed with chewing and local abrasion and then reforms. The sites are asymptomatic, and no treatment is required. Any mucosal surface may be involved as well as the oral cavity, but this is an occasional finding.

Papanicolaou-stained cytologic smears show a distinctive, perinuclear, pink halo (Fig. 23–13B) that mirrors the tonofibril condensation reported ultrastructurally. Biopsy is undertaken on occasion, and although the histology is characteristic, it is not pathognomonic. The significant features include the following:

- PARAKERATOSIS WITH PLUGGING
- ACANTHOSIS
- MARKED INTRACELLULAR EDEMA, GIVING A TYPICAL WASHED-OUT APPEARANCE AND VACUOLATED CELLS WITH PYKNOTIC NUCLEI
- DYSKERATOSIS

A histologic variant has been termed Oral Epithelial Nevus. The major features include the following:

- HYPERKERATOSIS
- PROMINENT GRANULAR CELL LAYER
- LITTLE, IF ANY, ACANTHOSIS

A number of conditions bear some resemblance to white sponge nevus, but the nevus can be differentiated from these on the basis of the clinical and histologic criteria:

1. Candidiasis
2. Leukoplakia
3. Lichen planus
4. Leukedema
5. Keratosis follicularis (i.e., Darier-White disease)
6. Pachyonychia congenita
7. Hereditary benign intraepithelial dyskeratosis (i.e., Witkop disease)
8. Congenital dyskeratosis (i.e., Cole-Rauschkolb-Toomey syndrome)
9. Icthyosiform dermatoses

Lesions of Salivary Glands

Mucous Extravasation Cyst

With the exception of the posterior lingual serous glands (i.e., von Ebner glands), which open into the trough of the vallate papillae, all other minor salivary glands are mucous or mixed (distal areas of the anterior lingual glands or the glands of Blandin and Nuhn); therefore, after obstruction or severance of the ducts, mucous retention and extravasation cysts may develop. Most of these cysts or mucoceles occur on the lower lip (Fig. 23–14A) and with their superficial position (Fig. 23–14B) may rupture and resolve spontaneously. More deeply placed lesions may reach 1 cm or more in diameter and, depending on their level within the tissues, will appear bluish or show no color change.

Lesions that are not covered by a thin tissue layer are treated most appropriately by surgical excision, including the underlying mucous glands.

The histology (Fig. 23–14C) depends on the history and duration of the lesion. A central mucous pool containing

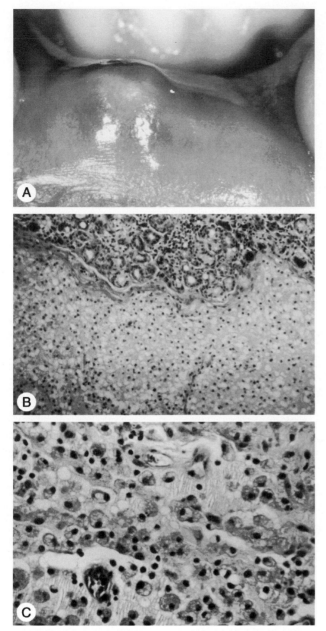

Figure 23–14. Traumatic lesions of the salivary glands. **(A)** Mucocele of the lower lip. The bluish lesions are freely movable and nonindurated. **(B, C)** A mucous extravasation cyst shows the distinct walling-off of the mucous pool and the presence of large numbers of macrophages and foam histiocytes.

varying numbers of macrophages, foam histiocytes, and polymorphonuclear leukocytes is surrounded by a nonepithelialized wall of compressed fibrous tissue. This is lined frequently by granulation tissue. The subjacent mucous glands show atrophic changes, ductal ectasia, and fibrosis.

These simple lesions are managed readily with the occasional complication of recurrence if the mucous glands are not removed or further damage is caused to adjacent glands. Rarely, mucous-producing tumors will mimic a mucocele clinically.

Necrotizing Sialometaplasia

Necrotizing sialometaplasia is a benign, self-limiting, inflammatory reaction, usually involving the minor mucous salivary glands of the posterior hard and soft palates, although any site containing these glands may be involved. The lesion is of considerable importance, because it may mimic malignancy both clinically and histologically, particularly squamous cell carcinoma or mucoepidermoid tumor.

Classically, the lesion presents as a deep ulcerative lesion (Fig. 23–15A) at the junction of the hard and soft pal-

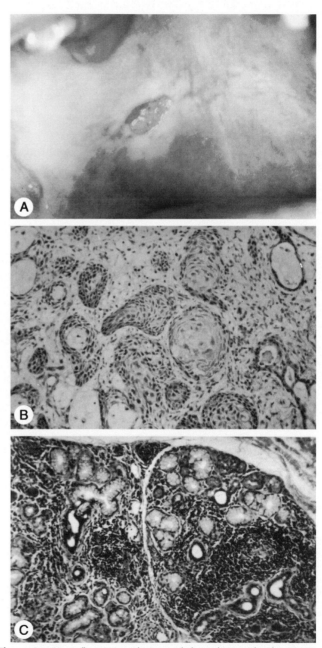

Figure 23–15. Inflammatory lesions of the salivary glands. **(A, B)** A lesion of necrotizing sialometaplasia shows marked squamous metaplasia of the acinar and ductal elements and pseudoepitheliomatous hyperplasia. **(C)** A minor mucous salivary gland from a patient with Sjögren syndrome shows extensive (grade 4) infiltration by lymphocytes and loss of acini.

ates. It is a presumed to be the result of local ischemia, and the histology and clinical appearance of a deep necrotizing ulcer that causes variable degrees of pain and heals spontaneously in 5 to 8 weeks supports this premise. Necrotizing sialometaplasia has been reported in all age groups except children, and although cases have been associated with vascular disease, this is a not a consistent finding.

The histologic appearance of necrotizing sialometaplasia is characterized by the following features:

- PSEUDOEPITHELIOMATOUS HYPERPLASIA ADJACENT TO THE ULCER
- ISCHEMIC OR COAGULATION NECROSIS OF THE GLANDULAR TISSUE IN A LOBULAR PATTERN
- RELEASE OF MUCUS AND A SUBSEQUENT INFLAMMATORY RESPONSE WHICH MAY BE INTENSE
- SQUAMOUS METAPLASIA OF ACINAR AND DUCTAL ELEMENTS
- PRESERVATION OF LOBULAR PATTERN

The treatment of necrotizing sialometaplasia is symptomatic; the use of topical or systemic antiinflammatory agents is valuable, although most lesions run the usual course of 5 to 8 weeks. The condition may be recurrent, and we have seen bilateral cases.

Stomatitis Nicotina

Commonly termed pipe-smoker's palate, stomatitis nicotina occurs on the posterior hard and anterior soft palate as a direct result of tobacco smoking. Initially, a surface hyperkeratosis forms, generally in association with local erythema, producing a diffuse, irregular, leukoplakic appearance. The openings of the minor mucous glands are erythematous, and as the condition progresses, they become partially occluded and peripherally hyperkeratotic, giving the typical appearance of the umbilicated papular lesion of stomatitis nicotina. If atrophy of the glandular elements is progressive, then in combination with the increasing hyperkeratosis of the tissues between the papules, the palate may become flatter, and the papules may present as small pits. This feature is particularly noticeable in some areas of India, where reverse smoking of chuttas is practiced.

The histology of the lesions of stomatitis nicotina is nonspecific but clearly the result of local irritation. The duct openings become closed with hyperkeratotic plugs, and the ducts show squamous metaplasia. The presence of atypia is variable, but it may be seen in the tissues surrounding the duct opening. The underlying mucous glands undergo atrophy, although an initial hyperplasia has been reported. The ductal components may become convoluted, and eventually, partial obstruction with subepithelial dilation caused by compression between the underlying bone and overlying hyperkeratotic epithelium occur. In severe cases, no evidence of the gland remains other than fibrosis.

Stomatitis nicotina is usually reversible. Most of the severe changes are seen only in long-term, heavy smokers.

In these patients, there is an increased risk of malignant transformation.

Sjögren Syndrome[21, 22]

Sjögren syndrome (SS) is a systemic autoimmune disorder and is the most prevalent connective tissue disease other than rheumatoid arthritis. Primary SS is based on the findings of dry mouth and eyes which, in combination with another connective tissue disorder, constitutes secondary SS. Both primary and secondary SS exhibit a range of changes and immunologic abnormalities other than xerostomia, xerophthalmia, and subsequent keratoconjunctivitis sicca. In the clinical workup of this patient group, a range of physical, hematologic and immunologic screens are required.

Of considerable value in making the diagnosis is the labial minor mucous salivary gland biopsy. The presence of focal sialadenitis is a reliable criterion to support the other diagnostic tests used in evaluating xerostomic patients suspected of having SS. The changes present in the minor glands reflect those in the parotid glands, in which there is a T-lymphocytic infiltrate, predominantly CD4+, that is responsible for direct injury to glandular tissues. There is a concurrent but less pronounced B-cell hyperactivity in which IgG-containing cells become dominant over the usual IgA-producing cells.

The glandular changes commence as focal periductal lymphocytic aggregations that, with progression, become punctate, nodular, and eventually diffuse. These changes are accompanied by acinar atrophy, ductal hyperplasia, and metaplasia, leading to epimyoepithelial cell islands and preservation of the overall glandular architecture. The epimyoepithelial cell islands are metaplastic epithelial cells and do not contain myoepithelial cells. They are present in the major glands only.

The glands should be evaluated for both the extent of acinar atrophy and destruction and the type and intensity of the cellular infiltrate. The major histologic features of SS (Fig. 23–15B) include the following:

- ACINAR ATROPHY
- LYMPHOCYTIC INFILTRATE WITH OCCASIONAL FORMATION OF GERMINAL CENTERS
- DUCTAL EPITHELIAL HYPERPLASIA AND METAPLASIA
- REPLACEMENT OF PARENCHYMA BY INFILTRATE

The grading standard designed by Chisholm and Mason is a useful gauge of glandular involvement. The number of foci, which consist of 50 or more lymphocytes, in 4 mm^2 of salivary gland tissue is counted. A grade of 0 indicates an absence of foci; 1 represents a slight infiltrate; 2 indicates a moderate infiltrate or less than one focus; 3 is assigned when there is one focus; and 4 indicates that there is more than one focus. Grade 4 is highly indicative of SS. Similar histologic features may be observed in bone marrow transplant recipients affected by graft-versus-host disease, in which cell-mediated cytotoxicity may be directed against epithelial targets.

Lesions of the Gingivae

The majority of both localized and generalized gingival enlargements are inflammatory in nature and are discussed under the general topic of gingivitis (Table 23–3). However, a small number of lesions are sufficiently distinctive in etiology, clinical presentation, and histology to warrant separate discussion.

Generalized Enlargement[14, 23]

- **DRUG-INDUCED**
    Dilantin (Phenytoin)
    Cyclosporine
    Nifedipine, Diltiazem
    Verapamil, Felodipine
    Oral Contraceptives
- **HEREDITARY**
    Fibromatosis Gingivae
    Tuberous Sclerosis
    Cherubism
    Fibromatosis Gingivae and
       Hypertrichosis
- **DEFICIENCY STATES**
    Avitaminosis A
    Avitaminosis C
- **LEUKEMIAS**
    Leukemic Infiltration
    Drug Toxicity
    Graft-Versus-Host Disease
    Marrow or Lymphoid Tissue
       Depression
- **ENDOCRINE**
    Puberty
    Pregnancy
    Hypothyroidism
    Cushing Syndrome
    Diabetes
- **CROHN DISEASE**

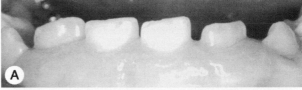

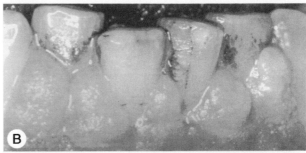

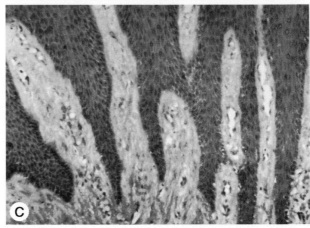

Figure 23–16. Gingival enlargement. **(A)** Bulky, dense, fibrous overgrowth of the gingivae occurs in fibromatosis gingivae, particularly around the lower anterior teeth. **(B)** Cyclosporin-induced gingival overgrowth occurred in a cardiac allograft recipient. The drug-related gingival overgrowth tends to involve the interdental papillae, in contrast to fibromatosis gingivae. **(C)** Phenytoin-induced gingival overgrowth shows a dense, fibrous tissue mass with elongation of rete pegs in a test-tube pattern. The latter is not an invariable finding.

Table 23–3. COMMON LESIONS OF THE GINGIVAE

CONDITION	IMMUNOPHENOTYPE AND HISTOPATHOLOGY	MICROORGANISMS IMPLICATED
Normal/healthy gingiva	T-cell–dominated, stable lesion Sparse infiltrate Epithelium intact	*Streptococcus* sp *Actinomyces* sp
Gingivitis	T-cell–dominated, stable lesion Perivascular infiltrate Neutrophils in epithelium Intercellular edema	As for normal/healthy
Periodontitis	B-cell–dominated, progressive lesion Plasma cells present Apical epithelial migration Epithelial ulceration Bone resorption	*Porphyromonas gingivalis* *Actinobacillus actinomycetemcomitans* *Eikenella corrodens* *Fusobacterium nucleatum* *Bacteroides intermedius*
Rapidly progressive periodontitis	As for periodontitis, but with acute neutrophil response superimposed in response to possible tissue invasion	As for periodontitis
Localized juvenile periodontitis	As for periodontitis, with tissue invasion by organisms	*Actinobacillus actinomycetemcomitans* *Capnocytophaga* sp
Acute necrotizing ulcerative gingivitis	Necrosis of epithelium and connective tissue Dense neutrophil infiltrate Lymphocytes and plasma cells Marked tissue invasion	*Fusobacterium* sp Spirochetes *Bacteroides intermedius*

The two most interesting and distinctive gingival conditions are fibromatosis gingivae (FG) and phenytoin gingival overgrowth. FG may be either idiopathic or hereditary with an autosomal dominant pattern of inheritance, with onset early in life so that delayed eruption, particularly in the permanent dentition, is common. Dense fibrous overgrowth (Fig. 23–16A) covers the dentition, either partially or wholly, in a lobular manner. Histologically, there is a dense, noninflammatory, fibrous hyperplasia covered with normal epithelium. Phenytoin gingival overgrowth differs from FG in that it is caused by the use of phenytoin, and that there is involvement of interdental papillae initially (Fig. 23–16C). The gingival effects of phenytoin seem to be dependent on the presence of plaque and other local irritants and on individual susceptibility rather than on the dosage or duration of use of the drugs. Histologically (see Fig. 23–16C), there is a bulk of uninflamed fibrous tissue with little obvious vascularity. The area of progressive expansion is chronically inflamed secondary to local irritants and plaque toxins. The surface is covered by a thickened epithelium that is keratinized and often shows elongated test-tube rete pegs. Other drug-related gingival overgrowths, such as that induced by cyclosporin (Fig. 23–16B), have features similar to those of phenytoin gingival overgrowth.

As with all drug-related gingival overgrowths, withdrawal of the offending agent usually produces an acceptable aesthetic result. Some gingival surgery may be required in a minority of cases. FG is more difficult to manage, and occasionally the teeth are removed to prevent recurrence of the condition.

Localized Enlargement

There are several categories of localized gingival enlargements.

- NEONATAL
  Congenital Epulis of the Newborn
  Melanotic Neuroectodermal Tumor
    of Infancy
  Dental Lamina Cysts (i.e., Bohn
    nodules)
- CHILDHOOD AND ADOLESCENCE
  Eruption Cysts
  Pericoronitis
  Odontogenic Tumors
- OTHERS
  Gingival Cyst of the Adult
  Epulis Fissuratum or Denture
    Hyperplasia
  Epulis Granulomatosum
  Tumors
- MOST SIGNIFICANT GINGIVAL
  ENLARGEMENTS
  Peripheral Odontogenic Fibroma
  Pyogenic Granuloma or
    Angiogranuloma
  Peripheral Giant Cell Lesion

The last category of epulides form a significant group, as they all appear to originate from the periodontal membrane and occur as an overexuberant response to local irritation.

The peripheral fibroma or peripheral odontogenic fibroma, the most frequently encountered localized gingival enlargement, presents as a firm, smooth-surfaced, sometimes lobulated mass growing from an interdental papilla (Fig. 23–17A). Histologically (Fig. 23–17B), these lesions vary in the degree of both cellularity and fibrosis, but the diagnosis hinges on the presence of fibroblastic tissue. This feature is characteristic and in many lesions, is accompanied by ossification, cementum formation, or irregular calcifications (hence the term peripheral fibroma with calcification).

The pyogenic granuloma, which is also a reactive lesion, is more correctly termed an angiogranuloma, because there is no pyogenic component to the lesion. This lesion is smooth surfaced, deep reddish blue in color, and characteristically ulcerated. Pyogenic granulomas tend to grow rapidly, cover the dental occlusal surfaces, and separate the teeth before reaching full size and becoming relatively static. The histology of pyogenic granuloma (Fig. 23–17C) is characteristically granulomatous with solid sheets of endothelial cells and small and large vascular channels separated by a variably inflamed, fibrous stroma. The surface of the lesion is ulcerated in at least some regions, but the deeper tissue levels may consist of a more mature fibrous tissue. This group of lesions is identical to the pregnancy epulis or tumor.

The peripheral giant cell lesion, or reparative granuloma, is similar in clinical appearance to the angiogranuloma, although the former is likely to be more cyanotic (Fig. 23–17D). This lesion occurs in a younger age group than the previously described conditions and occurs most frequently anterior to the molar teeth. This lesion is the most aggressive of the three epulides and causes local bone destruction and splaying of teeth. Histologically, the mass is nonencapsulated and consists of a cellular matrix containing fibroblasts, macrophages, and multinuclear giant cells that are in close association with vessel walls (Fig. 23–17E). Peripherally, the vascularity is prominent, but there are no associated giant cells. Surface ulceration and inflammation within the body of the lesion are variable and not of diagnostic importance. Many attempts have been made to separate the giant cell lesions into reactive and neoplastic categories, but there are no consistently reliable criteria to distinguish between the two types. A relatively uniform distribution of giant cells that are associated with stromal cells showing a nuclear preponderance in older patients is more likely to represent a neoplasm, but these lesions are reported only rarely in the jaw and are generally central rather than peripheral lesions. This group of lesions is aggressive in appearance and clinical behavior and deserves particular care in treatment.

Because all three epulides are distinctive in their deep-seated attachment to the periodontal ligament, growth potential, biologic behavior, and histology, they require more careful surgical treatment than do the reactive, soft fibrous epulis. Treatment involves local excision with thorough curettage of the subjacent alveolar surface and, if possible, primary coverage of the surgical bed. This technique reduces recurrence, which in some series is reported to be 30% but is much lower in our experience.

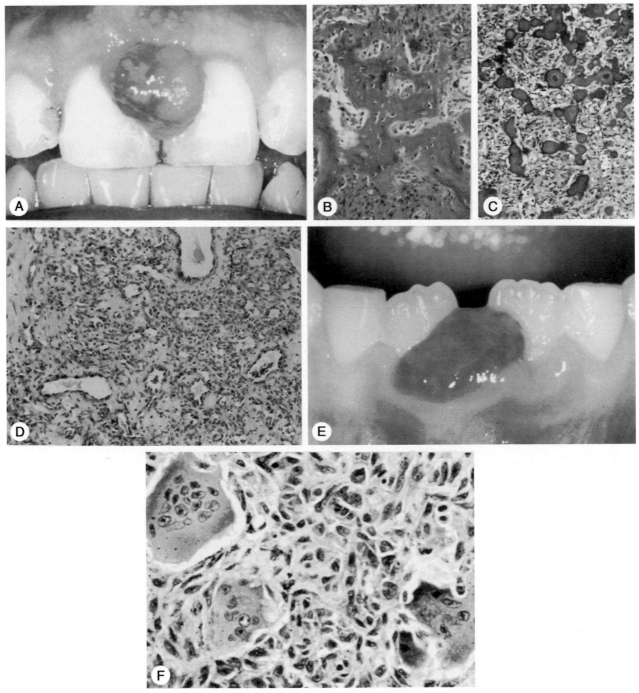

Figure 23–17. Localized gingival enlargements. **(A)** A peripheral fibroma extends from the gingival margin. The surface has been traumatized secondarily. **(B, C)** A peripheral fibroma shows the typical fibroblastic tissue response with the deposition of bone, calcific structures, and cementum spheres, some of which show concentric Leisegang rings. **(D)** This angiogranuloma consists of numerous small vascular channels and noncanalized endothelial cell clusters in variably inflamed connective tissue. **(E)** Typical cyanotic appearance of a peripheral giant cell lesion. This lesion has eroded the underlying alveolar bone and is causing displacement of the lower central incisor teeth. **(F)** A giant cell lesion contains a variable mononuclear cell component. Multinuclear giant cells are frequently seen in association with blood vessels.

Gingivitis[24–26]

Gingivitis is by far the most common condition that affects the oral mucosa. This condition is important not only because of its prevalence in the population, but because it may be superimposed on other entities that affect oral mucosa in the vicinity of teeth. Gingivitis is an inflammatory process that represents an immune response to the accumu-

lation of dental plaque. Thus, conditions that interfere with removal of plaque from the teeth (e.g., ulcerations of the gingiva, which make toothbrushing painful) will elicit gingivitis. Recognition of gingivitis is therefore essential when evaluating histologic material from any lesion located in close proximity to teeth.

Except for short periods immediately after performing oral hygiene (e.g., brushing), the hard surfaces of the teeth are colonized by organized masses of bacteria embedded in a matrix of bacterial products. These deposits of plaque, when removed regularly, are not thick enough to be seen by the unaided eye. Clinically, healthy gingivae are pink, firm, and display small surface undulations referred to as stippling.

If plaque is allowed to accumulate, clinically detectable inflammation develops over the ensuing 4 to 8 days, producing loss of stippling and edematous changes in the tissue (Fig. 23–18A). Production of fluid from the gingival crevice

is increased at this stage, and plaque deposits are clearly visible. Erythema does not develop in most individuals until relatively late (2-3 weeks) and is accompanied by gingival bleeding in response to brushing. These inflammatory changes resolve rapidly after plaque-removal measures are recommenced.

The oral epithelium of subjects with healthy gingivae is inflamed at the microscopic level, with small aggregations of lymphocytes present in the lamina propria and occasional

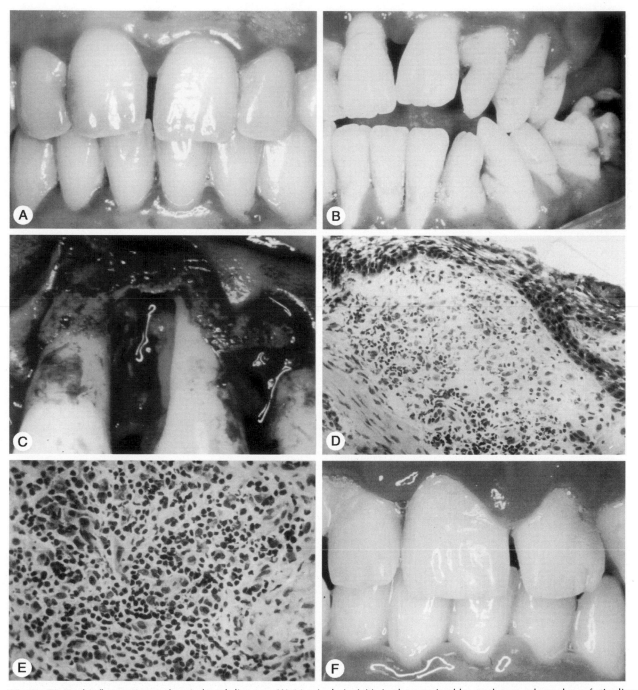

Figure 23–18. Gingival inflammation and periodontal diseases. **(A)** Marginal gingivitis is characterized by erythema, edema, loss of stippling, and bleeding in response to probing. **(B)** Progressive adult periodontitis shows extensive inflammation of the periodontal tissues and loss of tooth support. **(C)** Direct visualization of the supporting alveolar bone by raising a mucoperiosteal flap shows the extent of alveolar bone loss in a patient with adult periodontitis. **(D, E)** A histologic specimen from a patient with adult periodontitis shows extensive infiltration of the gingival connective tissues by mononuclear cells, particularly lymphocytes. **(F)** Acute necrotizing ulcerative gingivitis shows cratering of the gingival soft tissues.

intraepithelial lymphocytes. These aggregations persist despite repeated professional oral hygiene and therefore may be considered the background response to continuous exposure to bacterial products that diffuse through the epithelium. Immunohistochemical studies have established that this baseline entity is a T-cell dominated lesion that resembles a cutaneous delayed hypersensitivity response in phenotype and appears immunologically well controlled. This attribute and the fact that the connective tissue attachment of the tooth is not compromised by this condition has prompted use of the term ''stable lesion'' to describe the inflammatory response.

After plaque has accumulated for longer than 2 days, the bacteriologic composition of the plaque changes from predominantly gram-positive aerobes to gram-positive and -negative anaerobes. The resultant assault of bacterial products through the oral epithelium at first elicits a neutrophil response to the microorganisms. Intercellular edema of the oral epithelium and the presence of moderate numbers of neutrophils in the lamina propria and epithelium are conspicuous features of this stage. Over the ensuing 3 weeks, the lymphocytic infiltrate expands by recruiting additional cells from the circulation. Perivascular aggregates of T cells progressively enlarge and fuse to eventually occupy the bulk of the subepithelial tissue compartment. The essential immunologic nature of the lesion remains unchanged throughout this period; thus, the changes that occur can be thought of simply as expansion of the original stable lesion.

When plaque deposits persist for longer than 3 weeks, one of two scenarios may occur. The stable lesion may persist and the health of the dentition is not compromised. This occurs when the individual is resistant to the deleterious effects of plaque microorganisms because of a favorable host immunologic response, such as that which occurs in chronic gingivitis associated with the deciduous dentition in children. Alternatively, fundamental changes may occur in the nature of the lesion, and the resulting destructive changes may compromise the longevity of the dentition (Fig. 23–18B, C). This clinical entity, periodontitis, occurs in susceptible individuals and is associated with the conversion from a stable to a progressive lesion.

The time frame for the development of destructive inflammation from stable inflammation appears to vary among susceptible individuals; however, in the majority of cases, evidence of destruction can be found by the fourth decade of life. Although gingivitis responds readily to mechanical and chemical plaque control measures, treatment of periodontitis poses greater problems because of the difficulty in obtaining access to root surfaces for proper debridement.

Periodontitis[26]

The histopathology of periodontitis (Fig. 23–18D, E) is characterized by destructive alterations in the supporting tissues of the teeth (i.e., the connective tissue attachment and alveolar bone). The lesion is dominated by B lymphocytes and plasma cells. The latter produce predominantly IgG; however, because of polyclonal activation, the antibodies generated include many irrelevant specificities. Epithelial migration in the direction of the tooth apex is a conspicuous feature of the progressive lesion. The lesion is bordered by a fibrous band; beyond this band, osteoclastic resorption of alveolar bone occurs under the influence of soluble mediators, predominantly interleukin-1 and other proinflammatory cytokines released from the lesional cells.

Bacterial invasion into the connective tissue compartment does not occur in periodontitis; therefore, the cellular response that occurs is elicited by products derived from a number of specific gram-negative anaerobes. Periodontitis occurs in bursts; periods of progression and stability may be recognized. Each new burst corresponds with a conversion from a stable to a progressive lesion, with loss of supporting structures and partial regeneration occurring alternately, producing a net loss of tooth support over time. Local factors (e.g., emergence and subsequent elimination of specific bacteria) superimposed on a background of altered host response are probably responsible for the episodic nature of periodontitis.

Rapidly Progressive Periodontitis

In the gingivae, bacterial invasion into connective tissue occurs only in the presence of a defective host response, usually a defect in neutrophil number or function (e.g., diabetes mellitus, Down syndrome, cyclic neutropenia). In these conditions, an exaggerated neutrophil response is superimposed on the existing B-cell–dominated lesion of periodontitis, and suppuration occurs as a result of abortive phagocytosis. Extremely rapid bone resorption accompanies tissue invasion, hence the designation rapidly progressive periodontitis. Antibiotic therapy for this condition is of value in augmenting the effects of mechanical debridement and drainage. Chemotherapeutic approaches designed to correct the underlying phagocytic defect and thereby reduce the opportunity for tissue invasion are presently being evaluated.

Localized Juvenile Periodontitis

Localized juvenile periodontitis is a distinct entity characterized by circumpubertal onset, extensive bone loss at restricted sites (i.e., incisors and first molars only), a familial pattern of inheritance, and marked tissue destruction in the absence of gross deposits of plaque or overt clinical inflammation. Affected individuals usually display a neutrophil phagocytic defect. Unlike periodontitis and rapidly progressive periodontitis, in which a number of organisms have been implicated, localized juvenile periodontitis represents a specific infection by Actinobacillus actinomycetemcomitans. This organism produces a potent leukotoxin which probably contributes to an impaired host immune response in the gingival tissues. The lesion is dominated by plasma cells and B lymphocytes and shows a marked loss of collagen and bone resorption.

Although these histologic features resemble those described previously for periodontitis, the two conditions can be easily differentiated on clinical grounds. Treatment of localized juvenile periodontitis consists of mechanical debridement, the use of systemic tetracyclines, and where indicated, local irrigation with antimicrobials.

Acute Necrotizing Ulcerative Gingivitis[27]

Acute necrotizing ulcerative gingivitis (ANUG) occurs particularly in young adults and is almost invariably related to smoking, poor oral hygiene, preexisting gingivitis, and emotional stress. ANUG also occurs in individuals with AIDS, where it reflects an underlying perturbation in host immune defences. The clinical features of ANUG are diagnostic. The principal finding is necrotic lesions of the interdental and marginal gingiva (Fig. 23–18F) that have developed rapidly. The labial aspect of the gingiva is the most frequent site of involvement. These necrotic areas are covered by soft, yellow-white or grey pseudomembrane, which consists of fibrin, debris, masses of bacteria, and leukocytes. Adjacent unaffected gingival tissues are separated from necrotic areas by a well-demarcated erythematous zone. Affected individuals frequently complain of marked bleeding, considerable pain, and increased salivation. Lymphadenitis, fever, and malaise may occur in patients who have more advanced cases. The histopathology of ANUG is not pathognomic. Necrosis of the epithelium and superficial connective tissues are observed together with nonspecific inflammatory changes. The presence of microorganisms, especially spirochetes, in the tissues and a dense neutrophil infiltrate are the predominant changes. ANUG responds readily to systemic metronidazole and local debridement. Regrettably, cratered areas of gingiva are not restored during healing and predispose the patient to recurrence of the condition.

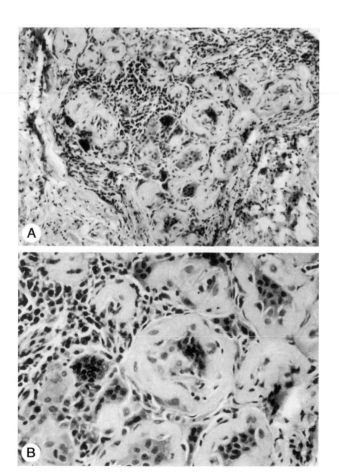

Figure 23–19. Pulse granuloma. **(A)** The pulse granuloma contains discrete, foreign-body giant cells and associated rings of hyalinized material. **(B)** Higher power shows the pale hyaline rings, some of which are incomplete and contain cellular connective tissue cores.

Pulse Granuloma[28, 29]

Pulse granuloma of the alveolus is a foreign-body granuloma that forms as a result of inclusion of food particles, particularly legumes, within the soft tissues or alveolus proper. Because of the apparent hyalinization of blood vessel walls, the condition is also called giant cell hyalin angiopathy. However, the histology of pulse granuloma closely resembles the granulomatous response seen in the lungs following aspiration of cooked leguminous foods, and the original hypothesis of a vascular lesion is no longer supported.

Pulse granulomas are always associated with a breach in the oral mucosa. Although most of these granulomas tend to be central bony lesions, several superficial lesions have been reported.

The major histologic features (Fig. 23–19) of pulse granuloma include the following:

- STARCH CONTAINING MESOPHYLL CELLS FROM LEGUME SEEDS (DIASTASE-SENSITIVE PAS- AND IODINE-POSITIVE)
- DISCRETE FOREIGN-BODY GIANT CELLS, EPITHELIOID CELLS, AND A ROUND CELL INFILTRATE
- RINGS OF HYALINIZED MATERIAL ARE FREQUENTLY ASSOCIATED WITH THE FOREIGN MATTER, AND CALCIFICATION OF THESE OCCURS IN SOME LESIONS
- LAKES OF AMORPHOUS AND GRANULAR MATERIAL REPRESENT LEGUMES IN VARIOUS STAGES OF BREAKDOWN

These lesions are treated by local curettage, and recurrence has not been reported.

Retrocuspid Papilla[15, 29]

Retrocuspid papilla is a small mucosal nodule on the gingiva associated with the lingual aspect of the mandibular cuspid teeth. This lesion is common in children but is seen much less frequently in adults. Histologically, the lesion represents a fibroepithelial hyperplasia. Retrocuspid papillae sometimes contain large stellate and multinucleated fibroblasts similar to those seen in giant cell fibroma. These lesions are developmental and do not represent a pathologic entity.

SELECTED REFERENCES

1. Savage NW, Seymour GJ, Kruger BJ. T-lymphocyte subset changes in recurrent aphthous stomatitis. Oral Surg Oral Med Oral Pathol 1985;60:175.
2. Savage NW, Seymour GJ, Kruger BJ. Expression of class I and class II MHC antigens on keratinocytes in recurrent aphthous stomatitis. J Oral Pathol 1986;15:191.
3. Walsh LJ, Savage NW, Ishii T, Seymour GJ. The immunopathogenesis of oral lichen planus. J Oral Pathol Med 1990;19:389.
4. Krutchkoff DJ, Eisenberg E. Lichenoid dysplasia: A distinct histopathologic entity. Oral Surg Oral Med Oral Pathol 1985;60:308.
5. Eisenberg E, Murphy GF, Krutchkoff DJ. Involucrin as a diagnostic marker in oral lichenoid lesions. Oral Surg Oral Med Oral Pathol 1987;64:313.
6. Vincent SD, Fotos PG, Baker KA, Williams TP. Oral lichen planus:

The clinical, historical and therapeutic features of 100 cases. Oral Surg Oral Med Oral Pathol 1990;70:165.

7. Eisen D, Ellis CN, Duell EA, et al. Effect of topical cyclosporine rinse on oral lichen planus. A double blind analysis. N Engl J Med 1990;323:290.

8. Schiodt M. Oral manifestations of lupus erythematosus. Int J Oral Surg 1984;12:101

9. Moy W, Kumar V, Friedman RP, et al. Cicatricial pemphigoid. J Periodontol 1986;57:39.

10. Williams DM, Leonard JN, Wright P, et al. Benign mucous membrane (cicatricial) pemphigoid revisited. Br Dent J 1984;157:313.

11. Okochi H, Nashiro K, Tsuchida T, et al. Lichen planus pemphigoides. J Am Acad Dermatol 1990;22:626.

12. Lang PG, Maize JC. Coexisting lichen planus and bullous pemphigoid or lichen planus pemphigoides? J Am Acad Dermatol 1983;9:133.

13. Lubow RM, Cooley RL, Hartman KS, McDaniel RK. Plasma-cell gingivitis. J Periodontol 1984;55:235.

14. Shafer WG, Hine MK, Levy BM. A textbook of oral pathology, 4th ed. Philadelphia: WB Saunders, 1983.

15. Savage NW, Monsour PJ. Oral fibrous hyperplasias and the giant cell fibroma. Aust Dent J 1985;30:405.

16. Eversole LR, Papanicolaou SJ. Papillary and verrucous lesions of oral mucous membranes. J Oral Med 1983;38:3.

17. Greenspan JS, Greenspan D, Lennette ET, et al. Replication of Epstein-Barr virus within the epithelial cells of oral hairy leukoplakia, an AIDS-associated lesion. N Engl J Med 1985;313:1564.

18. Fernandez JF, Benito MAC, Lizaldez EB, Montanes MA. Oral hairy leukoplakia: A histopathologic study of 32 cases. Am J Dermatopathol 1990;12:571.

19. Field EA, Tyldesley WR. Oral Crohn's disease revisited—a 10 year review. Br J Oral Maxillofac Surg 1989;27:114.

20. Paissaf DK. Oral submucous fibrosis. Int J Oral Surg 1981;10:307.

21. Holland D, Tan PLJ. Sjogren's Syndrome. Clinical spectrum, diagnosis and management. Curr Ther 1989;30:87.

22. Chisholm DM, Mason DK. Labial salivary gland biopsy in Sjogren's disease. J Clin Pathol 1968;21:656.

23. Savage NW, Seymour GJ, Robinson MF. Cyclosporin A induced gingival enlargement. J Periodontol 1987;58:475.

24. Seymour GJ, Gemmell E, Walsh LJ, Powell RN. The immunohistology of experimental gingivitis in humans. Clin Exp Immunol 1988;71:132.

25. Walsh LJ, Armitt KL, Seymour GJ, Powell RN. The immunohistology of chronic gingivitis in humans. Pediatr Dent 1987;9:26.

26. Seymour GJ, Powell RN, Davies IR. The immunopathogenesis of progressive chronic inflammatory periodontal disease. J Oral Pathol 1979;8:249.

27. Johnson BD, Engel D. Acute necrotizing ulcerative gingivitis. A review of diagnosis, etiology and treatment. J Periodontol 1986;57:141.

28. McMillan MD, Kardos TB, Edwards JL, et al. Giant cell hyalin angiopathy or pulse granuloma. Oral Surg Oral Med Oral Pathol 1981;52:178.

29. McCarthy PL, Shklar G. Diseases of the oral mucosa. 2nd ed. Philadelphia: Lea & Febiger, 1980.

24
Dermatopathology of the Ocular Adnexa

Kenneth L. Piest, William C. Lloyd, III, and Allan E. Wulc

INTRODUCTION

The ocular adnexal region is anatomically complex because it contains skin, muscle, fat, connective tissue, and glandular tissues. Nearly any type of tumor may develop in this area. The primary purpose of the eyelids is to provide protection for the eye; thus, the eyelids have both dynamic and functional roles. In the treatment of lesions in this area, any alteration of the anatomic structure must not disturb the functional and protective role of the eyelids, or significant ocular complications may occur. The anatomy of the eyelids and lacrimal system are reviewed in this chapter, and this review serves as a base for appreciating the origins of the diverse array of pathologic lesions that arise in the eyelids. Although many of the lesions described in this chapter are similar dermatopathologically to lesions elsewhere in the body, they are included because their appearance in the eyelids is occasionally distinct. Rare lesions that are unique to the eyelids are also described in this chapter, but these are not seen as often in practice.

This chapter focuses on the dermatopathology of lesions of the external eyelid and adnexae. Diseases that arise from the conjunctiva (i.e., mucous membrane), lacrimal system, or orbit and ocular surface disorders are beyond the scope of this chapter.

ANATOMY

The eyelids consist of six basic structural layers: (1) skin and subcutaneous tissue; (2) orbicularis muscle; (3) orbital septum; (4) muscles of retraction; (5) tarsus; and (6) conjunctiva. Part of the complexity of understanding the adnexal region is due to the fact that the underlying anatomy

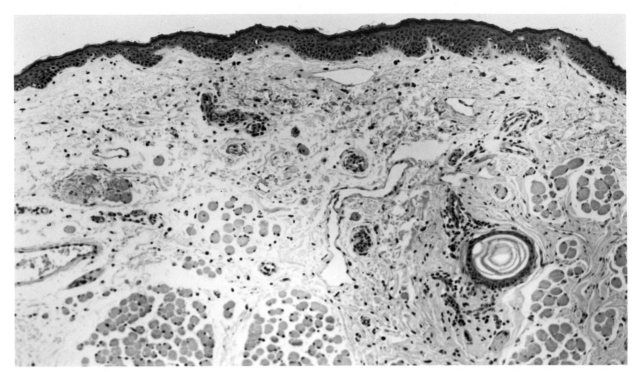

Figure 24–1. Normal adult eyelid skin. The epidermis is thin, and the dermis contains blood vessels, lymphatics, and nerves. Glandular structures are present in the subcutaneous layer.

changes with the distance from the eyelid margin. This knowledge is critical to anyone operating or involved in diagnostic pathology in the eyelid region. Understanding the structures involved in the surgical site, and therefore the tissues that require reconstruction, is fundamental to accurate diagnosis and treatment.

The skin of the eyelid is the thinnest in the body (<1 mm; Fig. 24–1). The eyelid epidermis is only six to seven cell layers thick. The dermis of the eyelid contains blood vessels, lymphatics, nerves, and elastic fibers. The thin subcutaneous layer of the eyelid contains the bulbs of hair follicles and pilosebaceous glands but essentially no fat. The nasal portion of the eyelid contains the highest number of sebaceous glands. They are also associated with the follicles of the eyelashes. Eccrine glands are diffusely located throughout the lid. Apocrine glands are concentrated near the lid margin.

The upper eyelid crease is found at the upper border of the tarsus (Fig. 24–2). It is formed by projections of the levator aponeurosis to the skin, allowing the skin to firmly adhere to the tarsal surface. The skin above the tarsus is mobile, which allows it to overhang the crease and form the lid fold. The lower lid crease is less defined, but it marks the inferior border of the tarsus.

Contraction of the orbicularis muscle closes the eye. This muscle is divided into three relatively distinct areas: the pretarsal orbicularis, the preseptal orbicularis, and the orbital orbicularis. These divisions have both anatomic and physiologic significance, because different portions of the muscle are involved in forced eyelid closure, involuntary closure (i.e., blink), and the lacrimal pump mechanism.

Directly beneath the orbicularis muscle is the tarsus (Fig. 24–3A), which consists of dense connective tissue that

gives the eyelid structural integrity. The tarsus is about 1 mm thick. The vertical height of the tarsus is about 10 mm and 3 to 4 mm in the upper and lower lids, respectively. Contained within the tarsus are the vertically oriented meibomian glands, which are sebaceous glands. The orifices of the glands are located at the lid margin (Fig. 24–3B).

Beyond 10 mm from the upper lid margin, or 4 mm from the lower lid margin, the structure directly beneath the

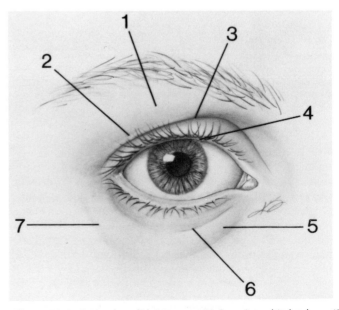

Figure 24–2. External eyelid anatomy. (1) Superior orbital sulcus. (2) Upper lid fold. (3) Upper lid crease. (4) Highest point of lid curve. (5) Nasojugal fold. (6) Lower lid crease. (7) Malar fold.

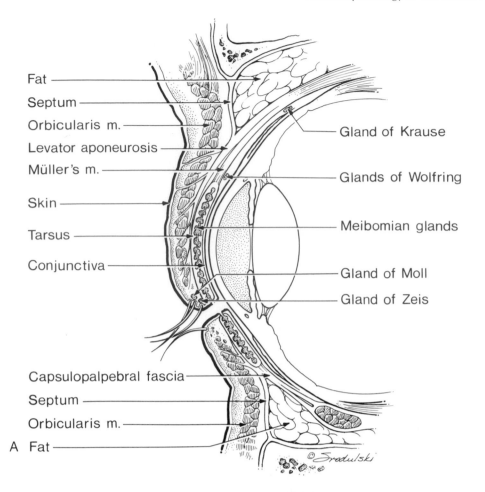

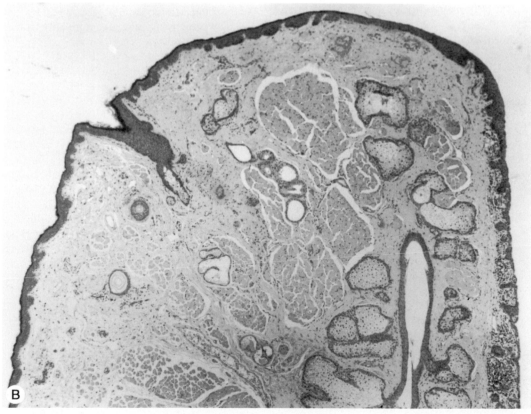

Figure 24–3. (A) Cross-sectional anatomy of the normal eyelid. **(B)** Cross section of the normal eyelid.

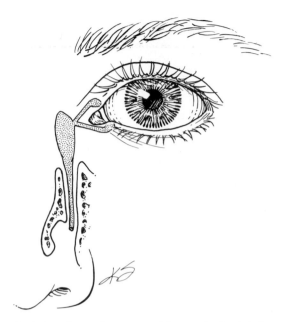

Figure 24–4. Location and anatomy of the nasolacrimal drainage system.

orbicularis is not the tarsus but the orbital septum. The orbital septum is a thin sheet of fibrous tissue that originates from the orbital rim and fuses with the retractors of the lid. This septum serves as a barrier between the orbit and the eyelid. Directly beneath the orbital septum lies anterior orbital fat.

In the upper eyelid, the retractors consist of the levator muscle, which distally turns into the levator aponeurosis, and the superior tarsal muscle, or Mueller muscle, on the posterior surface of the levator aponeurosis. The orbital septum fuses with the aponeurosis, which then inserts onto the anterior surface of the tarsus. In the lower lid, the capsulopalpebral fascia is the anatomic analog of the levator.

The conjunctiva forms the posterior layer of the eyelid and covers part of the external surface of the globe. It is composed of nonkeratinizing squamous epithelium and contains mucin-secreting goblet cells. Located in the superior and inferior fornix of the eyelids are the accessory lacrimal glands of Krause and Wolfring. The secretions from these glands form the major portion of basal tear secretion.

Medially and laterally, the eyelids are attached to the bony rims by the canthal tendons. Disinsertion of these tendons will cause significant functional problems. The lacrimal drainage system is found in the medial canthus. In general, disruption of the drainage system or the medial one third of the eyelid produces chronic troublesome tearing (Fig. 24–4).

EPITHELIAL TUMORS

Benign Lesions

Squamous Papilloma

Squamous papilloma is a broad classification that contains benign lesions caused by a hyperplasia of the epidermis,

which are the most common benign lesions of the eyelids. These neoplasms exhibit a variable clinical appearance; they can be sessile or pedunculated and are often multiple (Fig. 24–5A).

Histologically, squamous papillomas exhibit acanthosis, hyperkeratosis, and parakeratosis of the epithelium, which overlies a fibrovascular core (Fig. 24–5B, C).

Pseudoepitheliomatous Hyperplasia and Keratoacanthoma[1]

Pseudoepitheliomatous hyperplasia (PEH) and keratoacanthoma represent an epithelial hyperplasia that is often confused with a neoplastic process. These lesions can arise anywhere in the adnexal area, are typically of short duration (i.e., weeks to months), and may show surface ulceration or crusting resembling that of a true carcinoma. However, the clinical course of these lesions is self-limited. An underlying chronic dermal inflammatory reaction can incite an overlying hyperplastic epithelial proliferation. Two specific forms of PEH are the keratoacanthoma and the inverted follicular keratosis (Fig. 24–6A, B).

Keratoacanthoma is a specific variant of PEH. It occurs in sun-exposed areas of the body. Clinically, keratoacanthoma appears as a dome-shaped lesion with a keratin-filled central crater (Fig. 24–7). The lesion develops rapidly, usually over a period of several weeks. Keratoacanthoma is benign, and the natural course is rapid growth followed by spontaneous resolution over a period of weeks to months. Aggressive forms do occur and may require excision.

Histopathologically, the epidermis is thickened by a hyperplastic proliferation of squamous epithelium. A central mass of keratin is usually present, and a chronic inflammatory response often surrounds the base of the lesion (see Fig. 24–7).

Seborrheic Keratosis

Seborrheic keratoses (SKs) are extremely common benign lesions of the eyelids and facial area. These lesions usually first appear in the middle and late decades of life and tend to increase in size and number with increasing age. SKs have a wide range of clinical appearances, varying in size, shape, and pigmentation; however, most of these lesions tend to be sharply demarcated, slightly to moderately pigmented, and have a raised, friable surface. SKs often have a waxy-appearing keratin surface, giving them a greasy, stuck-on appearance (Fig. 24–8A). Dermatosis papulosa nigra (DPM) is a variant of SK seen in people of African descent. DPM can occur at a younger age than SK and appears as darkly pigmented papillar lesions. Neither SK nor DPM have malignant potential.

The histopathologic appearance of SK is variable and may show different degrees of hyperkeratosis, acanthosis, and adenoid changes. The acanthotic pattern often forms keratin-filled inclusion cysts in the epidermis called cutaneous horns. Varying amounts of pigment cells are also present (Fig. 24–8B, C). Growth is generally confined to the epithelial layer and rarely involves the dermis unless the lesion is inflamed. In this situation, an inflammatory reaction may be present in the dermal tissues.

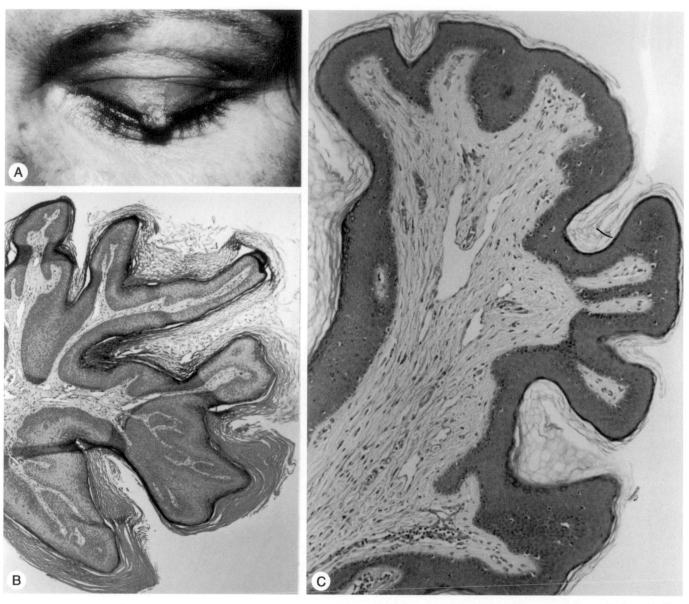

Figure 24–5. (A) Squamous papilloma of left upper eyelid. (B, C) A pedunculated skin growth exhibits hyperkeratotic and acanthotic epithelium, which surrounds a fibrovasular core.

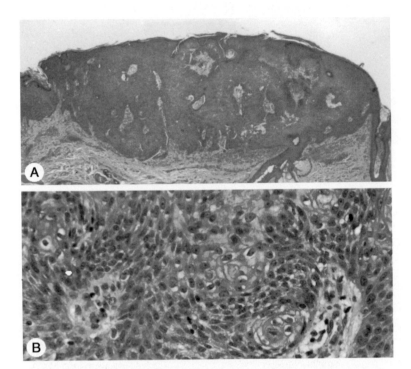

Figure 24–6. Inverted follicular keratosis. **(A, B)** Marked hyperkeratosis, parakeratosis, and basilar acanthosis are present. Note the flattened base of the lesion, which resembles a seborrheic keratosis. These lesions are sometimes referred to as irritated seborrheic keratosis.

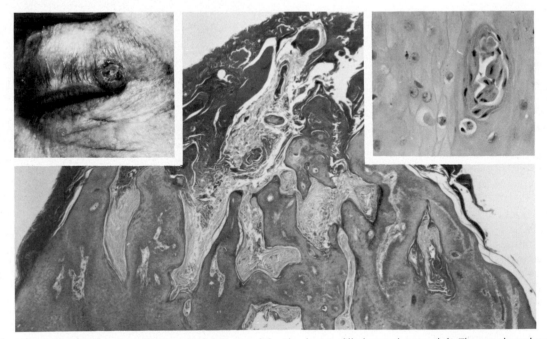

Figure 24–7. Keratoacanthoma. Dome-shaped lesion of the left upper lid with a keratin-filled central crater *(left)*. The cup-shaped mass is filled with keratin and lined by a hyperplastic proliferation of squamous epithelium. Higher magnification shows many atypical dyskertotic cells *(right)*.

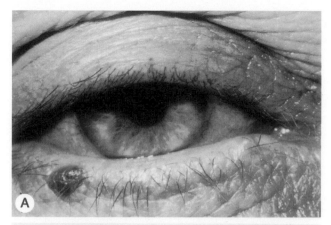

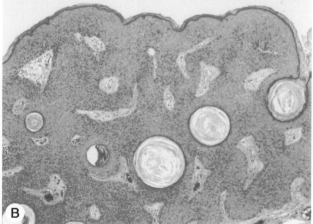

Figure 24–8. (A) Seborrheic keratosis. **(B)** This lesion is a variant of squamous papilloma that exhibits an additional finding—intraepithelial horn cysts. These lesions show varying degrees of pigmentation.

Premalignant and Malignant Lesions

Actinic Keratosis[2, 3]

Actinic keratosis is a precancerous lesion that occurs as a result of radiation damage to epidermal cells. The most common sites are sun-exposed areas of the body: usually the head, neck, and dorsa of the arms and hands. Fair-skinned, middle-aged or older individuals with a history of prolonged sun exposure without adequate protection are at high risk for developing actinic keratosis.

Clinically, these lesions are multiple in number, and they have a flat, scaly, erythematous appearance (Fig. 24–9A). Actinic keratoses are precursors of squamous cell carcinomas. It is estimated that 12 to 25% of affected patients eventually develop a malignancy. The prognosis for squamous cell carcinoma arising from an actinic keratotic lesion is good, because the metastatic rate is extremely low (1%).

Histopathologic changes of actinic keratoses are seen in both the epidermis and the dermis. Hyperkeratosis, parakeratosis, and dyskeratosis are evident in the epithelium. A chronic inflammatory response is usually present at the base of the lesion and involves the superficial dermis (Fig. 24–9B).

Intraepithelial Squamous Cell Carcinoma[2, 4–6]

Intraepithelial squamous cell carcinoma, also known as carcinoma in situ (CIN) or Bowen disease, is the earliest form of squamous cell carcinoma. It may arise from a precancerous lesion (e.g., actinic keratosis) or be de novo. These lesions appear as erythematous areas with scaly, fissured surfaces. They can occur in both sun-exposed and non–sun-exposed skin. CIN is associated with an increased incidence of other neoplasms; skin tumors may occur in up to 50% of cases and internal malignancies in up to 80% of cases. There is an association between Bowen disease and arsenic ingestion.

Histologically, the epidermis loses its cellular polarity, and evidence of hyperkeratosis and parakeratosis is evident. Abnormal mitotic figures are present. These changes occur throughout the epidermis and are confined to the epidermal layer by an intact basement membrane. If the basement membrane is violated, and the underlying dermis is involved, the lesion behaves as invasive squamous cell carcinoma.

Treatment is by local excision. As would be expected, excision does not prevent the occurrence of secondary malignancies.

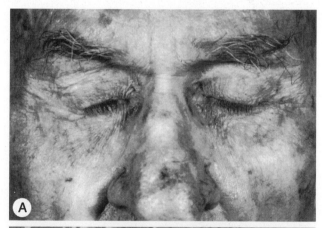

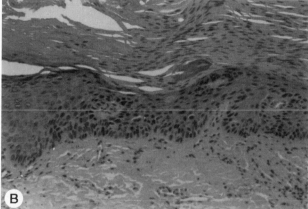

Figure 24–9. Actinic keratosis. **(A)** Multiple erythematous, flat, scaly, lesions cover the entire midface region. **(B)** This potentially precancerous skin lesion is characterized by hyperkeratosis, parakeratosis, dyskeratosis, and focally intense inflammation at the base of the lesion. The epithelial basement membrane is intact.

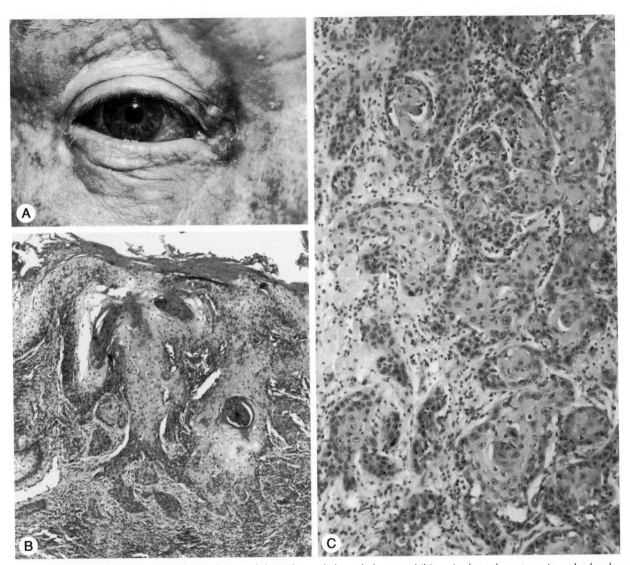

Figure 24–10. Squamous cell carcinoma. **(A)** This lesion of the right medial canthal area exhibits raised, erythematous, irregular borders with a central area of ulceration. Surface crusting is apparent over the inferior one half of the lesion. **(B, C)** The lesion is a centrally ulcerated mass with anaplastic squamous cells with abundant eosinophilic (i.e., keratin-filled) cytoplasm, dyskeratotic pearls, and circular aggregates of tumor cells.

Squamous Cell Carcinoma[7-12]

Squamous cell carcinoma (SCC) is a malignant tumor of the cells of the epidermis. Fewer than 5% of epithelial neoplasms of the eyelids are squamous cell carcinomas. SCC most commonly involves the lower eyelid but may occur in any location. When tumors involve the upper lid and lateral canthus, SCCs are more common than basal cell carcinomas in those locations. The same factors that promote the development of skin damage (e.g., actinic damage, fair complexion) predispose individuals to the development of SCC. Genetic conditions such as xerodermapigmentosa and albinism are well-known conditions associated with an increased risk of developing SCC. Immune suppression may also increase the risk of developing SCC, and the lesions primarily occur in sun-exposed areas. Previous radiation treatment is also another risk factor.

SCC usually arises in actinically damaged skin. These lesions usually present as elevated, indurated plaques or nod-

ules with irregular borders. As the tumor enlarges, ulceration, often covered by keratinaceous debris, may occur (Fig. 24–10A).

Histologically, there is loss of polarity of the epidermis, and the normal epidermis is replaced by haphazardly arranged dysplastic cells. Characteristic dyskeratotic cells with the formation of keratin pearls are common. The nuclei are prominent, and mitotic figures are seen. Invasion through the basement membrane and into the dermis occurs (Fig. 24–10B, C).

Treatment is by complete surgical excision. Use of frozen section or Mohs technique is recommended.

In eyelid lesions detected early, metastasis is rare (<1%). This is in contrast to SCC located in other anatomic sites, which may metastasize early in the course of disease. Advanced or neglected eyelid lesions do have the potential to spread both by local invasion and by metastasis. Dissemination to regional lymph nodes is more common than spread to distant organs. Also, direct perineural invasion into the central nervous system can occur. If local extension or orbital involvement is suspected, imaging studies should be obtained.

Although invasive SCC has metastatic potential, early eyelid lesions treated appropriately have an excellent prognosis. After treating a patient for SCC, regular follow-up examinations are imperative. All patients at risk of developing skin carcinomas should avoid excessive sun exposure and use sunscreens with a sun protective factor (SPF) greater than 15. Because sunscreens often contain ocular irritants, we suggest that patients at risk wear ultraviolet (UV) protective sunglasses.

Basal Cell Carcinoma[13-35]

Basal cell carcinoma (BCC) arises from the basal cells of the epidermis and generally occurs in areas of sun-exposed skin. In the ocular adnexal region, BCC is most common in the lower eyelid and medial canthal area. BCC is characterized by slow local growth, but the lesion is capable of extensive local invasion. Metastasis may also occur.

The most common clinical appearance of BCC of the eyelids is as a translucent nodule with superimposed telangiectatic vessels. Stromal tissue and a good blood supply are essential to the tumor's continued growth. As the tumor enlarges, central tumor necrosis may occur as growth surpasses the nutrient supply, producing a central ulcer in the nodule (Fig. 24–11A). When the lesion is on the eyelid margin, madarosis, or loss of normal lashes, may occur and is a strong indicator of cutaneous malignancy. Other clinical variations of BCC are possible. For example, the lesion may not have an elevated margin. The aggressive morpheaform variant may present as an indurated sclerotic plaque with ill-defined borders. Melanin may be present, producing varying degrees of tumor pigmentation.

Numerous subtypes of BCC have been described; those of the ocular area conform to those of basal cells elsewhere. Four basic types of BCC exist: nodular, ulcerative, morpheaform or sclerosing, and multicentric. The nodular form is the classic basal cell carcinoma. Growth of the tumor produces a localized mass. Tumor production of an angiogenic factor generates the characteristic superficial telangiectatic vessels. A pseudocapsule is formed as the tumor grows and compresses adjacent dermal tissues.

Histologically, the tumor nodule is composed of a uniform population of basaloid cells with peripheral cells that demonstrate a palisading pattern (Fig. 24–11B, C). Small-to-large cysts may form within the tumor nodule, which may make the diagnosis more difficult. If surface ulceration occurs, the pseudocapsule usually is not present; Instead, a chronic dermal inflammatory reaction is seen.

In the morpheaform or sclerosing type of BCC, elongated strands of basaloid cells are surrounded by a dense fibrous stroma. This appearance resembles scirrhous carcinoma of the breast. Morpheaform BCC is aggressive and deeply infiltrates adjacent tissue, making margins difficult to predict clinically and rendering complete excision difficult (Fig. 24–12A, B).

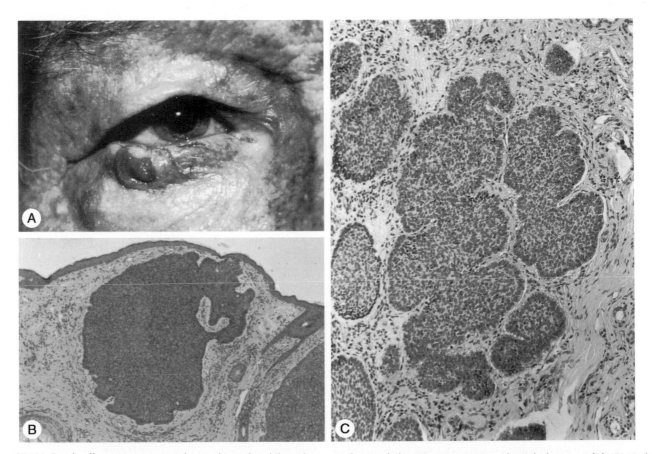

Figure 24–11. Basal cell carcinoma. **(A)** A large, elevated nodule with a central area of ulceration is present on the right lower eyelid. **(B)** Nodular basal cell carcinoma. **(C)** Nodular basal cell carcinoma demonstrating basaloid tumor cells and peripheral palisading.

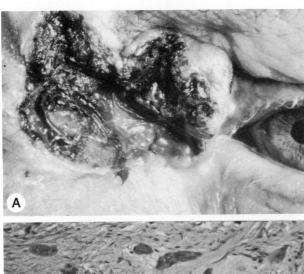

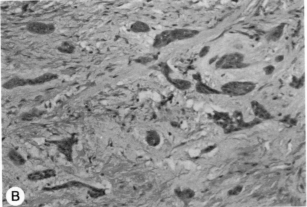

Figure 24–12. (A) Morpheaform basal cell carcinoma. **(B)** Strands and tendrils of tumor cells infiltrate the surrounding tissue. A discrete mass is not present.

The multicentric subtype of BCC has a more irregular surface than nodular BCC. As the name implies, diffuse multicentric involvement of the epidermis and superficial dermis by foci of basal cells and contiguous normal zones is seen.

The goal in management of BCC is the complete elimination of the tumor. With the nodular form, surgical excision of a small lesion with histologic confirmation is appropriate. The ulcerative, morpheaform, and multicentric types often extend beyond the area of apparent clinical involvement. In these cases, tumor excision with frozen section examination of all margins, including the tumor base, and Mohs micrographic surgery are the best available methods for complete tumor excision.

Even with the best techniques, evaluation of the margins may be quite difficult, especially with the morpheaform type or in a recurrence within scar tissue. Cryotherapy may be appropriate in situations in which multiple tumors are present or excision is not possible. With cryotherapy, a double freeze-thaw method with tissue temperatures to − 50°C is needed to destroy the tumor cells. Unfortunately, the surgeon is not assured of delivering the appropriate temperature to the malignant tissue; as a consequence, continued growth may occur, and uninvolved tissues may also be injured.

Metastasis from BCC is infrequent; incident estimates range from 0.028 to 1%. When metastases do occur, lymphatic spread to the regional lymph nodes and hematogenous spread to bone, lungs, and liver are the most common path-ways and sites. Despite its low metastatic rate, BCC is locally invasive. Orbital involvement with subsequent intracranial extension is the most common cause of death due to tumor spread. These tumors usually originate in the inner canthus; therefore, all lesions in this location are most appropriately managed by complete excision.

Disseminated disease from BCC is rare, but if suspected, a systemic workup is required. This workup includes a detailed history, physical examination with particular attention to the regional lymph nodes and sensory nerves in the individual area, and testing consisting of a complete blood count, liver profile, chest X-ray, bone scan, liver scan, and magnetic resonance imaging and computed tomography for periocular invasion if orbital or intracranial extension is suspected.

In cases in which orbital extension has occurred, exenteration is the recommended treatment. If the disease involves the regional lymph nodes, surgery and radiation therapy should be considered. Distant spread is associated with a poor prognosis, but chemotherapeutic treatments are available in these situations.

After treating a patient for BCC, regular follow-up examinations are imperative. Most recurrences develop within 5 years, but late recurrences are possible. New BCC lesions may also arise; 20 to 30% of these appear within 1 year of the original lesion. Patients with BCC may also be at risk for developing other malignancies. As recommended for SCC, all patients at risk of developing skin carcinomas should avoid excessive sun exposure, use sunscreens with a high SPF, and wear glasses with lenses that screen out UV rays.

MELANOCYTIC TUMORS

Ocular melanocytes are derived embryologically from neural crest cells. They are present in the eyelids, conjunctiva, and uveal tissues and pigment epithelium of the eye. In all of these locations, both benign lesions and malignant lesions can arise.

Nevi

Nevi are benign melanocytic lesions. Several types of nevi exist, and these vary in their clinical appearance (Fig. 24–13A). Nevi may be flat or elevated, and they may or may not be pigmented early in life. Hormonal factors during pregnancy or puberty may produce darkening or enlargement of nevi.

Junctional Nevi

Clinically, junctional nevi are usually flat, well circumscribed, and a uniform, pigmented, brownish color. The malignant potential of junctional nevi is extremely low. These are the most common and the most benign of the nevi.

Histologically, junctional nevi cells arise from the deeper layers of the conjunctival epidermis. The nests of nevoid melanocytes are confined to the deep epidermis and do not involve the underlying dermis.

Junctional nevi do have the potential of malignant trans-

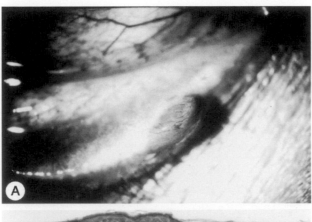

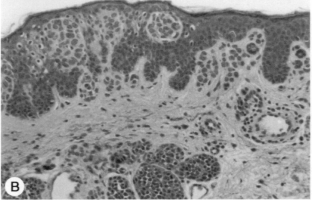

Figure 24–13. (A) A nevus of right lower lid margin is present. (B) Compound nevus. Nevus cells are present both within and beneath the epithelium. More mature nevus cells deep in the dermis lose cytoplasm, pigment, and nesting pattern and resemble lymphocytes.

formation; however, this potential is low. Malignant cells show more extensive cellular anaplasia, invasion into the dermis, and often, an associated dermal inflammatory reaction.

Intradermal Nevi

The surface of an intradermal nevus is usually elevated and often papillomatous. Hairs may be present on the surface, and pigmentation varies from almost amelanotic to deeply pigmented.

Histologically, intradermal nevus cells are located entirely within the dermis. Some cells may be seen extending into the deeper dermis; this does not imply a malignant transformation. Inflammatory cells are usually not present.

Compound Nevi

As the name implies, compound lesions have a combination of the features of junctional and intradermal nevi. Clinically, compound nevi are usually brownish in color.

Histologically, compound nevus cells in and near the epidermis are larger than the cells located in the dermis. The cells in the dermis show normal polarity by becoming smaller, darker, and more spindle shaped as they descend deeper into the dermis (Fig. 24–13*B*). The compound nevus does have low-grade malignant potential.

Miscellaneous Melanocytic Lesions

Other pigmented lesions that also occur in the ocular adnexal area include blue nevi, nevus of Ota or oculodermal melanocytosis, freckles or ephelicles, lentigo simplex, and lentigo senilis.

Malignant Melanoma[36]

Malignant melanomas account for approximately 1% of all primary eyelid malignancies. The clinical features, prognosis, and histology of malignant melanomas of the eyelid parallel those of the cutaneous melanomas elsewhere on the body. These lesions can arise from preexisting nevi, or they may occur spontaneously (Fig. 24–14*A, B*). The typical signs of malignant transformation should be familiar to all clinicians. These signs include changes in color, size, and surface consistency (e.g., friability, bleeding, ulceration). The different types of cutaneous melanomas that occur in the adnexal area also parallel those found elsewhere. These types include lentigo maligna melanoma, superficial spreading melanoma, nodular melanoma, and acral lentiginous melanoma.

Lentigo Maligna Melanoma[37–40]

Lentigo maligna melanoma occurs mainly in the elderly. The sun-exposed areas (i.e., facial, malar, and temporal regions) are the most commonly affected. Involvement of the adnexal area is relatively common. The chance of malignant transformation from the precursor lesion, lentigo maligna, is estimated to be about 25%, and the premalignant phase is quite long (10–20 years).

Superficial Spreading Melanoma

The superficial spreading melanomas arise from preexisting nevi approximately 50% of the time. These lesions occur in younger individuals than does lentigo maligna melanoma. The malignant cells are located throughout the epidermis, and there is dermal invasion.

Nodular Melanoma[41–49]

Nodular melanoma, as the name implies, is a more discrete lesion than the other types of malignant melanoma. These lesions develop in even younger populations (fourth to fifth decades of life) than the superficial spreading melanomas and are more common in men than in women. Nodular melanomas arise in both sun-exposed and non–sun-exposed areas, and they not only develop in cutaneous tissues but also occur in mucous membranes. Growth of these lesions is often quite rapid.

There is considerable histologic variation depending on the tumor type. In general, there is a loss of the normal cellular polarity. Invasion of the dermis occurs either concurrently or after epithelial invasion. The tumor cells demonstrate an increase in their nuclear-cytoplasmic ratio. Pigmentation can vary in different areas of the lesion. Often, there is an associated surrounding inflammatory reaction (Fig. 24–14*C*).

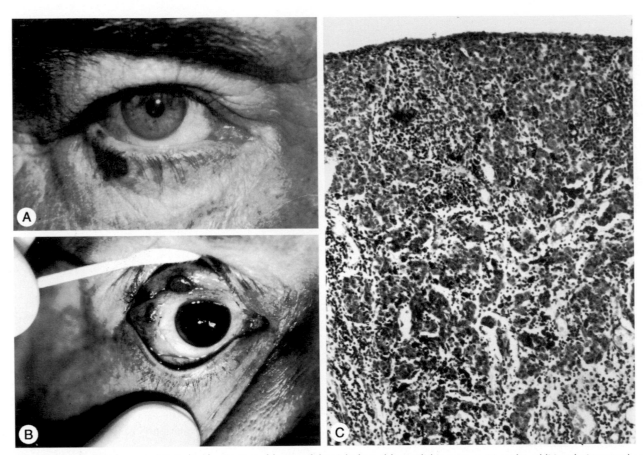

Figure 24–14. Malignant melanoma. **(A)** A deeply pigmented lesion of the right lateral lower lid is present. Note the additional pigmented area on the lid margin. (Courtesy of Charles R. Leone, M.D.) **(B)** This tumor invades the right upper lid margin and conjunctival surface. **(C)** Microscopic examination reveals a richly pigmented tumor composed of invasive, atypical melanocytes that arose from a preexisting junctional nevus that had been followed for many years.

The prognostic factors associated with ocular adnexal melanomas is similar to those of cutaneous melanomas elsewhere. Level of invasion according to the Clark classification, thickness of the tumor according to the Breslow method, and histologic type of the lesion influence the overall prognosis. The newer staging system adopted by the American Joint Committee on Cancer is based on tumor microstaging of the primary lesion and the known pattern of metastasis. In general, nodular melanoma has the worst prognosis, and lentigo maligna melanoma has the best prognosis.

GLANDULAR DISORDERS

Inflammations

Blepharitis

Blepharitis is a diffuse inflammatory reaction of the eyelid margin. Among the numerous causes are bacterial, viral, or fungal infections; allergies; and acne rosacea. Blepharitis may be acute, subacute, or chronic. Inflamed eyelids with a scaly debris along the base of the eyelashes and a foamy tear film that breaks up rapidly are common nonspecific findings. Exact treatment depends on the etiology, but good eyelid hygiene is necessary to treat all forms of blepharitis.

Hordeolum

Hordeolum is a purulent inflammation of an eyelid gland. These lesions are divided into two anatomic types: internal and external. An external hordeolum, or stye, is an infection of a hair follicle and the surrounding sweat and sebaceous glands. It often coexists with staphylococcal blepharitis. The eyelid develops a painful inflammation that localizes. After localization, it usually breaks through the skin and drains (Fig. 24–15A). Occasionally, if the infection does not localize, and spread continues to adjacent glands, cellulitis may develop. An internal hordeolum is the result of an infection of the meibomian glands of the tarsal plate. These too will usually localize, rupture, and drain on the inner conjunctival surface of the lid. In either case, warm compresses hasten resolution. Observation for cellulitis is warranted, but uncomplicated resolution is the rule.

Chalazion

Chalazion is a discrete, chronic, granulomatous inflammation of the sebaceous glands of the lids. This lesion presents as a firm, painless nodule located in the eyelid (Fig.

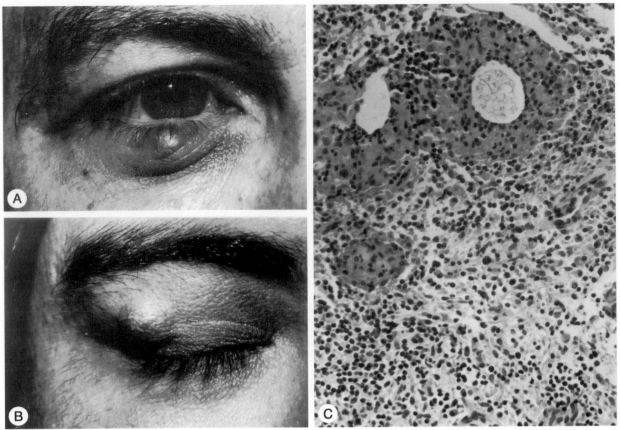

Figure 24–15. (A) External hordeolum. Note the erythema surrounding the lesion. It has already begun to localize and is beginning to point toward the skin surface. **(B)** In this chronic chalazion, no inflammation of the skin is present. **(C)** A chronic, noncaseating, granulomatous, inflammatory infiltrate surrounds lipid vacuoles in this chalazion.

24–15B). The more superficially located lesions probably involve the Zeis glands and the deeper nodules, the meibomian glands. If rupture through the tarsoconjunctival surface occurs, rapid growth of granulation tissue produces a pyogenic granuloma (see Fig. 24–21A). Pyogenic granulomas are painless, polypoid, and bleed easily because of the fragility of the tissue.

Histologically, the chalazion is a lipogranulomatous reaction centered around extravasated fatty globules from the eyelid glands. There is a noncaseating granulomatous reaction with epithelioid cells and multinucleated giant cells surrounded by a mixed cell inflammatory reaction (Fig. 24–15C). The fat globules are diagnostic for a chalazion and distinguish this disorder from other granulomatous conditions rarely seen in the eyelids (e.g., sarcoma, tuberculosis, fungal infection, leprosy, syphilis). Those physicians who are unfamiliar with the ocular pathology may confuse a chalazion with these other causes of granulomatous reactions.

Sebaceous Cell Carcinoma[50–59]

Sebaceous cell carcinoma of the eyelid accounts for 2 to 5% of epithelial eyelid malignancies. These lesions arise from the meibomian glands and Zeis glands of the eyelid or from sebaceous glands in the caruncle or brow. The upper eyelid contains approximately twice the number of meibomian glands as does the lower eyelid; this probably accounts for the fact that the upper lid is involved twice as often as the lower lid. Outside of the ocular area, the sebaceous cell carcinoma is an extremely rare tumor.

Sebaceous cell carcinomas are among the most malignant eyelid tumors, because they exhibit a broad spectrum of clinical presentations that lead to delay in diagnosis and definitive treatment. Sebaceous cell carcinoma frequently mimics inflammatory eyelid conditions. The term masquerade syndrome has been used to describe the situation in which sebaceous cell carcinoma masquerades as atypical or recurrent chalazion, unilateral blepharoconjunctivitis, or papillomas.

A sebaceous cell carcinoma most commonly presents as a firm nodule resembling a chalazion (Fig. 24–16A). However, a more diffuse thickening of the tarsus or a papillomatous growth pattern also may be observed (Fig. 24–16B). As the lesion involves the lid margin and the tumor invades the lash follicles, a loss of eye lashes occurs. Ulceration may also develop.

Sebaceous cell carcinoma tends to invade the overlying epithelium. It can form scattered nests of malignant cells (i.e., pagetoid invasion) or it may completely replace the epithelium (i.e., intraepithelial carcinoma) (Fig. 24–16C). The latter occurrence can give the clinical appearance of unilateral blepharoconjunctivitis. This clinical picture should immediately alert the clinician, because a true blepharoconjunctivitis is a bilateral condition. Another extremely important feature of sebaceous cell carcinoma is its tendency for

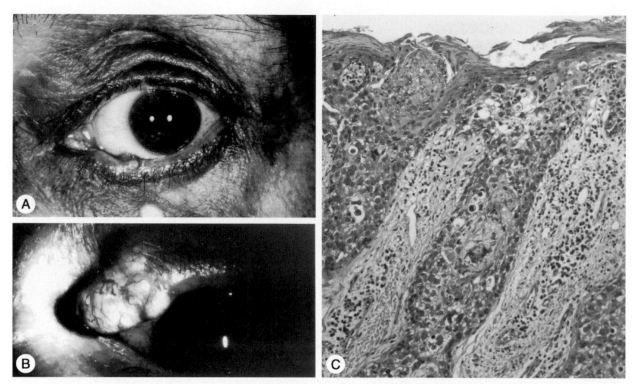

Figure 24–16. (A) Sebaceous cell carcinoma of the left lower eyelid, located at the medial one third of the lid margin, has a very nonspecific appearance. (Courtesy of Charles R. Leone, M.D.) **(B)** Sebaceous cell carcinoma of the lateral canthal area of the left lower lid is a large, yellowish lesion with a papillomatous-like growth pattern. Telangiectatic vessels are present on the surface, and there is a loss of eyelashes in the area of the tumor. **(C)** Histologic examination shows partial replacement of the eyelid epithelium by malignant cells.

multifocal sites of origin. Independent foci of tumor cells not only can involve multiple sites on the same eyelid but also can involve the upper and lower eyelid simultaneously. This occurs in 6 to 10% of cases, and it makes complete excision of the lesion extremely difficult.

Histologically, the tumor cells have abundant, vacuolated cytoplasm that gives the cell a foamy appearance. This vacuolated cellular appearance is the result of dissolved intracellular lipid. Varying degrees of mitotic activity and cellular differentiation can be seen (Fig. 24–17A, B). The malignant cells may invade the overlying epithelium, producing a change that resembles Paget disease and is referred to as pagetoid spread. Infiltrating cords rather than lobules of epithelial cells may be present, and occasionally these cords are arranged in single rows of malignant cells. Frozen sections stained for lipid are extremely useful in establishing the diagnosis. Even in cases with pagetoid invasion, intracytoplasmic lipid has been demonstrated.

The preferred treatment of sebaceous cell carcinomas of the eyelid is full-thickness excision with wide margins and with frozen section pathologic control. Despite these techniques, the recurrence rate after resection is approximately 30%. If the bulbar conjunctiva is involved, cryotherapy may be helpful to avoid loss of the globe. If the tumor has extended into the orbit, exenteration is recommended. In addition to local invasion, sebaceous cell carcinoma can spread through lymphatic or hematogenous routes. Regional lymph node metastases occur in up to 25% of patients. Vascular invasion can produce distant metastases with the primary distant metastatic sites (i.e., lung, liver, brain, skull). If distant metastases occur, they are almost always associated with a history of simultaneous involvement of regional lymph nodes. Thus, the patient should always be examined for palpable regional nodes.

The overall mortality rate from sebaceous cell carcinoma of the eyelid is estimated to be 20%. However, as a result of a higher index of suspicion and earlier diagnosis, the mortality rate is decreasing. Any suspicious lesion should be biopsied. Atypical chalazia should be treated appropriately, and the expressed debris or a biopsy specimen should be submitted for pathological evaluation. Unilateral blepharoconjunctivitis, especially if chronic, should be suspected and a scraping with cytological examination performed. If suspicious cells are found, an eyelid biopsy specimen should be performed to obtain the diagnosis.

Sweat Gland Tumors

Other lesions, both benign and malignant, can arise from the glands around the eye. Apocrine sweat glands are present in the eyelids and are known as the glands of Moll. The eccrine glands are located at the lid margin and in the dermis surrounding the eyelids. Most lesions that develop are not specific to the adnexal area and are similar morphologically and pathologically to lesions that occur elsewhere.

Syringoma

Syringomas are common benign lesions of eccrine origin that often occur in the adnexal region (Fig. 24–18). Most commonly found in young women, the lesions are generally multiple, waxy, 1- to 2-mm, yellowish nodules. Histologi-

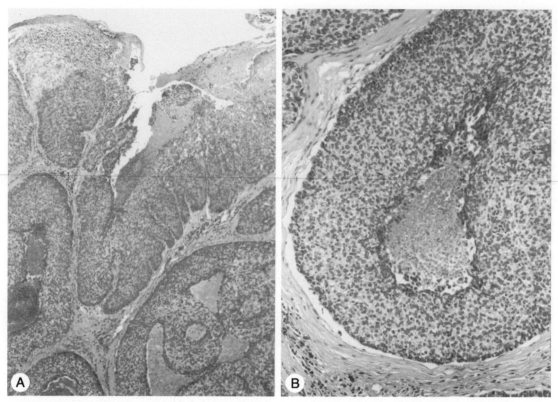

Figure 24–17. (A, B) Sebaceous cell carcinoma. Normal sebaceous elements are replaced by malignant epithelial cells. At first glance, the tumor lobules seem to have peripheral palisading. This appearance may falsely masquerade as a basal cell carcinoma.

cally, there is a proliferation of ductal elements within a fibrous stroma. The ducts commonly have a comma-shaped or tadpole configuration. The cystic ductules may contain a basophilic mucoid material or keratin, or they may undergo calcification.

Other Lesions

Other benign lesions that may occur in the eyelid region include pleomorphic adenoma and eccrine acrospiroma. Malignant tumors originating from the sweat glands are adenocarcinomas and may have mucinous or eccrine origins.

HAIR FOLLICLE TUMORS

There are four benign tumors that originate in the hair follicle: trichoepithelioma, trichofolliculoma, trichilemmoma, and pilomatrixoma. These lesions most commonly occur in the facial region, and all can involve the eyelid.

Trichoepithelioma[60, 61]

Trichoepitheliomas can arise as single or multiple lesions. The solitary lesion is a firm, flesh-colored nodule that tends to develop in the facial region but can occur elsewhere on the body. The solitary lesion usually arises late in life and has no inheritance pattern. The multiple nodular type has its onset in puberty, develops mainly in the facial region, and involves the eyelids. The multiple form is inherited in an autosomal dominant fashion and is sometimes referred to as a Brooke tumor. The lesions range from 2 to 8 mm in diameter and tend to slowly increase in size and number. Ulceration of the surface of the lesion is rare, but can cause these lesions to resemble BCC.

Histologically, lobules and strands of differentiated basaloid epithelial cells and horn cysts, composed of central keratin surrounded by basaloid cells are seen. The horn cysts are a characteristic finding in trichoepithelioma and represent immature hair structures. These differentiated basaloid epithelial cells can be difficult to distinguish from BCC, and horn cysts may be confused with the keratin pearls of SCC. However, the horn cyst shows complete and abrupt keratinization, whereas the keratin pearl shows a more gradual and incomplete keratinization.

Differentiation of the multiple trichoepithelioma from the basal cell nevus syndrome can be confusing. All data, both clinical and histologic, should be carefully evaluated to make the appropriate diagnosis. As previously mentioned, surface ulceration is rare in trichoepithelioma but is common in BCC. Trichoepitheliomas often involve the nasolabial folds in a symmetrical distribution and remain small. Malignant transformation of a trichoepithelioma is rare. In the basal cell nevus syndrome, lesions have a more random distribution, grow larger, may ulcerate, and invade adjacent tissue. Other systemic and ophthalmologic findings are associated with the basal cell nevus syndrome.

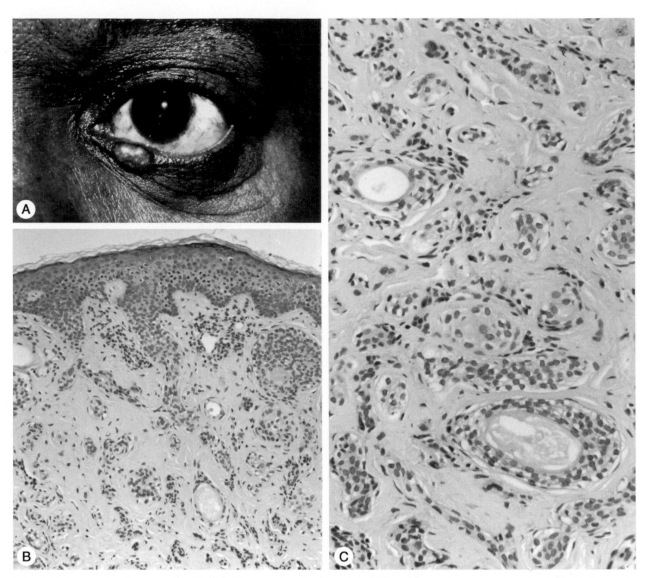

Figure 24–18. Syringoma. **(A)** A waxy, yellowish lesion is present on the lower lid of this middle-aged woman. **(B, C)** In this benign tumor of eccrine differentiation, there is a proliferation of cystic ductules and epithelial strands set within a fibrous stroma, showing a typical tadpole configuration.

Adnexal Carcinoma

Adnexal carcinoma is a nonspecific term used in ocular dermatopathology to describe a malignancy that resembles BCC and for which the origin (e.g., epidermis, hair follicle, sweat gland, sebaceous gland) cannot be determined.

NEUROGENIC TUMORS

Three neurogenic tumors are discussed in this section. The first two types, neurofibromas and neurilemmomas (schwannomas), are similar, because they are generally thought to be tumors of peripheral nerves. These are benign lesions, but they can be disfiguring in certain instances. Malignant transformation has been reported. The third type of neurogenic lesion, the neuroendocrine or Merkel cell tumor, is a malignant tumor of the skin mechanoreceptor responsible for the sensation of touch.

Neurofibroma

Neurofibromas may develop along any cranial nerve, peripheral nerve, or nerve root. They may occur as solitary or multiple lesions. Three different forms are recognized: plexiform, localized, and diffuse.

Plexiform neurofibromas usually occur in the eyelid and orbital regions and have the potential to cause massive deformity (Fig. 24–19A). This type of tumor is felt to be pathognomonic for neurofibromatosis. Histopathologically, a diffuse proliferation of Schwann cells, peripheral nerve axons, and endoneural fibroblasts is seen within a distinct perineural sheath (Fig. 24–19B).

Diffuse neurofibromas resemble plexiform neurofibromas, except they are less associated with neurofibromatosis. Diffuse neurofibromas lack a distinct perineural sheath on histologic examination. Both lesions are quite vascular.

The localized neurofibroma is a discrete mass that can occur anywhere in the body but often involves the face, ocular adnexal region, and orbit. This lesion is usually a distinct entity but can be associated with neurofibromatosis in approximately 12% of cases. Clinically, localized neurofibromas may be tender and painful. If excision is warranted, and the lesion is removed completely, they do not tend to reccur.

Neurilemmoma

Neurilemmoma, or schwannoma, occurs as single or multiple lesions along cranial or peripheral nerves. Grossly, they are firm, encapsulated, gray-white masses. Histologically, there are two patterns of neurilemmomas: Antoni A and Antoni B. The Antoni A type exhibits a fascicular cellular arrangement surrounded by a collagenous sheath (Fig. 24–19C). In contrast, the Antoni B pattern consists of a loose network of cells that lack a cellular pattern (Fig. 24–19D).

Merkel Cell Tumor[62–64]

Although rare, Merkel cell tumors, or neuroendocrine carcinomas, are commonly found on the face. The Merkel cells are located adjacent to the hair follicles and form the

mechanoreceptor complexes that mediate the sense of touch. Merkel cell tumors usually occur in the elderly. Clinically, these lesions appear as painless, cutaneous, reddish blue nodules. Telangiectatic vessels often cover the surface of the lesion (Fig. 24–20A).

Histologically, diffuse sheets of round or oval cells are seen. The nuclear-cytoplasmic ratio is high, as is the mitotic index (Fig. 24–20B). Immunohistochemical stains are helpful in confirming the diagnosis. Merkel cells contain metencephalon peptides and neuron-specific enolase. These staining properties may aid in identifying the tumor. Merkel cell tumors disseminate rapidly by deep local invasion, regional lymph node spread, and distant metastasis.

ANGIOMATOUS LESIONS
Pyogenic Granuloma

The pyogenic granuloma is a common lesion of the eyelid area. It usually develops after trauma or surgery (Fig. 24–21A). The name of this benign lesion is a long-standing, accepted term, yet it is an example of a classic misnomer. The lesion is neither pyogenic nor a granuloma. Clinically, the tumor appears as a rapidly growing, pedunculated, red-

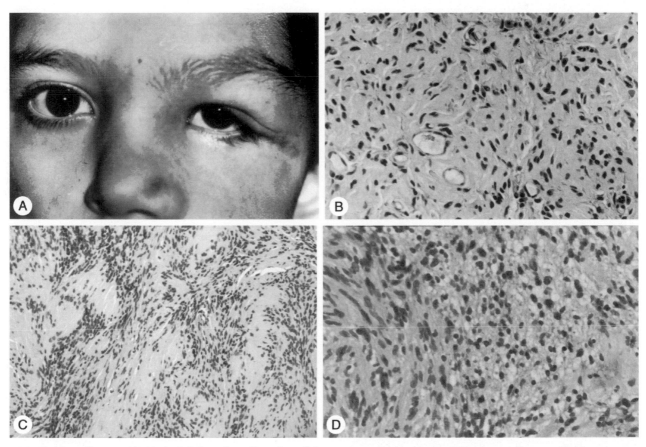

Figure 24–19. Neurofibroma. **(A)** Typical S-shaped configuration of the upper eyelid is characteristic of neurofibroma. **(B)** The tumor mass is composed of bland, spindle-shaped cells arranged in nerve bundles incorporating endoneurium and Schwann cells. Two different morphological patterns of neurilemmoma are found. **(C)** Antoni A pattern exhibits a fascicular arrangement surrounded by collagenous sheath. **(D)** Antoni B pattern is characterized by a loose network of cells with widened intercellular spaces.

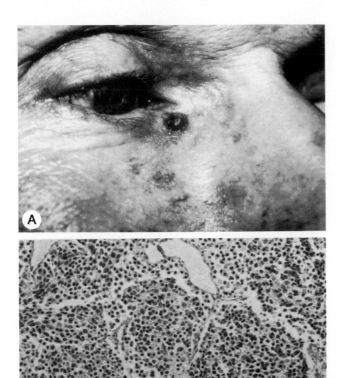

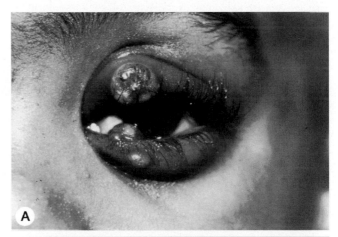

crease in fibrosis and replacement with adipose tissue occurs (Fig. 24–22*B*).

Cavernous Hemangioma

Cavernous hemangiomas are found much less frequently in the adnexal area than are capillary hemangiomas. Cavernous hemangiomas do not arise in infancy; they are most common in the second to fourth decades of life. These lesions show slow, progressive enlargement and have no tendency for spontaneous regression. Cavernous hemangiomas do not possess a prominent blood supply; therefore, the dilated vascular channels contain stagnant pools of blood which often thrombose and form phleboliths. The color of the lesion depends on the size and number of the vascular channels as well as the depth of the tumor. Superficial lesions exhibit a dark bluish color. Deeply situated lesions may only be detectable by their mass effect and produce no change in the overlying skin color.

Histologically, large, endothelial-lined, blood-filled vascular spaces separated by fibrous septae are seen. Malignant

Figure 24–20. Merkel cell tumor. **(A)** A small, reddish blue lesion is present in the right lower lid and medial canthal area. **(B)** Sheets of round and oval tumor cells featuring uniform nuclei and little cytoplasm are seen. Note the abundance of mitoses.

dish mass that bleeds easily. Histologically, pyogenic granuloma is composed of an exuberant proliferation of granulation tissue with prominent radiating vessels (Fig. 24–21*B*).

Capillary Hemangioma

Capillary hemangiomas are among the most common of the angiomatous lesions that occur in the eyelid and surrounding area. They usually appear in infancy as enlarging reddened masses commonly referred to as a strawberry birthmarks. Most of these lesions are superficial, but they can be deeply situated, resulting in a more violaceous hue. Capillary hemangiomas typically enlarge during the first year of life, diffusely infiltrating the adjacent tissue. Subsequently, most of these lesions begin to regress to varying degrees. The size of these lesions can range from a small localized area to extensive involvement of the midface and orbit. Capillary hemangiomas are raised lesions and they blanch with pressure and worsen with crying (Fig. 24–22*A*).

Histologically, capillary hemangiomas form lobules of capillaries separated by thin fibrous septae. The endothelial proliferation crowds out most of the capillaries' luminal spaces. Mitotic figures are not unusual, but these lesions are not malignant. As capillary hemangiomas regress, an in-

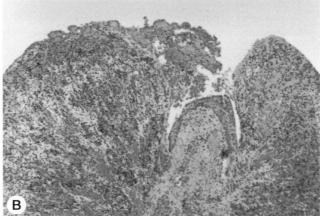

Figure 24–21. Pyogenic granuloma. **(A)** Multiple pyogenic granulomas of all four eyelids occurred following multiple recurrent chalazion. On the right lid, all of the lesions are on the inner aspect (not shown). The left lid has lesions on both the external and internal surfaces. **(B)** This benign, reactive mass is an exuberant proliferation of granulation tissue with a chronic inflammatory infiltrate. Capillaries, endothelium, fibroblasts, plasma cells, and lymphocytes are present.

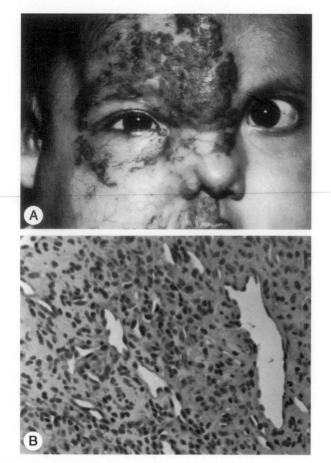

Figure 24–22. Capillary hemangioma. **(A)** Extensive involvement of the facial area is seen in this patient. **(B)** The lesion removed from the eyelid exhibits incomplete regression. The bulk of this hamartoma is a monotonous proliferation of capillaries, larger collecting vessels, and fibrosis.

transformation does not occur, but most lesions do require removal. Excision is usually curative.

Lymphangioma

Lymphangiomas are hamartomatous growths that have a predilection for the head and neck area. These lesions are usually apparent in infancy. Approximately 50 to 65% of lymphangiomas are noted at birth, and 90% are evident by 2 years of age. These tumors experience slowly progressive growth and have no tendency for regression. Lymphangiomas are unencapsulated tumors that have an infiltrative growth pattern. Lesions affecting the adnexal area often involve the eyelids, conjunctiva, and orbit. Spontaneous hemorrhages within the tumor are common and can present as a subconjunctival hemorrhage, diffuse hematoma of the eyelid, or severe ocular proptosis. The hemorrhages tend to form blood-filled cysts (i.e., chocolate cysts), which are usually resorbed. Total resection of these tumors is not possible, but debulking procedures can be performed for vision-threatening or severe deformities.

Histologically, lymphatic channels lined with a single layer of endothelial cells are present. Chronic nongranulom-

atous inflammation and lymphoid follicular germinal centers are interspersed between the lymphatic channels.

CYSTIC LESIONS

Hidrocystoma

Hidrocystomas originate in sweat glands and are of two types: apocrine and eccrine.

Apocrine Hidrocystoma

Apocrine hidrocystomas are common in the facial and eyelid area and appear as translucent, cystic nodules. In the adnexal area, they originate from a blocked excretory duct from the glands of Moll, which are concentrated along the eyelid margin. These lesions are fluid filled and are usually between 1 and 3 mm in size (Fig. 24–23A). Histologically, a clear, arborizing cyst lined with a bilayer of cuboidal epithelium is seen. The innermost cells secrete their products by apical decapitation (Fig. 24–23B).

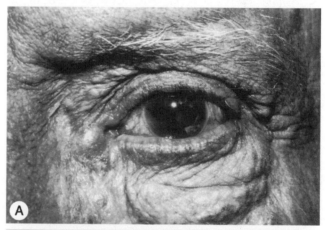

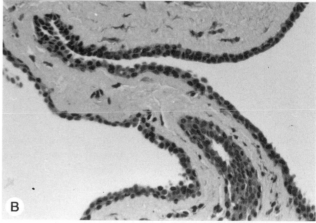

Figure 24–23. Apocrine hidrocystoma. **(A)** There is a translucent, cystic nodule adjacent to the lid margin in the left medial canthal area. **(B)** A clear, arborizing cyst is lined by a bilayer of low cuboidal epithelium. The inner cell layer elaborates its products by apical decapitation secretion.

Eccrine Hidrocystoma

Eccrine hidrocystomas also tend to occur on the face and commonly involve the eyelids. These lesions have a similar appearance to the apocrine cysts. Eccrine hidrocystomas are ductal retention cysts, and they secrete their products through an intact cell membrane. Histologically, a clear, cystic structure with a cuboidal epithelial bilayer but without apical decapitation is seen.

Epithelial Inclusion Cyst

Epithelial inclusion cysts, or epidermoid cysts, are extremely common lesions. They may be congenital, but they more commonly occur as a result of even minor trauma, including surgical trauma. Epithelial inclusion cysts are firm, mobile, painless, slowly enlarging lesions located in the subcutaneous tissue. Histologically, there is a cystic structure lined with keratinizing squamous epithelium. Keratinaceous debris fills the cyst lumen.

Dermoid Cyst

Dermoid cysts are thought to occur as a result of the sequestration of ectodermal tissue during embryonic development. These lesions are common in the adnexal area, especially in the superior temporal quadrant. Dermoid cysts are thought to be present at birth, but their size varies greatly, and these tumors may not be diagnosed until adulthood. Their growth is slow but is probably better characterized as intermittent with periods of dormancy. Dermoids may be located entirely in the subcutaneous tissue, may be attached to the periosteum of the orbital rim, or may have an intraorbital component (Fig. 24–24A). Rupture of the cyst provokes an intense foreign-body inflammatory response. Most lesions are usually removed (Fig. 24–24B).

Histologic examination demonstrates a cystic mass lined by stratified squamous epithelium. Adnexal structures are present in the cyst wall communicating with the cyst cavity. The cyst cavity is filled with the secreted debris (Fig. 24–24C).

MISCELLANEOUS LESIONS

Xanthelasma

Xanthelasma is the commonest form of cutaneous xanthoma. It occurs usually in middle-aged to elderly individuals and typically is located bilaterally in the medial canthal area. Xanthelasma presents as a slightly raised, soft, yellowish plaque of variable size (Fig. 24–25). Histologically, histocytes can be seen ingesting extravasated lipid (i.e., foamy histocytes). The plaques are located in the dermis. Most patients that develop these lesions have normal lipid levels, but these tumors do occur in patients with essential hyperlipidemia and disorders associated with increased lipid levels (e.g., diabetes).

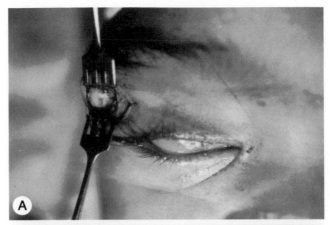

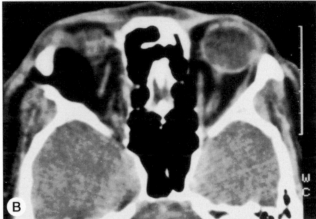

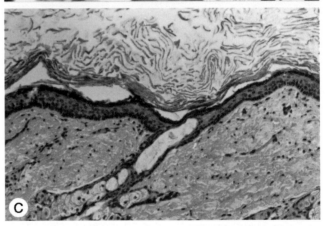

Figure 24–24. Dermoid cyst. **(A)** Gross appearance of the lesion at time of removal. Dermoid cysts are generally firm, encapsulated, ovoid, yellowish white lesions. **(B)** Computed tomographic scan demonstrates a dermoid cyst of the right orbit extending through the frontozygomatic suture area and giving off an external component, which renders it dumbbell shaped. There is an air density mass in the temporal aspect of the right orbit. **(C)** A choristomatous cystic lesion is lined by cutaneous epithelium that rests on dermal tissue containing skin appendages such as hair follicles, sebaceous glands, and sweat glands. These structures communicate with the cyst lumen and fill it with debris.

SUMMARY

Carcinomas of the eyelid are by far the most common malignant entities involving the ocular adnexal area, but vir-

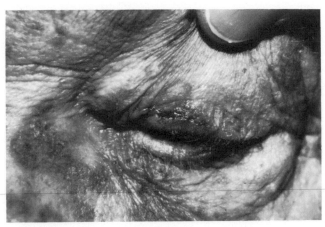

Figure 24–25. Xanthelasma. A yellowish, flat plaque is seen in the medial portion of the right upper eyelid. Lateral to the xanthelasma, near the lid margin, is an ulcerated basal cell carcinoma. In the surrounding tissue, there are multiple areas of erythematous, scaly, actinic keratotic lesions.

tually any other soft tissue or bony, benign or malignant neoplasm can occur in or around the eyelid. Treatment should be based primarily on early recognition and early diagnosis, by biopsy or excision if necessary, to maximize the patient's prognosis if a neoplastic process is suspected. If excision of any lesion, even small lesions, is required, reconstructive efforts should plan to restore both the form and function of the eyelid to protect the globe.

Acknowledgments

The authors wish to thank Krystyna Srodulski, medical illustrator, for her outstanding work in preparing the illustrations in this chapter. This work was supported in part by an unrestricted grant from Research to Prevent Blindness, Inc.

SELECTED REFERENCES

1. Requena L, Romero E, Sanchez M, et al. Aggressive keratoacanthoma of the eyelid: ''Malignant'' keratoacanthoma or squamous cell carcinoma. J Dermatol Surg Oncol 1990;16:564.
2. Graham JH, Helwig EB. Premalignant cutaneous and mucocutaneous diseases. In: Graham JH, Johnson WC, Helwig EB, eds. Dermal Pathology. Hagerstown, MD: Harper & Row, 1972:561.
3. Lund HZ. How often does squamous cell carcinoma of the skin metastasize. Arch Dermatol 1965;92:635.
4. Font RL. Eyelids and lacrimal drainage system. In: Spencer WH, ed. Ophthalmic Pathology: An Atlas and Textbook, vol. 3. Philadelphia: WB Saunders, 1986:2161.
5. Graham JH, Helwig EB. Bowen's disease and its relationship to systemic cancer. Arch Dermatol 1959;80:133.
6. Graham JH, Mazzanti GR, Helwig EB. Chemistry of Bowen's disease. J Invest Dermatol 1961;37:317.
7. Kwitko ML, Boniuk M, Zimmerman LE. Eyelid tumors with reference to lesions confused with squamous cell carcinomas. Arch Ophthalmol 1963;69:693.
8. Reifler DM, Hornblass A. Squamous cell carcinoma of the eyelid. Surv Ophthalmol 1986;30:349.
9. Lutzner MA. Skin cancer in immunosuppressed organ transplant recipients. J Am Acad Dermatol 1984;11:891.
10. Rao NA, Dunn SA, Romero JL, Stout W. Bilateral carcinomas of the eyelid. Am J Ophthalmol 1986;101:480.
11. Smith SP, Konnikov N. Eruptive epidermal cysts and multiple squamous cell carcinomas after therapy for cutaneous T cell lymphoma. J Am Acad Dermatol 1991;25:940.
12. Howard GR, Nerad JA, Carter KD, Whitaker DC. Clinical characteristics associated with orbital invasion of cutaneous basal cell and squamous cell tumors of the eyelid. Am J Ophthalmol 1992;113:123.
13. Miller SJ. Biology of basal cell carcinoma (part I). J Am Acad Dermatol 1991;24:1.
14. Miller SJ. Biology of basal cell carcinoma (part II). J Am Acad Dermatol 1991;24:161.
15. Lyles TW, Freeman RG, Knox JM. Transplantation of basal cell epitheliomas. J Invest Dermatol 1960;34:353.
16. Van Scott EJ, Reinertson RP. Modulating influence of stromal environment on epithelial cells studied in human autotransplants. J Invest Dermatol 1961;36:109.
17. Sexton M, Jones DB, Maloney ME. Histologic pattern analysis of basal cell carcinoma. Study of a series of 1039 consecutive neoplasms. J Am Acad Dermatol 1990;23:1118.
18. Wolf JE, Hubler WR. Tumor angiogenic factor and human skin tumors. Arch Dermatol 1975;111:321.
19. Downes RN, Walker NP, Collin JR. Micrograph (MOHS') surgery in the management of periocular basal cell epitheliomas. Eye 1990;4:160.
20. Doxanas MT, Green WR, Iliff CE. Factors in the successful surgical management of basal cell carcinoma of the eyelid. Am J Ophthalmol 1981;91:726.
21. Frank HJ. Frozen section control of excision of eyelid basal cell carcinomas: 8½ years experience. Br J Ophthalmol 1989;73:328.
22. Monheit GD, Callahan MA, Callahan A. MOHS micrographic surgery for periorbital skin cancer. Dermatol Clin 1989;7:677.
23. Gunnarson G, Larko O, Hersle K. Cryosurgery of the eyelid for basal cell carcinoma. Acta Ophthalmol 1990;68:241.
24. Farmer ER, Helwig EB. Metastatic basal cell carcinoma: A clinicopathological study of seventeen cases. Cancer 1980;46:748.
25. Lo JS, Snow SN, Reizner CT, et al. Metastatic basal cell carcinoma: Report of 12 cases with a review of the literature. J Am Acad Dermatol 1991;24:715.
26. Glover AT, Grove AS. Orbital invasion by malignant eyelid tumors. Ophthalmol Plast Reconstr Surg 1989;5:1.
27. Wilder RB, Shimm DS, Kittelson JM, et al: Recurrent basal cell carcinoma treated with radiation therapy. Arch Dermatol 1991;127:1668.
28. Baxter DL, Joyce AP, Feldman BD, Lynch JW. Cis-platinum chemotherapy for basal cell carcinoma: The need for post-treatment biopsy—report of a case. J Am Acad Dermatol 1990;6:1167.
29. Luxerberg M, Guthrie T. Chemotherapy of basal cell and squamous cell carcinoma of the eyelids and periorbital tissues. Ophthalmology 1986;93:504.
30. Morley M, Finger PT, Perlin M, et al. Cis-platinum chemotherapy for ocular basal cell carcinoma. Br J Ophthalmol 1991;75:407.
31. Epstein E. Value of follow-up after treatment of basal cell carcinoma. Arch Dermatol 1987;108:798.
32. Robinson JK. What are adequate treatment and following care for nonmelanotic cutaneous cancer? Arch Dermatol 1987;123:331.
33. Robinson JK. Risk of developing another basal cell carcinoma: A five year prospective study. Cancer 1987;60:118.
34. Schrieber MM, Moon TE, Fox SH, Davidson J. The risk of developing subsequent nonmelanotic skin cancer. J Am Acad Dermatol 1990;23:1114.
35. Lindelof B, Sigurgeirsson B, Wallberg P, Eklund G. Occurence of other malignancies in 1973 patients with basal cell carcinoma. J Am Acad Dermatol 1991;25:245.
36. Grossniklaus HE, Mclean IW. Cutaneous melanoma of the eyelid. Ophthalmology 1991;98:1867.
37. McGovern VJ, Mihm MC, Bailly C, et al: The classification of malignant melanoma and its histological reporting. Cancer 1973;32:1146.
38. Rodriguez-Sains RS, Jakobiec FA, Iwamoto T. Lentigo maligna of the lateral canthal skin. Ophthalmology 1981;88:1186.
39. Blodi FC, Widner RR. The melanotic freckle (Hutchinson) of the lid. Surv Ophthalmol 1968;12:23.
40. Clark WH, Mihm MC. Lentigo maligna and lentigo malignant melanoma. Am J Pathol 1969;55:39.
41. Breslow A. Thickness, cross-sectional areas and depths of invasion in the prognosis of cutaneous melanomas. Ann Surg 1970;172:902.
42. Breslow A. Tumor thickness, level of invasion and node dissection in stage I cutaneous melanoma. Ann Surg 1975;182:572.

43. Breslow A. Problems in the measurement of tumor thickness and level of invasion of cutaneous melanoma. Hum Pathol 1977;8:1.

44. Breslow A. Melanoma thickness and elective node dissection. Arch Dermatol 1978;114:1399.

45. Clark WH, From L, Bernardino EA, Mihm MC. The histogenesis and biological behavior of primary human malignant melanomas of the skin. Cancer Res 1969;29:705.

46. Clark WH, Ainsworth AM, Bernardino EA, et al. Developmental biology of primary human malignant melanomas. Semin Oncol 1975;2:83.

47. Clark WH, Mastrangelo MJ, Ainsworth AM, et al. Current concepts of the biology of human cutaneous malignant melanomas. Adv Cancer Res 1977;24:267.

48. Zoltie N, O'Neill TJ. Malignant melanoma of the eyelid skin. Plast Reconstr Surg 1989;83:994.

49. Ketcham AS, Balch CM. Classification and staging systems. In: Balch CM, Milton GW, eds. Cutaneous melanoma: Clinical management and treatment results worldwide. Philadelphia: JB Lippincott, 1985:55.

50. Boniuk M, Zimmerman LE. Sebaceous gland carcinoma of the eyelid, eyebrow, caruncle, and orbit. Trans Am Acad Ophthalmol Otolaryngol 1968;72:619.

51. Doxanas MT, Green RW. Sebaceous gland carcinoma: Review of 40 cases. Arch Ophthalmol 1984;102:254.

52. Khan JA, Doane JF, Grove AS. Sebaceous and meibomian carcinomas of the eyelid: Recognition, diagnosis, and management. Ophthalmol Plast Reconstr Surg 1991;7:6.

53. Rulon DB, Helwig EB. Cutaneous sebaceous neoplasma. Cancer 1974;33:82.

54. Brownstein S, Colere F, Jackson WB. Masquerade syndrome. Ophthalmology 1980;87:259.

55. Margo CE, Lessner A, Stern GA. Intraepithelial sebaceous cell carcinoma of the conjunctiva and skin of the eyelid. Ophthalmology 1992;99:227.

56. Rao NA, Hidayat AA, McLean IW, Zimmerman LE. Sebaceous gland carcinoma of the ocular adnexa: A clinicopathological study of 104 cases with five year follow-up data. Hum Pathol 1982;13:113.

57. Epstein GA, Putterman AM. Sebaceous adenocarcinoma of the eyelid. Ophthalmic Surg 1983;14:935.

58. Colak A, Aickurt C, Ozcan OE, Onol B. Intracranial extension of meibomian gland carcinoma. J Clin Neuro Ophthalmol 1991;11:39.

59. Char DH. Adult and pediatric lid tumor diagnosis. In: Char DH, ed. Clinical Ocular Oncology. New York: Churchill Livingston, 1989.

60. Wolken SH, Spivey BE, Blodi F. Hereditary adenoid cystic epithelioma (Brooke's tumor). Am J Ophthalmol 1968;68:26.

61. Gorlin RJ, Sedano HO. The multiple nevoid basal cell carcinoma syndrome revisited. Birth Defects 1971;7:1940.

62. Mamalis N, Medlock RD, et al. Merkel cell tumor of the eyelid: A review and report of an unusual case. Ophthalmic Surg 1989;20:410.

63. Rubsamen PE, Tanenbaum M, Holds JB, et al. Merkel cell carcinoma of the eyelid and periocular tissues. Am J Ophthalmol 1992;113:674.

64. Searl SS, Boynton JR, Markowitch W, diSant'Agnese PA. Malignant Merkel cell neoplasm of the eyelid. Arch Ophthalmol 1984;102:907.

25

Comparative Dermatopathology

Michael H. Goldschmidt

INTRODUCTION[1, 2]

Veterinary dermatopathology is an evolving discipline that covers a wide range of species. Dermatopathology of animals is not a recognized subspeciality, as it is in humans; it remains part of the broader discipline of veterinary pathology. However, the field of veterinary dermatopathology has evolved as a specialty, and the number of veterinarians with expertise in this area continues to grow.

The range of diseases in veterinary dermatopathology is extensive, as are the number of species in which these diseases occur. In experimental dermatopathology, the mouse and rat are the most commonly used species. However, the dog and the cat display the greatest diversity of diseases and afford the pathologist the largest number of specimens for histopathologic evaluation.

This chapter represents a very brief and general overview of the skin of the dog and cat and provides examples of the complex responses of their skin to injury. Additional information on specific diseases and their pathology is provided in other sources.

STRUCTURE OF CANINE AND FELINE SKIN

Canine and feline skin vary in thickness, which is inversely proportional to the degree of hairedness. Haired skin is often much thinner than nonhaired sites such as the footpads and planum nasale.

The basal cell layer of canine and feline skin is interspersed with melanocytes. The cells are cuboidal to columnar and may show occasional mitoses. The stratum spinosum is two to five cells thick in haired skin and thicker in nonhaired areas. The stratum granulosum may often be indistinct in normal haired skin. The stratum corneum is commonly four to nine cells thick but is thicker and more compact on the footpads and planum nasale. Melanocytes often have long dendritic processes with a variable number of melanin granules in their cytoplasm. Langerhans cells can only be visualized by electron microscopy; these cells lack the typical Birkbeck granules seen in human skin.

There are no rete ridges in haired skin; the numerous hairs serve to anchor the epidermis to the dermis. However, in the footpads and planum nasale, rete ridges are very prominent. In normal canine and feline skin, the basal lamina is indistinct.

Because of the lack of epidermal rete, the subdivision of the dermis into papillary and reticular sections is not possible. The terms superficial and deep dermis are substituted. In the superficial dermis, the collagen fibers are fine and fibrillar, whereas the deep dermis has larger, coarser collagen bundles. Elastin fibers are small and inconspicuous. Three vascular plexuses exist in the skin: the superficial plexus in the upper dermis, the middle plexus at the level of the sebaceous glands, and the deep plexus at the level of the dermis and panniculus adiposus.

Hairs are arranged in a compound manner. Each large primary hair is surrounded by a corona of smaller secondary hairs. Associated with each primary hair are sebaceous glands, apocrine glands, and an errector pili muscle, whereas the secondary hair may have only an associated sebaceous gland. Primary hairs emerge through separate infundibula, whereas secondary hairs share a common infundibulum.

Sebaceous and apocrine glands are found in haired skin; their ducts enter the infundibulum of the hair follicle. Eccrine glands are found only in the footpads. Modified sebaceous glands, found primarily in the perianal area, are referred to as perianal glands or hepatoid glands; the individual cells of these glands have an abundant eosinophilic cytoplasm, thus morphologically resembling hepatocytes. Modified apocrine glands include the ceruminous glands, which are found in the external ear canal; the anal glands, which open directly onto the perianal skin; and the anal sac glands, which open into the two anal sacs located on the ventrolateral aspect of the anus. The anal sac communicates with the skin through a duct.

REACTION PATTERNS[2, 3]

Since the publication of A.B. Ackerman's book, *Histologic Diagnosis of Inflammatory Skin Disease,* veterinary dermatopathology has followed the reaction patterns described in this text. This chapter is organized in terms of the reaction patterns that have proved useful in veterinary dermatopathology.

HISTOLOGY OF SPECIFIC DISORDERS

Diseases of the Epidermis

Pustular Diseases[4]

Pemphigus foliaceus is the most common autoimmune skin disease of the dog and cat. This condition affects haired skin primarily on the face, ears, feet, footpads, and groin but rarely involves mucous membranes. The clinical appearance is that of a vesicopustule that rapidly ruptures or degenerates (Fig. 25–1A). The histopathology of early intact pustules shows separation of the epidermis beneath the stratum corneum, exocytosis of neutrophils and eosinophils into the pustule, and extensive acantholysis; in some cases, rafts of acantholytic cells may be present (Fig. 25–1B). The infundibulum may be involved. Recornification of the base of the pustule is commonly seen. Within the superficial dermis, there may be vascular dilation with exocytosis of granulocytes and a perivascular lymphoplasmacytic infiltrate.

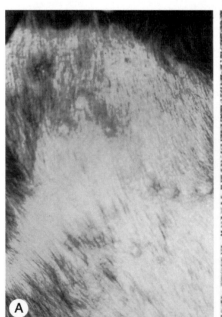
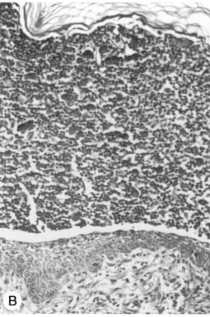

Figure 25–1. Pustular diseases: Canine pemphigus foliaceus. **(A)** Clinically there are multiple intraepidermal pustules that bridge several hair follicles. **(B)** Subcorneal pustules contain numerous acantholytic cells, neutrophils, and eosinophils.

The histopathologic differential diagnosis of pemphigus foliaceus should include superficial pyoderma and superficial folliculitis. Differentiation of pemphigus foliaceous from both of these diseases, which clinically appear as a superficial pustular dermatitis, is often difficult. In pemphigus foliaceous, the pustule is larger and usually bridges two or more hair follicles, and it contains significantly greater numbers of acantholytic cells and rafts of acantholytic cells.

Vesiculobullous Disorders

Dermatomyositis is a heritable disease seen primarily in the dog. Affected breeds are mainly collies and Shetland sheepdogs, and the disease often affects several individuals in a family. Lesions arise at sites of trauma or on pressure points, and early cutaneous changes are small pustules, papules, and plaques that often are ulcerated. Although the disease may regress, in most cases, it persists resulting in a scarring alopecia.

A biopsy specimen of affected skin shows vacuolar changes in the basal cells, dyskeratosis of individual keratinocytes, dermoepidermal separation that also involves the hair follicles, and perifollicular fibrosis with atrophy. A mild perivascular lymphoid infiltrate is present. Muscle degeneration and necrosis occurs in deep biopsy specimens taken from the head, but this is not a consistent finding. Lesions of muscle are best seen in specimens from sites where electromyographic changes have occurred.

Necrotizing Diseases

Erythema multiforme is relatively uncommon. Most cases occur secondary to administration of drugs, particularly trimethoprim sulfate antibiotics. The disease may involve haired skin and mucous membranes, and it presents as an erythematous, annular, arcuate, polycyclic lesion (Fig. 25–2A). Vesicles are infrequently seen.

Histologically, there is diffuse and variable dyskeratosis involving individual cells, primarily in the basal cell layer but extending into the upper epidermis (Fig. 25–2B). A superficial dermal lymphoid infiltrate with extension into the epidermis is seen, with a variable degree of superficial dermal edema and epidermal spongiosis. The infundibulum of hair follicles is often involved and destroyed. In cases in which dyskeratosis and epidermal spongiosis are severe, ulceration is often present. The very severe forms of erythema multiforme probably represent a spectrum of diseases that overlaps with toxic epidermal necrolysis.

Spongiotic Dermatitis and Exudative and Ulcerative Disorders

Allergic miliary dermatitis of the cat encompasses a number of hypersensitivity reactions to a variety of allergens, including atopy, food, intestinal and external parasites (primarily fleas), and drugs. Clinically, there is a papular, crust-

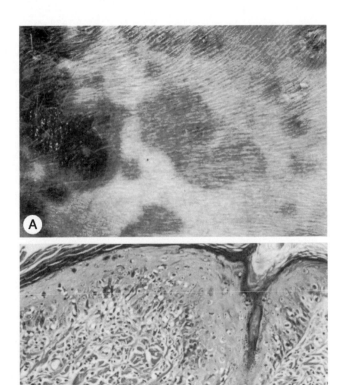

Figure 25–2. Necrotizing diseases of the epidermis. **(A)** Erythema multiforme is present in a dog with severe erythema and occasional target-like lesions. **(B)** The epidermis is hyperplastic with parakeratosis, diffuse dyskeratosis, and spongiosis, and there is a mild lymphoid infiltrate of the epidermis and dermis. Early vacuolar changes are seen within the basal cell area.

ing dermatitis (Fig. 25–3A), which may progress to foci of epidermal erosions and ulcers.

Histologically, these lesions vary with the stage of development of the condition. Early lesions are characterized by a perivascular infiltrate of eosinophils and increased numbers of mast cells, with moderate superficial dermal edema and spongiosis of the epidermis. There is exocytosis of the inflammatory cells into the epidermis, and a serocellular crust often occurs on the epidermis (Fig. 25–3B). Ulceration, which is often secondary to self-traumatization, evokes a proliferation of granulation tissue in the superficial dermis, and a hyperplastic epidermis is evident on re-epithelialization. The histopathology is merely an indication of an underlying hypersensitivity dermatitis that requires further clinical evaluation for the cause.

Hyperplastic Diseases

Acral lick dermatitis mimics prurigo nodularis in humans and is the result of constant irritation and self-traumatization of the skin, particularly the anterior aspect of the limbs. A specific etiology is not known. Allergic and other pruritic diseases and central or peripheral neurologic diseases are factors in initiating the itch-lick cycle that produces the

lesion. Clinically, the lesions are thick, firm, alopecic plaques with central ulceration and peripheral epidermal hyperplasia with alopecia (Fig. 25–4A). Most lesions are found on the carpus, tarsus, or radius.

The histologic changes include marked epidermal hyperplasia with acanthosis, compact orthokeratotic hyperkeratosis, focal parakeratosis at sites of recent self-trauma, hypergranulosis, and rete formation in areas of hair loss. The normal dermal collagen is often replaced by maturing granulation tissue. A perivascular infiltrate composed of lymphocytes and plasma cells is seen (Fig. 25–4B). The act of self-traumatization causes the hair shafts to break and perforate the follicular wall, allowing hair and keratinous material to enter the dermis, where they act as potent antigens and evoke a pyogranulomatous response that is rich in eosinophils (Fig. 25–4C).

Hyperkeratotic Diseases

Hepatocutaneous syndrome refers to an entity analogous to superficial necrolytic dermatitis in humans. The majority of affected dogs have an underlying hepatic disease rather than a pancreatic glucagonoma or diabetes mellitus. Clinically, the disease is a crusting, hyperplastic dermatitis affecting the skin of the periocular, perioral, genital, elbow, and footpad areas (Fig. 24–5A). Clinical signs of hepatic disease may not be seen initially.

The histologic changes include epidermal hyperplasia with marked parakeratosis. Spongiosis is severe and is limited to the upper portion of the epidermis. The keratinocytes in this area also show severe intracellular edema and necrosis. The deeper parts of the epidermis are mildly hyperplastic (Fig. 25–5B). A variable degree of lymphoid cell infiltration into the superficial dermis may be present.

Diseases of the Dermis

Perivascular Disorders

Atopy, also referred to as allergic inhalant dermatitis, is common in the dog and has a heritable basis. Affected animals are sensitized to inhaled environmental allergens and exhibit cutaneous disease as a result of the large number of mast cells within the skin. The disease may be seasonal or nonseasonal. Clinical signs include pedal and facial pruritus with secondary self-trauma and pyoderma or seborrhea involving the face, feet, and ventrum (Fig. 25–6A).

Biopsy specimens taken from dogs with atopy reveal a variable degree of superficial perivascular dermatitis which is predominantly mononuclear in type. Increased numbers of mast cells, as well as neutrophils and eosinophils, may be seen around these vessels. In long-standing cases, epidermal hyperplasia and spongiosis (Fig. 25–6B), as well as secondary superficial pyoderma, may be present.

Vascular Disorders

Vasculitis, whether immune mediated or associated with septicemia, is uncommon. The diagnosis of vasculitis is seldom made.

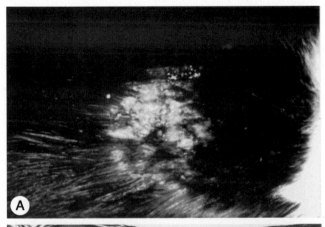

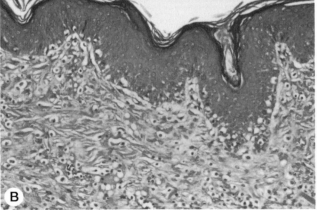

Figure 25–3. Exudative and ulcerative diseases of the epidermis. **(A)** Multifocal papular, pustular, and crusting dermatitis characterizes this allergic condition in a cat. **(B)** Epidermal hyperplasia is seen, with infiltration of the epidermis and dermis by mast cells and superficial dermal linear fibrosis.

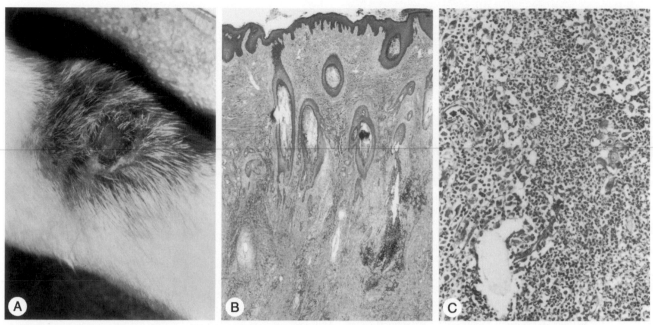

Figure 25–4. Hyperplastic diseases of the epidermis. **(A)** Acral lick dermatitis is present with a central ulcer and marked peripheral skin thickening. (Courtesy of Kevin Shanly, D.V.M.) **(B)** Epidermal hyperplasia, dermal fibrosis, periadnexal inflammation, and a perforating folliculitis are seen. **(C)** Naked pieces of hair have evoked an infiltrate of neutrophils and eosinophils.

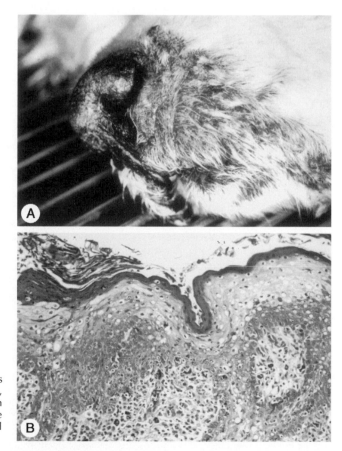

Figure 25–5. Hyperkeratotic diseases of the epidermis. **(A)** Hepatocutaneous syndrome (i.e., superficial necrolytic dermatitis) has produced an extensive, hyperplastic, crusting dermatitis involving the nasal skin. (Courtesy of Kevin Shanly, D.V.M.) **(B)** Parakeratosis, spongiosis of the upper portion of the epidermis, and epidermal hyperplasia with melanin drop-off and dermal inflammation are seen in this cross section.

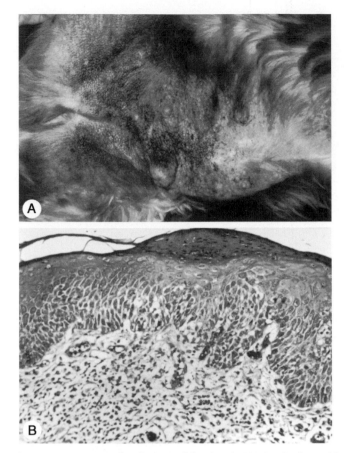

Figure 25–6. Perivascular diseases of the dermis. **(A)** Atopic dermatitis is seen, with hyperemia, hyperpigmentation, and thickening of the epidermis in the inguinal area. **(B)** Superficial parakeratosis at the site of self-induced trauma, epidermal and dermal edema, vascular dilation with margination of granulocytes, and perivascular infiltration by lymphocytes, plasma cells, and mast cells are seen.

Lichenoid Dermatitis

Vogt-Koyanagi-Harada–like syndrome is a depigmenting granulomatous dermatitis and uveitis primarily seen in akitas and other arctic breeds. The periorbital, perioral, nasal, and footpad skin is primarily affected (Fig. 25–7A).

The histologic findings include lichenoid dermatitis with little basal cell vacuolation. The dermal inflammatory cell infiltrate consists of histiocytes with lesser numbers of lymphocytes and plasma cells. Melanocyte destruction results in extensive accumulation of melanophages within the superficial dermis (Fig. 25–7B). My colleagues have been able to demonstrate retinal S-antigen by enzyme-linked immunosorbent assay of the serum of several affected animals.

Infectious Nodular and Diffuse Granulomatous and Pyogranulomatous Diseases[5]

An unusual manifestation of *Microsporum canis* infection in the cat is the formation of deep dermal and subcutaneous pseudomycetomas. The initial clinical manifestation is one or several intradermal nodules (Fig. 25–8A). In untreated cases or in cases in which treatment is discontinued, the

fungus deeply invades the underlying muscle and bone, with metastatic spread to regional lymph nodes and internal organs.

Evaluation of the lesions shows two different histologic appearances. One is a dense aggregate of fungal hyphae surrounded by a pyogranulomatous inflammatory response that includes numerous giant cells, some of which have intracytoplasmic fungi (Fig. 25–8B). The other histologic appearance is that of a dense central aggregation of hyphae surrounded by an eosinophilic Splendore-Hoeppli reaction and a peripheral pyogranulomatous inflammation with giant cells.

The diagnosis of *Microsporum canis* infection requires culture of the pseudomycetoma. No fungi can be cultured from the overlying epidermis and hair, nor can they be demonstrated in these sites with special stains.

Noninfectious Nodular and Diffuse Granulomatous and Pyogranulomatous Diseases[6]

Canine juvenile sterile pyogranulomatous dermatitis and lymphadenitis, also known as juvenile cellulitis, is a vesiculopustular disease (Fig. 25–9A). Most lesions are found

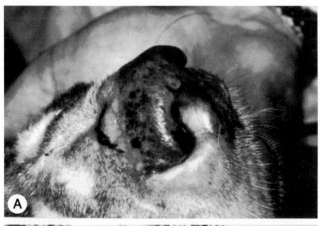

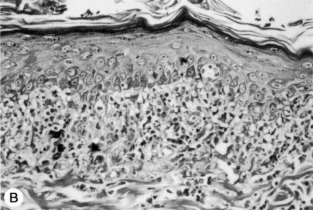

Figure 25–7. Lichenoid (i.e., interface) diseases of the dermis. **(A)** Nasal depigmentation is present in a case of Vogt-Koyanagi-Harada–like disease. (Courtesy of James Jeffers, V.M.D.) **(B)** Interface lichenoid dermatitis with melanin drop-off is seen; the cellular infiltrate consists of histiocytes and melanophages, with fewer lymphocytes and plasma cells.

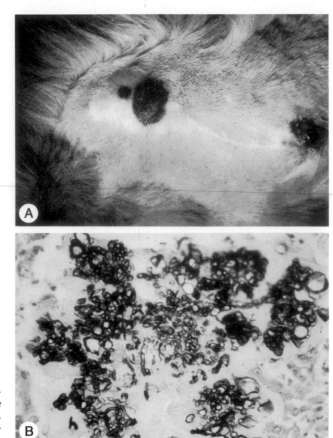

Figure 25–8. Infectious nodular granulomatous and pyogranulomatous disease of the dermis. **(A)** The large, erythematous, intradermal masses are the aggregates of *Microsporum canis* infection. (Courtesy of William Miller, Jr., V.M.D.) **(B)** Fungal pseudomycetoma and the associated granulomatous inflammation are present in the dermis.

around the face and head, and there may be fever, anorexia, and depression.

Histologically, there is a severe pyogranulomatous infiltrate in the dermis and panniculus adiposus (Fig. 29–9B). Similar pyogranulomatous foci can be seen in both regional and distant lymph nodes. Special stains for infectious agents are always negative. Electron microscopic examination of tissue from the skin and lymph nodes also fails to identify an infectious agent, and all cultures are negative. However, affected animals do respond to corticosteroid therapy, leading

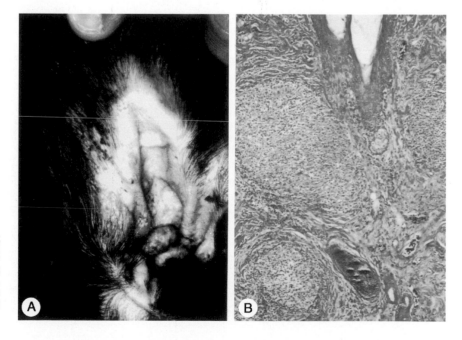

Figure 25–9. Noninfectious nodular and diffuse, granulomatous and pyogranulomatous diseases of the dermis. **(A)** Swelling, hyperemia, vesicles, and pustules involve the outer ear of this young dog with juvenile cellulitis. (Courtesy of James Jeffers, V.M.D.) **(B)** Numerous pyogranulomatous foci are seen within the dermis and are often associated with adnexa.

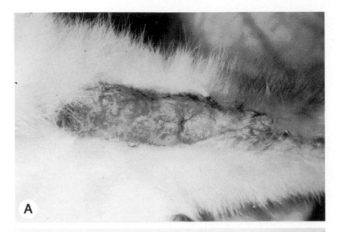

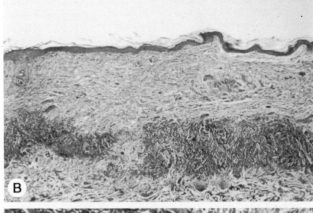

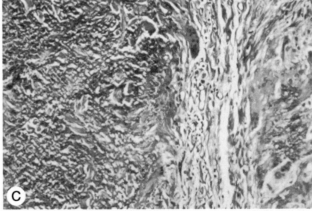

Figure 25–10. Nodular and diffuse diseases of the dermis with prominent eosinophils and plasma cells. **(A)** Collagenolytic granulomas involve the rear leg of a cat. (Courtesy of James Jeffers, V.M.D.) **(B)** A large band of degenerate collagen is seen in the deep dermis, and a small focus is present in the superficial dermis. A marked infiltrate by multinucleated giant cells surround these foci. **(C)** Higher magnification shows degenerate collagen surrounded by giant cells.

some researchers to speculate that this disease may represent an aberrant immunologic response to a common circulating antigen.

Nodular and Diffuse Infiltrates with Plasma Cells and Eosinophils

Collagenolytic granulomas commonly involve the skin or mucous membranes of the oral cavity; this disorder occurs more frequently in cats than in dogs. The cause of the lesion

is unknown, but there is some evidence that it may represent a hypersensitivity reaction to an allergen such as fleabites, food, or inhaled allergens.

Clinically, the lesions are firm, raised plaques that may have a linear appearance. Extensive swelling of the tissue may occur and is most noticeable on the face, particularly in the lips, and the caudal aspects of the rear legs (Fig. 25–10A). Ulceration is common on the skin and the mucous membranes.

Histologically, the most notable features of collagenolytic granulomas is a severe perivascular and interstitial infiltrate composed of eosinophils. There is alteration of dermal collagen, and degranulation and degeneration of eosinophils produces flame figures. In long-standing cases, these foci of altered collagen are surrounded by histiocytes and giant cells, and few eosinophils are seen (Fig. 25–10B, C). Occasionally, transepidermal or transfollicular elimination of the altered collagen may be evident. The histologic appearance of this lesion is very similar to that of Wells syndrome in humans.

Dysplastic and Depositional Disorders of Connective Tissue

Calcinosis cutis is a relatively common disease that is seen in association with hyperadrenocorticism in the dog

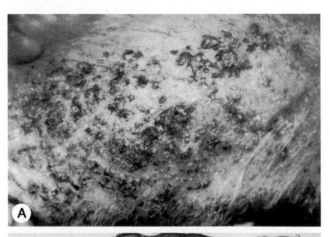

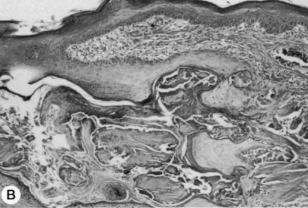

Figure 25–11. Dysplastic and depositional diseases of dermal connective tissue. **(A)** Alopecia, multifocal epidermal hyperplasia, and numerous pustules characterize this case of calcinosis cutis due to hyperadrenocorticism. (Courtesy of Kevin Shanly, D.V.M.) **(B)** The mineralized foci are being surrounded by the outer root sheath of the hair follicle, allowing the material to be removed from the dermis.

(Fig. 25–11*A*). This disorder is most often the result of iatrogenic rather than naturally occurring hyperadrenocorticism.

Dystrophic mineralization of the dermal collagen, which elicits a foreign-body response on the part of the dog, leads to infiltration by histiocytes and giant cells. In some long-standing cases, there is ossification of the mineralized collagen, which produces thick bands of intradermal bone, or transepidermal and transfollicular elimination of the foreign material takes place (Fig. 25–11*B*).

Diseases of Adnexal Appendages

Pustular and Nodular Diseases with and without Follicular Destruction

Canine demodicosis is caused by the mite *Demodex canis*. In small numbers, the mite is a normal inhabitant of the hair follicle, but in large numbers, these organisms produce disease. This situation is unlike that encountered in humans, in whom a large number of demodectic mites within a follicle is not considered abnormal. The mite is transmitted from the bitch to her pups early in neonatal life, while they nurse.

The clinical disease may be localized or generalized. The localized form of the disease is a small, erythematous, alopecic, circumscribed dermatitis that most often involves the head (Fig. 25–12*A*) and forelimbs. Most of these cases resolve spontaneously. Generalized demodicosis may be juvenile or adult in onset, and as the name implies, it affects large areas of the skin, particularly that of the head and forelimbs.

The histopathologic findings are variable. In cases of localized demodicosis, numerous mites are present in a dilated hair follicle with little or no intrafollicular or perifollicular inflammatory cell infiltrate. As the disease becomes more severe, neutrophils infiltrate into the follicle, which becomes dilated as a result of keratin accumulation from plugging of the infundibular orifice. Perifollicular lymphoid cells may be found. In the most severe form of the disease, there is a perforating folliculitis with release of keratin and *Demodex* mites into the dermis, where they evoke a severe pyogranulomatous response (Fig. 25–12*B, C*). These granulomatous foci may persist for a considerable time and resemble those seen in humans with acne rosacea.

Microsporum canis may produce intradermal and subcutaneous granulomas, as noted previously (see Infectious Nodular and Diffuse Granulomatous and Pyogranulomatous Diseases). The disease is more commonly seen as ringworm or dermatophytosis in the dog and cat. Exposure to the dermatophyte does not always result in the establishment of infection and disease; this may depend on the age of the

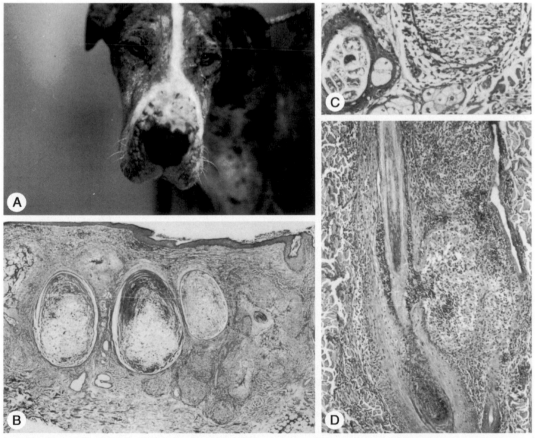

Figure 25–12. Pustular and nodular diseases, with and without follicular destruction. **(A)** Canine demodecosis is localized to the head of this dog. **(B)** Canine demodecosis with severe follicular hyperkeratosis, numerous *Demodex* mites within the dilated infundibulum, and several perifollicular granulomas are seen. **(C)** Higher magnification demonstrates intrafollicular mites and perifollicular granuloma with a central mite. **(D)** Dermatophytosis is present in a dog with a perforating folliculitis and numerous arthroconidia around the hair shaft.

animal, the young being more prone to infection, and the pathogenicity of the strain of fungus. Immunosuppression increases the likelihood of infection.

Lesions appear as a rapidly expanding, circular area of alopecia, with broken hairs and a variable degree of erythema. On occasion, the entire body may be denuded. Folliculitis is present in most cases, and papules and pustules involve the hair follicle.

Diagnosis is by microscopic examination (KOH or chlorophenolac preparations) of affected hairs for hyphae and conidia. A definitive diagnosis requires culture of the fungus *from affected hairs.*

Histopathologic findings are variable. Most cases show arthroconidia surrounding the hair shaft with no folliculitis and minimal perifollicular inflammation. This histology is often seen in cats. Folliculitis is characterized by an infiltrate of neutrophils into the follicular wall and lumen. Lesions seen clinically as kerions show rupture of the follicular wall with naked hair shafts in the dermis surrounded by a pyogranulomatous inflammatory response (Fig. 25–12D). Arthroconidia surround the hair shaft, and in some cases a Splendore-Hoeppli reaction may be seen around the hair. The presence of neutrophils and absence of eosinophils is useful in differentiating this lesion from a nonfungal perforating folliculitis.

Microsporum canis infection is the most common zoonosis seen in veterinary dermatology. Individuals who work with cats infected with the more virulent strains of the fungus have infection rates approaching 100%.

Atrophic Disorders of the Hair Follicle

Canine endocrine disorders induce severe atrophic diseases of the hair follicle resulting in noninflammatory, nonscarring alopecia. The development of the alopecia is caused by a failure of hair growth due to a deficiency or excess of a hormone or an abnormality of a receptor site for a hormone. In many cases, normal hair growth resumes when the underlying deficiency or excess is corrected. The most common

causes of canine endocrine alopecia are hyperadrenocorticism (Fig. 25–13A), hypothyroidism, hyperestrogenism associated with testicular Sertoli cell tumor, and imbalance, deficiencies, or excesses of male and female sex hormones.

The most consistent histopathologic findings are orthokeratotic hyperkeratosis with marked infundibular hyperkeratosis, alopecia, excessive numbers of telogen hairs, and the absence of any inflammatory cell infiltrate (Fig. 25–13B). Some cases may show epidermal hyperpigmentation and sebaceous gland atrophy. The definitive diagnosis of endocrine alopecia requires the biochemical identification of the underlying defect.

Dysplastic Disorders of the Hair Follicle[7]

Color dilution alopecia, also referred to as color mutant alopecia, is an inherited disease in which dilution of the coat color causes a partial alopecia. The disease is most often recognized in the doberman pinscher (Fig. 25–14A), but a recently recognized syndrome in the Rhodesian ridgeback associates the alopecia with cerebellar hypoplasia. Dogs that subsequently develop color dilution alopecia are born with a normal coat, but because they carry the gene for the defect, they begin to develop alopecia at 6 to 12 months of age. Hair loss is progressive, and little regrowth occurs in the affected areas. Follicular plugging and pyoderma or folliculitis occur secondary to the hair loss.

Histopathologic changes found in biopsy specimens from affected areas include large, irregularly shaped, dense melanin granules within melanocytes in the epidermis and hair matrix (Fig. 25–14B). This melanosomal abnormality results in melanin clumps within the hair shaft. Aggregates of melanophages are also present in peribulbar areas of the dermis and panniculus adiposus (Fig. 25–14C).

Diseases of the Panniculus[8]

Postvaccination alopecia is a lesion of the dog that occurs secondary to the subcutaneous administration of rabies

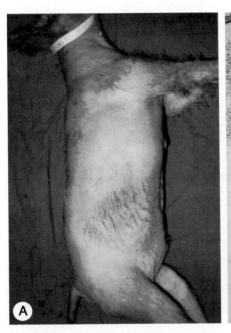
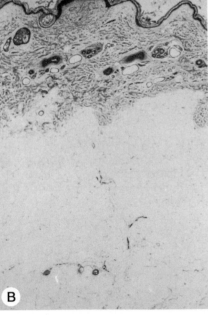

Figure 25–13. Atrophic diseases of the hair follicle. **(A)** Canine hyperadrenocorticism. This dog shows extensive alopecia and a pendulous abdomen. **(B)** The histologic appearance of hyperadrenocorticism includes epidermal thinning, hyperkeratosis and infundibular hyperkeratosis, decreased dermal collagen, and a lack of any inflammatory cells. Note the difference in histologic appearance in Figure 25–11 A, B, which also are caused by hyperadrenocorticism.

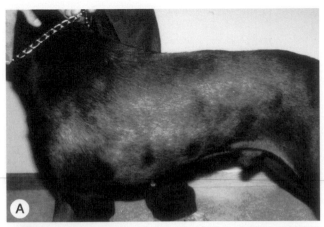

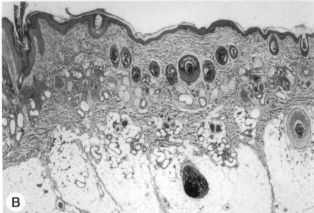

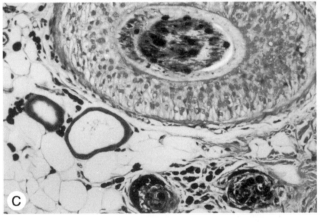

Figure 25–14. Dysplastic diseases of the hair follicle. **(A)** Color dilution alopecia involves the thoracic and abdominal area. (Courtesy of Richard Long, D.V.M.) **(B)** Hair loss and aggregation of melanin within the bulbar region, shaft of the hair, and within melanophages around hair follicles are apparent. **(C)** Higher magnification of **B**.

vaccine. The lesions, which arise 3 to 6 months postvaccination are hyperpigmented, alopecic macules that are 2 to 5 cm in diameter (Fig. 25–15A).

The primary histologic finding consists of intense perivascular aggregates of lymphocytes in the panniculus adiposus and deep dermis (Fig. 25–15B). In many cases, an accompanying infiltrate of eosinophils may be found, and in long-standing cases, germinal follicle formation may be evident. Necrosis of fat with a minimal infiltrate composed of

neutrophils and macrophages may be found, but granuloma and pyogranuloma formation are not features of this disease. In the dermis, perivascular lymphoid cuffs and, in some instances, an arteriolitis may be observed. Follicular and adnexal atrophy are common (Fig. 25–15C). Because these lesions arise at sites of prior rabies vaccinations, it has been speculated that the disease is the result of a host-antigen interaction at the site of massive antigen deposition.

Neoplasms

Cutaneous neoplasms are extremely common in the dog and cat. The incidence of specific neoplasms within the population is not known and is dependent on several factors. Some breeds have a predisposition for developing certain skin tumors. Environmental factors, such as the intensity of ultraviolet (UV) light, can significantly affect the incidence of specific neoplasms. Overall, the majority of epithelial, mesenchymal, and melanocytic neoplasms in the dog are benign, whereas many of the neoplasms in the cat are malignant. The following section provides a brief overview of these neoplasms in the dog and cat. Emphasis is placed on the histopathologic appearance of these neoplasms and on tumors that are unique to these species. A more comprehensive description of the clinical and histologic appearance of these tumors is provided elsewhere.

Basal Cell Tumor

Basal cell tumors are common in the dog and cat. This lesion is thought to arise from pluripotent epithelial cells of the skin and adnexa, not from the epidermis. The morphology of the tumor cell resembles that of a basal cell of the epidermis. There is no differentiation to either squamous or adnexal epithelium. The individual cells have little cytoplasm, are often columnar and palisaded, and may appear ovoid or fusiform. The tumor is subdivided into multiple lobules by connective tissue trabeculae; this stroma is usually collagenous. Mucinous ground substance and retraction spaces are not seen. Melanocytes are often found interspersed between the tumor cells. Central cystic degeneration of tumor lobules with aggregation of pigmented necrotic material is often seen in feline basal cell tumors.

A number of histologic patterns of basal cell tumor occur in the dog. These include solid, garland, medusoid, adenoid, cystic, and granular cell varieties. Often, more than one pattern is present in a tumor. The histologic pattern has no prognostic significance. Basal cell tumors in the dog and cat are benign masses that are cured by surgical excision.

Basal Cell Carcinoma

Basal cell carcinomas are found primarily in the cat. The majority of the lesions are solitary; however, they occasionally may be multicentric, they are often ulcerated, and histologically, there is invasion by cords of basophilic basaloid cells into the deep dermis and subcutis (Fig. 25–16A). A modest desmoplastic response may be associated with this tumor (Fig. 25–16B). Despite its infiltrative nature, metastases are rarely encountered.

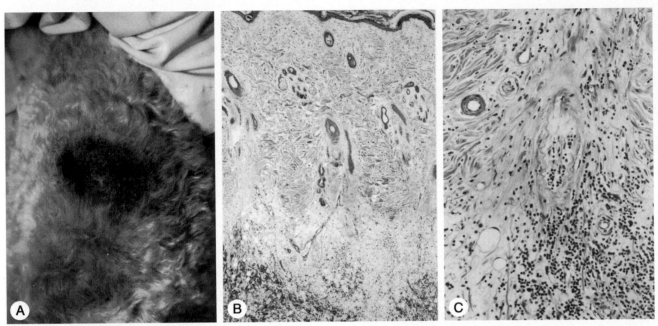

Figure 25–15. Diseases of the panniculus. **(A)** Alopecia and hyperpigmentation occurred at the site of a rabies vaccination. **(B)** Alopecia and dermal fibrosis are seen, particularly around the remnants of hair follicles. A marked lymphoid infiltrate obliterates the panniculus adiposus. **(C)** The inflammatory infiltrate of lymphocytes and plasma cells surround the remnants of the hair follicle.

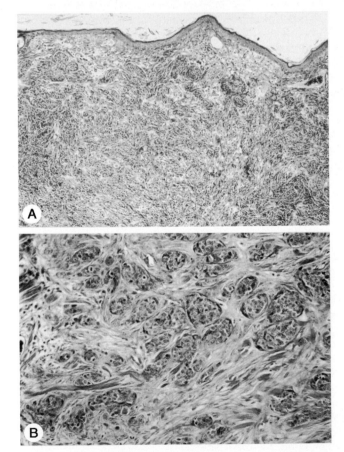

Figure 25–16. Basal cell tumor. **(A)** Feline basal cell carcinoma extends from the superficial to the deep dermis. **(B)** The deep edge of **A** shows infiltrating carcinoma cells and a modest desmoplastic host response.

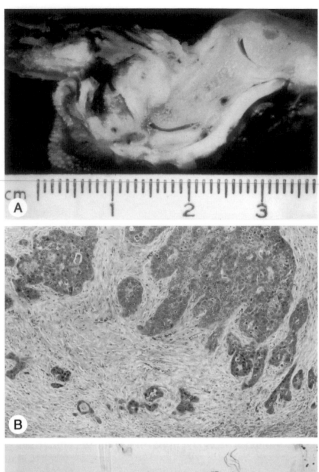

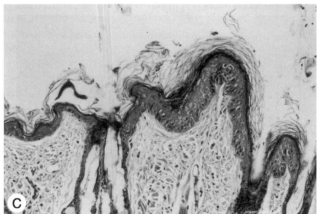

Figure 25–17. Squamous cell carcinoma. **(A)** Subungual squamous cell carcinoma with destruction of the third phalanx in a dog. **(B)** Infiltrative squamous cell carcinoma with desmoplasia. **(C)** Bowen disease in a cat.

Squamous Cell Carcinoma

In the dog and cat, there is often an association between squamous cell carcinoma and prolonged exposure to UV light. Thus, the tumor usually develops in areas where the hair and skin lack pigmentation and where the hair is short or absent and therefore provides little protection to the epidermis. Squamous cell carcinoma is usually seen in the pinnae, planum nasale, and eyelids of white cats. In dogs that sunbathe, the ventral abdomen and scrotum are involved, whereas the pinnae and dorsal trunk are more commonly affected in breeds that lack epidermal pigment or have a short hair coat. The subungual area is the most common site of origin of squamous cell carcinoma in the dog (Fig. 25–17*A*). The histopathology of this neoplasm is as described in humans and shows variable degrees of squamous differentiation (Fig. 25–17*B*).

I have only seen Bowen disease in cats. The lesions are often multicentric; they occur in cats that have both pigment and hair for protection from UV light (Fig. 25–17*C*). Invasion along the external root sheath of the hair follicle is a prominent histologic feature.

Sebaceous Tumors

Sebaceous tumors are common in the dog and are less common in the cat. The majority of sebaceous tumors are benign. In the dog, they arise most often on the head. There is a marked variation in the histopathology of the benign tumors which does not correlate with the prognosis. Well-differentiated tumors consist primarily of lobules of large cells with abundant sebaceous differentiation. Other tumors show extensive proliferation of reserve cells, which are small and have basophilic nuclei, little cytoplasm, and a large number of mitotic figures, with single cells or groups of cells showing sebaceous differentiation (Fig. 25–18*A*). Many of these lesions have areas of ductal differentiation, which are lined by an attenuated squamous epithelium.

In sebaceous carcinoma, the tumor cells often have an abundant, foamy cytoplasm and exhibit nuclear and cellular pleomorphism and variable numbers of mitotic figures. Metastasis to regional lymph nodes is occasionally found.

Sebaceous hyperplasia is usually a senile change in which the sebaceous proliferation occupies the superficial dermis and produces an exophytic growth. These lesions may be single or multiple.

Hepatoid Gland Tumors

Hepatoid gland tumors are modified sebaceous glands found only in the dog. These lesions are responsive to stimulation by androgens and androgen-like hormones produced by the testes and adrenal glands. The hepatoid glands continue to enlarge following the onset of sexual maturity. Tumors arising from the hepatoid are located primarily in the perianal area (Fig. 25–19*A*), but they may also arise on the

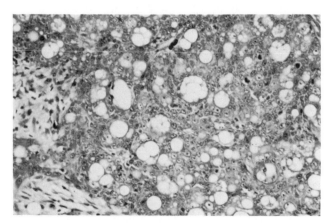

Figure 25–18. Sebaceous adenoma. There is marked mitotic activity but little nuclear pleomorphism associated with the reserve cells.

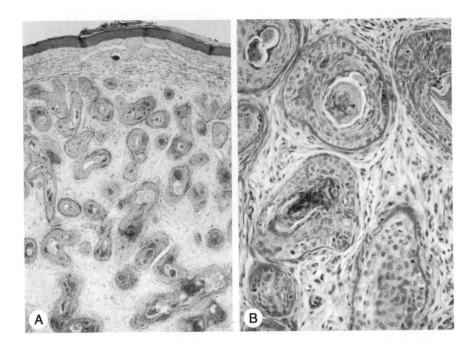

Figure 25–22. Trichoepithelioma. **(A)** The multiple islands of neoplastic cells show differentiation to the external root sheath and a central aggregation of shadow cells. **(B)** Higher magnification of **A.**

small basophilic cells, which often demonstrate considerable mitotic activity, occurs. An outer thickened basal lamina, differentiation of the neoplastic cells toward the various components of normal hair, and accumulation of small aggregates of shadow cells within the tumor are features of the canine trichoepithelioma (Fig. 25–22A, B). Only occasionally will these tumor cells have intracytoplasmic trichohyalin granules. Infiltrative and malignant trichoepitheliomas are less well differentiated; malignant tumors will metastasize to the regional lymph nodes and lungs.

Pilomatrixoma

The pilomatrixoma is similar to that seen in humans and often presents as a multilobulated dermal mass extending into the panniculus adiposus. This tumor may be variably pigmented. At the periphery of the lobules, the basophilic cells show an abrupt change to shadow cells (Fig. 25–23A, B). Ossification and infiltration by multinucleated giant cells is common. Occasional cases of malignant pilomatrixoma with lymph node and pulmonary metastases may be seen.

Melanocytic Tumors

Melanocytic tumors are common in the dog and uncommon in the cat. Nevi are not found in these species, although occasional cells resembling nevus cells may be seen in the epidermis of the nipple in the dog. The differentiation of benign from malignant melanocytic tumors in the dog is greatly influenced by the site of origin of the tumor. The

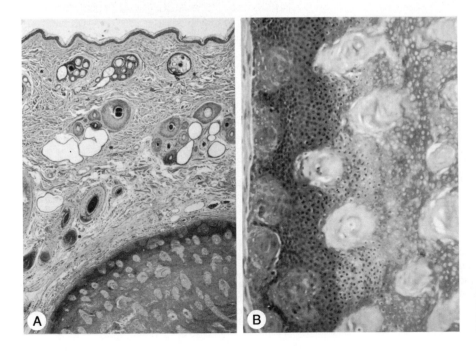

Figure 25–23. Pilomatrixoma. **(A)** Pilomatrixoma in the deep dermis has a peripheral rim of basophilic cells and large central aggregates of shadow cells. **(B)** Higher magnification of **A.**

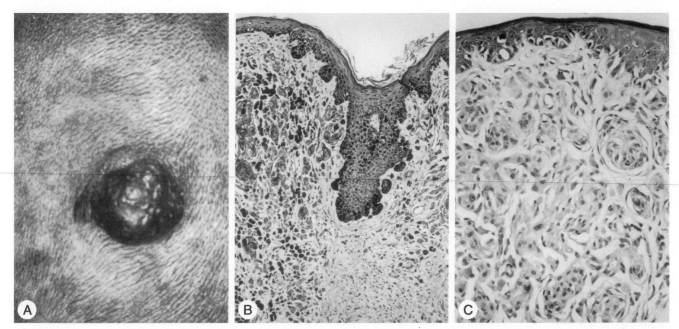

Figure 25–24. Melanoma. **(A)** A dermal melanoma arising on the haired skin of a dog. **(B)** This dermal melanoma in a dog with minimal junctional activity, a population of highly pigmented round cells in the upper dermis, and sheets of poorly pigmented tumor cells in the deeper zones. **(C)** Higher magnification of the upper portion of **B**.

majority of melanocytic tumors arising from the haired skin and the eyelid are benign. All melanocytic tumors arising from mucocutaneous junctions, especially the lip (Fig. 25–24D), and from the subungual area are malignant. The diagnosis of malignant melanoma arising within the haired skin requires careful histopathologic evaluation for evidence of nuclear pleomorphism and mitotic activity. *The criteria used for the diagnosis of malignant melanoma in humans are not applicable to the dog or cat.*

Dermal melanomas, which are benign, are often highly pigmented masses that occupy the dermis and extend into the panniculus adiposus (Fig. 25–24A). An intraepidermal component with junctional activity may be seen (Fig. 25–24B). Tumor cells vary from fusiform to oval, and the later often have an abundant amount of melanin in their cytoplasm; this melanin obscures the nucleus (Fig. 25–24C). Fusiform cells may exhibit neuroidal differentiation. Mitotic figures are uncommon.

Malignant melanomas have a variable degree of pigmentation. Tumor cells vary from fusiform to epithelioid. An intraepidermal or intramucosal proliferation of tumor cells may be seen in association with the dermal or submucosal component of the mass (Fig. 25–25B–D). Mitotic activity exceeds 3 mitoses per 10 high-power fields and is accompanied by nuclear pleomorphism. Metastases to regional lymph nodes and lungs are common.

Fibroma and Fibrosarcoma[9]

Both fibroma and fibrosarcoma are common in the dog. Their histopathologic appearance is similar to that seen in humans. In German shepherds, there is a heritable syndrome characterized by the development of multiple dermal fibromas, uterine leiomyomas, and renal cystadenocarcinomas.

Fibrosarcomas develop in cats; however, fibromas do

not. In cats younger than 5 years of age, the tumor may be multicentric and caused by the feline sarcoma virus (FeSV), which is a retrovirus. My colleagues and I have also recently described the development of fibrosarcomas at sites of prior vaccinations in the cat; these tumors often develop in association with a severe granulomatous inflammatory response.

Canine Hemangiopericytoma

Canine hemangiopericytoma is commonly seen on the limbs and thorax of old dogs. On gross evaluation, the mass is often multilobulated and may be myxomatous or sclerotic. On microscopic evaluation, the majority of the tumor cells are fusiform, and they form concentric whorls around a capillary lumen or a storiform pattern (Fig. 25–26A), with collagen deposition by the tumor cells. Some cells have a more abundant eosinophilic cytoplasm, and occasionally, multinucleated cells may be present. Mitotic activity is variable. Perivascular aggregates of lymphoid cells may be seen. These tumors commonly recur at the surgical site, but metastases are uncommon.

Giant Cell Tumor of Soft Tissues

Giant cell tumors of soft tissues, which are more common in the cat than in the dog, are located in the dermis and subcutis. The tumor cells vary from fusiform to epithelioid interspersed by numerous multinucleated giant cells. Recurrence of the tumor at the surgical site is common.

Lipoma and Liposarcoma

Lipomas are common in both the dog and the cat, but they have a predisposition to occur in aged, overweight bitches. Many of these tumors are large, and they may ex-

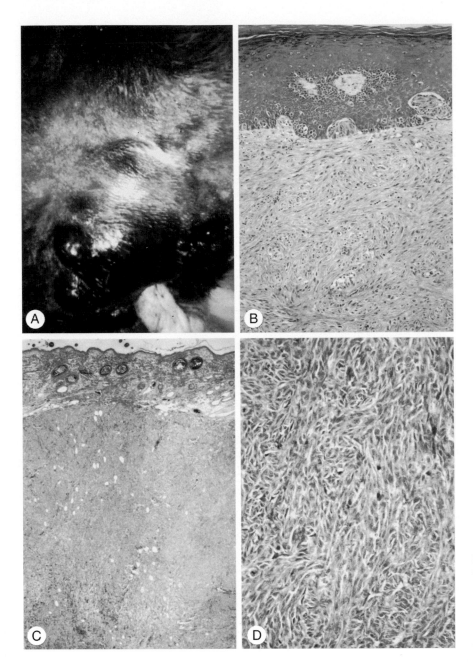

Figure 25–25. Melanoma. **(A)** Malignant melanoma arising at the mucocutaneous junction of the lip. **(B)** Malignant melanoma of the lip with nest of neoplastic cells in the epithelium and extensive invasion of the subepithelial tissue. **(C)** Malignant melanoma arising as a nodular mass in the skin. **(D)** Higher magnification of **C** reveals proliferation of spindle-type melanoma cells.

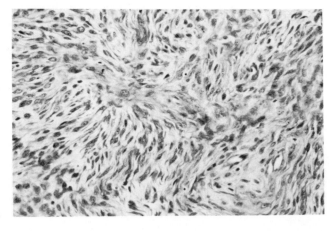

Figure 25–26. Canine hemangiopericytoma, storiform pattern.

hibit central necrosis. Infiltration of the surrounding muscle and connective tissue may be seen, often making surgical excision difficult and resulting in recurrence of the tumor.

Liposarcomas are uncommon. The well-differentiated, round cell, myxoid and pleomorphic types described in humans also occur in the dog.

Hemangioma and Hemangiosarcoma

Hemangiomas often arise as solitary or multiple, intradermal and subcutaneous masses. Both the capillary and cavernous types are seen in dogs and cats.

Hemangiosarcomas located within the dermis and subcutis may represent primary tumors or metastases from internal organs, especially the spleen, liver, and right atrial appendage of the heart. The vascular channels vary in diameter, and the lining neoplastic endothelial cells are often plump and pleomorphic and protrude into the luminal spaces.

Canine Cutaneous Histiocytoma

The canine cutaneous histiocytoma is a common tumor seen only in the dog. The clinical appearance of this tumor is that of an elevated, alopecic, red, intradermal nodule (Fig. 25–27A). The majority of cases occur as single tumors in dogs younger than 3 years of age. Many of these lesions occur on the head, particularly the ears.

Histologically, this tumor often shows epidermal hyperplasia with prominent rete, and the remnants of hair follicles are destroyed by the proliferating tumor cells (Fig. 25–27B, C). Occasionally, intraepidermal tumor cells may be found either singly or in small groups. The majority of the tumor cells are histiocytic in appearance, with central vesicular nuclei and pale eosinophilic cytoplasm (Fig. 25–27D). Numerous mitotic figures may be present. There are areas of necrosis with perivascular and periappendageal aggregates of lymphocytes and some plasma cells. Many of these tumors show spontaneous regression, whereas others require surgical excision and histopathologic evaluation for a definitive diagnosis.

Mast Cell Tumor

The mast cell tumor is common in the dog and cat. This lesion may be solitary or multicentric (Fig. 25–28A), and some cases may show metastatic spread, primarily to regional lymph nodes and the spleen. The intradermal and subcutaneous nodules may be extremely large. Most of these tumors are found on the rear legs and abdomen in the dog and on the head and neck in the cat.

In cats, the histologic appearance of this tumor is of round to polygonal cells with central nuclei, abundant eosinophilic cytoplasm, distinct cell borders, and few mitotic figures. In dogs, the histologic appearance of the tumor is ex-

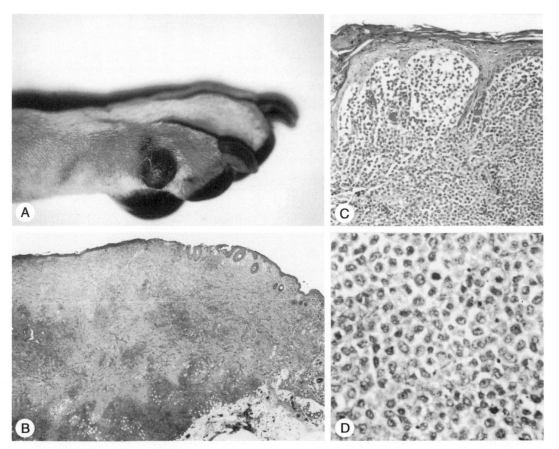

Figure 25–27. Canine cutaneous histiocytoma. **(A)** The lesion appears as an elevated, erythematous mass on the digit of a dog. (Courtesy of Barbara Kummel, D.V.M.) **(B)** Tumor cells infiltrate the dermis and panniculus adiposus, with extensive lymphoid infiltration into the tumor. **(C)** Sheets and cords of neoplastic cells are present in the dermis. **(D)** Neoplastic cells have ovoid nuclei, some of which have nuclear clefts. Mitoses are numerous.

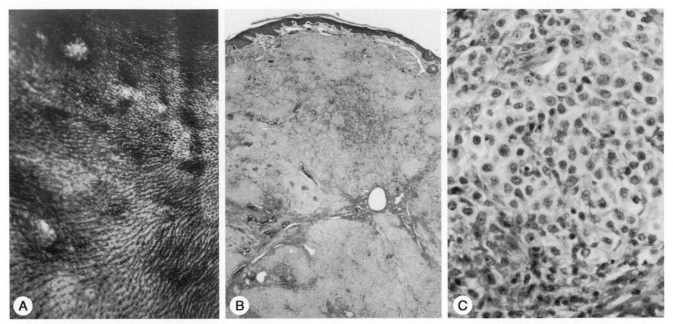

Figure 25–28. Mast cell tumor. **(A)** Multiple nodular intradermal masses are present in a dog. (Courtesy of Barbara Kummel, D.V.M.) **(B)** Dermal collagen has been obliterated by sheets of tumor cells. **(C)** High magnification reveals tumor cells and eosinophils.

tremely variable. The neoplastic cells infiltrate between the dermal collagen, forming cords, nodules, and sheets of neoplastic mast cells (Fig. 25–28B). The cytoplasm of these cells varies from eosinophilic to granular and basophilic. Eosinophils are diffusely scattered throughout the tumor (Fig. 25–28C). The presence of eosinophils is useful in helping to diagnose the malignant and anaplastic variants of this tumor, in which a few intracytoplasmic metachromatic granules are seen with special stains. Other helpful histopathologic features of this tumor are interstitial edema, perivascular hyalinization, foci of collagenolysis, and cystic dilation of apocrine glands.

Cutaneous Lymphosarcoma

Cutaneous lymphosarcoma is uncommon in both species but is less so in the dog than in the cat. The clinical appearance is similar to cutaneous T-cell lymphoma in humans; animals may present in the erythematous (Fig. 25–29A), plaque, nodular, or tumor stage of the disease. The latter two stages of presentation are the most common.

With regard to histopathology, two patterns of tumor infiltration may be seen: epidermotropic (Fig. 25–29B, C) and nonepidermotropic (Fig. 25–29D, E). In most instances, the neoplastic cells are monomorphous, large, lymphoblastic cells that show extensive mitotic activity and may invade the panniculus adiposus. The epidermotropic form shows the formation of intraepidermal aggregates resembling Pautrier microabscesses (see Fig. 25–29C), as well as involvement of the external root sheath of the hair follicle and the apocrine gland epithelium. Further subclassification into B- and T-cell tumors is not undertaken because of the lack of commercially available reagents. Cutaneous lymphosarcoma is an excellent animal model of a human disease which awaits further collaborative investigation.

Cutaneous Plasmacytoma

A recently recognized entity that occurs primarily in old dogs, cutaneous plasmacytoma has many clinical characteristics similar to the canine cutaneous histiocytoma. A predilection for the lips (Fig. 25–30A), digits, and oral mucosa has been found. The tumor occupies the dermis and extends into the panniculus adiposus, but it spares the epidermis (Fig. 25–30B). Sheets of tumor cells are often subdivided by a fine, fibrovascular, connective tissue stroma. Cells have peripheral nuclei, a variable amount of brightly eosinophilic cytoplasm, and distinct cell borders. Multinucleated tumor cells are not uncommon. Amyloid deposition by the tumor cells is rare and is associated with a greater incidence of tumor recurrence.

Cutaneous, Systemic, and Malignant Histiocytosis

Cutaneous histiocytosis is considered a non-neoplastic proliferative disorder. These lesions appear as plaques or nodules that wax and wane or may regress. Histologically, large histiocytes occupy the dermis and extend into the panniculus adiposus. The cells are monomorphous, often have a high mitotic rate, and may have abundant vacuolated cytoplasm. Another histologic pattern is more perivascular and periappendageal in its orientation, with a pleomorphic cell infiltrate that includes lymphocytes, plasma cells, and neutrophils.

Systemic histiocytosis is a heritable histiocytic proliferation seen in the Bernese mountain dog. Skin lesions are nodular and large, have a predilection for the facial and scrotal skin, and are accompanied by lymphadenopathy. Histologically, the masses comprise a perivascular infiltrate by large histiocytes in the skin and at the dermal-epidermal

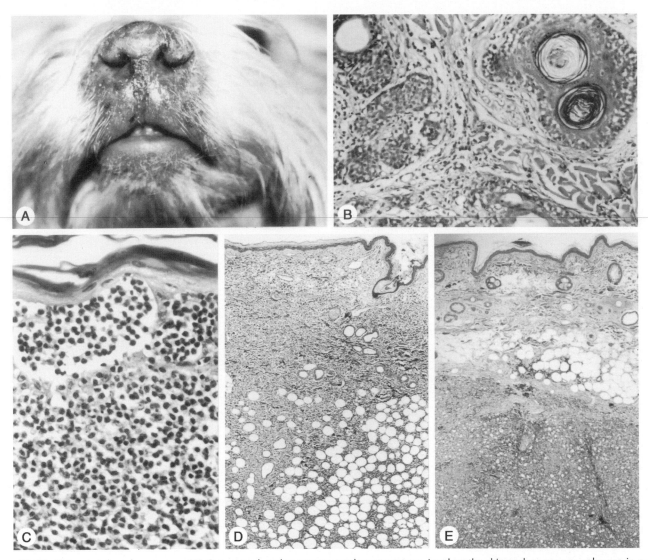

Figure 25–29. Cutaneous lymphosarcoma. **(A)** Cutaneous lymphosarcoma, erythematous type, involves the skin and mucous membranes in a dog. (Courtesy of Barbara Kummel, D.V.M.) **(B)** Cutaneous lymphosarcoma, epidermotropic type, with extensive involvement of the follicular epithelium. **(C)** Cutaneous lymphosarcoma with Pautrier microabscesses. The tumor cells appear plasmacytoid. **(D)** Cutaneous lymphosarcoma, nonepidermotropic type. **(E)** Cutaneous lymphosarcoma, subcutaneous nodule, Burkitt type, with numerous tingible-body macrophages in the tumor.

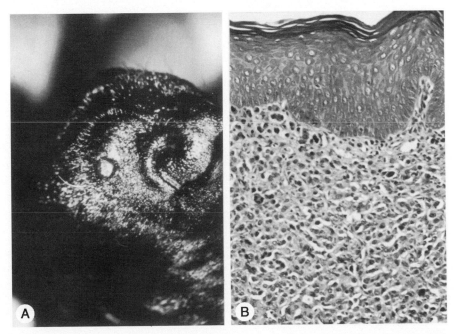

Figure 25–30. Cutaneous plasmacytoma. **(A)** Cutaneous plasmacytoma on the lip. (Courtesy of Barbara Kummel, D.V.M.) **(B)** There is extensive infiltration of dermal tissue by tumor cells.

junction. Invasion of the vessel walls results in vascular occlusion and necrosis.

Malignant histiocytosis is a multisystemic disorder that may involve the skin, but primarily involves the spleen, liver, and lungs. The neoplastic cells are pleomorphic with large, hyperchromatic folded nuclei, multiple nucleoli, and an abundant eosinophilic cytoplasm. Multinucleated cells are common, as is phagocytosis of erythrocytes and neutrophils by tumor cells.

Cysts

Cysts are common in the dog and cat, and include epidermal cysts; follicular cysts, which contain keratin and hair shafts; apocrine cysts; and ceruminous cysts, which contain an inspissated secretion, giving a dark appearance that may be mistaken for a melanoma. Dermoid cysts are congenital defects most often found in the midline on the neck and back of the Rhodesian ridgeback dog.

Tumor-like Lesions

Tumor-like lesions are common in the dog but uncommon in the cat. Calcinosis circumscripta resembles tumoral calcinosis seen in humans. These masses arise in young, large-breed dogs in the skin over joints but may also involve the tongue and ligamentum nuchae. On cut surface, the multilobulated mass has a chalky consistency. Histologically, there are islands of amorphous basophilic material with peripheral aggregates of histiocytes. The lesion may undergo mineralization and ossification.

Fibroepithelial polyps (i.e., skin tags) often arise on the limbs and ventral abdomen. Larger lesions are prone to trauma and ulceration.

Adnexal nevus is a term used to describe a congenital or acquired defect involving the adnexa. These elevated dermal masses are composed of excessive proliferation and enlargement of the adnexa and are arranged in a disorganized, haphazard manner. There is an accompanying dermal fibrosis.

SELECTED REFERENCES

1. Goldschmidt MH, Shofer FS. Skin Tumors of the Dog and Cat. Oxford, England: Pergamon Press, 1992.
2. Gross TL, Ihrke PJ, Walder EJ. Veterinary Dermatopathology: A Macroscopic and Microscopic Approach to the Diagnosis of Small Animal Skin Disease. St Louis: Mosby–Year Book, 1992.
3. Ackerman AB. Histologic Diagnosis of Inflammatory Skin Diseases. Philadelphia: Lea & Febiger, 1978.
4. Kuhl KA, Shofer FS, Goldschmidt MH. A comparative study of the histopathologic features of pemphigus foliaceous and superficial folliculitis in the dog. Vet Pathol 1994;31:19.
5. Miller WH Jr, Goldschmidt MH. Mycetomas in the cat caused by a dermatophyte: A case report. J Am Animal Hosp Assoc 1986;22:255.
6. Reimann KA, Evans MG, Chalifoux LV, et al. Clinicopathologic characterization of canine juvenile cellulitis. Vet Pathol 1989;26:499.
7. Miller WH Jr. Colour dilution alopecia in doberman pinschers with blue or fawn coat colours: A study on the incidence and histopathology of this disorder. Vet Dermatol 1990;1:113.
8. Wilcock BP, Yager JA. Focal cutaneous vasculitis and alopecia at sites of rabies vaccination in dogs. J Am Vet Med Assoc 1986;188:1174.
9. Hendrick MJ, Goldschmidt MH, Shofer FS, et al. Postvaccinal sarcomas in the cat: Epidemiology and electron probe microanalytic identification of aluminum. Cancer Res 1992;52:5391.

Index

Note: Page numbers in *italics* refer to illustrations. Page numbers followed by t indicate tables.